Hearing Impairment in Children

Edited By
Fred H. Bess, Ph.D.

This book was manufactured in the United States of America. Typography by Brushwood Graphics Studio, Baltimore, Maryland. Printing and binding by Maple Press, York, Pennsylvania. Cover design by Joseph Dieter, Jr.

Proceedings of the Third International Symposium on Childhood Deafness held July 28–30, 1986 at Nashville, Tennessee, co-sponsored by the Bill Wilkerson Hearing and Speech Center and Vanderbilt University School of Medicine.

Library of Congress Catalog Card Number 87-51659
ISBN 0-912752-13-0

Contents

Preface

The First International Symposium on Childhood Deafness was held in May of 1966 and was co-sponsored by Vanderbilt University School of Medicine and the Bill Wilkerson Hearing and Speech Center. Under the leadership of Freeman E. McConnell that conference was structured to provide a multidisciplinary update from both medical and nonmedical personnel on childhood deafness. The papers from that Symposium culminated in the now seminal textbook, *Deafness in Childhood* (McConnell and Ward 1967). Ten years following, the Second International Symposium was given at Central Michigan University, June 15–18, 1976, in Mt. Pleasant, Michigan. Once again, a proceedings from this conference was published in the text *Childhood Deafness: Causation, Assessment and Management* (Bess 1977).

This effort marks the proceedings from the Third International Symposium, and similar to its predecessors the book is designed to provide a multidisciplinary update on hearing impairment in children. The Symposium was sponsored by the Bill Wilkerson Hearing and Speech Center and the Division of Hearing and Speech Sciences at Vanderbilt University School of Medicine. The conference, held in Nashville, Tennessee July 28–30, 1986 brought together over 300 participants representing a variety of scientific and clinical disciplines. The book is organized into three sections. Part I deals with etiology/auditory disorders; Part II considers our most current information on identification and assessment, and Part III addresses the issue of management.

It is of interest to examine and contrast the three books that have resulted from these symposia. To some extent, the changes reflect our progress in understanding the complexities of hearing loss in children. For example, the text *Deafness in Childhood* (McConnell and Ward 1967) placed considerable emphasis on the pathology and medical treatment of such devastating complications as erythroblastosis fetalis, maternal rubella, and ototoxicity. Today, none of these conditions are looked upon as major causes of hearing impairment. Only four chapters from this book were specifically concerned with educational and audiologic management. Although the text *Childhood Deafness: Causation, Assessment and Management* (Bess 1977), reviewed many of the disorders covered by McConnell and Ward, greater focus occurred in the area of identification and assessment. New innovative approaches were being proposed for the screening and evaluation of auditory disorders. Between 1966 and 1977 we learned much about the behavioral assessment of hearing sensitivity among young children, the potential use of auditory evoked responses, and the application of acoustic immittance. Interestingly, it was in this book that one of the first references was made about our need to look closer at the milder forms of hearing impairment (Downs 1977).

The emphasis in this third text, *Hearing Impairment in Children*, appears to have shifted more toward management, as evidenced by the eleven chapters devoted to this topc. We have witnessed during this past decade significant changes in the provision of amplification to hearing-impaired children, and we have seen the development of alternative modes for stimulating the auditory system. Furthermore, our knowledge base with regard to approaches advocated in the management of this population has shown a marked increase, not just for the severe to profoundly hearing impaired but also for those with milder forms of hearing loss. In fact, the recognition that even mild hearing losses can produce complications in communication and psychoeducational progress prompted the use of the title *Hearing Impairment in Children* rather than Childhood Deafness. Appropriately, this book has also placed greater emphasis on the parent by including a discussion of hearing impairment from a parent's perspective as well as a chapter on parent counseling. It is hoped that these discussions will sensitize all professionals to the importance of dealing not only with the hearing-impaired child but the problems and frustrations of parents as well.

It is noteworthy that two of our contributors to *Hearing Impairment in Children*, namely LaVonne Bergstrom and Marion Downs, also contributed to the two previous books, *Deafness in Childhood* (1966) and *Childhood Deafness: Causation, Assessment and Management* (1977). We salute both of these distinguished scholars for their longstanding dedication, their munificent professional contributions, and their ever-present high standard of excellence in the pursuit of serving hearing-impaired children.

Numerous individuals contributed to the success of the International Symposium as well as this book. First and foremost is the staff of the Bill Wilkerson Hearing and Speech Center and the faculty and students within the Division of Hearing and Speech Sciences at Vanderbilt University School of Medicine, who provided constant encouragement, support, and enthusiasm for organizing and developing the Symposium. Particularly helpful were the contributions of Dottie Adams, Bertha Smith Clark, Jolie Fainberg, Susan Logan, Sally Meadows, Charlotte Prentice, Kathy Rhody, and Paulette Shanks. Finally, the Symposium and resulting publication would not have been possible without the generous support of Maternal and Child Health Services, Bureau of Community Health, U.S. Public Health Services.

F.H.B.

References

Bess, F. H. 1977. *Childhood Deafness: Causation, Assessment and Management*. New York: Grune & Stratton, Inc.

Downs, M. P. 1977. The expanding imperatives of early identification. *In* Bess, F. H. (ed.). *Childhood Deafness: Causation, Assessment and Management*. New York: Grune & Stratton, Inc.

McConnell, F., and Ward, P. H. 1967. *Deafness in Childhood*. Nashville: Vanderbilt University Press.

" . . . the management and care of deaf children is a combined operation calling for the whole-hearted cooperation of many disciplines—one that does not delegate to any discipline the automatic right to leadership."

Sir Terrence Cawthorne, 1966

Introduction

Early childhood is the fiery crucible in which we become molded into the essentials that we forever will be. To understand how to utilize that crucible in the best way for those who are hearing-impaired was the goal of the Third International Symposium on Childhood Deafness. It is a worthy goal, for it will improve the quality of life for the hearing-impaired while allowing society to reap the benefits of the resultant increased productivity. This is no idle dream as evidenced by Levitt's chapter (22), which confirms the inevitable correlation between early intervention and later speech and language abilities. With such a goal, this International Symposium was organized to place us at the cutting edge of the field.

It has been ten years since the last Symposium on Childhood Deafness, twenty since the first one. None of the members of those symposia, including myself, could have foreseen the rapid acceleration of techniques, instrumentation, or the shifts in the demographics of deafness that have occurred. As Dr. Bettye Caldwell's keynote paper expressed, "(We have) Come a Long Way . . . ." The "Way" is not always forward however. There have been enough negative concerns to dispel complacency. In brief, the chapters from this book have told us the following:

ADVANCES have been numerous and gratifying. Auditory brain stem response testing (ABR) has become a routine clinical tool rather than an experimental one. Our contributors inform us that we know the best signals to use, who should be monitored, and that children's responses differ in constant ways. This technique has affected pediatric audiological assessment as dramatically as the CT scan has altered medical diagnosis. If any prediction can be made it is that improved instrumentation will permit the ultimate in newborn screening: the application of ABR to every newborn child in the nursery.

Also honed to a fine point have been the techniques of acoustic immittance and acoustic reflex, which were still investigative tools 10 years ago. Northern (Chapter 12) points out that most of the earlier problems voiced then have been overcome: babies under 7 months can be validly tested by using a combination of tests with a 1400 Hz signal. Structural guidelines are now accepted but can be tailored to meet the criteria of special programs.

Certainly the most exciting of all advances has been cochlear implantation, which was just a gleam in the eyes of Drs. Blair Simmons and William House 20 years ago. With succeeding new generations of devices for implantation this innovative procedure may move from being a device only for the few profoundly deaf to a possible replacement for hearing aids for the partially impaired.

Other remarkable strides that are reported in this book include new frontiers in vibro-tactile instrumentation, the increased use of FM systems, VRA audiometry, and hearing aid fittings for milder hearing losses. An interest in milder losses in general is being seen.

No advance has been as gratifying as the changes in the demographics of deafness and hearing loss. Rubella as a cause of deafness is disappearing due to the increasing success of the rubella vaccine. Bacterial meningitis is beginning to decline because the new HIB vaccine is becoming increasingly effective. And few cases of deafness from hyperbilirubinemia are seen since the advent of photo-therapy and exchange transfusions. Medical advances are swift and telling.

CONCERNS are present, of course, and many members of the symposium have voiced alarms: Some new ototoxic drugs are lurking in every corner, as exemplified by the ototoxic effects of the new drug Cisplatin. And otitis media (OM) in infants seems to have escalated by crowding of the kind found in child care centers. The concern over this escalation is heightened by the reports of language learning problems resulting from early recurrent OM. As 50 percent of OM is silent, it must be identified by zealous monitoring. Other than tympanostomy tubes, low dosage of prophylactic antibiotics appears to be the most promising treatment.

In the realm of newborn screening, doubts are voiced over the ability of high-risk programs to identify the desired number of affected babies. It may be time to re-evaluate these programs, especially in the light of the possible availability of economical instrumentation that may permit ABR to be applied to all newborns. We may be moving toward the goal of cost-effective comprehensive neonatal screening. Such intensive monitoring may be required due to the increase in deafness from cytomegalovirus (CMV), which may take the place of rubella as the new scourge.

Attention must also be given to the management of children with unilateral deafness shown now by Bess and Tharpe, and Matkin (Chapter 8), to result in significant educational problems. Their intimations that right-ear deafness may be more virulent than that of the left ear opens up a brave new world of investigations. It follows that we can no longer be sanquine about mere recommendations for preferential seating in school for these children—it is not enough.

THE FUTURE will see vistas beyond our poor powers to visualize. Shaver (Chapter 2) has given us glimpses of the possibilities: Gene therapy and genetic engineering may one day open the way toward reduction of genetic deafness, once the gene of deafness is mapped. Prenatal and carrier tests may then be available, and the approximate 50 percent of congenital deafness attributable to heredity may gradually disappear. Even now, genetic counseling and new immunological developments are making inroads and will expand their effects. Improved prenatal care and control of infections will also be influential.

We are deeply indebted to Drs. Fred Bess and Freeman McConnell for their visions in initiating and perpetuating these important conferences. They have given us a glance at the past and a view of the future that will exhilarate us for another ten years.

Marion P. Downs, M.A., D.H.S.
Professor Emerita of Otolaryngology
University of Colorado Health Sciences Center
Denver, Colorado

Contributors

LaVonne Bergstrom, F.A.C.S., M.D.
Division of Head and Neck Surgery
UCLA Center for the Health Sciences
Los Angeles, California

Fred H. Bess, Ph.D.
Division of Hearing and Speech Sciences
Vanderbilt University School of Medicine
and
Bill Wilkerson Hearing and Speech Center
Nashville, Tennessee

Ingrid Blood, Ph.D.
Department of Communication Disorders
College of Health and Human Development
The Pennsylvania State University
University Park, Pennsylvania

Jamie A. Costello, M.A.
Division of BioelectroDiagnosis and Neural Monitoring
University of Pennsylvania Medical Center
Philadelphia, Pennsylvania

Julia M. Davis, Ph.D.
Department of Speech Pathology and Audiology
University of Iowa
Iowa City, Iowa

Allan O. Diefendorf, Ph.D.
Department of Audiology and Speech Pathology
University of Tennessee
Knoxville, Tennessee

Marion P. Downs, M.A., D.H.S.
Department of Otolaryngology
University of Colorado School of Medicine
Denver, Colorado

Rebecca E. Eilers, Ph.D.
Departments of Psychology and Pediatrics
Mailman Center for Child Development
University of Miami
Miami, Florida

Lynne Feagans, Ph.D.
Department of Individual and Family Studies
College of Health and Human Development
The Pennsylvania State University
University Park, Pennsylvania

G. Scott Giebink, M.D.
Departments of Pediatrics and Otolaryngology
University of Minnesota School of Medicine
Minneapolis, Minnesota

Michael E. Glasscock, III, M.D., F.A.C.S.
Department of Otology and Neurology
Vanderbilt University School of Medicine
Nashville, Tennessee
and
Department of Otolaryngology
University of Tennessee College of Medicine
Memphis, Tennessee

Karen M. Gollegly, M.A.
Section of Otolaryngology/Audiology
Dartmouth-Hitchcock Medical Center
Hanover, New Hampshire

Lincoln Gray, Ph.D.
Department of Otolaryngology—Head and Neck Surgery
University of Texas Medical School
Houston, Texas

Jens Grogaard, M.D.
Department of Pediatrics
Vanderbilt University School of Medicine
Nashville, Tennessee

James W. Hall, III, Ph.D.
Department of Otolaryngology—Head and Neck Surgery
University of Texas Medical School
Houston, Texas

David B. Hawkins, Ph.D.
Department of Communicative Disorders
University of South Carolina
Columbia, South Carolina

Robert A. Jahrsdoerfer, M.D.
Department of Otolaryngology—Head and Neck Surgery
University of Texas Medical School
Houston, Texas

Jeannette Seloover Johnson, Ph.D.
Hearing Health Care Program
3M Company
St. Paul, Minnesota

Laura Knox, M.A.
Parent Involvement Project
Nashville, Tennessee

Laura W. Kretschmer, Ed.D.
Department of Communication
University of Cincinnati
Cincinnati, Ohio

Richard R. Kretschmer, Jr., Ed.D.
Department of Special Education and Early Childhood
University of Cincinnati
Cincinnati, Ohio

Samuel C. Levine, M.D.
Department of Otolaryngology
University of Minnesota
Minneapolis, Minnesota

Harry Levitt, Ph.D.
Center for Research in Speech and Hearing Sciences
City University of New York
New York, New York

Stanley J. Maliszewski, Ph.D.
Guidance and Counseling
Omaha Public Schools
Omaha, Nebraska

Noel D. Matkin, Ph.D.
Department of Speech and Hearing Sciences
University of Arizona
Tucson, Arizona

Nancy S. McGarr, Ph.D.
Center for Research in Speech and Hearing Sciences
City University of New York
New York, New York

Kevin X. McKennan, M.D.
Department of Otolaryngology
University of California-Davis
and
Otology and Neurotology
The Sacramento Ear, Nose, and Throat Surgical and Medical Group
Sacramento, California

Mary Pat Moeller, M.S.
Center for Childhood Deafness
Boys Town National Institute
Omaha, Nebraska

Frank E. Musiek, Ph.D.
Section of Otolaryngology/Audiology and Section of Neurology
Dartmouth-Hitchcock Medical Center
Hanover, New Hampshire

Jerry L. Northern, Ph.D.
Department of Otolaryngology
University of Colorado School of Medicine
Denver, Colorado

D. Kimbrough Oller, Ph.D.
Departments of Psychology and Pediatrics
Mailman Center for Child Development
University of Miami
Miami, Florida

Wayne O. Olsen, Ph.D.
Department of Otolaryngology
Mayo Clinic
Rochester, Minnesota

William F. Rintelmann, Ph.D.
Department of Audiology
Wayne State University School of Medicine
Detroit, Michigan

Mark Ross, Ph.D.
Department of Communication Sciences
University of Connecticut
Storrs, Connecticut

Daniel M. Schwartz, Ph.D.
Division of BioelectroDiagnosis and Neural Monitoring
University of Pennsylvania Medical Center
Philadelphia, Pennsylvania

Richard H. Schwartz, M.D.
Child Health and Development
George Washington University School of Medicine
Washington, D. C.
and
Private practice of pediatrics
Vienna, Virginia

Richard C. Seewald, Ph.D.
Department of Communicative Disorders
Elborn College, University of Western Ontario
London, Ontario

Kathleen A. Shaver, Ph.D.
Genetic Services Center
Gallaudet Research Institute
Gallaudet University
Washington, D. C.

Jonathan G. Tubman, M.S.
Department of Individual and Family Studies
College of Health and Human Development
The Pennsylvania State University
University Park, Pennsylvania

Bruce A. Weber, Ph.D.
Center for Speech and Hearing Disorders
Duke University Medical Center
Durham, North Carolina

IN DEDICATION TO:
T. Shandy Holland
Freeman E. McConnell
T. Dean Clack

Issues on Etiology/Auditory Disorders

Chapter 1

Differential Diagnosis of Sensorineural Hearing Loss in Children

Michael E. Glasscock, III, *Kevin X. McKennan*, and *Samuel C. Levine*

INTRODUCTION

It should be stated at the outset that hearing loss is a symptom of a disease process and not the diagnosis. As with all other patient complaints, it represents a single clue to help us solve the medical puzzle. Too often in the past, "nerve deafness" was considered the final step in evaluation of hearing loss; this is clearly not the case today. In addition, many uninformed lay people and even some physicians have previously considered nerve deafness hopelessly untreatable. This pessimistic view, we know now, is far from the truth. The first step in treating hearing loss is to determine the cause.

There are many reasons to search conscientiously for the cause of hearing loss. (1) Early detection of hearing loss is crucial in order to minimize the adverse effects on cognitive, socioeconomic, and speech development. (2) Correctly diagnosing the patient's condition gives him a readily identifiable label that can be used by all health-care providers. It enables us to increase our understanding of hearing problems through retrospective and prospective studies. (3) Identification of a specific genetic syndrome allows us to conduct accurate genetic counseling. It is generally recognized that between one-quarter and one-half of all congenital hearing loss is genetic in origin. In the majority of these cases the inheritance patterns are fairly well established. Accurate genetic counseling of parents of a deaf child is one of a physician's most important roles. (4) In approximately one-third of the cases of sensorineural hearing loss in children the hearing loss is actually part of a larger constellation of problems that collectively are called a syndrome. Often the hearing loss is the initial or

This paper is based on research sponsored by The E.A.R. Foundation, Nashville, TN prime indication of a physical abnormality. It is vital that these syndromes are identified so that the non-auditory problems can also be managed. (5) For many of the classic hearing loss syndromes the long term prognosis for both hearing and other organ function is well established. Often the first question from parents is whether or not their child's condition will deteriorate further. It is impossible to discuss accurately these concerns until the hearing loss syndrome is identified.

Who Should Be Tested

The Joint Committee on Infant Hearing (1982) established guidelines to help health care providers identify infants at risk for hearing loss. These are: (1) a positive family history for childhood sensorineural hearing loss; (2) perinatal infection such as syphilis, rubella, toxoplasmosis, or cytomegalic inclusion virus infections; (3) malformations of the head or neck, especially auricular deformities; (4) low birth weight, i.e., less than 1500 grams; (5) severe hyperbilirubinemia; (6) bacterial meningitis; (7) low Apgar scale, especially those children with an Apgar less than three; (8) anoxia. The Joint Commission's guidelines are good rules to follow but they are not all inclusive. In Pappas and Schaibly's (1984) review of the etiology of childhood sensorineural hearing loss, they found that 46% of these patients did not have any of the risk factors cited above. It is clear that otolaryngologists, pediatricians, nurses, audiologists, and especially parents must be keenly aware of the possibility of hearing loss in our children and the devastating results if early diagnosis and treatment are not instituted.

Evaluation

The cornerstone of the diagnostic evaluation for childhood sensorineural hearing loss is a thorough history. Key questions must be asked regarding the time of onset of the hearing loss, suspected causes, and associated medical abnormalities, and a comprehensive family history must be taken. In the majority of cases the history alone will direct one to the correct diagnosis. Physicians must perform a careful physical examination. Special attention should be given to auricular or external auditory canal deformities, ocular disorders, and to the neurologic examination. One should be on the lookout for possible associated physical abnormalities. A clinical assessment of the child's hearing is helpful in corroborating the audiometric results.

The type of initial assessment depends on the age of the patient and the severity of the suspected hearing loss; behavioral audiometry for the infant, play audiometry for the young child, and standard pure-tone audiometry for the mature child will give an accurate estimation of the child's hearing thresholds. Tympanometry should be performed to rule out middle ear effusions and tympanic membrane perforations. In addition, acoustic reflex testing can be used to estimate hearing loss. Auditory evoked response testing has become the most reliable objective measurement of a child's hearing with virtually no age limit for this technique. Neonatal intensive care units throughout the United States perform this test on all high-risk neonates prior to discharge from the hospital.

After the history is taken and physical examination and audiometric testing are performed, a battery of blood tests are necessary. We routinely obtain a complete blood count, multiphasic chemistry panel (serum electrolytes, BUN, glucose, creatinine, cholesterol, triglycerides, and liver enzymes), thyroid hormone assay (serum thyroxine), FTA/VDRL, sedimentation rate, and routine urinanalysis. Although these tests are usually normal, they are inexpensive, reliable and at times, the only indication of an underlying metabolic abnormality. An electrocardiogram is not routinely performed unless there is a clinical suspicion of a cardiac disorder. If the child has had any fainting spells, drop attacks, seizure disorder, pulse or blood pressure abnormalities, or there is a family history of cardiac disease, then an electrocardiogram is performed to rule out cardioauditory syndromes such as Jervell-Lange-Nielsen.

Opinions have differed about the best way to study radiographically patients with sensorineural hearing loss. In a review of over 100 cases Pappas and Schaibly (1984) used polytomography to detect anatomic deformities of the cochlea in 10% of his patients studied. It now appears to many otologists, however, that the newer generation high resolution CT scanning of the otic capsule is more accurate. In an article in early 1986, Zalzal and co-workers (1986) encouraged otolaryngologists to use CT scanning to evaluate these patients. He described a 7% incidence of anatomic cochlear abnormalities using the CT scan. Unfortunately, in all but the most cooperative children, both the CT scan and polytomography must be performed under heavy sedation or general anesthesia.

In certain select cases, additional testing is indicated. Electronystagmography (ENG) is performed in those children with clinical nystagmus or a history of vertigo or loss of balance. Except in the mature child, it is difficult to perform this test reliably. Sedation cannot be used because it nullifies the test results. In patients with suspected autoimmune diseases, such as juvenile rheumatoid arthritis, serum lupus erythematosus or dermatomyositis, autoimmune tests such as an RA, ANA, LE prep, and sedimentation rate are performed. In children with coarse facial features, urine should be collected to rule out mucopolysaccharidosis. A lumbar puncture is not routinely performed but is indicated in cases of encephalitis or meningitis. Viral titers are useful only during the early course of the disease. Acute and convalescent viral titers must be obtained three or four weeks apart during the initial stage of the disease. If several years have passed since the disease, these studies are of little use. As the differential diagnosis is narrowed down to more and more obscure disorders, additional testing may be necessary.

CLASSIFICATIONS

In order to clarify the sometimes confusing array of diagnoses, several classifications have been developed. Each classification has certain advantages, although no system is clearly superior.

Konigsmark and Gorlin (1976) made many outstanding contributions to the field of classification. Their book on genetic disorders associated with hearing loss is a classic text. They noted that the majority of the syndromes of sensorineural hearing loss had, in addition to the inner ear, one prominent organ system affected. As a result, they classified sensorineural hearing loss syndromes according to the organ system most dramatically affected. For instance, all syndromes that affected both the eye and ear were classified under an ophthalmology heading. All those that affected both the heart and ear were placed under the cardiac subheading, and so on. This system is easy to use as long as there is one predominant organ system affected. When there are several organ systems equally affected, classification becomes difficult.

A pathological classification of the causes of sensorineural hearing loss has also become popular. This system is based on postmortem temporal bone findings. The various deformities in the otic capsule range from complete agenesis as seen in the Michel deformity to the cochleosaccular dysplasia of the Scheibe deformity. Between the two lie numerous other variants; the most notable being Mondini's deformity in which the cochlea does not have its normal two and one-half turns. This classification has enabled us to provide accurate anatomical correlations to the clinical findings in patients with sensorineural hearing loss. Unfortunately, only postmortem studies are available for proper classification. As a result, it is difficult to use this classification on a day-to-day basis.

The two more widely used classifications are the genetic-non-genetic and congenital-acquired systems. Although both are in wide use today, each system has certain disadvantages. In the first system, patients are categorized as having either a genetic (hereditary disorder) or a spontaneously occurring one. Since many of the dramatic hearing loss syndromes have distinct hereditary components, this system is useful most of the time. Unfortunately, the system breaks down occasionally. In some cases, the parents of the child simply do not know if other family members have had childhood hearing loss. There are undoubtedly disorders that appear to arise spontaneously, but are in fact genetically based. Some of the very rare autosomal recessive conditions occur so infrequently that it is difficult to determine if they have arisen spontaneously or are the result of the combination of rare recessive genes. Only after other offspring are affected, is the true genetic nature appreciated.

The second classification system categorizes the patient according to the time of onset. Hearing loss detected at birth is considered congenital while loss occurring after birth is considered delayed. This system is easy to use in most cases but even it fails at times. Neonates, especially those who are ill with other serious systemic disease, are not often recognized as having a significant hearing loss until long after they are discharged from the hospital. Although actually congenital, their hearing loss may be misclassified as acquired.

As a result of inadequacies of all of the systems, several authorities have combined these two systems into one larger classification. Congenital disorders and delayed onset disorders are divided into genetic and non-genetic subheadings. Overlaps occur because of the variation in presentation of different sensorineural hearing loss patients. This system, however, is a starting point.

Congenital Non-Genetic Group

RH INCOMPATIBILITY

Prior to the use of RhoGam(R) in the 1960s, Rh incompatibility was an all-too-frequent cause of erythroblastosis fetalis. This condition occurs when the blood type of the mother is Rh negative and that of the father Rh positive. Fifty percent of the time the child that is the product of this couple will have Rh positive blood. When the fetal blood mixes with the Rh negative maternal blood, the mother generates disruptive antibodies to the infant's Rh negative red blood cells. As a result, an immune-mediated hemolysis occurs in the infant, resulting in severe anemia. Multiple organ systems of the fetus are severely affected by this process, bilateral deafness being one of a number of serious sequelae. It is now standard practice to prevent the mother with Rh negative blood from generating these antibodies to fetal Rh positive blood by treating with RhoGam(R). As a result of this practice, it is now rare to see a child with deafness caused by Rh incompatibility.

HYPOXIA/ANOXIA

During fetal life and especially during delivery, the fetus may sustain a severe hypoxic injury from a number of causes. In the more severe cases, mental and physical retardation and bilateral deafness or significant sensorineural hearing loss result. With the advent of highly trained pediatricians, neonatologists, and high technology resuscitation equipment, more and more infants, who previously would have died, are being saved. As a result, there is a larger number of infants who have survived a premature or traumatic birth. It is imperative that all of these children be screened for hearing loss prior to being discharged from the hospital.

NEONATAL JAUNDICE

In the neonatal period, elevated bilirubin levels can result in a severe encephalopathy with many significant sequelae including bilateral deafness. Prior studies have shown that elevated serum bilirubin levels in access of 20mg percent places the neonate at significant risk. Since this condition is readily treatable, early detection and treatment can prevent any damage from occurring.

SYPHILIS

Syphilis has ravaged mankind for hundreds of years and continues to cause significant morbidity to this day. Syphilitic infections in fetuses can cause either congenital or delayed onset of sensorineural hearing loss. Congenital cases are usually much more serious than the delayed onset ones. A high index of suspicion is necessary to make the diagnosis. Routine screening with a VDRL or an FTA are performed by state laboratories throughout the country. A busy otologist can usually identify no more than two or three cases each year.

RUBELLA

Rubella, commonly referred to as German measles, is still with us despite widespread immunization programs. The last major epidemic was in 1964. The effects of rubella on the fetus are usually confined to the first trimester of fetal life. After the mother contracts rubella, a viremia occurs resulting in transplacental transmission of the rubella virus to the fetus. The fetus can be dramatically effected. Multiple problems, including cataracts, ventriculoseptal defects, patent ductus arteriosus, pulmonic stenosis, chorioretinitis, mental retardation and bilateral deafness can result. The sensorineural hearing loss can be unilateral or bilateral but is characteristically a flat type of hearing loss.

Conceivably, these cases could be totally eliminated by assuring that all women of childbearing age are immunized against the rubella virus. It is important, however, that the potential mother not be immunized during the three months before she becomes pregnant. Cases have occurred in which an immunization shortly before pregnancy was thought to have caused a rubella syndrome.

OTOTOXIC POISONING

There are many medications presently in use that have the potential for causing sensorineural hearing loss in children. The effects of specific drugs on the auditory system have been described elsewhere (Hawkins 1977).

RADIATION

Although the effects of low dose x-rays administered to a pregnant mother during the first trimester of pregnancy are not completely known, it is well known that therapeutic radiotherapy places a fetus at high risk for multiple congenital malformations including bilateral deafness. Prevention is the main treatment.

HYPOTHYROIDISM

In geographic areas where iodine is grossly deficient (the so-called goiter belts), severe fetal hypothyroidism can result. Inadequate levels of thyroid hormone typically result in a mixed sensorineural and conductive hearing loss. Although the full blown cases have a typical cretin appearance, milder cases may only be detectable by thyroid hormone laboratory analysis.

Congenital Genetic Group

Whether the genetic disorders of sensorineural hearing loss are classified as congenital depends on how carefully one analyzes these patients at birth. Unfortunately, many of the genetic manifestations are difficult to appreciate and, as a result, are not detected until the children are much older. The same syndrome may be considered as congenital in one patient but as a delayed onset in another patient.

Genetic syndromes (Hughes 1985; Konigsmark and Gorlin 1976; Paparella and Shumrick 1982) that fall into this category are so numerous that no list can be considered 100% complete. This list will concentrate on the more common and important disorders.

CHROMOSOMAL ABNORMALITIES

Trisomy 21 (Down syndrome), Trisomy 13 and Trisomy 18 are the three most common chromosomal hearing loss syndromes. The latter two involve multiple organ systems so severely affected that they are often fatal. Trisomy 13 patients typically have low set ears, deformed pinnae, optic nerve aplasia, cleft lip and palate, severe sensorineural hearing loss, and mental retardation. Trisomy 18 patients have similar deformities of the auricles, hand deformities, sensorineural hearing loss, and severe mental retardation. The most common trisomy abnormality is Down syndrome. Most authorities estimate that there are 1.5 Down syndrome children born out of each 1000 births. Although they typically have mild or a moderate conductive hearing loss secondary to middle ear effusions, sensorineural hearing loss has also been reported in 10 to 50% of the cases.

KLIPPEL-FEIL DISEASE

Children with this disease have multiple vertebral deformities. Typically, several cervical vertebrae are fused resulting in a short neck. In addition, spina bifida is fairly common. A mixed sensorineural and conductive hearing loss typically occurs in many of the patients. An autosomal recessive inheritance pattern exists.

MARFAN'S DISEASE

This syndrome is difficult to identify in infants and young children. Older children and adolescents typically become quite tall and have a ectomorphic appearance. Long spindly fingers, a pigeon breast deformity, hammer toes, and a mixed sensorineural conductive hearing loss are present. Serious cardiac and vascular abnormalities also occur secondary to the connective tissue disorder that underlies this condition. An autosomal dominant inheritance pattern exists.

HALLGREN'S SYNDROME

Individuals with Hallgren's syndrome have retinitis pigmentosa, ataxia, and sensorineural hearing loss. Some also have mental retardation. An autosomal recessive inheritance pattern is typical.

WAARDENBURG'S SYNDROME

Individuals with this disease account for one to seven percent of all cases of genetic sensorineural hearing loss. The full blown syndrome includes patients with a laterally displaced medial canthus, a broad nasal root, hyperplasia—with the eyebrows often meeting in the midline—and heterochromia irides. In 50% of the cases, sensorineural hearing loss occurs. An autosomal dominant inheritance pattern with variable expressivity is characteristic.

ALPORT'S SYNDROME

This syndrome causes approximately 1% of all hereditary deafness. The two main characteristics are a chronic glomerulonephritis and sensorineural hearing loss. In most cases, males are more severely affected. Typically, the sensorineural hearing loss has its onset during adolescence and is usually preceded by the glomerulonephritis by several years. In 10% of the individuals, cataracts are also present. An autosomal dominant pattern of inheritance is usually reported.

PENDRED'S SYNDROME

The presence of childhood thyroid enlargement and sensorineural hearing loss constitutes this syndrome. It is one of the common causes of genetic hearing loss. An autosomal recessive inheritance pattern exists.

MUCOPOLYSACCHARIDOSES SYNDROME

Although there are many types of mucopolysaccharidoses, Hunter's and Hurler's are the two more common varieties. As a result of inborn errors in mucopolysaccharide metabolism, an accumulation of mucopolysaccharides occurs in the soft tissues of the body. As a result, very coarse facial features, characterized as gargoylism, occur. In addition, these patients have mental retardation in varying degrees, skeletal deformities, liver hypertrophy, hypersplenism, and sensorineural hearing loss. Inheritance patterns vary with the particular syndrome.

CROUZON'S SYNDROME

This syndrome is also referred to as craniofacial dysostosis. As a result of premature closure of numerous cranial suture lines, these patients have marked facial and cranial deformities. Characteristically, they also have exophthalmos, auditory meatus atresia, and a mixed sensorineural conductive hearing loss. Typically, this is an autosomal dominant disorder.

USHER'S SYNDROME

Usher's syndrome causes approximately 10% of hereditary deafness. It consists of a combination of retinitis pigmentosa and congenital sensorineural hearing loss. Typically, visual difficulties occur during early childhood, often progressing to total blindness by the age of 20 to 30. Some of these patients will, in addition to the retinitis pigmentosa, have cataracts. An autosomal recessive pattern of inheritance is thought to be present.

REFSUM'S SYNDROME

This condition is also referred to as heredopathia atactica polyneuritiformis. It is characterized by ataxia, retinitis pigmentosa, a peripheral neuropathy, and progressive sensorineural hearing loss. In some patients, a skin condition referred to as ichthyosis is also present. Refsum's is a neuronal lipid storage disease. The diagnosis can often be confirmed by markedly elevated levels in the serum phytanic acid.

ALSTROM'S SYNDROME

This condition consists of retinitis pigmentosa, diabetes melitis, and progressive sensorineural hearing loss. The patients are often blind by the age of 20. This syndrome is inherited through an autosomal recessive pattern.

FAMILIAL HYPERLIPIDEMIA SYNDROME

This metabolic disorder of fat metabolism results in markedly elevated levels of blood lipids. Although categorized here under one name, there are multiple subgroupings. More accurate diagnosis is possible using electrophoretic analysis of blood lipids. The inheritance pattern can be either autosomal dominant or recessive. It is important that the children of all patients with this disorder be screened because prompt treatment of the lipid disorder will prevent many of the disabling consequences, including sensorineural hearing loss.

JERVELL-LANGE-NIELSEN SYNDROME

Although this syndrome accounts for less than 1% of all cases of hereditary deafness, it has received much notoriety in the otolaryngologic literature because these children have Stokes Adams attacks not infrequently resulting in sudden death. Typically, the patients have a profound sensorineural hearing loss with electrocardiographic abnormalities. Usually, a prolonged A-T interval, and enlarged T waves are present, although a large variety of electrical disorders are possible. These patients can present with either deafness or fainting spells. Sudden death has been reported as a complication of the cardiac abnormalities.

SICKLE CELL ANEMIA SYNDROME

Sickle cell anemia is a relatively common disorder in the black population affecting as many as 1 in 400 individuals. Reports of sensorineural hearing loss in these children are as high as 20% incidence. It is felt that the patients undergo ischemic damage to the cochlea as a result of blood cell sickling. Although sensorineural hearing loss is not uncommon, total deafness is unusual.

DELAYED ONSET NON-GENETIC GROUP

The causes for childhood sensorineural hearing loss in this category are legion, (Hughes 1985; Paparella and Shumrick 1982). Our discussion will be confined to common conditions and only those that produce "significant" hearing loss.

MENINGITIS

Meningitis is the most common intracranial complication from suppurative otitis media. Despite the advent of antibiotics, it is still a relatively common cause for serious infection in the pediatric age group. A recent paper by Baldwin et al. (1985) examined 54 patients discharged from the hospital with a diagnosis of meningitis. Seventy percent of these children had Haemophilis influenza meningitis and an alarming 40% of them tested audiometrically were determined to have sensorineural hearing loss. What is even more worrisome is that he found that 53% of those patients who were discharged with a diagnosis of meningitis were not referred for subsequent audiologic work-up. A major oversight is occurring in our health care system if the pattern they discovered is prevalent throughout the United States. Clearly, all patients with meningitis should have a hearing evaluation prior to and also after discharge from the hospital. Follow-up over a period of three to six months is mandatory since the hearing loss, especially if unilateral, may be difficult to detect and the consequences of missing the diagnosis are so grave.

CYTOMEGALOVIRUS INFECTION

Cytomegalovirus is now felt to be the most common cause of congenital viral induced deafness. The consequences of this viral infection are often not detected for months afterwards. CMV is a ubiquitous virus that is present in many healthy individuals. In the pregnant woman, who is nearly always subclinically infected with CMV, transplacental transmission of this virus commonly occurs. Fortunately, most infants will successfully fight off the infection but a small minority develop cytomegalic inclusion disease. These children are systemically quite ill. Once cytomegalic disease occurs, it is estimated that between 20 and 65% of the children will develop sensorineural hearing loss (Strauss 1985). At the present time there is no specific antiviral therapy for this condition. Vaccines are now under development.

MUMPS

In the past, mumps was the most common cause of unilateral sensorineural hearing loss. Typically, this occurred either during or shortly after the onset of mumps parotitis. With the current widespread use of measles, mumps, and rubella vaccination programs, the incidence of this condition has dropped dramatically.

MISCELLANEOUS VIRAL INFECTIONS

Cases of severe sensorineural hearing loss have been reported from most viral illnesses that affect children. Infectious mononucleosis, roseola (measles), varicella (chicken pox), and influenza all have been reported to cause sensorineural hearing loss.

FUNGAL DISEASES

With the increasing number of organ transplants being performed in the United States today, it is anticipated that an increasing number of patients will be undergoing immuno-suppressive therapy. As a result, infections with unusual and pathogenic organisms will become increasingly common. Mucormycosis, a fungal infection previously restricted to diabetics and cancer patients, is being reported in transplant patients. Other fungal organisms, including Aspergillus and Cryptococcus, have become potential pathogens. In one of the few reports on fungal meningitis, Nadol (1978) reported three of seven patients subsequently developed sensorineural hearing loss.

TUBERCULOSIS

An increasing number of immigrants from the Far East has resulted in a upsurge in the number of cases of tuberculosis in the United States. In a minority of these cases, chronic otitis media or tuberculosis meningitis may develop. The resulting chronic infection is seldom treated surgically with success unless antituberculous agents are also used.

CHRONIC OTITIS MEDIA

Paparella and his colleagues (1982) have demonstrated significant sensorineural hearing loss associated with chronic otitis media. Any practicing otolaryngologist who sees a moderate number of chronic otitis media cases has undoubtedly witnessed numerous cases of severe sensorineural hearing loss as a result of chronic infections.

PSEUDOHYPOACUSIS

Older children and especially adolescents will occasionally complain of functional or non-organic hearing loss. These patients can usually be reliably identified using standard audiometric techniques, tympanometry, and auditory brainstem response testing. Psychiatric counseling is important because "faked" hearing loss can occasionally be a signal of a serious mental and emotional problem.

NEOPLASTIC DISEASE

Leukemia and other serious blood dyscrasias can result in sudden or progressive deafness. Screening tests, including a complete blood count, readily identify these patients.

TRAUMA

Serious head injuries that produce basilar skull fractures can rupture the delicate cochlea, resulting in sudden partial or complete deafness. Approximately 70% of traverse and 10% of longitudinal bone fractures result in significant sensorineural hearing loss. Fortunately, this loss is usually unilateral.

MENIERE'S DISEASE

Episodic vertigo, sensorineural hearing loss, and a roaring tinnitus constitute the Meniere's triad of symptoms. Although it typically occurs in adults, recent reports attest to its presence in children and, especially, adolescents.

PERILYMPH FISTULA

Usually resulting from trauma, perilymph fistula typically causes sensorineural hearing loss and vertigo. In a child, vestibular complaints may be manifested only by an unsteady gait or stumbling. Exploratory tympanotomy is necessary in order to eliminate the symptoms and prevent progressive deafness.

OVERLAPPING CATEGORIES

Ototoxic drugs, infections, metabolic abnormalities, and many other conditions that cause sensorineural hearing loss are also described in the congenital non-genetic section.

UNKNOWN

Unfortunately, despite a most thorough evaluation, we will fail to diagnose a sizable percentage of these children.

Delayed Onset Genetic

Most delayed-onset genetic disorders (Hughes 1985; Paparella and Shumrick 1982) have been previously discussed in the section entitled congenital-delayed. Two conditions deserve special mention.

VON RECKLINGHAUSEN'S DISEASE—CENTRAL FORM

These patients, often young adults or adolescents, present with unilateral or bilateral tinnitus, hearing loss, or imbalance. Many of these patients have bilateral acoustic neuromas. Early detection and surgery is the only hope in preventing total bilateral deafness. Approximately one-half of these patients have a positive family history.

OTOSCLEROSIS

Although otosclerotic patients usually have a conductive hearing loss, some develop severe mixed hearing losses. Typically, onset is in the teen years or twenties. Surgical and medical treatment is effective in alleviating most symptoms.

Conclusion

The differential diagnosis of sensorineural hearing loss includes myriad causes, both genetic and non-genetic, congenital and delayed-onset.

It is not reasonable to commit to memory the extensive list of syndromes that can cause sensorineural hearing loss. The list is too long and too infrequently used. What *is* reasonable is to realize that a vast number of entities exist. Once a syndrome is identified, standard texts and the medical literature can be reviewed to obtain updated information. After a thorough diagnostic evaluation is made the appropriate treatment can be started.

REFERENCES

Baldwin, R. L., Sweitzer, R. S., and Freind, D. B. 1985. Meningitis and sensorineural hearing loss. *Laryngoscope* 95:802–804.

Hawkins, J. E. 1977. Ototoxicity in infant and fetus. *In* F. H. Bess (ed.) *Childhood Deafness: Causation, Assessment and Management.* New York: Grune and Stratton.

Hughes, G. B. 1985. *Clinical Otology*. New York: Thieme-Stratton.

Joint Committee on Infant Hearing *ASHA*. December, 1982, 1017–1018.

Konigsmark, B. W., and Gorlin, R. J. 1976. *Genetic and Metabolic Deafness*. Philadelphia: W. B. Saunders Co.

Nadol, J. B. 1978. Hearing loss as a sequelae of meningitis. *Laryngoscope* 88:739–755.

Paparella, M. M., and Shumrick, D. A. 1982. *Otolaryngology* Philadelphia: W B. Saunders Co.

Pappas, D. B., and Schaibly, M. 1984. A two-year diagnostic report on bilateral sensorineural hearing loss in infants and children. *American Journal of Otology* 5(5):339–342.

Strauss, M. 1985. A clinical pathologic study of hearing loss in congenital cytomegalo virus infection. *Laryngoscope* 95:951–961.

Zalzal, G. H., Schott, S. R., Towkin, R., and Cotton, R. T. 1986. Value of CT scan in the diagnosis of temporal bone diseases in children. *Laryngoscope* 96(1):27–32.

Chapter 2

Genetic Causes of Childhood Deafness

Kathleen A. Shaver

Introduction

Recent advances in the field of genetics have greatly increased the ability to diagnose and, potentially, to treat genetic disease. Within the past ten years, new techniques in molecular genetics have greatly expanded the diagnostic capabilities of geneticists. Carrier testing for diseases such as Tay Sachs, sickle cell anemia, and phenylketonuria have been widely available for some time and new tests for such genetic disorders as cystic fibrosis and Huntington's disease are on the horizon. Gene therapy to attempt to replace defective gene products may soon be a reality for some of the more common genetic disorders. These accomplishments are astounding considering that it was only in 1953 that Watson and Crick (1953) published their seminal paper describing the structure of DNA and shortly afterward that the correct number of chromosomes in man became known.

At least 50 percent of moderate to profound sensorineural hearing impairment present at birth or occurring in early childhood results from genetic factors (Rose, Conneally, and Nance 1977). Descriptive knowledge about forms of genetic deafness is continually expanding. As of 1983, from 150 to 175 different genetic syndromes have been described that involve hearing impairment as a major feature (Konigsmark and Gorlin 1976; McKusick 1983). The list continues to grow year by year as more hearing-impaired people are seen for diagnostic evaluation in genetic centers across the world and more is learned about specific types of genetic hearing loss through population studies; however, despite the increase in knowledge about many genetic diseases, very little is known about the chromosomal location or the biochemical nature of genes that cause deafness.

As health care providers and educators become aware of the importance of genetic factors in childhood deafness, the demand for genetic services by families and deaf individuals themselves has increased greatly (Freeman, Carbin, and Boese 1981). In spite of this, very few centers exist to provide genetic evaluation exclusively for the families of deaf children and knowledge of genetics among the deaf themselves is greatly lacking. It has been only within the past few years that genetic services and education in genetics for hearing parents of deaf children, for deaf adults, and for the medical and educational community have become more widespread.

Principles of Inheritance

Every cell of the body, other than the sex cells, contains an exact copy of deoxyribonucleic acid (DNA), the biochemical genetic material inherited from the parents. The DNA is organized in the nucleus of the cell into structures called chromosomes. There are 46 chromosomes, 23 pairs, in the nucleus of every human somatic cell. One of each pair of chromosomes is of paternal origin, the other of maternal origin. One pair of chromosomes is called the sex chromosomes. Females have two X chromosomes and males have an X and a Y chromosome. Each of the chromosomes is composed of thousands of genes—the biochemical instructions responsible for directing the body's growth and development. When considering the complexity of the organ of hearing, it is easy to comprehend the large number of genes necessary for the normal development and functioning of the sense of hearing. Hundreds of genes are involved in the biochemical pathway necessary to construct a normal ear. One change in a single gene in the pathway controlling the development or functioning of the hearing organ can result in deafness.

Because chromosomes come in pairs, the genes that control particular traits also come in pairs, one from each of the parents. A particular gene at each chromosomal locus (location) can exist in several slightly different molecular forms. An individual who has one copy of an altered gene for deafness and one normal gene is called a "heterozygote." Persons who have two identical genes for a trait such as deafness are called "homozygotes." When only one copy of a gene is required for a particular trait to be expressed, that trait is called dominant (the heterozygous state). When two copies of the gene are required (the homozygous state), that trait is called recessive. Deafness can be inherited in either of these ways. Occasionally, recessive genes for deafness are located on the X-chromosome and the trait is inherited as X-linked recessive.

Approximately two-thirds of genetic hearing impairment is not associated with other physical traits or disease. One-third of genetic hearing impairment occurs as part of a "syndrome" in which it is associated with other physical

Table I

Konigsmark's Classifications of Genetic Hearing Loss*
1. No Associated Abnormalities
2. External Ear Abnormalities
3. Eye Disease
4. Musculoskeletal Disease
5. Integumentary System Disease
6. Renal Disease
7. Nervous System Disease
8. Metabolic and Other Abnormalities

*Konigsmark and Gorlin 1976

features caused by the same gene. These syndromes can involve deafness with accompanying visual impairments, renal disease, skin disease, and metabolic disease among others (table I). Many types of deafness may also be distinguished by age of onset and audiometric characteristics including stability, progression, and severity.

DOMINANT INHERITANCE

Dominant inheritance is estimated to account for at least 20% of genetic types of deafness (Rose, Conneally, and Nance 1977). In dominant deafness, only a single copy of a gene for hearing impairment is required and is usually inherited from one of the parents. As shown in figure 1, a person with dominant

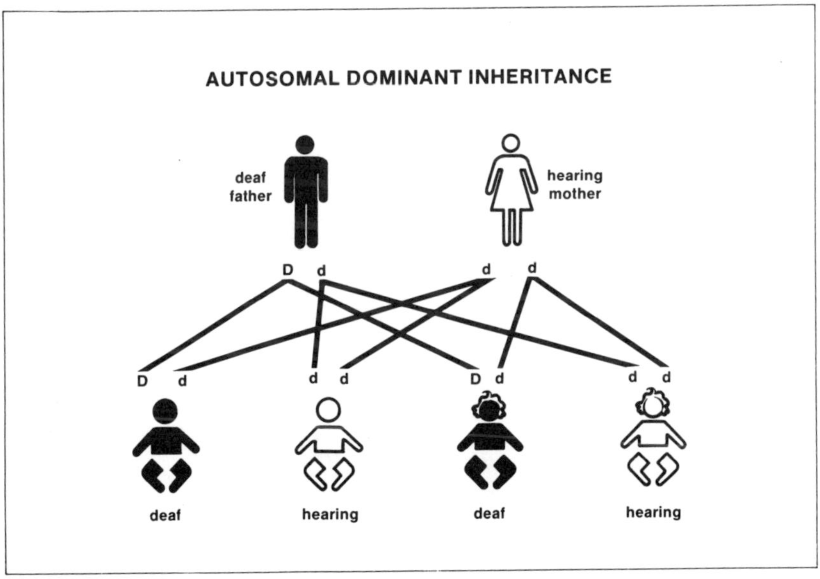

Figure 1. Persons with dominant deafness have one dominant gene (D) and a corresponding normal gene (d). Each child has a 50/50 chance to inherit the deafness gene (D) from the parent who has this trait.

deafness is usually heterozygous for the deafness gene. The chance that a person with a dominant type of deafness will have a deaf child is 50% if the other parent is not also heterozygous for a dominant gene for deafness. The hearing status of the first child has no bearing on the hearing status of subsequent children: the chance that each child will be deaf is always 50/50 if only one of the parents is heterozygous for a dominant gene. A child with a dominant type of genetic hearing impairment usually has a family history of deafness in several successive generations. Figure 2 illustrates a family in which the dominant gene for deafness was passed through seven generations. The proband, or index case, is indicated by the arrow. The dominant deafness in this family was also associated with albinoidism (a pigment disorder that manifests itself in the hair, skin, and fundus), so that the family members were always able to accurately predict the hearing status of a child at birth by observing the hair, skin, and eye color.

Dominant types of hearing loss are sometimes characterized by variable expression and/or reduced penetrance. One of the most frequent types of dominantly inherited hearing loss is Waardenburg syndrome—an alteration of the cells of the pigment epithelium derived from the neural crest—which causes bilateral or unilateral hearing loss, pigment anomalies such as white forelock, early greying, and different colored irides, and the appearance of widely spaced eyes, a condition called dystopia canthorum (Smith 1982). As with many dominantly inherited syndromes, Waardenburg syndrome exhibits variable expression in individuals who carry the gene, meaning that a person may have one,

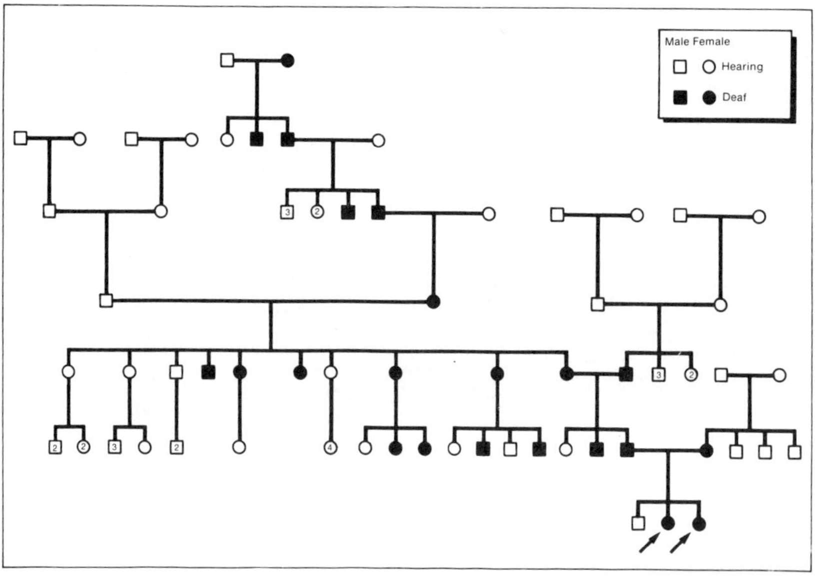

Figure 2. Pedigree illustrating dominant inheritance of deafness in seven generations. Arrows indicate the probands (index cases).

several, or all of the features of this syndrome. Only 20% of people who have Waardenburg syndrome are deaf, but a hearing parent with the syndrome can have a deaf child. Dominant genes may also exhibit reduced penetrance, meaning that some family members who have the gene may not be deaf or exhibit any features of the syndrome. This phenomenon often leads some families to believe that the gene is "skipping generations." Reduced penetrance is illustrated in the family shown in figure 3. This family was diagnosed as having a dominant form of progressive hearing impairment. However, reduced penetrance occurs in the paternal grandmother and is assumed in one of the great-grandparents. Audiological assessment of the paternal grandmother revealed the presence of a mild high-frequency hearing loss of which she was never aware.

Other dominantly inherited syndromal types of deafness include Treacher Collins syndrome (conductive or mixed hearing impairment associated with facial malformations), branchial-oto-renal syndrome (ear pits, branchial clefts, kidney malformations, and deafness), osteogenesis imperfecta (brittle bones and conductive hearing impairment), and Alport syndrome (progressive hearing impairment and nephritis).

RECESSIVE INHERITANCE

In recessively inherited hearing impairment, a person must receive a double dose of the gene, one copy from each parent, in order for the trait to be expressed. Recessive genes account for the major proportion of genetic hearing

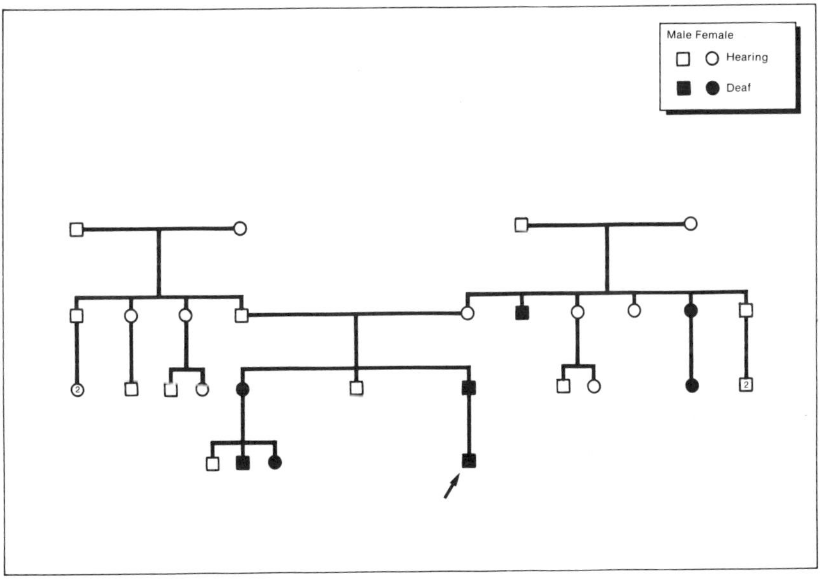

Figure 3. Pedigree illustrating dominant inheritance of deafness with reduced penetrance in the proband's grandmother and one of the great-grandparents.

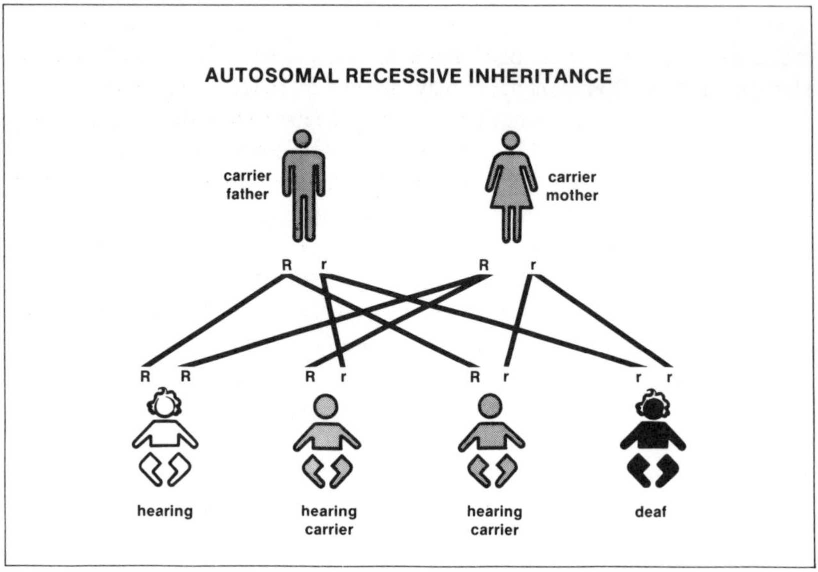

Figure 4. Persons with recessive deafness have a double dose of the deafness gene (r), one inherited from each of the parents. The parents are hearing carriers and have a 25% chance to produce a deaf child with each pregnancy.

loss, with up to 80% of these deaf children having a recessively inherited type of disorder. In recessive inheritance, the chance that two heterozygous carriers will have a homozygous (deaf) child is one in four or 25%, as shown in figure 4. Again, this risk applies to all pregnancies: chance has no memory. Because family size is limited in many modern families, there may, by chance, be only one deaf child in the family. Both parents must be heterozygous for the recessive gene: although they both "carry" one copy of the gene they have normal hearing.

Approximately one in eight people in the general population is a carrier of a gene for deafness, however, there are many different types of recessive genes for hearing loss, and a mating between two individuals who both carry the exact same gene for hearing loss is extremely rare. It is much more common for this to occur in a mating where the parents are related to one another. The more closely the parents are related, the more likely it is that they both inherited the gene from their common ancestor. This "consanguinity" or mating between blood relatives is the hallmark of recessive deafness. Figure 5 illustrates the pedigree of a Canadian family in which consanguinous matings occurred several times, resulting in deaf children. The fathers of the deaf children in the proband's generation were brothers and all of the mothers were related to one another (two were sisters and the mother of the proband was their second cousin).

One of the more commonly occurring recessive genetic syndromes involving

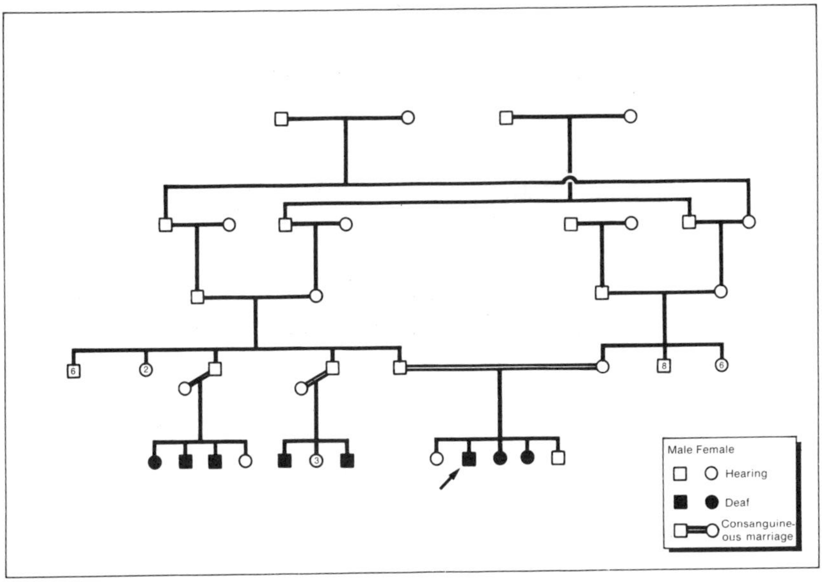

Figure 5. Pedigree illustrating recessive inheritance. Deafness in this family resulted from consanguineous marriages. The mothers of the proband's deaf cousins are sisters and the mother of the proband is their second cousin.

deafness is Usher syndrome, which occurs in 3 to 5% of children in residential schools for the deaf. Usher syndrome is the association of congenital sensorineural deafness with the eye disease, retinitis pigmentosa. This progressive disease of the rod cells located on the periphery of the retina symptomatically involves first the loss of night vision and then a slowly progressive tunnel vision. Usher syndrome is an excellent example of a genetic disease that occurs more frequently in certain ethnic groups. Only 1 in 100 people in the general population are heterozygous (carriers) for the gene for Usher syndrome; however, among a group of people of French-Canadian extraction in Louisana (Cajuns), the frequency of heterozygotes is much higher. The high rate of inbreeding in this population accounts for the greatly increased number of deaf-blind persons in the state of Louisiana (Boughman, Vernon, and Shaver 1983). Other syndromal types of recessively inherited hearing impairment include the Jervell Lange-Nielsen syndrome (congenital deafness and a conductive heart problem which often leads to death in young adulthood), and Pendred syndrome (congenital sensorineural deafness associated with goiter).

X-LINKED INHERITANCE

One of the 23 pairs of chromosomes is referred to as the sex chromosomes. Females have two X chromosomes and males have an X chromosome which they inherit from the mother and a Y chromosome inherited from the father.

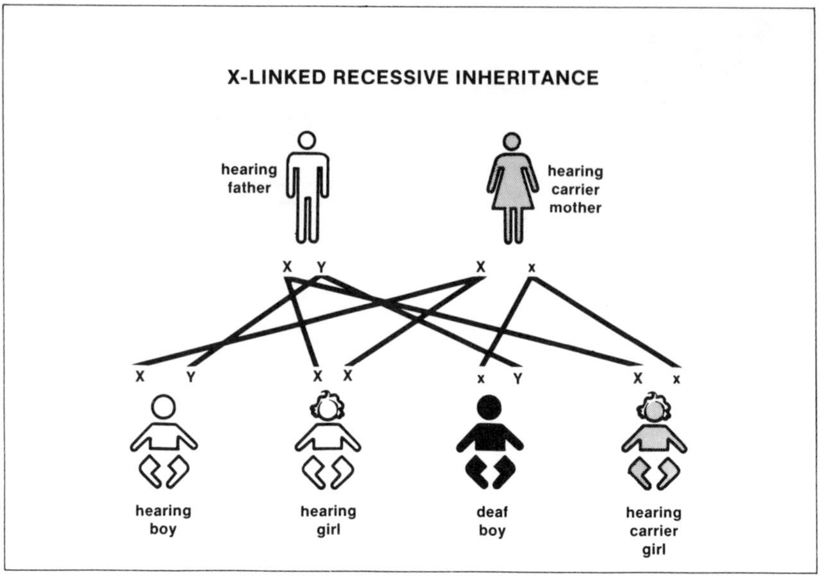

Figure 6. X-linked recessive deafness is caused by a gene on the X chromosome and occurs only in males. The sons of a woman who is a carrier of X-linked deafness have a 50% chance to be deaf and the daughters have a 50% chance to be carriers.

Occasionally, genes for deafness are located on the X chromosome. Although a female who has a recessive gene for deafness on one of her X chromosomes does not exhibit hearing impairment, each of her sons has a 50% chance of being deaf and each of her daughters has a 50% chance to be a carrier (see figure 6). An affected male (with a mate who is *not* a carrier) can have two types of children: all of his daughters will be carriers and all of his sons will be normal since they receive the Y chromosome from their father. An example of a family in which deafness occurs as an X-linked recessive trait is shown in figure 7. Affected males sometimes occur in multiple generations and are always related through carrier females.

Genetic Evaluation and Counseling

Genetic counseling is defined as "the process of communication between a genetic counselor and the client concerning information about the nature of a disorder and available options open to a couple who are found to be at risk of transmitting a genetic disorder" (Emery 1984). Genetic counseling is essentially a process of education although, as Emery states, an effective genetic counselor (communicator) must recognize the emotional state of the family and their attitudes toward the disorder and assist them in dealing emotionally with the affected family member. Genetic counseling is never directive: the role of

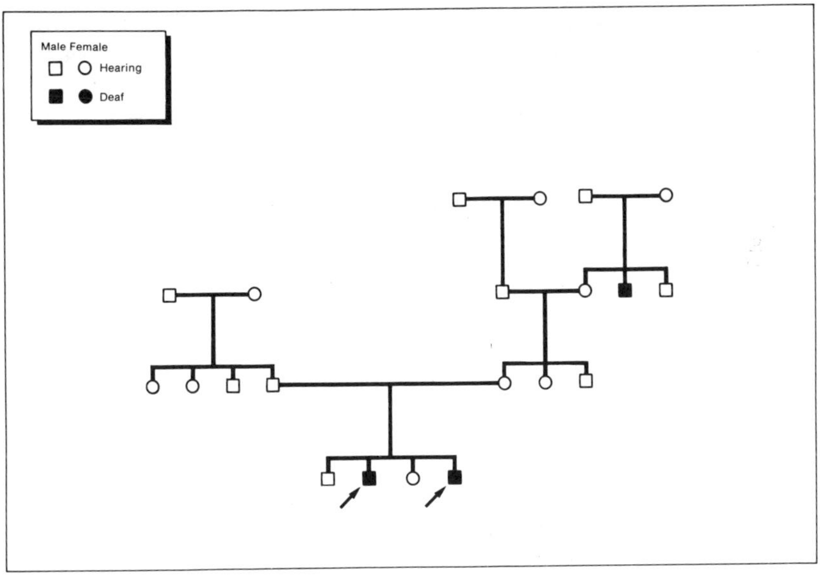

Figure 7. Pedigree illustrating X-linked recessive inheritance. The mother, grandmother and great-grandmother of the probands are obligate carriers.

the counselor is not to tell the client what to do, but rather to educate, inform, and provide emotional support. These concepts become especially important when counseling deaf clients who often have language and cultural differences that make their perspective much different from that of a hearing couple with a deaf child.

The need for genetic counseling for deafness can be easily documented. Table II shows data collected by the Center for Assessment and Demographic

Table II

Major Causes of Hearing Loss Reported to
Annual Survey of Hearing Impaired Children and Youth*, 1984–1985

Cause	Number	Percent of Total
Heredity	6,087	12.0%
Maternal Rubella	5,350	10.5%
Meningitis	4,147	8.2%
Prematurity	2,158	4.3%
Otitis Media	1,769	3.5%
High Fever	1,621	3.2%
Complications of Pregnancy	1,601	3.2%
Trauma	1,549	3.1%
Infection	1,394	2.7%
Rh Incompatibility	576	1.1%
Other	3,692	7.3%
Unknown	10,812	21.3%
Data Not Available	9,975	19.6%
TOTAL	50,731	100.0%

*Center for Assessment and Demographic Studies, Gallaudet Research Institute

Studies at Gallaudet College taken from the 1984–1985 Annual Survey of Hearing Impaired Children and Youth. Data was collected on over 50,000 deaf children from schools and special education programs for deaf children, concerning the cause of hearing loss as listed in school records. Previous experience indicates that many students are improperly placed in categories of environmental or acquired etiology. Heredity is listed as the cause of the hearing loss in only 12% of the cases, while the expected figure should be approximately 50%. This very low number reflects partly the difficulty of making a diagnosis of recessive genetic deafness when there may be only one deaf child in the family and no other family history of deafness, and partly the lack of genetic diagnostic work-ups available for deaf children. Although the situation has improved somewhat during the past ten years, a 1977 survey of schools and programs for the deaf (Nance et al. 1977) indicated that only 49 of the 421 (11.6%) programs responding reported that genetic counseling services were provided for students and their families. The individual responsible for genetic counseling was reported to be a geneticist in only about half of these cases. In a similar survey at Gallaudet College by the same group of researchers, only 7% of the participating parents of 555 students identified hereditary causes for deafness in their children, even though 58% of the deaf students showed clear evidence of genetic etiology in their family history. Even in families where both parents and all the siblings were deaf, the cause of deafness in the student was stated to be hereditary in only 14% of the cases. Hearing parents and the deaf themselves are often unaware of a genetic etiology of hearing impairment even when there are several affected family members or when a specific genetic syndrome has been diagnosed. Our recent experiences at Gallaudet College indicate that, in 80 cases where our evaluation found the cause of deafness to be genetic, only 20% of the parents originally thought that the cause might be genetic. In a majority of these cases another immediate family member was also deaf. A dramatic example of this discrepancy was a large family in which Waardenburg syndrome was documented in three successive generations. Various environmental causes of the hearing losses were reported by the family for each affected individual, ranging from "fell in a hole" to "stuck behind the ear with a pair of scissors." The family was astonished to learn that the hearing loss resulted from the same genetic cause in each of the seven deaf members of the family.

Proper diagnostic evaluations by qualified geneticists could greatly increase the number of identified cases of genetic hearing impairment. Some of the patients seen in the Gallaudet Genetic Services Center knew their diagnosis, but were not aware of how it was inherited or the implications of this for their own children. This was especially a problem with the patients with Usher syndrome: although most of these patients had been previously diagnosed and knew they had this entity, an explanation of the genetics of this disorder had never been provided to them.

The genetic counseling process begins with the collection of family and medical history information which assists in leading to an accurate diagnosis. The most critical information often comes from the family history or from physical features found on examination of the proband and other family members. Since genetic tests for carrier status for even the more common types of deafness do not exist and most deaf children do not have recognizable syndromic forms of deafness, diagnoses of genetic hearing loss must often be inferred from information obtained from the family history. Even when a mode of inheritance can be identified, in most cases an exact type of genetic deafness cannot be specified. Other information, including complete medical and prenatal history and audiological data from many family members, is often helpful in making a more specific diagnosis.

When the exact etiology of the deafness cannot be determined and specific probabilities about the expected risks for deaf or hearing children cannot be given, empiric risk figures obtained from statistical analysis of population data are used. Table III is compiled from the results of pedigree analysis on approximately 14,000 matings collected from the Annual Survey of Hearing Impaired Children and Youth conducted by the Center for Assessment and Demographic Studies at Gallaudet College and from the national deafness survey conducted by Professor E. A. Fay at Gallaudet College at the turn of the century (Bieber and Nance 1979). The statistical method used to estimate the proportions of genetic deafness attributable to various modes of inheritance and the overall proportion of genetic versus acquired deafness is called segregation analysis (Nance 1980). This method was used to estimate that 50 to 60% of moderate to profound prelingual deafness is genetic in etiology (Rose, Conneally, and Nance 1977). It was also used to obtain empiric risk figures for hearing-by-hearing matings with and without a family history of deafness outside of the immediate family, deaf-by-hearing matings, and deaf-by-deaf matings.

The most common situation in genetic counseling is the birth of a deaf child to normal hearing parents. If more than one child is deaf or if the parents are

Table III

Recurrence Risk of Subsequent Deaf Offspring in Various Matings

Mating Type	Number of Deaf Offspring	Number of Tested Offspring (s) 0	1	2	3	4	5
Hearing-by-hearing:							
Positive family history	1	NA[a]	0.200	0.187	0.172	0.156	0.138
Negative family history	1	NA	0.098	0.082	0.067	0.054	0.043
Rubella cohort	1	NA	0.058	0.029	0.022	0.017	0.013
Deaf-by-hearing:							
All hearing children	0	0.067	0.043	0.026	0.016	0.010	0.006
At least one deaf child	>0	NA	0.408	0.408	0.408	0.408	0.408
Deaf-by-deaf:							
All hearing children	0	0.097	0.041	0.029	0.020	0.014	0.010
All deaf children	S	0.097	0.617	0.799	0.918	0.966	0.990
Deaf and hearing children	>0,<S	NA	NA	0.325	0.325	0.325	0.325

Note: Adapted from Bieber and Nance, 1979.
[a]NA = Not applicable

found to be close relatives (consanguinous), recessive inheritance can be assumed with reasonable confidence and a recurrence risk of 25% given; however, if only one child is deaf and the parents are unrelated, either this represents an environmental form of deafness with a recurrence risk of close to zero, or it represents a case of recessive deafness with a recurrence risk of 25%. In this situation, table III is used to provide the family with a more accurate recurrence risk figure based on the number of hearing children in the family (hearing-by-hearing mating type). The more hearing children there are in the sibship, the more likely it is that an environmental (acquired) etiology is responsible for the deafness. This is reflected in table III by a decrease in the risk of a second deaf child. As an example, if the first-born child of hearing parents is deaf and there is no family history of deafness, the chance that the next child will be deaf is approximately 10%. If a relative other than a parent or sibling is deaf, this increases the chance that the deaf child has a genetic form of deafness, thereby giving the parents a higher risk of recurrence. If hearing parents have a first-born deaf child and there is even a remote family history of deafness, the chance that the next child will be deaf is 20%.

Deaf children can result from a deaf-by-hearing mating if the deaf parent has a dominant form of hearing impairment, in which case the chance for deaf children would be 50%. If the deaf parent has a recessive form of hearing impairment and the hearing parent is a heterozygous carrier for the same recessive type of hearing impairment, then there is also a 50% chance for a hearing-impaired child with every pregnancy. If the deaf parent has an environmental or acquired hearing impairment, the chance for deaf offspring is essentially zero. Table III shows that the probability that the first child will be deaf in this type of mating is between 6 and 7%. When only hearing children are born, the chance for a deaf child continues to fall. If a deaf child is born, it is assumed that the deaf parent has a genetic form of deafness, and the chance that all subsequent children will be deaf is 40%. This figure takes into account the reduced penetrance that occurs in many types of dominant deafness.

Deaf-by-deaf matings often present extremely complex counseling situations because the two parents may have two different types of genetic hearing impairment. If one parent has a dominant form of deafness, then the chance for deaf children is 50%. If both parents have the same or different dominant forms of deafness, the chance for a deaf child increases to 75%. If both parents have the same recessive type of deafness caused by identical genes at the same chromosomal location, then all the children will be deaf. However, this situation is infrequent because there are so many types of recessive deafness. If the two parents have different types of recessive deafness, then all of the children will be hearing, although they will be carriers of two different types of genetic deafness. Figure 8 illustrates a family with matings of various types. It is assumed that the parents of the proband have the same recessive type of deafness because both sets of grandparents were hearing, the mother's parents were third cousins, and all the children from the deaf-by-deaf mating were also deaf.

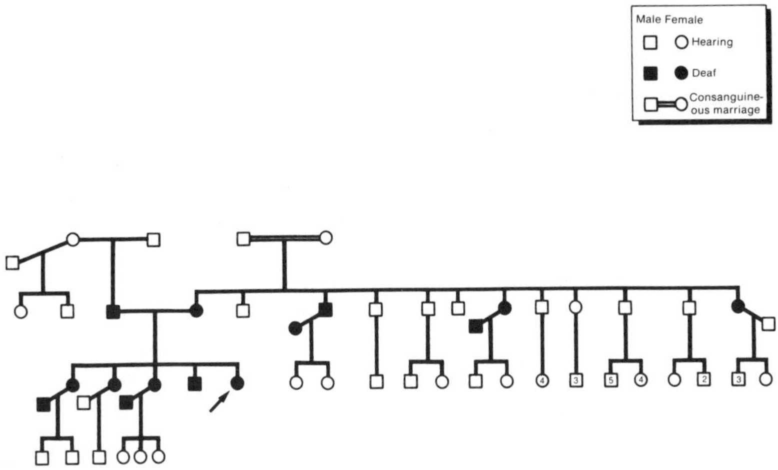

Figure 8. Pedigree illustrating various types of marriages among the deaf. Deafness in the proband's sibship is assumed to have resulted from a recessive by recessive marriage.

Some of the older siblings of the proband married deaf individuals with other types of genetic and environmental hearing impairments, and all of their children were hearing.

Table III incorporates all of the different possibilities of a deaf-by-deaf mating into an overall risk figure. This table is used only when the cause of deafness in either of the parents cannot be determined. The probability that the first child of a deaf couple will be deaf is less than 10%. This figure decreases substantially with the birth of hearing children. If the first child is deaf, the chance that the next child will be deaf increases to 62% and continues to approach 100% with the birth of more deaf children. In the family shown in figure 8, the probability for the sixth child to be deaf is greater than 99%. If there are both deaf and hearing children in the family, the probabilities are much different (32% for subsequent children).

A large proportion of deaf adults now seeking genetic counseling include those individuals born deaf as a result of maternal rubella. Most of these individuals will marry another deaf person who may have a genetic type of deafness. The estimate of 50% environmental versus 50% genetic has been made using populations that include deaf individuals born during the rubella cohort. It has been estimated that 85% of deaf individuals born during 1964 or 1965 have environmentally caused deafness, accounted for mostly by the dramatic increase in deafness caused by the rubella epidemic during those years (Bieber 1981). Table III also includes recalculated estimates for those individuals born during the rubella epidemic (Boughman and Shaver 1982).

CULTURAL DIFFERENCES/ISSUES IN GENETIC COUNSELING

During genetic counseling, effective genetic information can be given to the family to assist them in dealing with powerful emotions that arise naturally and with the coping process. When counseling the hearing parents of deaf children in whom a recessive etiology is confirmed or suspected, it is often helpful to inform them of the frequency of abnormal genes in the general population. Hearing parents very often feel tainted by being carriers of "bad" genes. This heightens the guilt they feel about having a deaf child. In reality, every person is a carrier of at least three to five recessive genes that would cause serious diseases when present in a double dose. In addition, one in eight persons in the general population is a carrier of a recessive gene for deafness. However, the probability of mating with a person who is also a carrier of the exact same recessive gene is quite low. It is also helpful to tell the parents about the frequency of birth defects. In the United States, 3 to 4% of all newborns have a serious birth defect. This information concerning the high frequency of mutant genes in the population can help relieve parents of guilt and shame and help them adjust and plan for the future rationally (Nance 1971).

Genetic counseling of deaf couples and individuals is often quite different from other genetic counseling. Because of the existence of a deaf culture with its own language and social system, some deaf couples do not consider their "risk" that of having a deaf child, but rather that of having a hearing child with whom they may not be prepared to cope. Deaf parents often prefer deaf children and are very curious about their reproductive possibilities. In the past, genetics has been viewed by the deaf community as very threatening. This came as a result of the emphasis in genetic counseling on "curing" a disease and the "normal" or "abnormal" state. The study of genetics is rooted in the eugenics movement in the late 1800s. Individuals such as A. G. Bell believed that preventing deaf persons from marrying one another would greatly reduce the incidence of deafness (Bell 1883). Population studies of deafness have made it clear that less than 10% of deaf couples have deaf children. Much education concerning the true goals of genetic counseling is required within the deaf community to overcome these factors. Education of genetic counselors themselves is also continuing to promote understanding of the cultural and language differences in the deaf community (Boughman and Shaver 1982; Boughman and Shaver 1983a).

To assist in communication with deaf clients, manual signs have been developed and standardized for some of the specialized vocabulary used by geneticists (Boughman and Shaver 1983a; Boughman and Shaver 1983b). These signs were developed in cooperation with native deaf signers, certified interpreters of American Sign Language, linguists and professionals in the area of deafness, and geneticists fluent in sign language, and are now in wide circulation. It is also hoped that more genetic counselors who are fluent in sign language can be trained in the future. As with any other language, the use of sign language by the counselor with deaf clients, rather than interpreters, greatly improves the rapport and expression of feelings by the clients, and in general leads to a more open counseling session.

The counseling of deaf individuals is a process that is greatly improved with early education in the basics of human genetics. Education in genetics for deaf students at the high school level is not widespread, and discussions of the genetics of hearing impairment are virtually absent. This is a topic that would be highly appropriate for deaf students. New high school curricula in genetics have been written and are being distributed to programs for the deaf (Cunningham 1986; Doblmeier 1985). As an additional aid to genetic counseling, written material about genetics, especially written for deaf people and the parents of deaf children, have been developed and are now available through the Gallaudet College Press (Nance et al. 1981; Roehrig 1983; Boughman and Shaver 1983b).

COMPUTER DATA SETS AS AN AID IN COUNSELING

Other techniques have also been used to optimize the information that can be given to a family during genetic counseling. Computerized pedigree linkage of family data is now being developed at the Genetic Services Center at Gallaudet College. This is an attempt to improve the identification of mode of inheritance in individual cases of deafness by linking current pedigrees to a large, nationwide sample of deafness pedigrees collected at the turn of the century. It is possible to establish genealogical linkages in a small proportion of such cases, which can be very useful in confirming the genetic etiology of deafness in the proband. The hereditary deafness data base was initiated in 1900 by Dr. Edward Allen Fay, a professor at Gallaudet College and a protégé of Alexander Graham Bell, who himself had a deep interest in the hereditary nature of deafness long before the rediscovery of Mendel's work in 1901. With support from Bell, Fay collected detailed pedigree data—including names, birthdates, and birthplaces—on more than 30,000 individuals contained within families identified through 5,000 marriages among the deaf. Multiple ascertainment sources were utilized and Fay attempted to identify all marriages in North America that included at least one deaf partner. These data are much more complete and accurate than contemporary family histories are concerning ancestors living in the 19th century.

The computerized Fay data set is now being combined with other smaller data sets including pedigree information on all deaf students who attended the Clarke School for the Deaf in Massachusetts from 1930 through 1966 (Chung and Brown 1970). Contemporary family histories obtained at the Gallaudet Genetic Services Center are now entered routinely into the data set and the surnames of all individuals are matched against the Fay roster. Whenever a possible match is found, comparisons of birthdate, birthplace, spouse's name, and other identifying information is used to confirm the match. This data set will become even more useful as it is expanded with the entry of more current family histories and can be used not only as an aid to genetic counseling, but also to locate families for future DNA mapping studies.

An increase in genetic services to deaf people, use of manual signs for genetic terminology, and education of geneticists and medical personnel on the cultural aspects of deafness has greatly enhanced the utilization of genetic services by deaf individuals and their families. Moreover, the competence, quality, and cultural sensitivity of the services that are provided, and awareness of the cultural differences and special needs of deaf children and adults among health professionals has also improved.

Future Directions in Genetics and Deafness

The field of genetics has changed greatly during the past ten years. New products and screening tests are becoming available because of new genetic techniques. Molecular genetic engineering has led to increased availablity of such substances as human growth hormone, insulin, and interferon. New technology in molecular genetics has enabled the mapping of the exact location of individual genes to specific chromosomes. Over 400 human genes have been definitively mapped and almost 400 more have been tentatively mapped (McKusick 1985). This has led to the identification and mapping of more than 200 genes that cause human disease (Hall 1985). This has been accomplished by family studies in which molecular genetic methods are used to show that disease genes are linked closely with specific identifiable genes or DNA markers whose chromosomal location is known. Because of this new technology, new tests are now possible such as prenatal diagnosis of hemoglobinopathies, carrier tests and, prenatal diagnosis of Duchenne muscular dystrophy and some hemophilias, and potentially, prenatal and premorbid diagnosis of Huntington's disease. Recent developments have also made the actual change or replacement of genes a very real possibility in the next few years. Geneticists are on the verge of managing human disease at the biochemical or molecular level rather than merely treating symptoms.

Amniocentesis is now a standard prenatal diagnostic procedure used in many medical centers across the country (Charrow and Nadler 1984). The optimum time to perform amniocentesis is at 16 weeks of pregnancy and results are obtained within two to four weeks. Beginning in 1983, chorionic villus sampling was developed to provide first-trimester prenatal diagnosis (Simoni et al. 1983). This procedure involves sampling of the developing chorionic villi, which have the same genetic constitution as the fetus, by passing a catheter through the cervix into the placenta. A sample of chorionic tissue is obtained and can be used for direct chromosomal, biochemical, and DNA studies without tissue culture. The procedure is performed between the ninth and eleventh week of gestation and morphologic defects of the chromosomes can be detected within a few hours (Jackson 1985). As clinicians gain more experience with this procedure, it will become more widely available.

At present, there are no single gene defects that cause deafness that are amenable to prenatal diagnosis or carrier detection. For the rare instances of X-linked deafness it is possible to determine fetal sex, but direct testing for the genes in question is not available. Visualization of the fetus indirectly using sonography, or directly using a fetoscope (a fiber optic device) can be used to detect those fetuses with malformations of the limbs, face, or heart, or pigmentary abnormalities associated with deafness.

In combination with other types of investigations such as pathological studies, new genetic techniques will assist in understanding the biochemical nature of the defects that cause hereditary hearing impairment. Molecular genetic analysis of some of the more common types of hereditary deafness, such as Usher syndrome and Waardenburg syndrome, are already underway in some laboratories and will greatly expand in other laboratories within the next few years. These mapping studies will be used to answer questions of heterogeneity within various types of deafness. Eventually, it is hoped that prenatal and carrier tests will be available for some of the more common types of hereditary deafness. These developments may also lead to new avenues in the treatment or cure of these diseases.

References

Bell, A. G. 1883. Upon the formation of a deaf variety of the human race. *Memoirs of the National Academy of Science* 2:1–84.

Bieber, F. R. 1981. Genetic studies of questionnaire data from a residential school for the deaf. Doctoral dissertation, Medical College of Virginia, Richmond.

Bieber, F. R., and Nance, W. E. 1979. Hereditary hearing loss. *In* Jackson and Schimke (eds.). *Clinical Genetics: A Sourcebook for Physicians* (pp. 443–461). New York: John Wiley & Sons.

Boughman, J. A., and Shaver, K. A. 1982. Genetic aspects of deafness: Understanding the counseling process. *American Annals of the Deaf* 127:393–400.

Boughman, J. A., and Shaver, K. A. 1983a. Responsibilities in genetic counseling for the deaf (letter to the editor). *American Journal of Human Genetics* 5:1317–1319.

Boughman, J. A., and Shaver, K. A. (acknowledged) 1983b. *Signs for Genetic Counseling*. The National Academy, Division of Public Services, Gallaudet College Press.

Boughman, J. A., Vernon, M., and Shaver, K. A. 1983. Usher syndrome: Definition and estimate of prevalence from two high-risk populations. *Journals of Chronic Disease* 36:595–603.

Charrow, J., and Nadler, H. L. 1984. Prenatal diagnosis. *In* A. Emery and D. Rimoin (eds.). *Principles and Practice of Medical Genetics* (pp. 1458–1477). New York: Churchill Livingstone.

Chung, C. S., and Brown, K. S. 1970. Family studies of early childhood deafness ascertained through the Clarke School for the Deaf. *American Journal of Human Genetics* 22:630–644.

Cunningham, P. 1986. Gallaudet College—Personal Communication.

Doblmeier, J. 1985. Model Secondary School for the Deaf—Personal Communication.

Emery, A. E. H. 1984. Introduction—The principles of genetic counselling. *In* A. E. H. Emery and I. Pullen (eds.). *Psychological Aspects of Genetic counselling* (pp. 1–10). San Diego: Academic Press.

Freeman, R. D., Carbin, C. F., and Boese, R. J. 1981. *Can't Your Child Hear?* Austin, Texas: Pro-Ed, Inc.

Hall, J. G. 1985. Medical genetics. *Journal of the American Medical Association* 254:2296–2298.

Jackson, L. G. 1985. First-trimester diagnosis of fetal genetic disorders. *Hospital Practice* 20:39–48.

Konigsmark, B. W., and Gorlin, R. J. 1976. *Genetic and Metabolic Deafness*. Philadelphia: W. B. Saunders Co.

McKusick, V. A. 1983. *Mendelian Inheritance in Man* (6th ed.). Baltimore: The Johns Hopkins University Press.

McKusick, V. A. 1985. The Human Gene Map I December 1984. *Clinical Genetics* 27:207–239.

Nance, W. E. 1971. Genetic counseling for the hearing impaired. *Audiology* 10:222–233.

Nance, W. E. 1980. The genetic analysis of profound prelingual deafness. *Birth Defects: Original Article Series* 16(4):263–269.

Nance, W. E., Cunningham, P., Lloyd, E., Rikuris, E., and Shaver, K. A. (acknowledged) 1981. *What Every Person Should Know About Heredity and Deafness.* The National Academy, Division of Public Services, Gallaudet College Press.

Nance, W. E., Rose, S. P., and Conneally, P. M., and Miller, J. Z. 1977. Opportunities for genetic counseling through institutional ascertainment of affected probands. *In* Lubs and de la Cruz (eds.). *Genetic counseling*. New York: Raven Press.

Roehrig, A. (acknowledged) 1983. *A Deaf Person's Adjustment to Usher's Syndrome*. Hearing-Vision Impaired Programs, College for Continuing Education, Gallaudet College Press.

Rose, S. P. 1975. Genetic studies of profound prelingual deafness. Doctoral dissertation, Indiana University, Indianapolis.

Rose, S. P., Conneally, P. M., and Nance, W. E. 1977. Genetic analysis of childhood deafness. *In* Bess, F. H. (ed.). *Childhood Deafness* (pp. 19–35). New York: Grune and Stratton.

Simoni, G., Brambati, B., Danesino, C., Rossella, F., Terzoli, G. L., Ferrari, M., and Freccaro, M. 1983. Efficient direct chromosome analyses and enzyme determinations from chorionic villi samples in the first trimester of pregnancy. *Human Genetics* 63:349–357.

Smith, D. W. 1982. *Recognizable Patterns of Human Malformation*. Philadelphia: W. B. Saunders Company.

Watson, J. D., and Crick, F. H. C. 1953. Molecular structure of nucleic acids: A structure for deoxyribose nucleac acid. *Nature* 171:737.

Chapter 3

Infectious Agents That Deafen

LaVonne Bergstrom

Introduction

Infectious diseases capable of causing prelinguistic hearing loss are preventable. It would seem that cases due to these illnesses should be curiosities, anachronisms from the pre-antimicrobial era. However, failure to be immunized, to have one's children immunized, to have prenatal care, or to be delivered in a medical facility—even though one has had no prenatal care—have always been problems for our health delivery system. Families most in need of preventive medical care, especially the working poor and ethnic groups at increased risk, find that the basic needs of shelter and food use up most of their income. Homeless families are a new challenge that has not been well addressed by our institutions.

Bacterial Agents

Prior to the antibiotic era, acute and chronic otitis media were the major causes of deafness. "Common" complications of otitis media occurred in about 25% of cases and included persistent tympanic membrane perforation (frequently bilateral), ossicular erosion or even necrosis, cholesteatoma, acute mastoiditis, petrositis, septic thrombophlebitis of the sigmoid venous sinus, epidural or brain abscess, labyrinthitis, and meningitis. Without antibiotics, surgery was the only alternative, but myringotomy, mastoidectomy, and craniotomy were the main techniques available. The mortality rate for the central nervous system complications was high; for example, for meningococcal meningitis the death rate was 75%. Furthermore, meningococcal meningitis occurs in epidemics, fortunately at widely spaced intervals. One attack usually confers permanent immunity, but an occasional patient has relapses or recurrences (Bradford 1954). Deafness occurs in 10 to 12% of patients, but the degree of severity ranges from unilateral mild to bilateral severe to profound (Swartz 1984).

Pneumococcal meningitis caused deafness in 31% of the cases in a recent prospective study (Dodge et al. 1984); more than reported in earlier series. *Hemophilus influenzae* meningitis caused deafness in only 6% of patients. Recovery of hearing may occur; in one study 14 of 34 infants had no response to auditory brainstem response (ABR) testing, but at six months only one had persistent deafness (Munoz et al. 1983). Other studies show similar results (Vienny et al. 1984; Kaplan et al. 1984). However, Silkes and Chabot (1985) published an 11 year follow-up of a child who had *Hemophilus influenzae* at age 2½ and unremitting progressive hearing loss in the absence of otitis media. Their report did not mention a CT scan of the temporal bone which might have revealed another lesion that might have contributed to the further loss of hearing.

Spread of meningitis organisms to the labyrinth may occur retrograde from the subarachnoid space along eighth nerve fibers, the periotic duct, or cochlear aqueduct. Direct spread of otitis media organisms from the middle ear to the labyrinth may occur also. The most likely pathogenesis is spread through the blood stream which precedes and accompanies meningitis, as suggested by Schuknecht in a personal communication to Dodge and co-workers (1984).

Other bacteria that can cause meningitis include *Staphylococcus aureus* and gram negative organisms such as *E. coli*. The latter may be seen in the sepsis following premature rupture of fetal membranes, delay of onset of labor, ascending infection of membranes and of the infant. Generalized sepsis and neonatal meningitis ensue. This sequence of events may be prevented by prompt admission to the hospital and vigorous treatment of the mother during labor with triple antibiotic drugs until cultures and sensitivities are available. As soon as the baby is born cultures of its cavities and fluids are taken and the baby given triple drug therapy until the organism or organisms are identified.

Recurrent otitic meningitis may be due to a relapse, but the possibility of a pre-existing anatomic route for re-contamination of the meninges should be investigated. CT scan is helpful in this regard, but surgical exploration of the mastoid and middle ear, looking for an abnormal opening or a cerebrospinal fluid leak might be necessary. A number of papers have been published showing the pathology or operative findings in such cases. Repeated episodes of meningitis may eventually kill the patient. Congenital defects of the stapes or otic capsule are often found (Barr and Wersall 1965; Rice and Waggoner 1967; Hipskind, Lindsay, and Jones 1976).

Studies of the temporal bones, the labyrinthine structures, and middle ear show variable pathology. If the patient dies of tympanogenic meningitis, the middle ear may contain leukocytes and dead bacteria. Occasionally the round window membrane is infiltrated with inflammatory cells. On the scala tympani

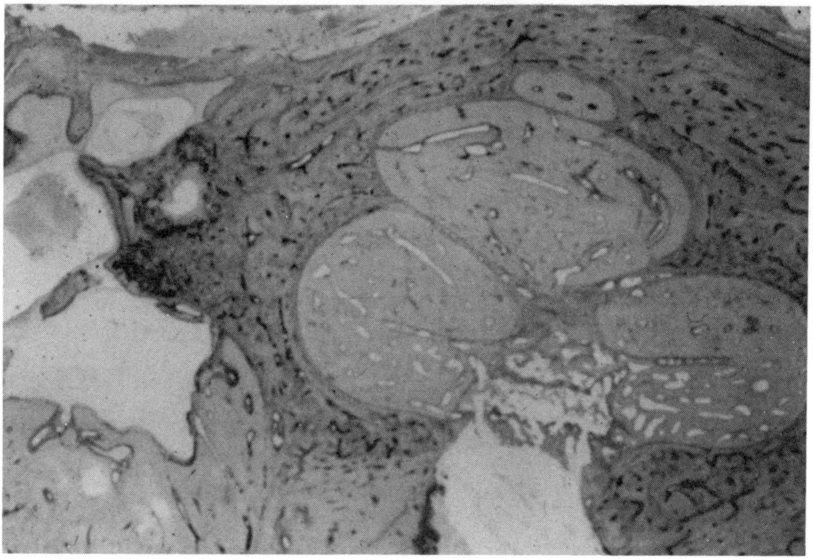

Figure 1. Labyrinthitis ossificans of the cochlea resulting from meningitis many years before. (From F. Black et al., 1971. Used with permission from Colorado Associated University Press, Boulder, Colorado)

side of the membrane there may be leukocytes and a dense fibrous response. The round window niche may be obliterated by fibrous granulation tissue (Paparella, Goycoolea, and Meyerhoff 1980). After some time the cochlear spaces may be filled with bone (figure 1). In other instances the cochlea is nearly empty except for torn and drooping membranes (figure 2).

One other type of otitis media and meningitis deserves mention, although in most areas of North America it is rare. Primarily a disease of children, tuberculous otitis media is generally characterized by chronic, painless otorrhea unresponsive to the usual antibiotics. The discharge is foul and generally thin. Multiple tympanic membrane perforations may be seen and granulation tissue may be present. Vertigo, ataxia, multiple cranial nerve palsies, temporal bone erosion, and intracranial abscesses may be seen concomitant with tuberculous meningitis. The source of infection used to be bovine tuberculosis acquired from drinking unpasteurized milk, but now pulmonary and generalized infections are the major causes of *Mycobacterium tuberculosis* cases (Jeang and Fletcher 1983; Kearns et al. 1985). Groups at risk include American Indians and Eskimos, some immigrant groups, immunosuppressed and immunoincompetent patients. Tuberculosis has been reported in patients having acquired immune deficiency syndrome (Sunderam et al. 1986).

Chronic bacterial otitis media itself may cause progressive sensorineural hearing loss, usually in the high frequencies. This can be differentiated from

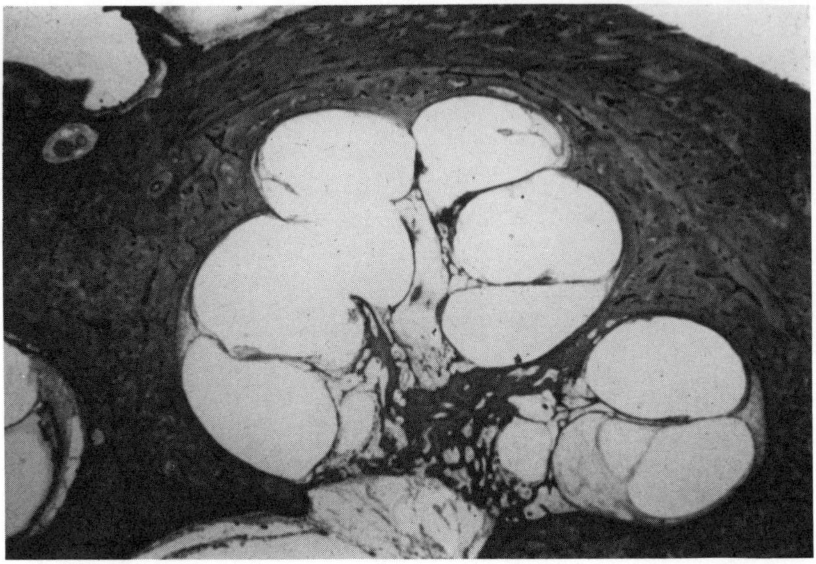

Figure 2. Meningitis with some fibrosis in the basal coil. Note the almost total destruction of the structures in the endolymphatic duct but persistence of spiral ligament and stria vascularis in the basal coil; also note complete neural atrophy.

the aging processes, as was demonstrated by Paparella et al. (1980) in 32 patients who had unilateral chronic otitis media and mastoiditis. It is not uncommon to see children who become unsteady or ataxic during a bout of acute suppurative otitis media—which usually clears, but suggests the possibility of serous labyrinthitis. In her classic book, *The Deaf Child,* Edith Whetnall noted severe partial deafness in 24 children who had chronic suppurative otitis media, 34 cases of moderate deafness, and 25 cases who had slight deafness. This represents 10.5% of her cases reported in 1953. Her patient load also included 130 cases of meningitis, an additional 16%, approximately (Whetnall and Fry 1964).

One would think then—her cases probably having had their onset prior to the antibiotic era—that otitis media and meningitis would be less likely to be a cause of deafness in children today. In a series of somewhat more than 1000 prelinguistically hearing-impaired individuals, 23 multihandicapped children, 7 of whom had clefts, had mixed hearing loss and a drop in the high frequencies in one or both ears. Nineteen others had chronic otitis media or cholesteatoma which was the direct cause of their hearing impairment or which added further decrement to a pre-existing congenital loss. Seven had unilateral otitis media, always in the same ear, 3 due to cholesteatoma. There were 29 who had meningitis: 16 of unspecified type, one of whom also had craniotomy for abscess; 6 *H. influenzae;* 2 meningococcal, one of whom also had *H. influenzae* meningitis; one *D. pneumoniae;* 2 measles meningitis; one viral; and one due to *E. coli.* Four had abnormal temporal bone x-rays, including one who had concomitant skull fracture. Four had normal CT scans and polytomograms of the temporal bone. One had a mild cranial abnormality. Finally 88 patients have or had recurrent or chronic otitis media without apparent effect on their hearing after their first visit. In all, this totals 153 individuals whose hearing is at risk or has been affected by otitis media or its sequelae (Bergstrom, unpublished data).

Congenital syphilis does not cause pre-linguistic hearing loss, although other congenital abnormalities may present at birth or in early childhood. The incidence of sexually transmitted disorders is escalating in this country. A recent article advocated screening of semen used for artificial insemination and screening of the donor as well. Because all the necessary tests cannot be completed at the time of donation, only screened, frozen semen should be used (Mascola and Guinan 1986). Childhood hearing loss due to congenital syphilis has been described as follows: "Congenital cases may present with otological manifestations from childhood to old age. . . . In most congenital cases the onset of deafness is bilateral and the progression symmetrical" (Booth 1982). "Congenital syphilis exists in two forms, early (infantile) and late (tardive). Infantile congenital syphilis is often severe and fatal . . . onset in early childhood is often characterized by sudden, bilateral, severe deafness. Vestibular manifestations are uniformly present but are often poorly documented by the parents" (Schuknecht 1974).

Goodhill (1939) described the temporal bone findings in eight congenital (infantile prenatal) cases. Four had positive serologies. (About half of syphilitic neonates have a weak or negative serology.) The pathology of the middle ear showed vascular congestion, infiltrations of cells in the antrum or mastoid, purulent otitis, bony distortion of the stapes footplate or crura, and mucosal slough of the tympanic membrane. The inner ears showed hemorrhage in the perilymphatic spaces of cochlea and vestibular labyrinth; atrophy of the organ of Corti, spiral ganglion and vestibular ganglion cells; periostitis causing irregular bony contour of the posterior and superior semi-circular canals; early gummata; and liquefaction of the bone marrow. General physical findings included icterus, bulging fontanelles, palatal ulcers, hepatosplenomegaly, skin eruption, scaling of the epidermis of palms and soles, snuffles, pneumonia, fever, convulsions, fissured lips, and bleeding or bruising.

All of the preceding entities are treatable or preventable. Appropriate oral antibiotics will clear most acute cases of otitis media. Culture can be obtained by tympanocentesis or myringotomy if desired. Certain "at risk" populations require special consideration. One such group is premature or sick neonates who may be colonized with gram negative or commensal organisms. Some *Hemophilus* species are non-typable. *Branhamella* (formerly Neisseria) *catarrhalis* is more frequently seen in cultures. *Klebsiella pneumoniae* and *Pseudomonas aeruginosa* may also infect the middle ear. Some strains of *S. pneumoniae* and *H. influenzae* have become resistant to penicillin G, am-

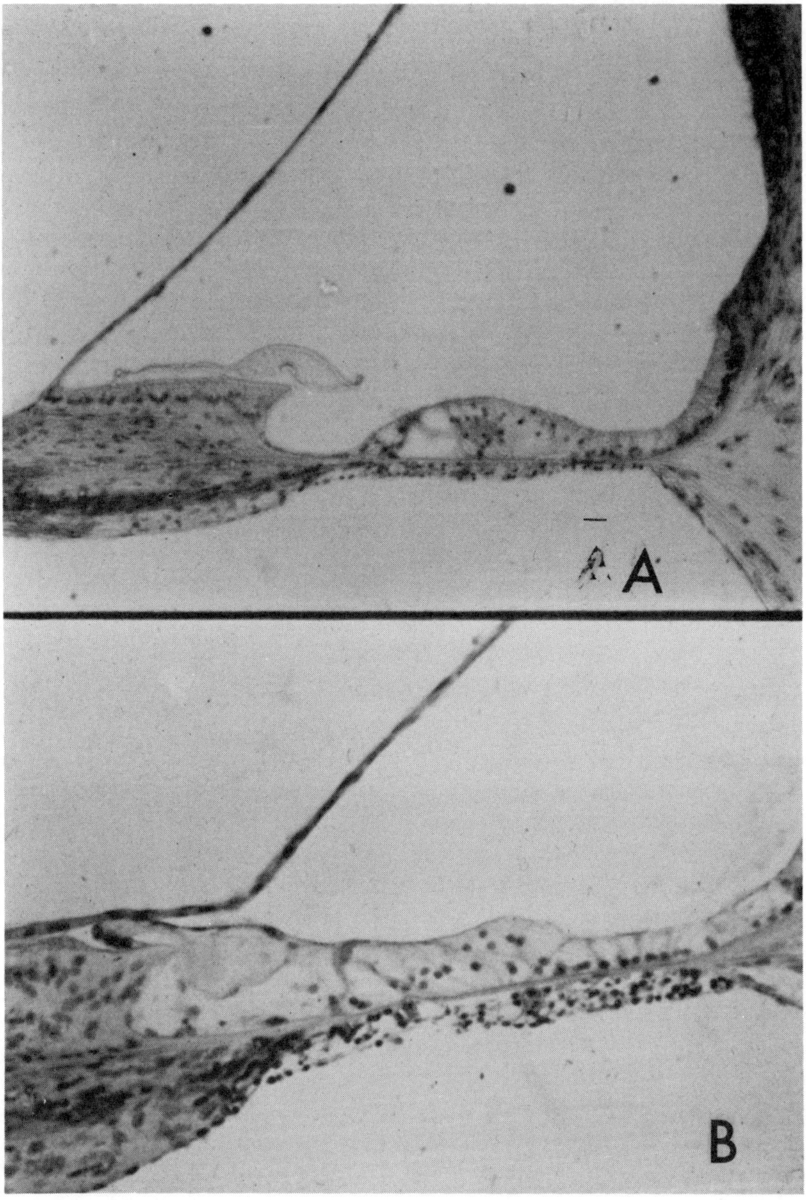

Figure 3. (A) Normal cochlear structures and organ of Corti (OC). (B) Organ of Corti showing only supporting cells. Hair cells are atrophic. Tectorial membrane is retracted into the limbus and encased in epithelial cells. (C) Bulky stapes with minimal cartilaginous fixation of the anterior annulus. (arrow) Note the organ of Corti atrophy (c) and the saccular membrane collapse (S). (From Hemenway et al. 1969. Used with permission of the authors and the publisher)

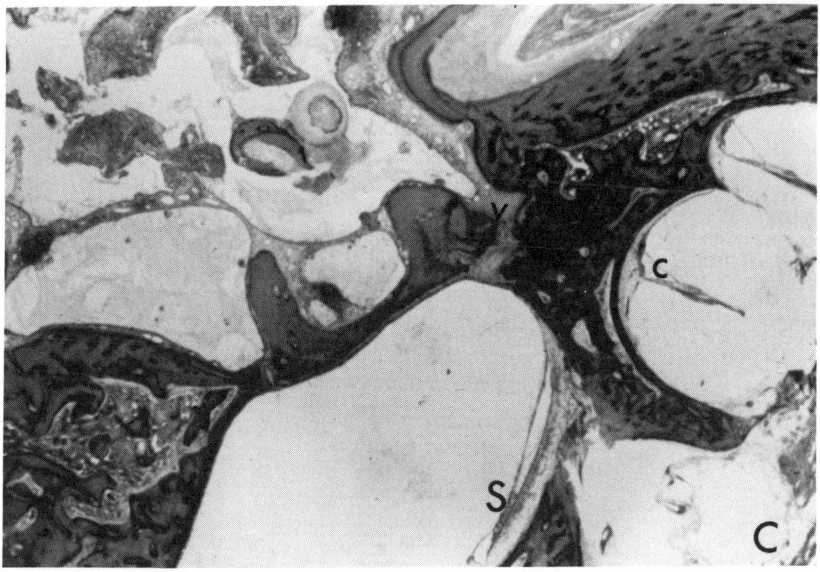

picillin, and amoxicillin by producing beta lactamase which degrades beta lactam (Klein and Daum 1985). A new antibiotic, amoxicillin clavulanate, has been developed to circumvent this mechanism. One group of investigators has even devised and used a protocol to prevent infection of the middle ear and cochlea for cochlear implant surgery (Clark et al. 1980).

Myringotomies and tubes ventilate the middle ear and provide temporary or long-term return to normal middle ear status and hearing. Various types of morbidity may be associated with their use, ranging from postoperative infection or premature extrusion of the tube to rare instances of keratoma cyst on the tympanic membrane or frank cholesteatoma.

However, several studies, using the child as his own control during interims when the tube is not in the eardrum, have shown a statistically lower rate of acute otitis media when the tube is in place than when it is out. This provides relatively short-term relief. A pioneer study was that of Gebhart (1981). Antibiotic prophylaxis on a long-term basis may also be efficacious; recent practice is to use for long-term prophylaxis a once-or-twice-a-day regimen of antibiotics that are usually used therapeutically. Short-term bursts of nasal or systemic corticosteroids have also been tried, with mixed results, to clear the Eustachian tube and middle ear of fluid. Gottschalk has described a technique of "controlled middle ear inflation" to empty the Eustachian tube and middle ear of fluid after adenoidectomy, and the placing of anterior and posterior myringotomy incisions in the tympanic membrane. He rarely uses tubes (Gottschalk 1984). Decongestants and antihistamines are rarely effective; antihistamines may interfere with the surfactant-like substance in the Eustachian tube.

Vaccines for *S. pneumoniae* and *H. influenzae* have been produced which are approximately 50% effective in children over the age of two years. Type 6A pneumococcus is a major cause of pneumococcal otitis media but the response to this vaccine by Type 6A is very poor (Lim 1985; Peltola et al. 1984).

Specific genetic immunoglobulin markers have been found in families prone to otitis media. Low antibody levels to pneumococcal polysaccharide antigens have been observed in children (Prellner et al. 1985).

Congenital syphilis is also preventable. Both premarital and prenatal screening blood tests are available; however, there are no tests given to detect venereal disease in the unmarried couple or that contracted through casual sexual contact. Undocumented alien women may never go to a doctor or hospital for prenatal care or delivery, and in the latter case, if the infant is infected, it will not receive treatment or will receive it too late. Many of today's first-time pregnant women are very young and may seek care late in the pregnancy or only when they are in labor. Ideally, women at risk should have appropriate serologic testing early in pregnancy, and even if the test is negative it should be repeated in the third trimester of pregnancy (Mascola et al. 1984).

A disconcerting observation is that the standard regimen of penicillin may not protect the fetus. The reasons for this phenomenon are unknown, but should be the subject of intense research.

Viruses

The fetus and infant are particularly vulnerable to certain viruses, for example, rubella, especially if the mother is not immune, either naturally or from immunization during her childhood.

VIRAL CHARACTERISTICS

Viruses, seldom visible by ordinary light microscopy, can be seen with the electron microscope. Two broad categories of viruses are known: riboviruses that contain ribonucleic acid (RNA), and deoxyriboviruses that contain deoxyribonucleic acid (DNA). Table I lists the viruses that cause hearing loss and the clinical and pathologic aspects of each virus. Their important chemical constituents include structural proteins; enzymes (their own or those absorbed from host cells); lipids (also derived from host cells in which the virus grew); and nucleic acids. Viruses grow and replicate and attach to receptor sites on the host cell, penetrate into the cytoplasm of that cell, and divest themselves of their coat (uncoating). This ingenious process makes them very difficult to detect and easy for them to seem to have disappeared, a process called eclipse. Actually during this time the virus is synthesizing nucleic acids and viral proteins and maturing while hiding in the host cells. After a period of hours of assembling these components, the mature virus is released from the cell either slowly or in an explosive burst that destroys the cell. During their intracellular

Table I

Viruses Known to Cause Hearing Loss		
DNA Viruses	Clinical Picture	Otopathology
Adenoviruses	Upper respiratory infection, Otitis Media, Sudden sensorineural deafness (occasional)	Cochleosaccular degeneration
Herpes viruses		
Varicella-	Congenital facial defects[1]	None
Zoster-oticus	Sudden deafness, vertigo, facial palsy	Neuropathic findings in geniculate ganglion and facial nerve
Cytomegalovirus	Congenital deafness	Inclusion bodies on cochlear membranes, destruction of organ of Corti
EB virus	Infectious mononucleosis Sudden sensorineural hearing loss	Unknown
Poxvirus	Smallpox	Abortion, stillbirth, premature delivery
RNA Viruses		
Rhinoviruses	Upper respiratory infection, Otitis media, occasional sudden sensorineural deafness	Cochleosaccular degeneration
Togaviruses		
Rubella	Congenital deafness	Cochleosaccular degeneration
Coronaviruses	Upper respiratory infection, otitis media, rarely sudden sensorineural deafness	Unknown
Retrovirus		
Human Immuno-Deficiency Virus	Sudden deafness Opportunistic infections: Cryptococcal meningitis	Cryptococcal invasion of the cochlear and vestibular labyrinths
Orthomyxovirus		
Influenza viruses	Sudden deafness	Cochleosaccular degeneration
Paramyxoviruses	Sudden deafness Mumps, measles Parainfluenza	Cochleosaccular degeneration

[1]Paryani and Arvin 1986; Siegel 1973

existence the viruses induce the host cell to produce aberrant materials and develop abnormal properties that cause clinical and pathological effects in the host. After this the virus may die, transform, or survive, leaving evidence of its sojourn.

The virion, or virus particle, and "naked" viral nucleic acid, which is not neutralized by a specific viral antibody, may also be infective; the latter to a lesser degree than the virion. When the virus is outside the host cell, structural proteins protect its viability and structure. These structural proteins are antigenic when they attach to susceptible host cell surfaces, evoking immunologic "memory" and alerting specific antibodies to inactivate the virus if the host has previously encountered that virus. The resulting antigen-antibody reaction protects the normal individual from being infected again with mumps, measles or rubella (Jawetz, Melnick, and Adelberg 1987; Real, Thomas, and Gerwin 1987; Illis 1975; and Sever 1973). Both humoral and cellular immune mechanisms participate in the host's response to viral infection. At least two types of anti-virus antibody are produced: neutralizing antibodies which block viral attachment to susceptible cells by binding to the viral surface and hemagglutination antibodies which help to make the virus susceptible to lysis. Cellular immune defenses include cytotoxic T cells, helper T cells, and T cells mediating delayed-type sensitivity that can be stimulated to manufacture lymphokines after interacting with the virus. Some lymphokines—for example, gamma interferon—can increase production of natural killer cells. However, viruses may affect the nature of the immune responses by infecting macrophages or lymphocytes, cells that can eat and digest viruses (Sharpe and Fields 1985).

Viral vaccines act in a similar way, but since they are made from dead or attenuated (weakened) live viruses they do not provide permanent immunity, and booster doses are required. Immunoincompetent hosts who have congenital diseases such as DiGeorge's thymic aplasia, thymic dysplasia, or dysgammaglobulinemia; immunocompromised individuals, such as irradiated, transplant, or AIDS patients; persons on immunosuppressants such as anti-cancer chemotherapy, high-dose corticosteroids, or azothiaprine are susceptible to a variety of viruses.

The fetus does not make immunoproteins during the first three months of intrauterine life and is most vulnerable then. In the second trimester antibody production begins; if the fetus has been infected with a virus his immune globulin M (IgM) in the serum will be elevated. Specific fractions of IgM can be isolated and titrated so that the infecting virus can be identified. If the mother is immune to a particular virus the fetus will have no need to make antibodies and will, in fact, be protected by his mother's antibodies to about six months of extrauterine life. After that time he becomes susceptible and will make his own antibodies if his immune system is normal. Patients who have had congenital rubella may not have permanent immunity and can contract rubella in childhood. They should be immunized if their anti-rubella titers drop to non-immune levels.

Congenital rubella stimulates fetal IgM production, but has the capability of producing a curious paralysis of this system allowing the live virus and antibody to coexist in the unfortunate individual for several years. Defects in the immune system have been detected in some instances (Hardy 1973).

CLINICAL FEATURES

Congenital Viral Infections: Rubella. Congenital rubella continues to be a problem because of insufficient immunization of susceptible children and women. Non-immune status needs to be documented in women of child-bearing age, including teenagers, because other mild viral illnesses may closely resemble rubella, but of course do not protect against it. The risk of the fetus acquiring congenital rubella syndrome from the newer vaccine strain RA 27/3 is calculated to be 0–2.4%, but no actual case has been observed, although virus isolation from the products of conception is only 3% (*Morbidity and Mortality Weekly Report* 1986). The virus isolation rate for the older Cendehill or HPV-77 vaccine strains is 20%, but no cases of rubella virus syndrome have been seen from these vaccines either. Spontaneous abortions and stillbirths were at a low rate, and about 9% of women whose immune status was unknown or who were susceptible underwent induced abortions. Earlier studies of the older vaccines indicated an overall infection rate of 5–10%, but no rubella syndrome (*Morbidity and Mortality Weekly Report* 1986; Larson et al. 1971; Modlin et al. 1976).

A susceptible mother is usually infected via the respiratory route. Other sources may infect the nurse or laboratory technician who handles specimens or diapers. The virus stays in the throat and urine for about seven days, during which time the susceptible person is infectious. Virus is also carried in the bloodstream from which it can easily infect the placenta, and, in about one-third of cases, also infect the fetus. It is not known why the other two-thirds of fetuses escape infection. The mother's infection may resemble a mild cold and rash may not be apparent. The first clinical step is lymph node enlargement in the neck and behind the ears, followed by respiratory symptoms and then a discrete or confluent rash beginning on the face and disappearing rapidly over about a three-day period. Temperature, headache, malaise, and joint swelling may also occur. A rare, but serious complication, is encephalitis.

What are the chances for the fetus to escape congenital rubella defects? In the first month of pregnancy, 50% are affected, 22% in the second, and in subsequent months the incidence drops to 6–10%. In the second and third trimesters there is a small incidence of deafness (Hardy 1973) (See table II). Early rubella has four effects on the fetus: teratogenic (producing a malformation), infectious, immunologic, and growth retardation due to inhibition of mitoses, causing fewer numbers of cells as well as loss of infected cells (Naeye and Blanc 1965). Late intrauterine rubella shows no teratogenic effects, but has viral effects on the inner ear closely resembling those seen in postnatally acquired viral infections (Hardy 1973).

The severely involved rubella infant is small for gestational age, has a "blueberry muffin rash" due to deficiency in platelets (blood clotting cells); enlarged liver and spleen; jaundice; microcephaly; heart, kidney, muscle, bone, and central nervous system lesions; cataracts; is deaf and developmentally retarded. Rubella virus also damages the endothelial lining of blood vessels, causing clogged vessels and, in some cases, ischemic damage. Chromosome breakages may also be seen. Virus may persist in body tissues and fluids for many months. Cataract fluid from one reported case persisted for more than three years after birth. Another unusual case known to the author was still shedding virus near age six, but had none of the common lesions of central nervous system, eye, ear, or heart. Delayed progressive encephalopathy may begin in late childhood in some instances and eventually causes a vegetative state. This illustrates a "slow virus" capability of the rubella virus.

Table II

The Johns Hopkins Rubella Study: Status of Surviving Children with Congenital Rubella at 4 to 5 Years of Age

Intelligence (IQ Score)	No.	Percent	H/O Maternal Rubella	Birth Weight <2,501 gm	Other Abnormalities						
					Cardiac	Auditory	Visual	CNS	Other Minor	Small Head	None
Above average ⩾110	20	11.7	13	3	7	15	1	3	6	11	4
Average 90–190	49	28.6	20	7	15	21	. . .	7	12	22	11
Low normal 75–89	31	18.1	14	12	14	17	4	10	9	20	1
Borderline 70–74	22	12.0	6	10	8	12	7	9	6	21	. . .
Defective <70	49	28.6	24	25	23	28	21	30	2	38	(1)
Total No.	171	. . .	77	57	67	93	33	59	35	112	16¢(1)
%		100.0	45	33	39	54	19	34	20	65	9

Distribution of defects in 171 children with congenital rubella by IQ score at 4 to 5 yr of age. The Stanford-Binet was used where possible—other tests such as the Merril Palmer, Leiter, and Cattell were given where the child was deaf or otherwise unable to take the Binet.

From the Archives of Otolaryngology Vol. 98, October, 1973, page 233, copyright 1973, American Medical Association and with the permission of Janet Hardy.

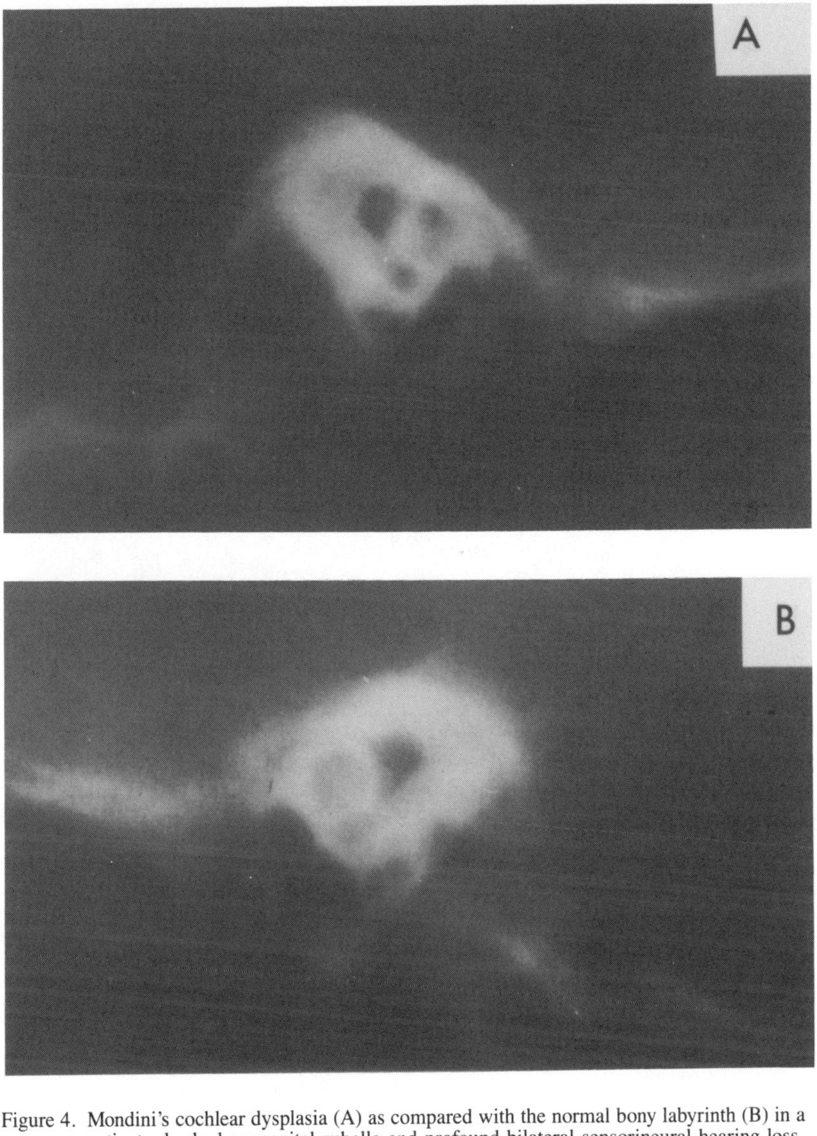

Figure 4. Mondini's cochlear dysplasia (A) as compared with the normal bony labyrinth (B) in a patient who had congenital rubella and profound bilateral sensorineural hearing loss. (From F. Black et al. 1971. Used with permission from Colorado Associated University Press, Boulder, Colorado.)

The hearing loss may be flat, basin shaped, or profound with hearing only in low frequencies. Hearing loss may fluctuate, and occasionally an ear will be useless for speech discrimination.

Less severely involved rubella children may have congenital conductive hearing losses and facial abnormalities, usually mild. One severely affected boy had unilateral microtia, partial facial paralysis, and a Mondini cochlear malformation (figure 4). Several well-documented rubella cases have been observed that show normal hearing from birth to the second year of life, then rapid onset of progressive hearing loss and cessation of progress in speech and language. Rubella virus may cause chronic arthritis in children (Chantler, Tingle, and Petty 1985).

In one case, a female infant was born at term. Maternal rubella had been suspected at birth. Although neither maternal rubella titers nor viral studies on the baby had been obtained, the consulting ophthalmologist found unmistakable rubella retinopathy. For this reason, she was followed with hearing tests. Tests remained normal through the 18th month of life, by which time speech had developed normally. At 24 months of age a sensorineural hearing loss averaging 75 dB in the speech frequencies was detected, and a hearing aid was fitted at the age of three years. Family history was negative for hearing loss.

Cytomegalovirus (CMV). This organism is now more commonly seen in neonates than rubella, but resulting deafness, which earlier was thought would equal that due to rubella, seems now to be less frequent than in rubella. The loss is sensorineural and may be sloping, flat, or even a corner audiogram. Congenital cytomegalovirus passes through the bloodstream, crosses the placental barrier and may cause devastating effects in the fetus, while the mother is unaware of having been ill. Cytomegalovirus infection may also be acquired from an intrauterine transfusion to treat erythroblastosis fetalis, which is an extremely rare event. The mother may continue to shed virus in her saliva, urine, breast milk, feces, or tears.

An estimated 33,000 infants are born with CMV in the United States each year, but only 10% are symptomatic at birth. Five to 15% more are at risk for development of abnormalities within the ensuing two years. The children symptomatic at birth have a potential mortality of 20 to 30% due to hepatomegaly, splenomegaly, microcephaly, direct hyperbilirubinemia, and hemorrhagic complications. Ninety percent of the survivors have late complications: hearing loss, mental retardation, delayed psychomotor development, chorioretinitis, optic atrophy, seizures, expressive-language delays, learning disabilities, and dental defects. The 5 to 15% of infants who appeared normal at birth are at risk to develop sensorineural hearing loss (5–10% of cases), bilateral in 50% of cases. The loss may be progressive (Stagno and Whitley 1985). CMV has been isolated from the perilymph of a deceased infant, using micropipette technique, through a tiny hole in the footplate (Davis et al. 1979).

CMV is of low-grade virulence. Placental barrier prevents in utero transmission in primary cytomegalovirus infection in about 60% of fetuses, and only

11% of infants infected have clinical manifestations at birth. Maternal immunity to CMV does not prevent reactivation. Congenital infections from reinfection seem less likely to cause fatal damage. The presence of CMV in the mother's genital tract at birth and in breast milk is likely to result in transmission to the infant. A pregnant woman with a mononucleosis-type syndrome but a negative heterophile titer is suspect for primary CMV (Stagno and Whitley 1985).

Other Congenital Viral Infections. Prospective studies compared number and time of onset of fetal deaths following maternal mumps, rubella, hepatitis, chicken pox, measles, and similar events for controls (Siegal, Fuerst, and Peress 1966). There was a statistically significant increase in early fetal death after rubella and mumps and an increase in perinatal deaths after rubella and hepatitis. Fetal death from hepatitis was linked to severity of maternal hepatitis and to early infection of the fetus in intrauterine rubella. Fetal deaths from mumps were due to gonadal infection and to placental and hormonal changes early in pregnancy (Siegel et al. 1966). There was no increase over controls in another study of gestational chickenpox, measles, mumps, hepatitis, and congenital malformations (Brown 1970). A study of pregnant women who had chickenpox showed that some had pneumonia and premature labor, but fetal infection also occurred. If the mother died before the fetus was viable the fetus also died (Siegel 1973). Varicella-zoster was not associated with fetal malformations, but one of two infants had microcephaly; the other had a cataract. Another had the cutaneous scarring, bony defects, and atrophy of a lower limb seen in congenital varicella (Paryani and Arvin 1986). None of the fetuses or infants had ear defects or hearing loss, but the sample sizes were relatively small.

DIAGNOSIS

Congenital viral disorders can be diagnosed by taking swabs of the infant's body fluids and cavities and by taking two serologies at six to eight week intervals or a single specimen if an earlier specimen was not collected. Cultures for multiple viral entities should be submitted, including the TORCH organisms: Tissues such as the placenta, surgical specimens, biopsies or autopsy tissues could also be examined for viruses.

PATHOLOGY IN THE EAR

One of the first descriptions of the inner ear pathology in congenital rubella was reported by Lindsay, Caruthers, Hemenway, and Harrison (1953). In 1969, Hemenway, Sando, and McChesney described the temporal bone findings in a well-documented rubella case who lived for several months. She had hearing responses at about 80 dB. One temporal bone showed cartilaginous fixation of the stapes, in addition to classical cochleosaccular degeneration (figure 3C). In 1954 Lindsay and Hemenway described the pathology in the inner ear of an

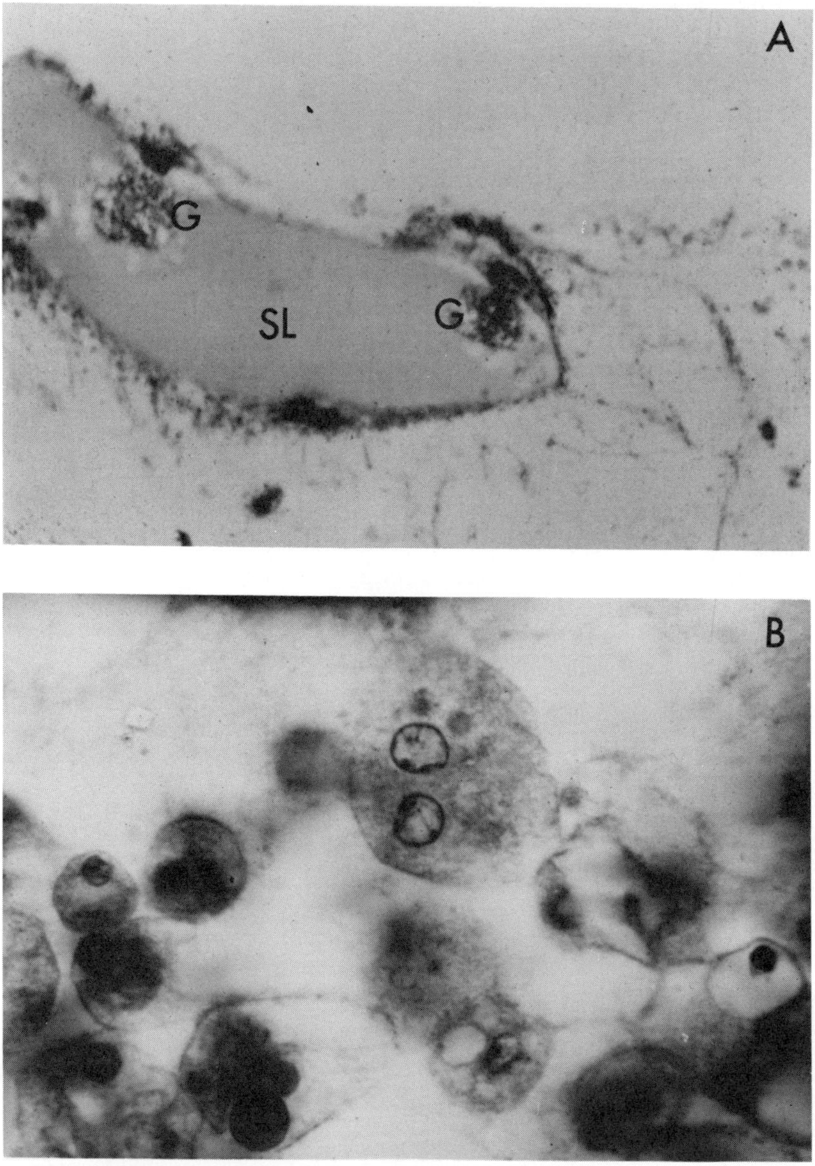

Figure 5. (A) Serous labyrinthitis (SL) and Warthin-Finkeldy granulomata (G) in the lumen of the utricle in an infant who died of measles complications (Case One). This is a subacute lesion. (B) High magnification view of loose stria vascularis cells in endolymph. (C) Degenerated crista (C) in infant who died of measles complications. Note the serous labyrinthitis. (D) Saccular collapse and neural atrophy. (From Lindsay and Hemenway 1954 Reprinted by permission of *Annals of Otology, Rhinology and Laryngology.)*

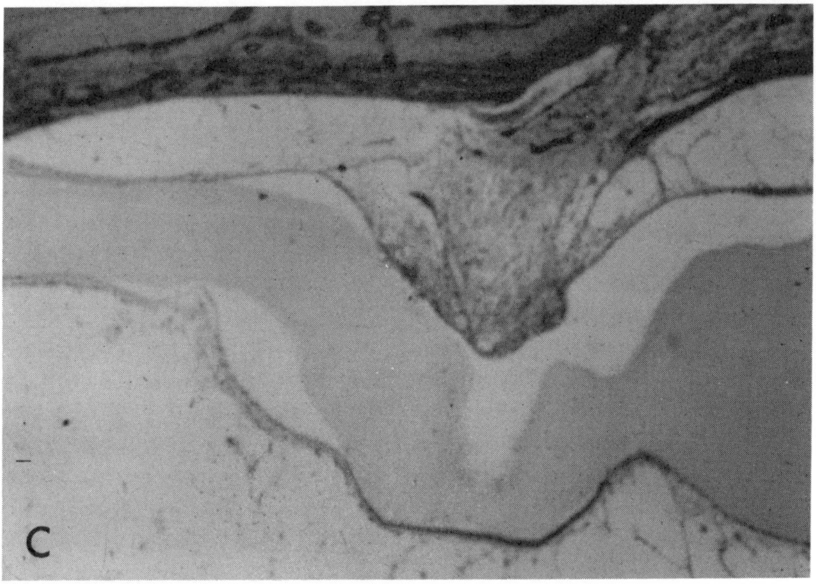

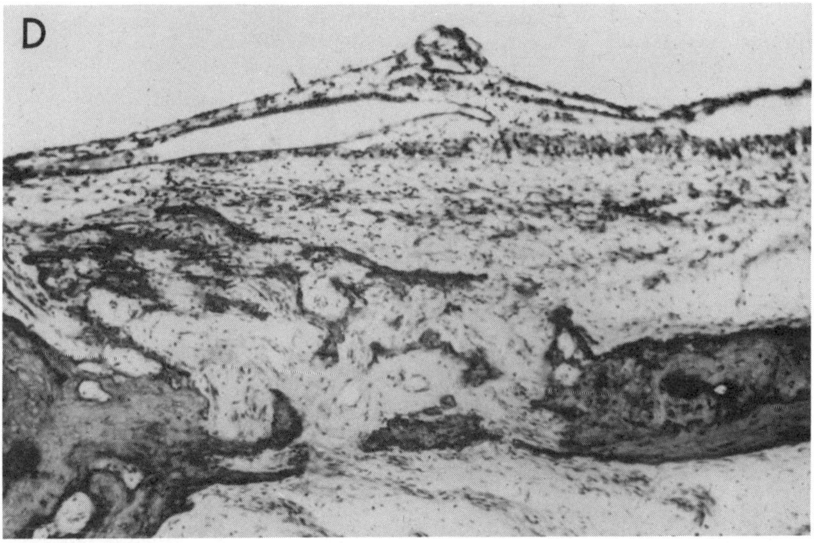

infant who died of complication of measles (figure 5). Lindsay, Davey, and Ward (1960) gave a detailed study of the general pathology and the temporal bone pathology of a young child who developed bilateral profound sensorineural hearing loss after a prolonged bout of mumps. (figure 6) He lived three years after that and died of renal failure.

In 1967 Hemenway and Bergstrom reviewed these temporal bone studies and other specimens, correlating the clinical and pathologic findings with the char-

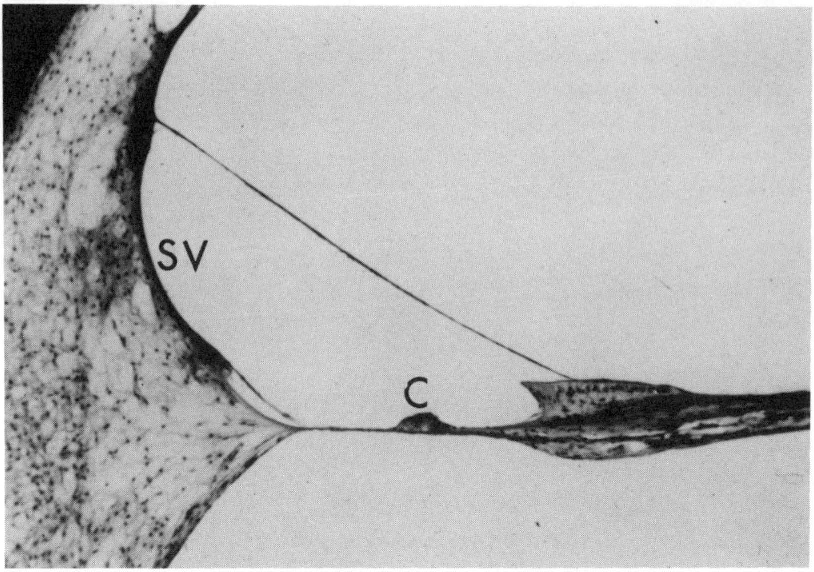

Figure 6. Changes in the cochlear duct due to severe mumps deafness (Case Three). Note the mound of undifferentiated cells representing the organ of Corti (C). The tectorial membrane is absent and the stria vascularis (SV) is atrophic. (From Lindsay, Davey, and Ward, 1960. With permission from the Annals Publishing Co., St. Louis, Mo.)

acteristics of the viruses. A total of 19 ears were analyzed, including five cases of sudden deafness (Schuknecht et al. 1962). A similar pattern of cochlear pathology was found in all cases and vestibular abnormalities were seen in some. In four cases, one of subacute measles, the second the end result of severe measles endolabyrinthitis; the third, a healed mumps endolymphatic labyrinthitis, and the fourth with pathology compatible with either mumps or measles, a pattern resembling cochleosaccular pathology was delineated. The primary lesion was thought to be in the stria vascularis which generally was quite atrophic in the basal coil, less so in the middle coil, and nearly normal in the apical coil. The organ of Corti destruction paralleled the severity of strial atrophy. The most striking finding was detachment of the tectorial membrane from the organ of Corti. It characteristically appeared rolled up in the limbus and encased in an epithelial layer. At the apex the tectorial membrane was still attached and flattened out over the cochlea. The saccular membrane was collapsed and adherent to the macula whose sensory cells had degenerated. In case one the lumen of the utricle showed serous labyrinthitis. Case two showed additional degeneration of the utricle and the semicircular canal cristae. The vestibular system was normal in the mumps case. The neuronal population varies.

The sudden deafness cases showed very similar cochlear duct findings, but the vestibular endorgans were normal. The underlying pathogenesis of these lesions was thought to be related to the hematogenous dispersal of virus to various body sites, including the stria vascularis (Schuknecht et al. 1962). All of the cases resembled the congenital rubella temporal bone findings.

The pathology of deafness due to cytomegalovirus is quite different from that just described. Cytomegalic inclusion cells have been found on or in the epithelial membranes (Myers and Stool 1968) (figure 7). Sensory cells have not been involved generally. Hydrops and strial atrophy have been noted, but the tectorial membrane has been relatively normal. Inflammatory infiltrate surrounds nerves and has been found in the scala tympani and vestibuli. Electron microscopy has demonstrated viral particles in various inner ear epithelial cells.

Fungal and Parasitic Agents

These organisms tend to have devastating effects on the ear and hearing in that they may cause destructive labyrinthitis and meningitis. Their course may be indolent, and death may ensue in the neonatal forms, or in the child or adult after many months or even years.

Cryptocococcus neoformans (formerly called *Torula histolytica*) is a fungus that has a predilection for the lungs, central nervous system, and skin, and causes subacute or chronic disease. Disease can spread from the lung to the brain, causing meningitis or brain abscess. After weeks or months, increased cranial pressure, coma, and death may occur. A disseminated form may occur

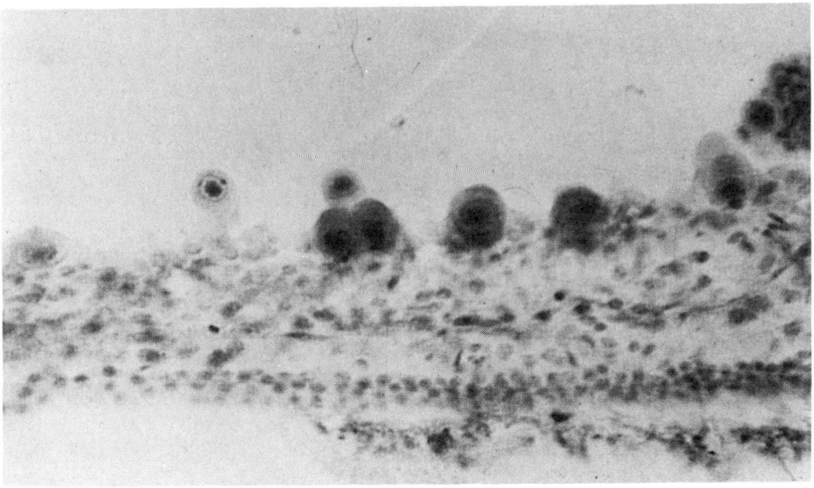

Figure 7. Cytomegalovirus. Large inclusion bodies in the saccular membrane. Similar bodies were also present in the cochlear duct. (From Myers and Stool, 1968. Reprinted by permission of *Laryngoscope*)

in the neonate, but the manifestations can be confused with those of cytomegalic inclusion disease or congenital toxoplasmosis, i.e., jaundice, hepatomegaly, splenomegaly, chorioretinitis, intracranial calcifications, hydrocephalus, and cerebral degeneration. The treatment of choice is intravenous amphotericin B, which may be nephrotoxic in some individuals. It also can be injected into the spinal fluid (Harris 1969).

At least two temporal bone studies have been reported in the literature. The first, reported by Igarashi et al. (1975) was that of a 19-year-old woman with symptoms appearing nearly a year before hospitalization and positive lumbar puncture. She was treated for 15 months with intermittent intravenous and cerebral ventricle infusions. One and one-half years after her first symptoms she noted progressive deafness in her right ear which was accentuated when she was receiving amphotericin B injected into the ventricles. Her audiogram showed progressive loss of hearing in the right ear until there was no response 20 days before her death. Acoustic reflexes were absent in both ears. In the left ear, responses at 4 kHz and 8 kHz were unobtainable. Electronystagmography showed direction-changing nystagmus with positioning. Autopsy of the temporal bones showed foci of demyelination of eighth nerve fibers and yeast-form fungi infiltrating to cochlear and vestibular end organs. Vestibular and cochlear neural and neurosensory epithelium destruction was extensive, and some perilymphatic and endolymphatic spaces contained dense eosinophilic precipitate (figure 8). Seventh nerve and geniculate ganglion were not affected. The left

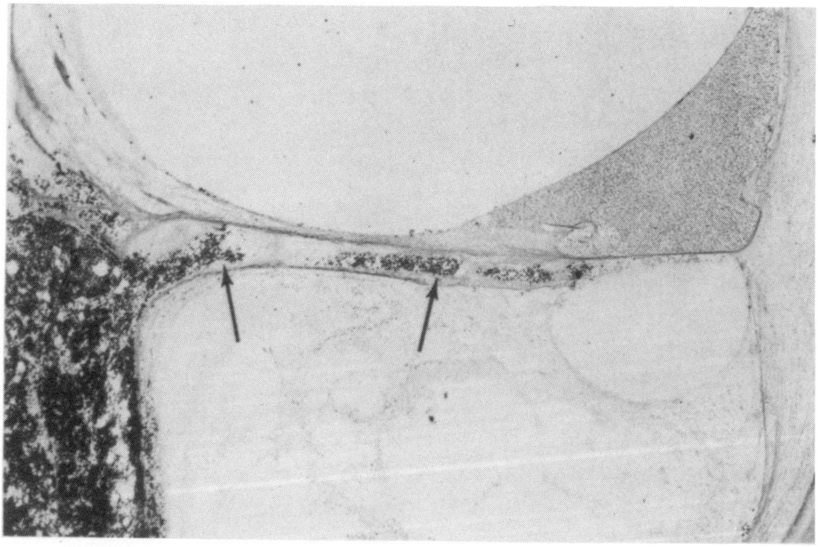

Figure 8. Temporal bone section showing cryptococcal infiltration within the osseous spiral lamina. (arrows) Stria vascularis atrophic, the organ of Corti destroyed, and the scala media filled with hemorrhage. Igarashi, M., Weber, S. C., Alford, B. R., Coats, A. C., and Jerger, S. 1975. Reprinted with permission of *Archives of Otolaryngology.* Used with permission.

ear was less severely involved. There were multiple cysts in the cerebrum and cerebellum. The investigators commented that the patient's hearing loss was probably due to the fungal infection rather than amphotericin B. McGill (1978) reported on a case of cryptococcosis in an alcoholic cirrhotic man who died two weeks after initial symptoms, one of which was progressive hearing loss in the right ear. The temporal bone findings were similar to but milder than those reported by Igarashi et al (1975) with the additional finding of multiple cryptococcal granulomata.

Mucormycosis in the temporal bone was first reported by Bergstrom, Hemenway and Barnhart (1970). The patient was a severe diabetic who presented with unilateral facial palsy. At mastoidectomy for facial nerve decompression, grey material was found in the mastoid. At pathology this tissue yielded a pure culture of non-septate hyphae typical of phycomycetes. Nasopharyngeal biopsy and culture were negative. The patient survived, even though he could not be treated with amphotericin B because of decrease in renal function shortly after beginning intravenous treatment.

McGill (1978) described a diabetic man with involvement of the base of the skull and multiple cranial nerves followed by death due to rupture of a mycotic aneurysm of the right internal carotid artery. Study of the temporal bones showed inflammation of the middle ears and mastoids and a destructive lesion of the right petrous apex. The inner ear endorgans and neuronal population were preserved. Pathologic examination of necrotic tissue from the skull base showed large, non-septate hyphae typical of mucormycosis.

Aspergillosis of the paranasal sinuses and middle cranial fossa in an alcoholic man also caused extensive involvement of the middle ears, infiltration of the nerve trunks in the internal auditory canal with septate hyphae, fibrinous precipitate in some perilymphatic spaces and in the right ear severe destruction of sensory and neuronal elements (McGill 1978).

Fungal infections may occur in immunocompromised hosts such as children born with combined immunodeficiency syndrome, those born with thymic dysplasia or aplasia syndrome, those on long-term corticosteroid treatment, those who have had organ transplants, children receiving anticancer or antileukemia drugs and children who have AIDS. Involvement of the temporal bone is probably quite rare but might be expected to increase somewhat as the number of immunosuppressed patients increases.

Toxoplasmosis gondii, an intracellular parasite, occurs in two clinical forms: congenital, acquired in utero from a mother infected during pregnancy, and postnatal. The latter is not apparent commonly, but when symptoms do occur any combination of the following may be seen: malaise, three-day fever, myalgia, maculopapular rash, generalized lymphadenopathy, hepatomegaly, encephalitis, pneumonia, myocarditis and, rarely, chorioretinitis, usually unilateral. The Sabin dye test is diagnostic, and complement fixation test and hemagglutination test may be useful.

Congenital infection may result in stillbirth, prematurity, and in addition to the postnatally acquired manifestations, the newborn may have hydrocephalus, microcephaly, chorioretinitis, psychomotor retardation, ocular palsies, and seizures. The full impact of developmental retardation may not be evident until weeks or months after the apparent cessation of infection. A few reports of patients having hearing or vestibular problems were summarized by Keleman who added the clinical and temporal bone pathology findings in two additional cases (Keleman 1968). Previous clinical reports were of severe sensorineural hearing loss in three family members who had acquired toxoplasmosis. A wandering type of nystagmus and otitis media were noted in one toxoplasmosis patient, but no evidence was found to implicate toxoplasmosis as the etiologic agent. Another report was of toxoplasma organisms being found in the mastoid processes at mastoidectomy. Autopsy revealed toxoplasmosis encephalomyelitis and toxoplasma organisms in the middle ear. One of Keleman's cases also showed otitis media, mesenchyme in the vestibular endolymphatic spaces, hemorrhagic destruction of the cupulas of the semicircular ducts, and absence of spiral ganglion cells in the middle and lower apical cochlear turns. The second case, a very premature hydrocephalic stillborn, had hemorrhagic otitis media and partial hemorrhagic destruction of the crista of the superior semicircular duct. Toxoplasma organisms were not found. One may conclude that *T. gondii* is rarely a cause of congenital hearing loss, when other etiologies are considered. Toxoplasmosis laboratory tests should be part of the TORCH investigation of infants born with central nervous system and ocular manifestations. Newborn screening using auditory brainstem response testing will identify infants who should be followed for being at risk for hearing loss and who have positive titers for toxoplasmosis.

EPILOGUE

What potentially deafening organisms will physicians be battling 10 years from now? Will there be new ototoxic medications to combat even more aggressive organisms? Will immunoincompetent and immunosuppressed individuals be treated on the moon in impregnable self-contained units? Will the otologist of the future "beam up" there to do otologic surgery in a germ-free environment? And finally, will all Eustachian tubes be working by then?

REFERENCES

Barr, B., and Wersall, J. 1965. Cerebrospinal otorrhea with meningitis in congenital deafness. *Archives of Otolaryngology* 81:26–28.

Bergstrom, L., Hemenway, W. G., and Barnhart, R. A. 1970. Rhinocerebral and otologic mucormycosis. *Annals of Otology, Rhinology and Laryngology* 79:70–81.

Booth, J. B. 1982. Medical management of sensorineural hearing loss. Part I: Late syphilis: Cardiovascular system; endocrine system; renal system. *Journal of Laryngology and Otology* 96:673–684.

Bradford, W. L. 1954. Bacterial infections. *In* W. E. Nelson (ed.). *Textbook of Pediatrics*. 6th edition. Philadelphia: W. B. Saunders Co.

Brown, J. C. 1970. Maternal virus infection and congenital anomalies. *Archives of Environmental Health* 21:362–365.

Chantler, J. K., Tingle, A. J., and Petty, R. E. 1985. Persistent rubella virus infection associated with chronic arthritis in children. *New England Journal of Medicine* 313:1117–1132.

Clark, G. M., Pyman, B. C., and Pavillard, R. E. 1980. A protocol for the prevention of infection in cochlear implant surgery. *Journal of Laryngology and Otology* 94:1377–1386.

Davis, L. E., James, C. J., Fiber, F., and McLaren, L. C. 1979. Cytomegalovirus isolation from a human inner ear. *Annals of Otology, Rhinology and Laryngology* 88:424–426.

Dodge, P. R., Davis, H., Frigin, R. D., Holmes, S. J., Kaplan, S. L., Jubelirer, D. P., Stechenberg, B. W., and Hirsh, S. K. 1984. Prospective evaluation of hearing impairment as a sequela of acute bacterial meningitis. *New England Journal of Medicine* 311:869–874.

Gebhart, D. E. 1981. Tympanostomy tubes in the otitis media prone child. *Laryngoscope* 91:840–866

Goodhill, V. 1939. Syphilis of the ear: A histopathologic study. *Annals of Otology, Rhinology and Laryngology* 43:676–707.

Gottschalk, G. H. 1984. Tympanostomy tubes: To be or not to be. *American Journal of Otology* 5:248–250.

Hardy, J. B. 1973. Clinical and developmental aspects of congenital rubella. *Archives of Otolaryngology* 98:230–236.

Harris, J. S. 1969. Mycotic infections. *In* W. E. Nelson, V. C. Vaughan III, and R. J. McKay (eds.). *Textbook of Pediatrics*. 9th Edition, 706–707.

Hemenway, W. G., and Bergstrom, L. 1967. The pathology of acquired viral endolabyrinthitis. *In* F. McConnell, and P. H. Ward (eds.) *Deafness in Childhood*. Nashville: Vanderbilt Press.

Hemenway, W. G., Sando, I., and McChesney, D. 1969. Temporal bone pathology following maternal rubella. *Arch. Klinische Exp. Ohr. Nas. Kehlkopfheilk* 193:287–300.

Hipskind, M. M., Lindsay, J. R., and Jones, T. D. 1976. Recurrent meningitis and labyrinthine gusher, related to congenital defects of the labyrinthine capsule and stapes footplate. *Laryngoscope* 86:682–689.

Igarashi, M., Weber, S. C., Alford, B. R., Coats, A. C., and Jerger, J. 1975. Temporal bone findings in cryptococcal meningitis. *Archives of Otolaryngology* 101:577–583.

Illis, L. S. 1975. *Viral Diseases of the Central Nervous System*. Baltimore: Williams & Wilkins Co.

Jawetz, E., Melnick, J. L., and Adelberg, E. A. 1987. *Review of Medical Microbiology, Ed. 17*. Norwalk, CT and Los Angeles: Appleton and Lange.

Jeang, M. K., and Fletcher, E. C. 1983. Tuberculous otitis media. *Journal of the American Medical Association* 249:2231–32.

Kaplan, S. L., Catlin, F. I., Weaver, T., and Feigin, R. D. 1984. Onset of hearing loss in children with bacterial meningitis. *Pediatrics* 73:575–578.

Kearns, D. B., Coker, N. J., Pitcock, J. K., and Jenkins, H. A. 1985. Tuberculous petrous apicitis. *Archives of Otolaryngology* 111:406–408.

Keleman G. 1968. Toxoplasmosis and congenital deafness. *Archives of Otolaryngology* 68:547–561.

Klein, J. O., and Daum, R. S. 1985. *The Diagnosis and Management of the Patient with Otitis Media*. New York: Biomedical Information Corp.

Larson, H. E., Parkman, P. D., Davis, W. J., Hopes, H. E., and Meyers, H. M. Jr. 1971. Inadvertent rubella virus vaccination during pregnancy. *New England Journal of Medicine* 284:870–873

Lim, D. (ed.). 1985. Recent advances in Otitis Media with Effusion. *Annals of Otology, Rhinology and Laryngology* Suppl. 116, Panel Report 4, 18–22.

Lindsay, J. R., Carruthers, D. G., Hemenway, W. G., and Harrison, S. 1953. Inner ear pathology following maternal rubella. *Annals of Otology, Rhinology and Laryngology* 62:1201–1218.

Lindsay, J. R., Davey, P. R., and Ward, P. H. 1960. Inner ear pathology in deafness due to mumps. *Annals of Otology, Rhinology and Laryngology* 69:918–935.

Lindsay, J. R., and Hemenway, W. G. 1954. Inner ear pathology due to measles. *Annals of Otology, Rhinology and Laryngology* 63:754–771.

McGill, T. J. I. 1978. Mycotic infection of the temporal bone. *Archives of Otolaryngology* 104:140–144.

Mascola, L., and Guinan, M. E. 1986. Screening to reduce transmission of sexually transmitted diseases in semen used for artificial insemination. *New England Journal of Medicine* 314:1354–1359.

Mascola, L., Pelosi, R., Blount, J. H., Binkin, N. J., Alexander, C. E., and Cates, W. Jr. 1984.

Congenital syphilis: Why is it still occurring? *Journal of the American Medical Association* 252:1719–1749.

Modlin, J. F., Herrmann, K., Brandlin-Bennett, A. D., Eddins, D. L., and Hayden, G. F. 1976. Risk of congenital abnormality after inadvertent rubella vaccination of pregnant women. *New England Journal of Medicine* 294:972–974.

Morbidity and Mortality Weekly Report, March 7, 1986 Vol. 35 No.9 pp 275–276, 281–284. Massachusetts Medical Society.

Muñoz, O., Benitez-Diaz, L. Martinez, M. C., and Guiscafre, H. 1983. Hearing loss after *Hemophilus influenzae* meningitis: follow-up study with auditory brainstem potentials. *Annals of Otology, Rhinology and Laryngology* 92:272–275.

Myers, E. N., and Stool, S. 1968. Cytomegalic inclusion disease of the inner ear. *Laryngoscope* 88:1904–1915.

Naeye, R. L., and Blanc, W. 1965. Pathogenesis of congenital rubella. *Journal of the American Medical Association* 194:1277–1283.

Paparella, M. M., Goycoolea, M. V., and Meyerhoff, W. L. 1980. Inner ear pathology and otitis media. *Annals of Otology, Rhinology and Laryngology* Suppl.68:249–253.

Paryani, S. G., and Arvin, A. M. 1986. Intrauterine infection with varicella-zoster virus after maternal varicella. *New England Journal of Medicine* 314:1542–1546.

Peltola, H., Käyhty, H., Virtanen, M., and Mäkelä, P. H. 1984. Prevention of *Hemophilus influenzae* type B bacteremic infections with the capsular polysaccharide vaccine. *New England Journal of Medicine* 310:982–984.

Prellner, K., Hallberg, T., Kalm, O., and Månsson, B. 1985. Recurrent otitis media: Genetic immunoglobulin markers in parents and their children. *Journal of International Pediatric Otorhinolaryngology.*

Real, R., Thomas, M., and Gerwin, J. M. 1987. Sudden hearing loss and acquired immunodeficiency syndrome. *Otolaryngology-Head and Neck Surgery* 97:409–412.

Rice, W. J., and Waggoner, L. G. 1967. Congenital cerebrospinal fluid otorrhea via a defect in the stapes footplate. *Laryngoscope* 77:341–349.

Schuknecht, H. F. 1974. *Pathology of the Ear* 263–266. Cambridge, MA: Harvard University Press.

Schuknecht, H. F., Benitez, J., Beekhuis, J., Igarashi, M., Singleton, G., and Ruedi, L. 1962. The pathology of sudden deafness. *Laryngoscope* 72:1142–1157.

Sever, J. L. 1973. Present status of vaccines for rubella. *Archives of Otolaryngology* 98:265–268.

Sharpe, A. H., and Fields, B. N. 1985. Pathogenesis of viral infections. Basic concepts derived from the Reovirus model. *New England Journal of Medicine* 312:486–496.

Siegel, M. 1973. Congenital malformations following chickenpox, measles, mumps and hepatitis. *Journal of the American Medical Association* 226:1521–1524.

Siegel, M., Fuerst, H. T., and Peress, N. S. 1966. Comparative fetal mortality in maternal virus disease. *New England Journal of Medicine* 274:768–771.

Silkes, E. D., and Chabot, J. 1985. Progressive hearing loss following *Haemophilus influenzae* meningitis. *International Journal of Pediatric Otorhinolaryngology* 9:249–256.

Stagno, S., and Whitley, R. J. 1985. Herpesvirus infections of pregnancy. Part I: Cytomegalovirus and Ebstein-Barr virus infections. *New England Journal of Medicine* 313:1270–1274.

Sunderam, G., McDonald, R. J., Maniatis, T., Oleske, J., Kapila, R., and Reichman, L. B. 1986. Tuberculosis as a manifestation of the Acquired Immunodeficiency Syndrome (AIDS). *Journal of the American Medical Association* 256:362–366.

Swartz, M. N. 1984. Bacterial meningitis. *New England Journal of Medicine* 311: 912–913.

Vienny, H., Despland, P. A., Lütschg, J., Deonna, T., Dutoit-Marco, M. L., and Gander, C. 1984. Early diagnosis and evolution of deafness in childhood bacterial meningitis: A study using brainstem auditory evoked potentials. *Pediatrics* 73:579–586.

Whetnall, E., and Fry, D. B. 1964. *The Deaf Child.* William Heinemann Medical Books Ltd.

Chapter 4

A Review of Syndromes That Deafen

Robert A. Jahrsdoerfer, James W. Hall, and *Lincoln Gray*

It would be presumptuous of us to attempt to review in this chapter the hundreds of syndromes that cause deafness. The differences in some of these syndromes may be subtle and include a single additional trait whose clinical impact may be insignificant except to identify the syndrome. It is therefore very difficult for one to be cognizant of all syndromes—difficult for the dysmorphologist, more difficult yet for those of us who narrow our field of interest to the ears and hearing.

We have chosen four syndromes for review here: congenital atresia/stenosis of the ear, Treacher Collins syndrome, Waardenburg's syndrome, and Cogan's syndrome. As a phenotype, congenital atresia of the ear represents a potpourri of syndromes in which failure of development of the external ear canal, and the associated hearing loss, is preeminent. This is in contradistinction to the many other craniofacial syndromes (hemifacial microsomia, Goldenhar's syndrome, for example) in which the facial features may take on a higher priority than the hearing.

Treacher Collins syndrome is chosen because it represents one of the most difficult syndromes to treat and demands the best talent and effort from those who try to help these patients.

Waardenburg's syndrome is unique because of its unusual and variable expressivity, and lastly, Cogan's syndrome, known to us for many years, is now recognized as an autoimmune disorder affecting children and young adults with potentially devastating audiovestibular consequences.

Congenital Aural Atresia/Stenosis

Congenital microtia and atresia/stenosis may be syndromic, or may represent a single malformation. A syndrome by definition implies that there is at least one other trait by which the malformation is recognized. We have seen cases of atresia/stenosis of the external ear canal which could be traced through five generations, yet, the external ear in the affected individuals had a normal appearance. In a situation such as this, a patient with a mild conductive hearing loss of 35–40 dB, and soft tissue atresia, may go undiagnosed for years. In our series, a patient with normal auricles and deep meatal pits, but with complete atresia, went 30 years before congenital atresia of the ear canals was diagnosed.

Other families in the series in whom a genetic transmission was noted had atresia and digital malformations, stenosis with preauricular pits and stapes ankylosis, and microtia/atresia with genitourinary findings. Most patients, however, represent isolated cases of atresia/stenosis with or without microtia. The collective experience of the authors includes over 600 patients with congenital ear malformations who were evaluated. Of this group, 250 patients had surgery.

Our standard protocol for evaluating patients with congenital ear or facial malformations (or high-risk registry patients) is auditory brainstem response (ABR) testing shortly after birth and at monthly intervals thereafter. If a hearing loss is diagnosed, or even suspected, a hearing aid is fitted early in life. There is no rationale for waiting six weeks, or six months, as has been recommended in the past.

At age three or four years, high resolution CT scanning of the temporal bone is performed to determine the surgical candidacy of the child. If surgery is indicated, every effort is made to operate on at least one ear prior to beginning school. The specifics of the preoperative evaluation and surgical technique have been reported in previous publications (Jahrsdoerfer et al. 1985) and will not be repeated here. It is worthwhile to reiterate that in carefully selected patients with atresia/stenosis, the postoperative speech reception threshold (SRT) is 15–25 dB routinely.

TREACHER COLLINS SYNDROME

Treacher Collins syndrome (mandibulofacial dysostosis) is an autosomal dominant genetic disorder that affects primarily the region of the head and neck. The systemic manifestation of the syndrome is bilateral and usually symmetrical. There is full penetrance, but the expressivity is variable. The syndrome is thought to be responsible for 300 new cases annually in the United States.

The facial features of Treacher Collins syndrome are characteristic. These include an antimongoloid slant to the palpebral fissures, hypoplasia of the mandible, hypoplasia of the malar bones, colobomata of the lower eyelids, cleft palate occasionally, and malformation of the ears. The external ears in patients with Treacher Collins syndrome may range from being well-formed but almost always smaller than normal, to Grade III microtia, representing little more than amorphous nubbins of skin and cartilage on the lateral face. Congenital atresia is present in over 50% of patients with this syndrome. The hypoplastic mandible predisposes to a small oral cavity which makes endotracheal intubation both difficult and hazardous. Rarely, a patient with severe mandibular hypoplasia who requires general anesthesia may need to have a tracheotomy performed to secure the airway.

The hearing loss encountered in patients with Treacher Collins syndrome is usually conductive, but on rare occasions may include a sensorineural component. Even when the ear canal is open and an ear drum can be visualized, a severe conductive hearing loss may be present. This attests to the many and varied ossicular malformations found in this syndrome.

In the recent past, literature pertaining to the diagnostic radiography of Treacher Collins syndrome stressed the use of multidirectional polytomography in the preoperative assessment of these patients (Lloyd and Phelps 1979; Phelps, Poswillo, and Lloyd 1981). While polytomography was considered state-of-the-art in the 1970s, and undoubtedly rendered valuable information, its performance pales when compared to the sophisticated technology of high resolution CT scanners.

A temporal bone protocol using computed tomography to study patients with congenital ear malformations has been in routine use at the University of Texas Medical School–Houston since 1982. The temporal bone imaging obtained in this manner has been of immeasurable help in determining whether or not a patient with Treacher Collins syndrome is a candidate for surgery. While this scanning technique is used in the preoperative evaluation of all patients with congenital ear malformations, it is of particular value in patients with Treacher Collins syndrome where the malformations are unusually severe. By utilizing a radiographic protocol that produces life-sized images without loss of resolution, the condition of the middle ear and other temporal bone structures can be routinely determined preoperatively. For example, a stapes can be identified, if present, and the course of the facial nerve can be traced—information which is of critical importance to the surgeon. This information was essentially unobtainable using polytomography.

While high resolution CT scanning can accurately identify the structural integrity of the middle and inner ear with a high degree of precision, regrettably, it tells us nothing of the hearing. As hearing is recognized as the most important parameter that needs to be measured early in the life of the individual, the advent of auditory brainstem response (ABR) testing has been of inestimable help. Our standard protocol for assessing hearing in neonates and young children with congenital ear malformations is to use simultaneous multichannel recordings of the ABR. By comparing ABR recordings for the electrode on the mastoid ipsilateral to the stimulus vs. the contralateral electrode, peripheral (VIII cranial nerve) auditory function can be routinely specified for each ear without the use of masking noise.

Despite the advances in the preoperative evaluation of patients with Treacher Collins syndrome, only a small percentage ever become candidates for ear surgery to improve hearing. The reason for this is that patients with Treacher Collins syndrome have the most bizarre middle ear malformations of any craniofacial group. The mastoid is almost never pneumatized. In place of air cells there are large islands of bone marrow which tend to bleed throughout the surgical procedure. The ossicles are often abnormal, particularly in those patients with atresia where a fused incus/malleus complex may be situated far from the stapes and oval window. A malformed stapes, although present, may be buried beneath thickened middle ear mucosa concealing its location and making the search dangerous. The middle ear cleft is often narrow, sometimes nothing more than a mere slit in the temporal bone. The labyrinthine windows may be absent and the facial nerve may be displaced and naked. Even fenestration of the horizontal semicircular canal is hazardous as the severely malformed temporal bone architecture makes this structure hard to find.

The reality of the situation is that fewer patients with Treacher Collins syndrome are operated on than any other patient group with congenital atresia. In the author's experience, of 42 patients with Treacher Collins syndrome who were studied, only 7 became surgical candidates for hearing rehabilitation.

There are other options, however. Even if the middle ear in Treacher Collins syndrome patients with atresia is unrepairable, a new tympanic membrane, and external ear canal, can be constructed to accommodate an ear level hearing aid. Additionally, technological advances in bone conducting hearing devices have recently given new hope to those patients who are not otherwise candidates for surgical repair. One technique involves a bone anchored hearing aid developed by Tjellstrom et al. (1983) which utilizes a titanium screw percutaneously imbedded into the mastoid. A second device is an implantable bone-conducting hearing device pioneered by Hough, Himelich, and Johnson (1986) in collaboration with the Xomed Corporation. Hough claims that a speech-reception threshold of 27 dB may be obtained by the implantable bone-conducting hearing aid.

There appears to be good potential for the implantable bone-conducting hearing aid to be of benefit to a specific subset of patients with ear malformations. Its use, however, should be restricted to those patients who are not otherwise candidates for the surgical repair of their congenital atresia. Of all the craniofacial groups, patients with Treacher Collins syndrome who have markedly hypoplastic middle ears appear to be the best candidates for the implantable bone-conducting hearing aid. In otherwise good surgical candidates, it makes little sense to insert an implantable device when surgery for the correction of atresia/stenosis can achieve normal or near normal hearing.

COGAN'S SYNDROME

Cogan's syndrome typically includes interstitial keratitis, audiovestibular symptoms, and a negative serologic test for syphilis. The audiovestibular symptoms may include sudden and progressive deafness, tinnitus, and vertigo.

Nausea and ataxia may also be part of the syndrome. The hearing loss may fluctuate or may progress to complete sensorineural deafness.

The audiovestibular findings in Cogan's syndrome often antedate the ocular symptoms (McDonald, Vollertsen, and Younge 1985), but may occur concomitantly, or even later. Although interstitial keratitis is the ocular hallmark of Cogan's syndrome, this condition is infrequently seen because patients developing redness of the eyes, photophobia, and other ocular inflammatory diseases are seen early and are often treated with topical steroids for a presumed viral conjunctivitis (Cobo and Haynes 1984). The symptoms thereafter tend to resolve and the true ocular presentation of Cogan's syndrome, namely, interstitial keratitis with vasculitis, is often masked. Only weeks or months later, when the audiovestibular symptoms first become evident, is the diagnosis of Cogan's syndrome considered.

Cogan's syndrome is usually a disease of young adults. The youngest reported patient is a child of 2½ years (Kundell and Ochs 1980) and the syndrome is being reported with greater frequency in children. There appears to be a female to male preponderance. While the audiovestibular symptoms may frequently progress to complete deafness, blindness is unusual. There is evidence to suggest that Cogan's syndrome is part of a systemic disease with a larger symptom complex. For example, a review of the English literature pertaining to 78 patients with Cogan's syndrome (Vollertsen et al. 1986) showed that one-third of the patients had abdominal findings (usually GI bleeding), one-fourth of the patients had cardiac involvement (most often aortic insufficiency), one-fifth of the patients had genitourinary problems, and one-fifth of the patients had symptoms of chest disease.

The diagnosis of Cogan's syndrome is not an easy one to make. Moreover, failure to make the diagnosis early may have grave sequelae. It is estimated that for treatment to be effective, parenteral steroids must be given within two to four weeks of the onset of the audiovestibular symptoms. The fact that a patient may be taking topical steroids for an eye problem has little or no effect on the development of audiovestibular symptoms. The initial recommended dose of systemic steroids is 2 mg prednisone/kg daily. However, it should be noted that despite seemingly adequate steroid therapy, the progressive hearing loss may not be reversed and the patient may develop permanent deafness.

The etiology of Cogan's syndrome is obscure despite evidence that one is dealing with an autoimmune reaction. Hughes et al. (1983) believe that the process is autoimmune and mediated through cellular pathways. They caution that systemic steroids may mask positive test results because maintenance doses of steroids are known to suppress cell-mediated immunity. They recommend that steroid treatment be stopped, if possible, a few days prior to testing. If steroids alone are unsuccessful in reversing the hearing loss, cyclophosphamide may be added after the method of McCabe (1979).

On the other hand, Arnold, Pflatz, and Altermatt (1985) demonstrated that the lymphocyte mitogen stimulation test failed to indicate the presence of cellular immunity in the fresh blood of patients with Cogan's syndrome, Meniere's disease, or progressive sensorineural hearing loss. They did show, however, that serum from two patients with Cogan's syndrome not only reacted with healthy inner ear tissue, but also demonstrated antibodies directed against epithelial cells of healthy human cornea. It is unclear, however, which patients, if any, were being treated with systemic steroids at the time of testing.

The ophthalmological literature (Cobo and Haynes 1984) tends to divide Cogan's syndrome into typical and atypical forms based on the involvement of the cornea (typical), or ocular/orbital inflammatory disease not involving the cornea (atypical). Both patient types exhibit audiovestibular disease which may be profound and irreversible if untreated in the first few weeks. Conversely, while the hearing may worsen, the keratitis tends to resolve spontaneously. Vision, therefore, appears to be at much less risk than hearing or balance.

The differential diagnosis of Cogan's syndrome includes syphilis with interstitial keratitis, other forms of autoimmune inner ear disease, viral infections involving the inner ear, Wegener's granulomatoses, sarcoidoses, polyarteritis nodosa and other systemic vascular diseases, and Vogt-Koyanagi-Harada syndrome.

In brief, Cogan's syndrome is a potentially devastating disease of children and young adults. Successful therapy depends on early recognition with prompt treatment of the audiovestibular symptoms with systemic steroids. Continued investigation into the immunology of the disease is necessary and should have our higher priority.

WAARDENBURG'S SYNDROME

Waardenburg's syndrome is an autosomal dominant disorder showing a high degree of variable expressivity. The clinical manifestations of this syndrome can be divided into three major categories: periorbital, pigmentary disorders, and cochleovestibular changes (Galich 1985). It is believed that the syndrome accounts for about 3% of all hearing impairment in children (Brookhouser and Smith 1986).

The most striking characteristics of this syndrome are the pigmentary changes. Heterochromia irides is the hallmark of this syndrome and should strongly suggest the diagnosis. When both irides are depigmented resulting in pale blue eyes, the appearance is less striking. Depigmentation may be incomplete and the color of the iris may show brown spots on a blue iris, or vice versa. Of interest is the finding that depigmentation in one iris tends to mirror the findings in the fundus (Goldberg 1966). For example, a depigmented blue iris would have a corresponding lack of pigmentation in the fundus of the same eye.

Other pigmentary changes involve the presence of a white forelock which is present in about 20% of patients. Additionally, the hair may be prematurely gray. Both of these signs may be masked by cosmetic alteration, namely, dyeing the hair. It is therefore essential that the interviewer specifically inquire into these traits.

The periorbital signs of Waardenburg's syndrome include dystopia canthorum, a broad nasal root, and confluent eyebrows (synophrys). It is important to note that hypertelorism is apparent and not real. While the medial canthi may be displaced laterally, the interpupillary distance is normal. The patient may also pluck the eyebrows to further disguise the syndrome.

The cochleovestibular findings are the most disabling aspect of Waardenburg's syndrome. Hearing loss occurs in only 20% of patients but the deafness may be profound and may involve one or both ears. Although only two temporal bone studies have been reported in the literature (Fisch 1959; Rarey and Davis 1984), the histopathology was similar. Fisch studied the temporal bones of a 3½ year old child with Waardenburg's syndrome and noted an absent organ of Corti and atrophy of the spiral ganglion. Rarey and Davis studied the temporal bones from a 22 month old Navajo boy (who also had Hirschsprung's disease) and found bilateral atrophy of the organ of Corti and the stria vascularis, and sparsity of spiral ganglion cells. Sections from the vestibular end organs showed degeneration and loss of Scarpa's ganglion cells.

Rarey and Davis (1984) believe that the association of inner ear abnormalities and Hirschsprung's disease supports the contention of a hereditary defect in neural crest cells. Neural crest cells, besides differentiating into spinal and cranial nerves, and autonomic ganglia, are also the precursors of pigmented cells. There is strong evidence to suggest a potential association between pigmentary defects elsewhere in the body and pigmented cells of the membranous labyrinth. While a cause and effect relationship is probable, the degree to which inner ear pigmentary changes in Waardenburg's syndrome are related to congenital deafness is conjectural and in need of further investigation.

References

Arnold, W., Pflatz, R., and Altermatt, H. 1985. Evidence of serum antibodies against inner ear tissues in the blood of patients with certain sensorineural hearing disorders. *Acta Otolaryngologica (Stockh)* 99:437–444.

Brookhouser, P. E., and Smith, S. D. 1986. Childhood hearing loss: Medical genetic considerations. *In* J. E. Bordley, P. E. Brookhouse, and G. F. Tucker (eds.). *Ear, Nose, and Throat Disorders in Children* (pp. 98–148). New York: Raven Press.

Cobo, L. M., and Haynes, B. F. 1984. Early corneal findings in Cogan's Syndrome. *Ophthalmology* 91:903–907.

Fisch, L. 1959. Deafness as part of an hereditary syndrome. *Journal of Laryngology and Otology* 73:355–382.

Galich, R. 1985. Temporal bone involvement in Waardenburg's Syndrome. *Ear, Nose and Throat Journal* 64:71–77.

Goldberg, M. 1966. Waardenburg's Syndrome with fundus and other anomalies. *Archives of Ophthalmology* 76:797–810.

Hough, J., Himelich, T., and Johnson, B. 1986. Implantable bone conduction hearing device: audiant bone conductor. *Annals of Otology, Rhinology and Laryngology* 95:498–504.

Hughes, G. B., Kinney, S. B., Barna, B. P., Tomsak, R. L., and Calabrese, L. H. 1983. Autoimmune reactivity in Cogan's Syndrome: A preliminary report. *Otolaryngology—Head and Neck Surgery* 91:24–32.

Jahrsdoerfer, R. A., Yeakley, J. W., Hall, J. W., Robbins, K. T., and Gray, L. C. 1985. High resolution CT scanning and auditory brain stem response in congenital aural atresia: Patient selection and surgical correlation. *Otolaryngology—Head and Neck Surgery* 93:292–298.

Kundell, S. P., and Ochs, H. D. 1980. Cogan Syndrome in childhood. *Journal of Pediatrics* 97:96–98.

Lloyd, G. A. S., and Phelps, P. D. 1979. Radiology of the ear in mandibulofacial dyostosis—Treacher Collins Syndrome. *Acta Radiologica Diagnosis* 20:Fasc. 1B, 233–240.

McCabe, B. F. 1979. Autoimmune sensorineural hearing loss. *Annals of Otology, Rhinology, and Laryngology* 88:585–589.

McDonald, T. J., Vollertsen, R. S., and Younge, B. R. 1985. Cogan's Syndrome: Audiovestibular involvement and prognosis in 18 patients. *Laryngoscope* 95:650–654.

Phelps, P. D., Poswillo, D., and Lloyd, G. A. S. 1981. The ear deformities in mandibulofacial dyostosis (Treacher Collins Syndrome). *Clinical Otolaryngology* 6:15–28.

Rarey, K. W., and Davis, L. E. 1984. Inner ear anomalies in Waardenburg's Syndrome associated with Hirschsprung's Disease. *International Journal of Pediatric Otorhinolaryngology* 8:181–189.

Tjellstrom, A., Rosenhall, U., Lindstrom, J., Hallen, O., Albrektsson, T., and Branemark, P. I. 1983. Five year experience with skin-penetrating bone-anchored implants in the temporal bone. *Acta Otolaryngologica* 95:568–575.

Vollertsen, R. S., McDonald, T. J., Younge, B. R., Banks, P. M., Stanson, A. W., and Ilstrup, D. M. 1986. Cogan's Syndrome: 18 cases and a review of the literature. *Mayo Clinic Proceedings* 61:344–361.

Chapter 5

High-Risk Neonates and Long-Term Outcomes

Jens Grogaard

Each year more than 100,000 newborn infants are admitted to intensive care nurseries, the majority facing life-threatening events during their first few days. Among these high-risk neonates we find a majority of preterm babies, but term babies with birth asphyxia, respiratory distress, infection, jaundice, metabolic problems, and severe congenital anomalies also require special care.

Major advances in medical care have enhanced survival rates for these infants, with increasing numbers of infants at risk for a host of adverse sequelae. The hospitalization can last from days to months and the discharge of a high-risk infant from the intensive care nursery does not always signify resolution of the infant's problem. Continuing care of the high-risk infant and follow-up programs for these babies are obviously necessary and extremely important.

In order to discuss long-term outcome of the high-risk neonates, it is necessary to review some of the most common problems these babies face during their neonatal period. The Neonatal Intensive Care Nursery (NICU) at Vanderbilt Hospital has an average number of 750 admissions per year. Two hundred of these babies are severely premature with birthweight ranging from 500 g to 1500 g. Forty percent of these babies have a birth-weight less than 1000 g and will be referred to as Very Very Low Birth Weight babies (VVLBW). Ten years ago, most VVLBW babies died within a few days of birth. Today, the survival rate is close to 50% for the babies between 500 and 750 gm and 80% for babies of 750–1000 gm birthweight. A multicenter survey (Sell 1986) on mortality data in infants with birth weight less than 1001 g showed a decrease in mortality for infants born from 1978 to 1983. The survey consisted of data from twenty-six centers with a total of 1623 infants from 1978 and data on 2351 infants born

Supported by SCOR Grant HL 14214

during 1983 in 40 different centers. However, the data should be interpreted with caution because of the heterogenous population and the wide range in mortality among centers (12.5% to 100%). Average mortality in 1978 for infants below 751 g was 79.1% compared to 63.9% in 1983. For infants weighing 751–1000 g, the figures were 49.6% in 1978 and 33.9% in 1983. These data indicate that we are facing an increase in the number of surviving VVLBW babies in the NICUs, requiring increased time and effort to achieve optimal long-term outcome. Mortality by gestational age was, as expected, highest in the lower gestational ages. The greatest change in mortality was found in babies with gestational ages of 28 weeks or above, while no change was to be found in babies below 26 weeks gestation. Being born 12–15 weeks prematurely, all these babies have very immature organs and organ function. The problems these babies face in the neonatal period are mainly due to immaturity of the lungs, central nervous system, gut, liver, kidneys, and the immune system.

Hyaline membrane disease (HMD) is still the most frequent respiratory disease of the newborn and the leading single cause of death in the premature infant. HMD begins at or within a few hours of birth as respiratory distress associated with a failure of oxygenation due to intra- and extra-pulmonary shunting. Lack of oxygen to the lung tissue and inadequate function of the surfactant system due to immaturity are thought to be involved as causes. The damage to the lung is at the peripheral level of the lung, e.g., respiratory bronchiole and alveoli, where the oxygenation takes place, with resulting remodeling and repair of that region. The majority of these infants need respiratory support, most often provided by additional oxygen and assisted ventilation.

Respirator-assisted ventilation may be required in Very Low Birth Weight (VLBW) infants also, primarily because of lung immaturity, often associated with pulmonary edema (wet lung syndrome). Problems with maintaining body temperature and adequate metabolism associated with inability to maintain caloric needs, especially orally, are also frequent in the VLBW babies. Once these babies have recovered from HMD or wet lung syndrome (in 3 to 5 days) and are on low levels of oxygen, they often begin to have episodes when they stop breathing (profound apnea) and the heart-rate slows (bradycardia). These difficulties may become life-threatening because they may produce marked oxygen-deficiency (hypoxemia). Frequently, these conditions seem to be reflex in origin, and are associated with a redistribution of blood flow, in the pattern of the diving seal, i.e., flow to brain, heart, and adrenals is maintained at the expense of flow to gut, kidney, skeleton, and skin. Blood may also be distributed away from the lung through fetal shunts (ductus arteriosus and foramen ovale). This condition is currently treated either pharmacologically or by continuous distending airway pressure (CDAP) delivered by nasal prongs or by assisted ventilation.

Studies have shown that, in premature newborns over 32 weeks gestation, HMD only occasionally fails to clear and leave normal lungs (Stahlman et al. 1982).The presence of severe prematurity, however, seems to have potential for increasing the chance of long-term lung dysfunction, especially when coupled with HMD. Oxygen therapy, which often is necessary in these infants, may produce oxygen toxicity and further damage to the lung resulting in scarring associated with long-term abnormalities in pulmonary function. In the last seven years the number of patients developing chronic lung disease or bronchopulmonary dysplasia (BPD) has increased markedly. The percentage of our survivors with birthweight less than 1500 g who developed chronic lung disease (BPD) increased from 3% to 28% over a ten year period. Two-thirds (69%) of these babies with BPD had HMD, implying that factors other than HMD might also lead to BPD.

A common problem in patients with respiratory diseases, whether acute or chronic, in the neonatal period, is to maintain adequate oxygenation of the different organs during the course of the disease. In addition, adequate nutritional supply is of supreme importance for normal growth and development of the immature organs, especially the central nervous system. The immature liver is not yet capable of metabolizing and detoxifying many nutritional and pharmaceutical products. The initial stormy clinical course of some of the very low birth weight babies often provides periods of inadequate oxygenation and nutrition. In addition, the immature gut may not tolerate oral feedings, and intravenous nutrition may be required. Periods of insufficient nutritional supply or of metabolic disorders due to immaturity are important factors that may well disturb normal growth and development in these babies, including that of the brain, and thus may affect the long-term outcome. Problems in babies with insufficient caloric supply during the neonatal period may resemble some of the problems of fetuses who have ceased to grow normally. Current studies suggest that this group of infants may remain abnormal in growth and development, including development of their brain. Even with extensive neonatal care with optimal nutrition, some intrauterine growth-retarded babies will already have suffered permanent damage and reveal neurodevelopmental sequelae similar to cerebral palsy and/or mental retardation.

The very low birth weight babies may be in a similar situation; they are born 3 to 3½ months prematurely, at a gestational age when they normally have an accelerated growth pattern. Both acute and chronic diseases during the neonatal period could, therefore, severely affect both short- and long-term outcome.

VLBW babies are also extremely sensitive to generalized infections, e.g., sepsis and meningitis, during the neonatal period. The skin and mucus membranes are thin and fragile. The risk of infection increases with the necessity of using foreign objects such as endotracheal tubes, central and peripheral intraarterial and intravenous lines, and chest tubes. An immature immune defense system combined with portals of entry less able to withstand bacterial invasion make the VLBW babies more prone to infection, even from bacteria of the normal human microbial flora. Group B beta-hemolytic streptococcal sepsis with shock lung, which is not restricted to premature infants, carries the highest morbidity and mortality in this group of infected infants. These infants may be seriously ill, and may rapidly develop cardiovascular collapse, apnea, and shock lung, similar to what one sees with generalized infection due to gram negative sepsis. We believe this organism (B streptococcus) is capable of producing toxin that can reproduce all the signs and symptoms associated with the whole organism (Hellerqvist et al. 1981). In these cases, the lung is the target organ. Early recognition with initiation of antibiotic therapy and shock management has changed the mortality of this disease from above 50% ten years ago, to 10 to 20% today.

The majority of infections in the neonatal period are treatable, but often the VLBW babies tend to be reinfected, which results in repeated courses of different antibiotics, repeated need for assisted ventilation, and periods of decreased or changed nutrition, all associated with the possibility of affecting growth and development. Infections within the central nervous system particularly increase the risk of neurodevelopmental sequelae.

Intraventricular hemorrhage (IVH) is a major problem in the NICU, both medically and ethically. This type of hemorrhage has been reported to occur in as many as one third of the VLBW babies and usually begins in the tissue surrounding the lateral ventricles of the brain (the germinal matrix). The hemorrhage may be confined to this area; it may rupture into the ventricles and leak through the ventricular system around the brain stem; or it may rupture into the brain parenchyma. Combinations of all three are likely to occur. Serial studies using ultrasound now allow us to differentiate among these types of IVH and to define their extent with considerable accuracy, so that prognosis may be better defined in the future.

Most infants who develop IVH are below 1500 g at birth, and most probably have suffered intrauterine, intrapartum, or early neonatal asphyxia. The peak incidence of the hemorrhage is between 30 and 40 hours after birth, and adverse neonatal events may precipitate the occurrence. It is thought that the infant who is at risk for IVH has lost autonomic control of the intracerebral vascular bed, and is thereby at the mercy of our management (Lou, Lassen, and Friis-Hansen 1979). This might include positive pressure ventilation and other events that may acutely increase arterial pressure. This is reflected immediately in changes in the cerebral vascular pressure and blood flow, secondary events that may be the immediate determinants of the hemorrhage.

As can be seen from this review of some of the neonatal problems of the high-risk neonate, several possibilities exist for an adverse outcome in these babies. The rapid development of neonatal intensive care during the last 10–20 years requires long-term follow-up in order to justify our treatment and changes of policy. Furthermore, we would like to identify neonatal risk factors, to predict outcome, and to identify our risk groups in a better way. NICU outcome studies may be difficult to compare because of heterogeneous patient populations, differences in treatment, differences in definition of the degree of handicapping conditions, and differences in evaluation methods.

Survival rate for the VVLBW babies with follow-up varies from 14 to 59% depending on a number of variables, such as birth weight, gestational age, birth asphyxia, year of birth, and place of birth. The year of birth is often an indicator of the developmental level of modern neonatal intensive care linked with available technologic supports available at that time (Sell 1986).

The number of NICU graduates that have been followed varies in different studies between 56 and 98% and the duration of follow-up ranges between 6 months and 18 years (Sell 1986). Normal outcome was seen in 35 to 81% of the follow-up patients. Three other studies showed normal outcome in only 28 to 45% of the children (Alden, Mandelhorn, and Woodrum 1972; Nickels, Bennett, and Larson 1982; Sell 1986). Severe or major handicaps were found in 6 to 32%. Sensorineural hearing loss ranged from 0 to 12% (Nickels et al. 1982; Alden et al. 1972; Stewart, Turean, and Rawlings 1977; Bennett, Robinson, and Sells 1983). Severe visual handicap was usually found in 3 to 8% of the follow-up babies, but one center reported 25% visual abnormalities.

The wide range in the results reflects different time periods (20 year range) during which modern perinatal care has been developing rapidly. Further, this survey shows several blank spots indicating the differences in the follow-up format.

The percentage of educational problems in the VVLBW children seems to be very high. However, as of today, there are only a few long-term follow-up studies completed. The studies of Nickels et al. (1982), Stewart et al. (1977) and Sell (1986) all have small numbers of children evaluated for educational problems (representing only 3 to 30% of the survivors). In Nickel's study (1982) of 25 school age children, 16 required educational assistance for learning disability, loss of vision or hearing, orthopedic or neurologic problem, or mental retardation.

These figures may at first look discouraging, but when put in a wider perspective there have been tremendous gains in perinatal care since 1960. Table I demonstrates a net change of 16,000 normal babies with birth weight below 1500 g in 1978 compared to 1960. Babies with moderate abnormality have decreased 25% during the same period while babies with severely abnormal outcome increased by 13%. Death rate has declined by 54%. Overall, the number of normal VLBW survivors has increased seven-fold and the number of abnormal children has decreased. However, there is a small shift within the abnormal group toward a slight increase in severe abnormals. Hagberg, Olow, and Hag-

Table I

Effect of Intensive Perinatal Care
A Comparison of the Outcome in VLBW* Infants Born 1960 and 1978

Outcome	# of infants in 1960	# of infants in 1978	# of infants Net Change
Normal	2.790	18.833	+ 16.043
Abnormal (moderate)	5.425	4.069	− 1.356
Abnormal (Severe)	2.596	2.945	+ .349
Dead	27.979	12.904	− 15.075

*VLBW—very low birth infants weighing < 1500g
Source: Office of Tech Assessment

berg (1973) have followed the spectrum of cerebral palsy in Sweden in five year periods from 1954, and demonstrated a decrease in incidence of cerebral palsy in the first part of the 1970s. A slight increase was noted in the weight group between 2000 and 2500 g which was thought to be of prenatal origin. In general, the severity of acquired cerebral palsy in the perinatal period has decreased with modern perinatal intensive care. Thus, we see less cerebral palsy today per 1000 live births compared to the 1950s and 1960s, and the clinical presentation of cerebral palsy seems to be less severe (Hagberg, Hagberg, and Olow 1975).

Our own long-term follow-up of preterm survivors of HMD started in 1961. Since 1972, the follow-up has also included VLBW-babies (< 1500 g) without HMD. Follow-up examination is done at 6 months, 1 through 7 years annually, and at 11 years. On each visit an interval history and physical examination is done by a pediatrician or a nurse clinician. A clinical psychologist carrys out a psychological test appropriate for age. Speech and hearing evaluation was included at 4 years and 8 years of age by the Bill Wilkerson Hearing and Speech Center. A variety of developmental tests are used. From ages 1 to 3 years, the Gesell Developmental Examination is given; at 3 years of age, a combination of the Leiter International Performance Scale and the Peabody Picture Vocabulary Test is used. For children 5 years and older, the Wechsler Preschool and Primary Intelligence Scale for Children is used. Test results at ages 5, 6 and 11 are expressed as IQ scores. The tests are grouped into preschool and school age categories for each patient. Results at ages 2 and 3 are designated as preschool scores. The school age period is defined as ages 5, 6, or 11 years. One hundred seventy four babies born from 1961 to 1971 were followed to age 11. Table II shows the distribution of birth weight and gestational age in these 174 children. This was a relatively mature population of preterm infants. Only 27 (15%) weighed less than 1500 g and 44 (25%) were under 32 weeks gestation. The mean birth weight was 2133 g (range: 960 to 4142 g) and the mean gestational age was 34.6 weeks (range: 27 to 40 weeks). Fifty (29%) of the 174 infants were inborn and the remaining 124 were referred outborns. Eighteen percent (31 babies) were small for gestational age. There were 52 infants requiring assisted ventilation, and the remaining 122 were treated with mask oxygen alone. Table III demonstrates the results of the developmental tests scores for preschool and school age. The test scores increased substantially by a mean of ten

Table II

Birth Weight and Gestation 1961–1971*

Birth Weight g	No.	Gestation wk	No.
<1000	2	<28	8
1001–1500	25	29–32	36
1501–2000	45	33–36	90
>2001	102	>37	40

*(Published courtesy of American Journal of Diseases of Childhood: Mayes et al. "Changing Cognitive Outcome in Preterm Infants with HMD." Vol. 139, pp. 20–24. Copyright 1986, American Medical Association).

Table III

Development Outcome in Preschool and School Age Test Groups (n = 174 children)*				
Preschool Scores		School Age Scores		
		IQ < 80	IQ = 81–110	IQ ⩾ 111
30	IQ⩽80	12	18	0
131	IQ = 81–110	8	83	40
13	IQ⩽111	0	3	10

*(Published by courtesy of American Journal Diseases of Childhood. Mayes et al. "Changing Cognitive Outcome in Preterm Infants with HMD," American Journal of Diseases of Children, 1985 Vol. 139, p. 20–24. Copyright 1986, American Medical Association).

points from preschool testing to school age. This change in the tests scores may reflect the different instruments used at preschool and school age or it may reflect true differences associated with the maturation of preterm infants.

Test scores and socioeconomic variables: Socioeconomic data were available for 63% of the children. Parental age was not an associated factor in patient outcome. Paternal education and employment correlated positively with IQ scores at school age. The higher the level of paternal education and employment, the better the intellectual outcome ($P < 0.004$).

Neurological handicaps: Two infants were diagnosed as having cerebral palsy. Both of these infants had school age IQ scores of less than 70. No infants developed hydrocephalus and no infant was believed clinically to have had a major intraventricular hemorrhage. No infant had permanent changes of retinopathy of prematurity. This may well be a reflection of the high death rate of infants with IVH and of infants of very low birth weight during this era. The most important predictor of better outcome in this sample was paternal educational and employment level and this effect was most notable for school age scores, which may reflect the importance of home environment, genetic background, or both.

The improved supportive technology for critically ill premature infants, including those of VLBW, is demonstrated in the increasing numbers of VLBW babies in our follow-up from 1972 through 1976 and 1977 through 1983 (table IV). This table reflects the low number of surviving VLBW babies during the first decade, 1961–1971, and the increase during the next two periods. This

Table IV

Low Birth Weight Infants 1961–1983 VUMC Survivors (Follow-up)					
	<1000g	1000–1500g	1501–2000g	Mean BW*	Mean GA*
1961–71	2	25	45	2133g	34.6 wk
1972–76	26	63	50	1960g	33 wk
1977–83	82	216	69	1295g	30.2 wk

Babies >2001 g are not included in the table. *Mean Birth Weight (BW) and Gestational Age (GA) are based on all follow-up infants eligible for follow-up. VUMC = Vanderbilt University Medical Center.

change is also reflected in the decrease in mean birth weight and mean gestational age for all infants eligible for follow-up. Several important management changes occurred during this time, including introduction of the Baby Bird Respirator, the use of constant distending airway pressure, and the use of parenteral nutrition. Our regionalized transport system began to function during the latter part of 1974, and had a significant influence on referral patterns. Two hundred four babies with HMD and 28 babies with non-HMD born from 1972 to 1976 were followed. No significant differences between the two groups were seen regarding gestational age or birth weight.

The developmental scores during preschool and school age showed the same pattern as during the first ten year period (1961–1971) with a shift to higher scores in the school age period. Birth weight or gestational age were correlated with developmental quotient (DQ) particularly at preschool age ($p < 0.001$), but after five years of age there was a stronger correlation between parental education level and infant developmental outcome ($p < 0.001$).

One hundred thirty-two VLBW follow-up infants with BW <1250g born from 1976 to 1982 show the same pattern with increasing or a shift in test scores from the first year to school age (table V). Thus, there seems to be a consistent pattern through the last 20–25 years with an increase in DQ from preschool to school age in our follow-up patients.

Hearing impairment: The incidence of hearing loss in infants with respiratory distress or extreme immaturity has been observed to exceed the 0.1% noted for normal newborns. Davis and Stewart (1975) suggested that the incidence of moderate to severe hearing impairment among very low birth weight survivors may be less than 2%. From 1980 to 1984 a total of 352 children were evaluated at the Bill Wilkerson Hearing and Speech Center for routine audiometric tests (Kenworthy et al. 1987). Air conduction thresholds were determined using age-appropriate behavioral audiometric techniques with facilities and instruments calibrated in accordance with applicable standards from the American National Standards Institute. Acoustic immittance measurements (tympanometry and acoustic reflexes) and speech recognition data were also obtained on each child. Incomplete data were obtained on 85 children who were therefore excluded. Table VI presents the percentage of children with hearing impairment. Hearing impairment was defined as the better ear average loss

Table V

Longitudinal Development Follow-up
Infants with Birthweight < 1250g VUMC 1976–1982

Age (yr)	Mean DQ (+ SD)*	n
1	73.3 (17.7)	79
2	76.3 (23.4)	52
3	80.6 (14.4)	57
5	88.8 (12.5)	21

*DQ–developmental quotient. n = # of infants tested
VUMC–Vanderbilt University Medical Center

Table VI

Follow-up Children with Hearing Impairment.

Criterion*	4 Year (181)	8 Year (55)	11 Year (30)
2 SD	37%	14.5%	13.3%
>25 dB HL	14.9%	5.5%	3.3%

*Classification based on better-ear pure-tone average for 1000, 2000, and 4000 Hz. SD = two standard deviations above the mean for normal, chronological-age matched samples reported in the literature.

(1000–4000 HZ) that exceeded the normative data for children at each age group by two standard deviations or more. Hence, it is seen that 37% of the 4 year old children exhibited hearing impairment. In the older age groups there was a decrease in the overall prevalence, with a 14.5% rate for the 8 year olds and 13.3% rate for the 11 year olds. The higher incidence of hearing impairment in the 4 year olds is most probably due to the prevalence of middle ear disease with effusion in this population, as reported by other investigators (Bergman et al. 1985 and Hubatch et al. 1985). None of the impairment exceeded a 45 to 50 dB hearing loss. When the definition of hearing loss was changed to a better ear average of >25 dB, the percentage of children with hearing loss substantially decreased in all three groups (table VI). These data are currently being evaluated further in order to try to identify independent predictors of hearing loss. Several variables including birth weight, asphyxia, episodes of extra-uterine hypoxia, use of ototoxic drugs, jaundice, IVH, and HMD will be analyzed.

In conclusion, the numbers of VLBW survivors are increasing and the overall long-term outcome seems to justify our neonatal (perinatal) intensive care. However, the need for well coordinated long-term follow-up is of great importance and ought to be mandatory for all NICUs in order to continue treatment and support for the graduated high-risk infant and his family. Several studies have confirmed that early detection of sequelae and possible abnormalities combined with individual optimal treatment is the key to the best outcome.

References

Alden, E. R., Mandelhorn, T., and Woodrum, D. E. 1972. Morbidity and mortality of infants weighing less than 1000 grams in an intensive care nursery. *Pediatrics* 50:40–49.

Bennett, F. C., Robinson, N. M., and Sells, L. J. 1983. Growth and development of infants weighing less than 800 grams at birth. *Pediatrics* 71:319–323.

Bergman, I., Hirsch, R., Fria, T., Shapiro, S., Holzman, I., and Painter, M. 1985. Cause of hearing loss in the high-risk premature infants. *Journal of Pediatrics* 106:95–101.

Davis, P. A., and Stewart, A. L. 1975. Low birth weight infants: Neurological sequelae and later intelligence. *British Medical Bulletin* 31:85–91.

Hagberg, B., Olow, I., and Hagberg, B. 1973. Decreasing incidence of low birth weight diplegia—an achievement of modern neonatal care? *Acta Paediatr. Scand* 62:199.

Hagberg, B., Hagberg, G., and Olow, I. (1975). The changing panorama of cerebral palsy in Sweden 1954–1970 II. Analysis of the various syndromes. *Acta Paediatr. Scand., 64*, 193.

Hellerqvist, C. G., Rojas, J., Green, R. S., Sell, S., Sundell, H., and Stahlman, M. T. 1981. Studies in Group B hemolytic streptococcus. *Pediatric Research* 15:892–898.

Hubatch, L., Johnson, C. J., Kistler, D., Burns, W., and Moneka, W. 1985. Early language abilities of high-risk infants. *Journal of Speech and Hearing Disorders* 50:195–207.

Kenworthy, O. T., Bess, F. H., Stahlman, M. T., and Lindstrom, D. P. 1987. Hearing, speech and language outcome of infants with extreme immaturity. *The American Journal of Otology* 8:419–425.

Lou, C., Lassen, N. A., and Friis-Hansen, B. 1979. Impaired autoregulation of cerebral blood flow in the distressed newborn infant. *Journal of Pediatrics* 94:118.

Nickels, R. E., Bennett, F. C., and Larson, F. N. 1982. School performance of children with birth weights of 1000 g or less. *American Journal of Diseases of Childhood* 136:105–110.

Sell, E. J. 1986. Outcome of very very low birth weight infants. In *Clinics in Perinatology* 13:2, 451–459.

Stahlman, M, Hedvall, G., Lindstrom, D., and Snell, J. 1982. Role of Hyaline Membrane Disease in production of later childhood lung abnormalities. *Pediatrics* (69)5:572–576.

Stewart, A. L., Turean, D. M., and Rawlings, G. 1977. Prognosis for infants weight 1000 g or less at birth. *Archives in Diseases of Childhood* 52:97–104.

Chapter 6

Epidemiology of Otitis Media with Effusion

G. Scott Giebink

It is appropriate for a book on childhood hearing impairment to consider otitis media since this middle ear disease often has profound effects on middle ear structures and thus, indirectly on inner ear function. Moreover, recent studies suggest that inflammation of the middle ear tissues may directly affect inner ear structure and function by passive diffusion or active transport of toxins and other inflammatory mediators through the round window membrane. The following discussion will focus on the epidemiology of otitis media.

A discussion of epidemiology focuses on understanding the relationships of various factors that determine the frequency and distribution of a disease. Before considering the epidemiology of otitis media, however, it is important first to define the disease, review its frequency and incidence rate, and understand etiologic factors and pathogenic mechanisms. These facts provide a framework for reviewing factors that affect the frequency and distribution of otitis media.

OTITIS MEDIA DEFINITIONS

Definitions and classifications of otitis media were considered extensively by panels at the three International Symposia on Otitis Media with Effusion (Bluestone 1984). Otitis media is an inflammation of the middle ear, which may or may not be of infectious origin, and often results in the accumulation of fluid in the middle ear space (middle ear effusion). The process may be acute, subacute, or chronic. Acute otitis media (AOM) is arbitrarily defined as the

Supported in part by grant number NS-14538 from the National Institute of Neurological and Communicative Disorders and Stroke, and grant number AI-17160 from the National Institute of Allergy and Infectious Diseases initial three weeks of middle ear inflammation and is generally, although not always, symptomatic with signs and symptoms of upper respiratory illness, fever, ear pain, and decreased hearing. Subacute otitis media is arbitrarily defined as inflammation persisting between the third and eighth week after onset, and chronic otitis media describes middle ear inflammation lasting longer than eight weeks. Otitis media can be further classified on the basis of clinical signs and symptoms, middle ear effusion characteristics, and middle ear histopathology.

Table I lists the clinical classification of otitis media and includes synonymous terms used by many clinicians. During the early phase of middle ear inflammation, effusion may be absent with the only clinical sign being tympanic membrane inflammation. Observations of otitis media in animal models suggest that upper respiratory viral infection frequently leads to middle ear inflammation without effusion (Giebink and Wright 1983). Acute otitis media is recognized when one or more of the following are present: ear pain or ear pulling, fever, recent onset of irritability, and a tympanic membrane that is bulging, opaque, and has limited mobility—indicative of middle ear effusion. Erythema of the eardrum is an inconsistent finding.

Middle ear effusion commonly persists for more than two weeks after antibiotic treatment of the acute episode, and the persistence of asymptomatic middle ear effusion has been called otitis media with effusion (OME). The most frequent otoscopic finding is opacification of the tympanic membrane with reduced eardrum mobility and often a retracted tympanic membrane. Because the eardrum is opaque, a visual assessment of effusion type—serous, mucoid, or purulent—is not possible.

Chronic otitis media defines intractable middle ear tissue pathology, such as granulation tissue, cholesterol granuloma, middle ear adhesions, and ossicular fixation. These conditions often occur with an eardrum perforation, but commonly are found behind an intact tympanic membrane.

Recent studies by Paparella et al. (1984) have focused attention on clinically silent otitis media. In a careful review of 366 temporal bones from 258 patients,

Table I

Clinical Classification

	Synonyms
Otitis Media Without Effusion	Myringitis
Acute Otitis Media	Suppurative Purulent Bacterial
Otitis Media With Effusion	Secretory Nonsuppurative Serous Mucoid
Chronic Otitis Media	Suppurative Purulent
[Silent Otitis Media]	

Table II

Silent Otitis Media

Histopathologic classification	No. of temporal bones	Average age	History of otitis media (% of cases)		Unresolved middle ear mesenchyme* (% of cases)
			Present	Absent	
COM	163	50	31	69	9
POM	79	40	9	91	33
SPOM	94	45	7	93	20
SOM	21	52	14	86	14
MOM	9	4	0	100	78
Average	366		19%	81%	20%

*All but 2 patients < 2 years
From Paparella M. M., et al. 1984

review of medical records revealed a past history of otitis media in only 19% of cases (table II). There was no history of otitis media in 81% of these cases; therefore, silent otitis media may be a significant clinical problem. Review of these temporal bones suggested that unresolved middle ear mesenchyme, which was present in 20% of cases, was a possible etiologic factor in the development of silent otitis media. These observations have also been confirmed recently by Marchant et al. (1980) in a prospective study of 70 infants who were observed frequently during the first year of life for middle ear disease; 77% of infants experienced one or more otitis media episode, and 13% developed chronic OME during the first year. However, onset of otitis media was asymptomatic (i.e., silent) in 46% of the episodes.

Otitis media can also be classified according to characteristics of middle ear effusion. This classification is, of course, possible only following myringotomy and aspiration of effusion or by trans-tympanic membrane needle paracentesis. Effusion is classified as purulent when it is thin, cloudy, and contains abundant leukocytes. Serous effusion is an amber colored, thin fluid. Mucoid effusion is a thick, highly viscous, often glue-like fluid, which is usually cloudy. Seromucoid, seropurulent and mucopurulent effusion describe fluids that have intermediate characteristics.

Studies at the University of Minnesota have classified effusion by these criteria since 1976. Acute otitis media is most often associated with a purulent effusion, but not always (table III). In a recent study, 21% of effusions obtained from 61 children (72 ears) with acute, symptomatic otitis media were mucoid in character (Giebink et al. 1984). In contrast, children who clinically appear to have chronic OME most often have mucoid effusion or no effusion when myringotomy is performed for tympanostomy tube placement (Giebink, Le, and Paparella 1982) (table III). The frequency of mucoid otitis media (MOM) was highest among infants and decreased significantly with increasing age, whereas serous otitis media (SOM) was least frequent among infants and increased significantly with age. The frequency of purulent otitis media (POM) and ears with no effusion did not change signficantly with age.

Table III

Middle Ear Effusion Classification in Children 6 Months–12 Years

Clinical classification	% of ears				
	Purulent	Serous	Seromucoid	Mucoid	No effusion
AOM[1] (n = 72)	68	10	—	21	1
Chronic OME[2] (n = 1,796)	—	9	7	48	36

[1]Giebink, Batalden, Russ, and Le. 1984.
[2]Giebink, Le, and Paparella. 1982.

Temporal bone studies of human patients with otitis media and animal models of POM, SOM, and MOM have permitted the development of a histologic classification of otitis media (Juhn 1982). Inflammatory changes in the subepithelial space of the middle ear mucosa are significant in all forms of otitis media, but especially in POM and SOM. Epithelial metaplasia to secretory cells is most common in MOM. The histopathologic process is dynamic and is consistent with a continuity of middle ear inflammation with transitions between SOM, POM, and MOM.

Biochemical characteristics of middle ear effusion reflect inflammatory changes in the middle ear cavity, and these characteristics are under intense investigation at several institutions (Juhn 1984). Progress to date indicates that a biochemical classification may be forthcoming which will characterize the nature of inflammation at a given time and predict future otitis media recurrence and middle ear sequelae.

FREQUENCY AND INCIDENCE OF OTITIS MEDIA

Otitis media is a worldwide health problem, particularly among infants and young children (Giebink and Quie 1978). Nearly 50% of children experience an acute otitis media episode by one year of age, 60 to 70% experience an episode before entering school, and approximately 35% experience recurrent acute otitis media during the first three years of life (Howie et al.; Teele, Rosner, and Klein 1980; Teele et al. 1983). A smaller proportion of children, who experience acute otitis media, approximately 5–10%, develop chronic OME (Howe et al. 1975; Schwartz, Schwartz, and Rodriquez 1981).

Middle and inner ear complications and sequelae of otitis media occur predominantly in individuals who have experienced chronic OME. Twenty-two publications have reported the prevalence of otitis media sequelae. However, most pathological entities are not clearly described or defined in these reports and demographic elements, such as patient age, OME duration, and years of follow-up, are rarely specified. Therefore, comparing these studies to determine the incidence of specific sequelae of chronic OME is difficult.

Twenty studies report the prevalence of sequelae after tympanostomy tube insertion for chronic OME; overall, approximately 20–40% of ears showed evidence of sequelae at follow-up (table IV). Among the reports that stated a percentage of ears with specific sequelae, tympanic membrane pathology included diffuse atrophy in an average of 9% of cases, diffuse tympanosclerosis in 9%, eardrum retraction in 15%, and chronic perforation in 1.3%. Middle ear space pathology, when described in these reports, included atelectasis in an average of 7% of cases, adhesions in 2.4%, ossicular disruption in 0.9%, a deep retraction pocket in 3.5%, cholesteatoma in 0.6%, and chronic otorrhea in 10%. The wide variation in the incidence of specific sequelae among the reports makes it impossible to determine whether the true incidence of sequelae increases or decreases with age. The problems encountered in analyzing these widely divergent data underscore the need for a carefully controlled prospective study using standardized diagnostic criteria and validated observers to describe accurately the incidence of otitis media sequelae.

The incidence of chronic OME sequelae not managed with tympanostomy tubes seems to be similar to the incidence of sequelae in intubated ears. Three controlled studies have investigated children with bilateral OME, in whom only one ear was intubated (Brown, Richards, and Ambegaokar 1978; Kilby, Richards, and Hart 1972; Kokko and Palva 1976; Lildholdt 1984). The incidence of chronic perforation and adhesive otitis media was somewhat greater in the non-intubated ears; whereas, the incidence of atrophy, diffuse tympanosclerosis, retraction, atelectasis, and cholesteatoma was somewhat greater in ears with tubes (table IV). These reports, although incomplete and generally noncomparable, indicate that the sequelae of chronic OME occur in both non-intubated and intubated ears.

A clinical study of middle ear pathology in 169 consecutive cases of chronic otitis media was recently completed at the University of Minnesota. Patients were 5 to 64 years of age at the time of exploratory or reconstructive surgery. Pathology included (in decreasing frequency) granulation tissue, mucosal thickening, ossicular erosion, keratoma (cholesteatoma), tympanosclerosis, ossicular fixation and cholesterol granuloma (figure 1). Figures 2 and 3 illustrate the prevalence of each type of pathology by patient age.

Hearing sensitivity has been measured in patients with chronic OME treated with and without tympanostomy tubes. Among ears treated with myringotomy but without tubes, two studies, one in Wales and one in Finland, reported a mild hearing loss with a pure-tone average of 12–14 dB after three to five years; these investigators found that the pure-tone averages of intubated and non-intubated ears were not significantly different one to five years postoperatively (Kokko and Palva 1976; Brown et al. 1978). Five studies have reported the incidence of hearing loss after tube insertion; mild hearing loss (15–30 dB) was observed in an average of 20% of ears, and moderate hearing loss (30–50 dB) in 3.4% of ears after one to eleven years of follow-up (table V). Therefore, mild to moderate hearing loss is not an uncommon sequelae of chronic OME disease irrespective of tube therapy.

Table IV

Incidence of Chronic OME Sequelae Managed with and without Tympanostomy Tubes

						Percentage of ears with designated sequelae										
						Tympanic membrane					Middle ear space					
First Author–Country (Year)	No. subjects	(ears)	Age (yrs.)	Follow-up (yrs.)	All OM Sequelae	Diffuse atrophy	Diffuse Tympanosclerosis	Retraction	Chronic Perforation	Granulation around tube	Atelectasis	Adhesions	Ossicular Disruption	Deep Retraction Pocket	Cholesteatoma	Chronic Otorrhea
NORMAL UNSELECTED CHILDREN																
Felding–Denmark	501	(1,001)	9	–	9.7	–	–	–	–		–	–	–	–	–	–
Virolaihen–Finland	1,207	(2,414)	7–8	–	0.9	–	–	–	0.1		0.7	–	–	–	0.1	–
Tos–Denmark (1984)	222	(263)	5	–	28.1	4.6	4.9	28.1	–		–	–	–	–	–	–
Tos–Denmark (1984)	222	(263)	6	–	46.1	13.4	7.4	46.1	–		–	–	–	–	–	–
Tos–Denmark (1984)	222	(263)	7	–	47.9	11.8	7.6	47.9	–		–	–	–	–	–	–
	1,930	(3,678)														
OME–NO TUBE																
Kilby–Wales	52	(52)	4–10	2	–	–	19.2	36.5	5.8		–	–	–	3.8	0	0
Kokko–Finland	17	(33)	–	$4^1/_2$	26.0	3.4	3.4	–	0		0	6.1	–	–	0	0
Brown–Wales	55	(55)	4–10	5	–	–	0	16.4	0		–	–	–	0	0	0
Lildholdt–Denmark	150	(150)	–	5	–	–	11.3	–	–		–	–	–	–	–	–
	222	(238)														
OME WITH TUBE																
McLelland–USA	307	(697)	<10	1	–	–	–	1.6	1.4	–	–	–	–	–	0.1	3.6
Tos–Denmark (1984)	–	(76)	4	1	14.4	7.9	14.4	7.9	–	–	–	–	–	–	–	–
Tos–Denmark (1984)	–	(76)	4	2	36.5	34.9	28.6	36.5	–	–	–	–	–	–	–	–

Tos–Denmark (1984)	–	(76)	4	3	49.2	31.1	36.1	49.2	–	–	–	–	–	–	–	–
Kilby–Wales	52	(52)	4–10	2	–	–	26.9	46.2	1.9	–	–	–	–	9.6	0	–
Kokko–Finland	164	(290)	–	3	34.5	7.6	10.0	–	1.7		4.1	0	–	–	1.4	1.7
Brown–Wales	55	(55)	–	5	–	–	41.8	18.2	0	–	–	–	–	5.5	0	–
Lildholdt–Denmark	150	(150)	–	5	–	–	52.0	–	0	–	–	–	–	–	0	30.0
Mawson–England	114	(202)	4–15	½–4	62.9	–	29.7	23.3	0.5	–	9.4	–	–	–	–	–
Pappas–USA	743	(1,460)	70%<9	½–5	–	–	–	–	0.9	–	–	–	–	–	0	–
Tos–Denmark (1976)	109	(184)	<14	1–5	38.5	–	–	–	–	–	–	4.9	–	–	1.0	–
Renvall–Sweden	210	(335)	7	3–4	25.0	–	–	–	–	–	3.9	–	–	–	0.3	–
Sakai–Japan	124	(152)	7½	5	29.0	–	–	21.7	5.9	–	–	–	–	0.7	0.7	–
MacKennon–England	165	(95)	<16	<6	–	–	13.0	–	3.0	–	–	–	–	–	4.8	–
Barfoed–Denmark	90	(173)	1–14	4½–7½	79.0	6.9	22.5	24.9	4.6	–	–	5.8	–	–	0	0.6
Hughes–USA	311	(838)	<13	5–7	–	–	–	–	1.6	–	–	–	0	–	0.5	–
Tos–Denmark (1976)	109	(184)	<14	5–8	33.0	–	13.6	–	1.6	–	25.0	3.3	–	–	1.1	–
Gunderson–Norway (1976)	100	(196)	1–14	7½	18.9	–	–	–	–	–	–	11.2	–	–	5.6	–
Gunderson–Norway (1984)	95	(179)	–	12½	28.4	–	–	–	–	–	–	17.3	–	–	–	–
Ohnishi–Japan	230	(512)	–	–	–	5.0	2.0	–	1.0	3.7	4.5	0.4	0.2	–	0.2	–
Birck–USA	736	(2,237)	<10	–	–	–	0.3	–	0.6	0.1	–	0.7	–	–	0	15.1
Muenker–Germany	631	(1,060)	–	–	17.6	–	–	–	2.5	1.8	7.2	–	2.0	–	1.2	2.9
Draf–Germany	385	(876)	–	–	–	–	–	–	0.3	–	–	–	–	–	1.6	12.5
	4,719	(9,767)			30.6*	8.8	8.5	15.3	1.3	1.1	7.3	2.4	0.9	3.5	0.6	10.1

*Average rate for all sequelae in 'OME with tube' reports

– = data not available

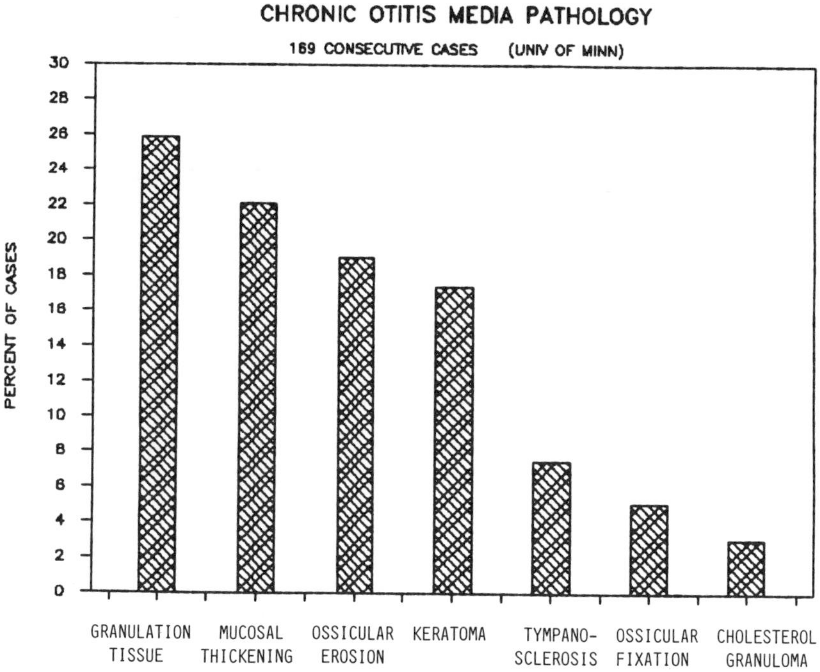

Figure 1. Prevalence of middle ear pathology in 169 consecutive cases of clinically manifest chronic otitis media classified at the time of exploratory or reconstructive surgery.

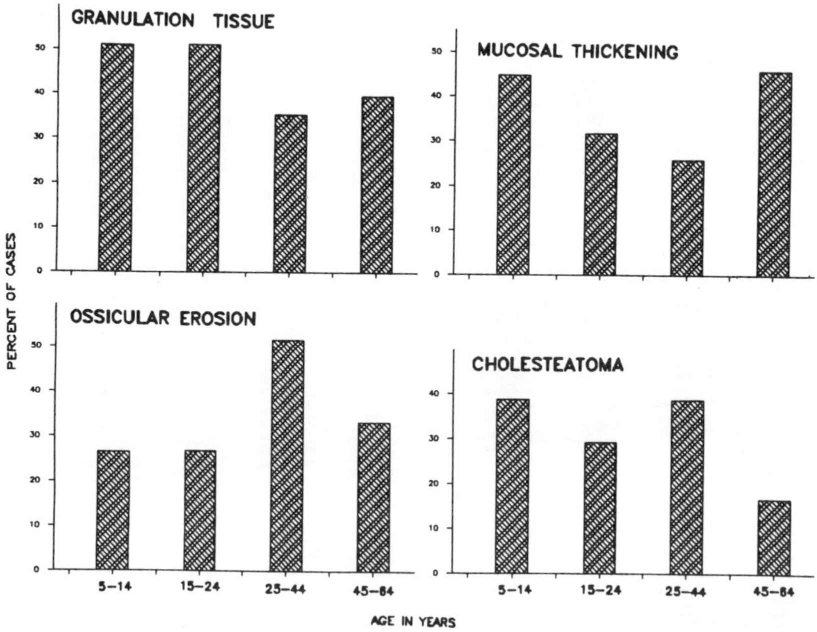

Figure 2. Prevalence of middle ear granulation tissue, mucoid thickening, ossicular erosion, and cholesteatoma (keratoma) in 169 consecutive cases of chronic otitis media by patient age at time of surgery. Group sizes were 5–14 yrs (n = 49), 15–24 yrs (n = 41), 25–44 yrs (n = 31), and 45–64 yrs (n = 48).

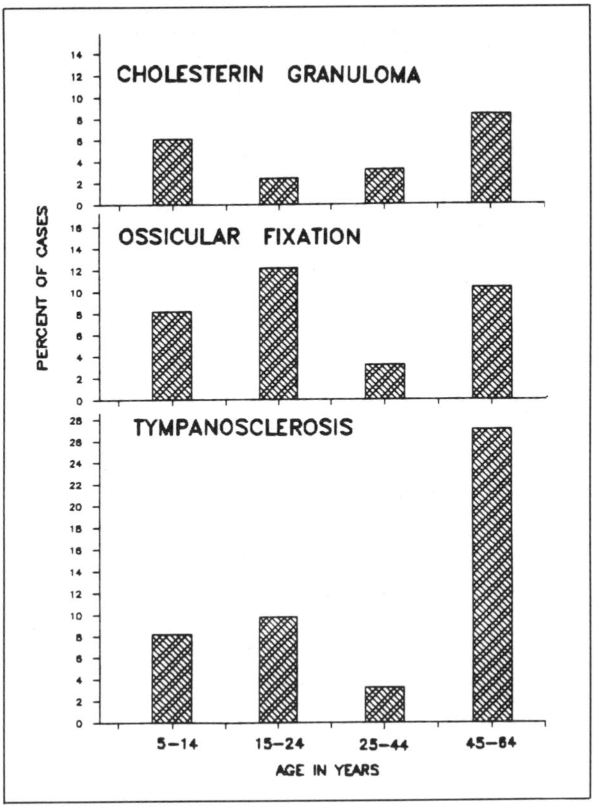

Figure 3. Prevalence of cholesterin granuloma, ossicular fixation, and tympanosclerosis in 169 consecutive cases of chronic otitis media (see figure 2 legend).

OTITIS MEDIA ETIOLOGY AND PATHOGENESIS

Researchers generally agree that eustachian tube dysfunction contributes to the pathogenesis of otitis media, although it is not clear whether the dysfunction is a primary etiologic factor or secondary to underlying upper respiratory tract inflammation. Several common respiratory viruses damage the cilia of nasal epithelial cells; these viral infections may lead to impaired mucociliary clearance and eustachian tube dysfunction (Carson, Collier, and Shih-chin 1985). The muscular opening function of the eustachian tube is poor in most children with OME and in children with histories of middle ear disease even when they are well (Berry et al. 1979; Bylander et al. 1984). Moreover, the frequency of poor eustachian tube opening is higher in healthy children than in healthy adults suggesting that tubal function matures with increasing age.

Bacteria play a major role in the pathogenesis of acute otitis media and OME. Bacteria are cultured in approximately 70% of middle ear effusion samples from children with acute otitis media (Giebink and Quie 1978), and in approx-

Table V

Hearing Loss after Tympanostomy Tube Insertion for Chronic OME in Children

First author	Years between tube insertion and testing	No. of ears tested	% of ears with specified hearing loss 15–30 dB	30–50 dB	> 50 dB
Mawson	½–4	199	25	7	1
Barfoed	4–7	102	41	1†	na
Tos (1984)	1–5	184	12	3	0
Tos (1984)	5–8	184	5	1.5	0
Gunderson	2–11	179	21#	na	na
Sakai	na	152	22#	na	na
Average		1,000	19.6	3.4	

na = not available
# = % of ears > 20 dB
† = % of ears > 30 dB

imately 35% of effusion samples from children with chronic OME (Giebink 1984; Juhn et al. 1982). Moreover, many effusion samples which do not yield bacteria on culture show evidence of recent bacterial infection by microscopic and immunochemical examination of the effusion (Giebink 1984; Juhn 1982, Leinonen 1980). The presence of viable bacteria and of their cell envelope substances in sterile effusion suggests that bacteria and their products are etiologic factors in chronic OME and may lead to sequelae.

The interaction of viral respiratory tract infection, bacterial infection of the middle ear space, and eustachian tube dysfunction leads to a release of inflammatory mediators in the middle ear space. In an attempt to understand the pathogenesis of otitis media and develop effective intervention strategies to prevent otitis media, several investigators have analyzed the biochemical composition of middle ear effusion. Events occurring within the middle ear space and tissues during inflammation include migration of inflammatory cells, release of enzymes from these cells as well as middle ear epithelial cells, diffusion of protease inhibitors, and change in the permeability of middle ear subepithelial capillaries (Juhn 1984).

Concentrations of specific enzymes and plasma components in effusion reflect the nature and degree of mucosal inflammation, and recent evidence suggests that the relative concentrations of these specific enzymes may be associated with otitis media chronicity. For example, ossicular destruction by proteases, leading to conductive hearing loss, is a well-described complication of chronic otitis media. Enzymes and cell mediators associated with bone resorption have been identified in middle ear effusion in cases of chronic OME. Collagenase, the tissue destructive protease, has been localized within middle ear granulation tissue at bone resorbing areas in ossicles from ears with chronic otitis media.

The host normally mounts an intense local and systemic immune response during otitis media. Specific antibodies are produced locally in middle ear tissues and secreted into effusion, thus promoting the clearance of infecting microorganisms. Differences among hosts in their local or systemic immune response to inflammation may lead to persistence of microorganisms or their antigens in the middle ear, and these stimulate a continued inflammatory response.

OTITIS MEDIA RISK DETERMINANTS

The foregoing discussion underscores the multifactorial nature of otitis media etiology and pathogenesis. Epidemiologic studies have attempted to describe relationships among many factors in an attempt to identify those factors that alter the frequency and distribution of otitis media. Studies have been conducted to determine risk factors for acute otitis media and chronic OME, but there have been no epidemiologic studies examining risk factors for otitis media sequelae.

Risk determinants for acute otitis media include young age at the time of the first otitis media episode, frequent otitis media episodes during infancy, the winter season, upper respiratory infection, and craniofacial developmental abnormalities (Giebink 1984). Risk determinants for recurrent and chronic OME include young age at the first otitis media episode, prior history of recurrent otitis media, white race, male sex, family history of otitis media, and day care attendance (Biles, Buffer, and O'Donnell 1980; Lundgren, Ingvarsson, and Olofsson 1984; Onion and Taylor 1977; Shurin et al. 1979; Teele, Rosner, and Klein 1980). In addition, bilateral otitis media, parental smoking, frequent symptoms of upper respiratory illness, and low birth weight have been implicated as risk determinants of chronic OME (Daly et al. in press; Kraemer et al. 1983; Marchant et al. 1980; Shurin et al. 1979; Stewart et al. 1984; VanCauwenberge and Kluyskens 1984).

Patient age is one of the most important determinants of otitis media risk. Otitis media is predominantly a disease of infants and young children. Two large studies of children followed from birth reported that nearly 50% developed an otitis media episode by age one year (Howie et al. 1975; Teele et al. 1980), and a more recent study employing several methods to detect effusion found that 77% of children experienced otitis media by their first birthday (Marchant et al. 1980). In that study, infants with bilateral chronic OME could be identified early: 53% of infants with bilateral otitis media at age two months subsequently had bilaterial chronic OME, compared to only 4% of infants without bilateral otitis media at age two months. The greater susceptibility of young children to otitis media may reflect the increased frequency of respiratory virus infection at this age, the immaturity of local and systemic immune responses, postural feeding practices—such as nighttime bottles—or less competent eustachian tube function.

The timing and number of previous otitis media episodes are principal factors in identifying the child who develops recurrent acute otitis media and chronic OME. A number of otitis media episodes during the first year and presence of otitis media by two months of age are clearly high risk conditions. In a recent study, the risk of chronic OME was increased nearly seven times in children with one or two prior otitis media episodes, and 165 times in children with more than six episodes (Kraemer et al. 1983).

Patient gender is also a factor in determining risk of otitis media since most studies indicate a somewhat greater frequency of otitis media among males (61–70% of cases) than among females. The basis for the male predilection has not been investigated and may relate to an overall gender difference in the rate of all childhood infections.

Considerable information has accumulated on the prevalence of otitis media in different racial groups. Eskimo, American Indian, and Hispanic children have an incidence of otitis media even higher than white American children, and chronic otorrhea has been especially prevalent in Eskimos and American Indians. Black American children have a lower incidence of otitis media than white American children. These racial differences may be explained by differences in the anatomy of the eustachian tube among different populations.

The seasonal distribution of otitis media, which peaks between October and April and declines markedly during summer months, is well known to clinicians and parents. The seasonal factor, however, is confounded by the occurrence of respiratory virus infection during the winter months (Henderson et al. 1982). Since nearly all epidemiologic studies of otitis media have been conducted in temperate climates, it is not possible to determine the importance of season as a risk determinant exclusive of the effect of respiratory virus infection and crowding of children in preschool and school settings.

Socioeconomic, cultural, genetic, and nutritional factors are closely interrelated. There is no doubt that factors that cause a delay in seeking medical attention, crowding, suboptimal nutrition, poor hygiene, inadequate treatment compliance, and inattention to symptoms may increase the incidence and severity of otitis media. Epidemiologic studies in urban settings have shown an inverse correlation between socioeconomic status and the incidence of otitis media. For example, a study in an Alaskan native community noted a reduction in the rate of chronic otitis media when living standards and medical care were improved (Kaplan, Fleshman, and Bender 1973). Genetic factors, however, may outweigh socioeconomic factors since another study reported no change in the prevalence of otitis media when American Indian children were adopted from low socioeconomic to middle class foster homes (Spivey and Hirschhorn 1977). Several case-control studies have identified family history of middle ear disease as a risk factor for otitis media. More extensive studies are required to define the apparent genetic predisposition to otitis media.

Environmental factors also contribute to the risk of otitis media. Studies in Denmark and the United States have shown a higher incidence of OME (Fiellau-Nikolajsen 1979), of chronic OME (Daly et al. in press) and of acute otitis media (Visscher et al. 1984) in children who attend day-care centers as opposed to children cared for at home. However, a group environment for preschool children intensifies exposure to respiratory viral pathogens, and confounds the analysis of these interdependent risk factors.

There is very little information on the importance of nutritional content and feeding practices relative to the risk for otitis media. Although breast fed Eskimo infants experienced a lower incidence of chronic otitis media than bottle fed infants in one study (Schaefer 1971), a similar relationship was not observed in American whites (Cunningham 1977). Urban black and white American children, however, were reported to clear their middle ear effusions more rapidly if they had been breast rather than bottle fed (Teele et al. 1980).

Certain disorders of craniofacial development increase the risk of otitis media. The universality of OME among children with cleft palate and the high prevalence of OME in children with Down syndrome has been described in many reports. Clinicians have suspected that allergy is a risk factor for otitis media, yet few biochemical studies substantiate the importance of respiratory inhalant allergens in the etiology of otitis media.

Occasional therapeutic intervention trials in patients with otitis media have explored demographic and clinical factors associated with treatment response. A study at the University of Minnesota reported that among 61 children with acute otitis media, treatment failure was significantly more common in children three years old and younger compared with those older than three years (Giebink et al. 1984). Children were also more prone to treatment failure if they had a history of more than five previous episodes of otitis media, had serous or mucoid middle ear effusion, or had bilateral middle ear disease.

CONCLUSION—GAPS IN KNOWLEDGE

Epidemiologic studies to date have characterized major risk factors for acute otitis media, recurrent otitis media, and chronic OME; studies have not been performed to investigate risk factors for chronic otitis media. The continuum of otitis media from acute to chronic and the multifactorial nature of otitis media are well documented; therefore, multivariate analyses must be used in future studies to distinguish important risk factors from confounding variables. A few recent studies have used the multivariate approach. For example, a study at the University of Minnesota examined relationships between chronic OME and demographic and OME-related variables in 359 children. All variables were included in a step-wise multiple logistic regression model with chronic OME as the dependent variable. Although four variables were significantly related to chronic OME, the best regression model included only three: bilateral OME, duration of OME of at least three weeks, and day care attendance. No other factors contributed significantly to the risk of chronic OME in this population (Daly et al. in press).

Major gaps persist in our understanding of otitis media epidemiology. It will be important to determine whether children at high risk for recurrent acute otitis media and chronic OME can be identified at a young age. Early identification would permit early intervention and prevention of sequelae. Detailed genetic investigations should be pursued to identify genetic risk determinants of middle ear disease and otitis media sequelae. Clinical and pathological features of otitis media that predict future sequelae should be identified. Since all epidemiologic studies are critically dependent on accurate diagnostic methods, noninvasive technology to identify OME, and especially middle ear sequelae accurately, should be refined.

REFERENCES

Barfoed, C., and Rosborg, J. 1980. Secretory otitis media: Long-term observations after treatment with grommets. *Archives of Otolaryngology* 106:553–556.

Berry, Q. C., Doyle, W. F., Cantekin, E. I., and Bluestone, C. D. 1979. Longitudinal assessment of eustachian tube function in children. *Laryngoscope,* 89:1,446–1,456.

Biles, R. W., Buffer, P. A., and O'Donnell, A. A. 1980. Epidemiology of otitis media: A community study. *American Journal of Public Health* 70:593–598.

Brick, H. G., and Mravek, J. J. 1976. Myringostomy for middle ear effusions: Results of a two-year study. *Annals of Otology, Rhinology and Laryngology* 85(Suppl 25):263–267.

Bluestone, C. D. 1984. State of the art: Definitions and classifications. *In* D. J. Lim (ed.). *Recent Advances in Otitis Media with Effusion* (pp. 1–4). Philadelphia: B. C. Decker, Inc.

Brown, M. J. K. M., Richards, S. H., and Ambegaokar, A. G. 1978. Grommets and glue ear: A five-year follow-up of a controlled trial. *Royal Society of Medicine Journal* 71:353–356.

Bylander, A., Tjernstruöm, Ö., Ivarsson, A., and Ingvarsson, L. 1984. Eustachian tube function in children with and without otologic history. *In* D. J. Lim (ed.). *Recent Advances in Otitis Media with Effusion* (pp. 56–58). Philadelphia: B. C. Decker, Inc.

Carson, J. L., Collier, A. M., and Shih-chin, S. H. 1985. Acquired ciliary defects in nasal epithelium of children with acute viral upper respiratory infections. *New England Journal of Medicine* 312:463–468.

Cunningham, A. S. 1977. Morbidity in breast-fed and artificially fed infants. *Journal of Pediatrics* 90:726–729.

Daly, K., Giebink G. S., Le, C. T., Batalden, P. B., Anderson, R. S., and Russ, J. N. In press. Determining risk for chronic otitis media with effusion.

Draf, W., and Schulz, P. 1980. Insertion of ventilation tubes into the middle ear: Results and complications, a seven-year review. *Annals of Otology, Rhinology and Laryngology* 89(Suppl 68):303–307.

Felding, J. U., Fiellau-Nikolajsen, M., and Højslet, P. E. 1984. Impedance as an indicator in irreversible otopathology and hearing loss in nine-year olds. *In* D. J. Lim (ed.). *Recent Advances in Otitis Media with Effusion* (pp. 357–359). Philadelphia: B. C. Decker, Inc.

Fiellau-Nikolajsen, M. 1979. Tympanometry in 3-year-old children. Type of care as an epidemiological factor in secretory otitis media and tubal dysfunction in unselected populations of 3-year-old children. *Otolaryngology, Rhinology and Laryngology* 41:193–205.

Giebink, G. S., and Quie, P. G. 1978. Otitis media: The spectrum of middle ear inflammation. *Annual Review of Medicine* 29:285-306.

Giebink, G. W., Le, C. T., and Paparella, M. D. 1982. Epidemiology of otitis media with effusion in children. *Archives of Otolaryngology* 108:563–566.

Giebink, G. S., Juhn, S. K., Weber, M. L., and Le, C. T. 1982. The bacteriology and cytology of chronic otitis media with effusion. *Pediatric Infectious Diseases* 1:98–103.

Giebink, G. S., and Wright, P. F. 1983. Different virulence of Influenza A virus strains and susceptibility to pneumococcal otitis media in chinchillas. *Infection and Immunity* 41:913–920.

Giebink, G. S., Batalden, P. B., Russ, J. N., and Le, C. T. 1984. Cefaclor vs. amoxicillin in the treatment of acute otitis media. *American Journal of Diseases of Children* 138:287–292.

Giebink, G. S. 1984. Epidemiology and natural history of otitis media. *In* D. J. Lim (ed.). *Recent Advances in Otitis Media with Effusion* (pp. 5–9). Philadelphia: B. C. Decker, Inc.

Gunderson, T., and Tonning, F. -M. 1976. Ventilating tubes in the middle ear: Long-term observations. *Archives of Otolaryngology* 102:198–199.

Gunderson, T., Tonning, F. -M., and Kveberg, K. H. 1984. Ventilating tubes in the middle ear: Long-term observations. *Archives of Otolaryngology* 110:783–784.

Henderson, F. W., Collier, A. M., Sanyal, M. A., Watkins, J. M., Fairclough, D. L., Clyde, W. A., Jr., and Denny F. W. 1982. A longitudinal study of respiratory viruses and bacteria in the etiology of acute otitis media with effusion. *New England Journal of Medicine* 306:1,377–1,383.

Howie, V. M., Ploussard, J. C., and Sloyer, J. 1975. The "otitis-prone" condition. *American Journal of Diseases of Children* 129:676–678.

Hughes, L. A., Warder, F. R., and Hudson, W. R. 1974. Complications of tympanostomy tubes. *Archives of Otolaryngology* 100:151–154.

Juhn, S. K. 1982. Panel discussion: Pathogenesis of otitis media. Studies on middle ear effusions. *Laryngoscope* 92:287–291.

Juhn, S. K. 1984. Biochemistry of middle ear effusion: State of the art. *In* D. J. Lim (ed.). *Recent Advances in Otitis Media with Effusion* (pp. 181–184). Philadelphia: B. C. Decker, Inc.

Kaplan, C. J., Fleshman, J. K., and Bender, T. R. 1973. Long-term effects of otitis media: A ten-year cohort study of Alaskan Eskimo children. *Pediatrics* 52:577–585.

Kilby, D., Richards, S. H., and Hart, G. 1972. Grommets and glue ears: Two-year results. *Journal of Laryngology and Otology* 86:881–888.

Kokko, E., and Palva, T. 1976. Clinical results and complications of tympanostomy. *Annals of Otology, Rhinology and Laryngology* 85(Suppl 25):277–279.

Kraemer, M.J., Richardson, M. E., Weiss, N. S., Furukawa, C. T., Shapiro, C. G., Pierson, W. E., and Bierman, C. W. 1983. Risk factors for persistant middle ear effusion. *Journal of the American Medical Association* 249:1022–1025.

Leinonen, M. K. 1980. Detection of pneumococcal capsular polysaccharide antigens by latex agglutination, counterimmunoelectrophoresis, and radioimmunoassay in middle ear exudates in acute otitis media. *Journal of Clinical Microbiology* 11:135–140.

Lildholdt, T. 1984. Consequences of ventilation tube treatment. *Acta Otolaryngologica* (Stockholm) 414(Suppl):170.

Lundgren, K., Ingvarsson, L., and Olofsson, B. 1984. Epidemiologic aspects in children with recurrent acute otitis media. *In* D. J. Lim (ed.). *Recent Advances in Otitis Media with Effusion* (pp. 22–24). Philadelphia: B. C. Decker Inc.

MacKennon, D. M. 1971. The sequel to myringotomy for exudative otitis media. *Journal of Laryngology and Otology* 85:773–793.

Marchant, D. C., Shurin, P. A., Rutczyk, V. A., Waskiowski, D. E., Tutihasi, M. A., and Kinmey, S. Z. 1980. Course and outcome of otitis media in early infancy: A prospective study. *Journal of Pediatrics* 104:826–831.

Mawson, S. R., and Fagan, P. 1972. Tympanic effusions in children. Long-term results of treatment by myringotomy, aspiration and indwelling tubes (grommets). *Journal of Laryngology and Otology* 86:105–119.

McLelland, C. A. 1980. Incidence of complications from use of tympanostomy tubes. *Archives of Otolaryngology* 106:97–99.

Muenker, G. 1980. Results after treatment of otitis media with effusion. *Annals of Otology, Rhinology and Laryngology,* 85(Suppl 68):308–311.

Ohnishi, T., Mochizuki, M., and Hongo, S. 1984. Complications of otitis media with effusion in Japanese children. *In* D. J. Lim (ed.). *Recent Advances in Otitis Media with Effusion* (pp. 360–362). Philadelphia: B. C. Decker, Inc.

Onion, O. K., and Taylor C. 1977. Epidemiology of recurrent otitis media. *American Journal of Public Health* 67:472-474.

Paparella, M. M., Jung, T. T. K., Mancini, F., Shea, D., and Agarwal, S. P. 1984. *In* D. J. Lim (ed). *Recent Advances in Otitis Media with Effusion* (pp. 78–84). Philadelphia: B. C. Decker, Inc.

Pappas, J. J. 1974. Middle ear ventilation tubes. *Laryngoscope* 84:1098–1116.

Renvall, U., Liden, G. Jungert, S., and Nilsson, E. 1978. Long-term observation of ears with reduced middle ear pressure. *Acta Otolaryngologica* 86:104–109.

Sakai, M., Shinkawa, A., and Saito, S. 1985. Late results of hearing in children treated with tympanostomy tube. (Abstract) Presented at Extraordinary International Symposium on Recent Advances in Otitis Media with Effusion, January 13–15 at Kyoto, Japan.

Schaefer, O. 1971. Otitis media and bottle feeding: An epidemiological study of infant feeding habits and incidence of recurrent and chronic middle ear disease in Canadian Eskimos. *Cana-*

dian Journal of Public Health 62:478–489.

Schwartz, R. H., Schwartz, D. M., and Rodriquez, W. J. 1981. (Abstract). Otitis media with effusion: Natural course in untreated children. *Pediatric Research* 15:556.

Shurin, P. A., Peltin, S. I., Conner, A., Donner, A., and Klein, J. O. 1979. Persistence of middle ear effusion after acute otitis media in children. *New England Journal of Medicine* 300:1121–1123.

Spivey, G., and Hirschhorn, N. 1977. A migrant study of adopted Apache children. *John Hopkins Medical Journal* 140:43–46.

Stewart, I., Kirkland, C., Simpson, A., Silva, P., and Williams, S. 1984. Some factors of possible etiologic significance related to otitis media with effusion. *In* D. J. Lim (ed.). *Recent Advances in Otitis Media with Effusion* (pp. 25–27). Philadelphia: B. C. Decker, Inc.

Teele, D. W., Rosner, B. A., and Klein, J. O. 1980. Epidemiology of otitis media in children. *Annals of Otology, Rhinology and Laryngology* 89(Suppl 68): 5–6.

Teele, D. W., Klein, J. O., Rosner, B., Bratton, L., Fisch, G. R., Mathieu, O. R., Porter, P. J., Starobin, S. G., Tarlin, L. D., and Younes, R. P. 1983. Middle ear disease and the practice of pediatrics. Burden during the first five years of life. *Journal of the American Medical Association* 249:1026–1029.

Tos, M., and Paoulsen, G. 1976. Secretory otitis media: Late results of treatment with grommets. *Archives of Otolaryngology* 102:672–675.

Tos, M., Stangerup, S. E., Holm-Jensen, S., and Sørensen, C. H. 1984. Spontaneous course of secretory otitis and changes of the eardrum. *Archives of Otolaryngology* 110:281–289.

VanCauwenberge, P. B., and Kluyskens, P. M. 1984. Some predisposing factors in otitis media with effusion. *In* D. J. Lim (ed.). *Recent Advances in Otitis Media with Effusion* (pp. 28–31). Philadelphia: B. C. Decker, Inc.

Virolainen, E., Puhakka, H., Aantaa, E., Tuohimaa, P., Ruuskanen, O., and Meurman, O. H. 1980. Prevalence of secretory otitis media in seven to eight year old school children. *Annals of Otology, Rhinology and Laryngology* 89(Suppl 68):7–10.

Visscher, W., Mandel, J. S., Batalden, P. B., Russ, J. N., and Giebink, G. S. 1984. *In* D. J. Lim (ed.). *Recent Advances in Otitis Media with Effusion* (pp. 13–15). Philadelphia: B. C. Decker, Inc.

Chapter 7

The Otitis-Prone Child: Considerations for the Patient, Parent, and Primary Care Physician

Richard H. Schwartz

Introduction

A child who has suffered three or more episodes of acute otitis media in a 12 month period is generally identified as otitis-prone (Howie, Ploussard, and Sloyer 1975). For the purposes of this paper, children who have liquid in their middle ear clefts for three months (chronic otitis media with effusion) (Senturia et al. 1980) or more, are also included in that category.

The Child With Frequent Episodes of Acute Otitis Media

Approximately 20% of all children will have three or more documented episodes of acute otitis media by their third birthday (Teele et al. 1980, 1983). A much smaller percentage will have three or more episodes of acute otitis media in an 12 month period (Howie, Ploussard, and Sloyer 1975).

The criteria for diagnosis of acute otitis media have been precisely defined, and include a combination of abnormal findings on otoscopic examination: (1) complete or partial bulging of the tympanic membrane with obliteration of the malleolar handle or the lateral (short) process of the malleus; (2) impairment of mobility of the tympanic membrane in both lateral (outward) and medial (inward) directions; (3) opacification (dullness) of the normally lustrous tympanic membrane, usually associated with a yellowish or pink to red coloration (Schwartz, Stool, and Rodriguez 1981). The presence of the third criterion, that of color change, in the absence of the more important first and second criteria, has *never been proven* to be sufficient for the diagnosis of "early acute otitis media," although anecdotes abound. Abnormal tympanic membrane color changes, i.e., redness, may be caused by variations in the brilliance and wavelength of the otoscopic light source, by vigorous crying by the child, and by inconsistencies in the observations of different otoscopists; that is, redness of the eardrum often lies in the eye of the beholder.

From a parent's prospective, an otitis-prone child represents a considerable investment in money, time, concern for the child, and frustration. In Northern Virginia communities, for example, an episode of acute otitis media will cost at least $55 for the initial and follow-up visits during regularly scheduled office hours (add $15 more for an after-hours visit and $30 to $50 more for an emergency room visit), and $10 for the least expensive antibiotic (add $10 to $20 more for alternative antibiotic medication). Parental time, concern for the frequently ill and occasionally suffering child, and frustration over disruptions in sleep, work, or leisure time are more difficult to quantify but certainly are not less important.

MANAGEMENT OF RECURRENT ACUTE OTITIS MEDIA

Chemoprophylaxis of the otitis-prone child may be effected by administration of one of several antimicrobial agents on a variety of dosage schedules. The least expensive and most studied method is the administration of a morning and a bedtime dose (or, alternatively, a bedtime dose only) of a single sulfonamide drug such as sulfisoxazole or sulfamethoxazole—30 to 40 mg per kg body weight per dose of medicine (Schwartz, Puglise, and Rodriguez 1982; Liston, Foshee, and Pierson 1983). Although the fixed combination of trimethoprim-sulfamethoxazole is also widely used for prophylaxis of the otitis-prone child, it has, at least in the United States, not been subjected to rigorous clinical investigation for that purpose.

The physician must decide on the duration of prophylaxis. If a mild upper respiratory infection with stuffy nose or rhinorrhea usually precedes, by several days, an episode of acute otitis media in a given otitis-prone child, chemoprophylaxis may be administered in pulse courses beginning at the onset of rhinitis and ending two or three days after the upper respiratory infection has cleared, usually a five- to seven-day treatment course (Biedel 1978). If there is no such history of predictable antecedent upper respiratory infection in the otitis-prone child, consideration should be given to continuous chemoprophylaxis, at least during the cooler months of the year (November through April or May in most areas of the United States and Canada).

DIAGNOSIS OF PERSISTENT OTITIS MEDIA WITH EFFUSION

The diagnosis of persistent OME is best made by pneumatic otoscopy using brilliant halogen light and aural speculum of a size and shape to allow penetration 10 to 15 mm into the external auditory canal. Tympanometry or acoustic reflectometry using an Acoustic Otoscope (Lampe et al. 1985; Schwartz and Schwartz 1986), are valuable techniques which improve objective detection of liquid in the middle ear cleft. A flat tympanogram (type B pattern) or a reflectance reading of 7–10 are strongly supportive of the diagnosis of AOM or persistent OME. The absence of pain, fussiness, or bulging of the tympanic membrane usually exclude the diagnosis of acute otitis media.

Otitis media with effusion simply means there is liquid in the middle ear cleft. Liquid or gel may be present in approximately 50% of all young children 10 to 14 days after a presumably successfully treated episode of acute otitis media. The tympanic membranes will usually be opaque, with loss of normal pearl-like lustre, and may be in a neutral position or retracted. Bulging of the tympanic membrane is a rare event in such cases because middle ear pathogenic bacteria, even if present, are almost always quiescent and of low virulence. The liquid is most often mucoid and gel-like, but may be thin and serous.

The natural history of otitis media with effusion has been well delineated (Shurin et al. 1979; Groothuis et al. 1979; Fiellau-Nikolajsen 1983; Schwartz, Rodriguez, and Grundfast 1984). Because the half-life of middle ear effusion is approximately two or three weeks, even without medical intervention, only 12% of children with otitis media with effusion will have persistent, chronic OME after 90 days of repeated observation. Although medical therapy, including antibiotics (Schwartz et al. 1982; Marks, Mills, and Shakien 1983), and/or oral corticosteroids (Schwartz, Puglese, and Schwartz, 1980; Mackin and Jones 1985; Berman and Grose 1986; Woodhead et al. 1986). has, on occasion, shown promise in controlled clinical trials, such therapy should be considered as under investigation at this time.

Children with persistent otitis media with effusion are usually without complaint, although they usually suffer a hearing deficit averaging 25 to 30 dB. However, such hearing losses may range from 15 dB to 40 dB (Friel-Patti et al. 1982; Hubbard et al. 1985; Fria, Cantekin, and Eichler 1985; Teele et al. 1984). Bothersome persistent symptoms such as disruption of sleep, of balance, and of temperament (irritability or petulance) demand definitive surgical intervention, without excessive delay. In the absence of such problems, a policy of watchful waiting seems advisable for otherwise normal children, in order to allow the natural history of OME to unfold.

The Re-evaluation Visit for Persistent Otitis Media With Effusion

Re-evaluation visits for persistent OME may be scheduled at six- to eight-week intervals in the absence of significant ear pain or notable hearing impairment.

Tympanometric and Audiometric Evaluation of the Child With Chronic OME

In an otherwise healthy child, tympanometry or acoustic reflectometry are valuable and important objective tests to support or rule out a diagnosis of persistent OME because of opacity and retraction of the tympanic membrane with diminished cone of light reflex and impaired mobility of the eardrum to positive pressure applied by means of the pneumatic otoscope. However, it is helpful to obtain a tympanogram and, when possible, an audiogram as well. If these tests support a diagnosis of persistent OME, photocopies of each test, and of the pertinent medical record may be sent to the otologist. It is occasionally possible to obtain a pure-tone audiogram on three year old children; more often, children are at least four years old before they will be cooperative and give consistent and valid responses to pure-tone audiometric tests in our pediatric office. A pure-tone hearing loss of greater than 35 dB in both ears merits consideration of prompt referral for an otologist's opinion.

Medical Management of a Child With Subacute or Chronic OME

During the several months over which they may observe a child with chronic OME, primary care physicians may offer several suggestions to the parents of such children:

1. Infants who have persistent OME should not be fed milk in the supine position because milk may enter the patulous eustachian tubes of some infants and contribute to the middle ear pathology (Nelson 1971).
2. Elimination diets which exclude dairy products, citrus fruits, eggs, peanut butter (in older children), and possibly soy, wheat, or corn products may be worth a trial, particularly if there is documented history of atopic disease in the child or parents (Chan, Logan, and McBean 1967; Kraemer et al. 1983).
3. Parents who smoke cigarettes or other tobacoo products should be counseled to smoke only outdoors, since cigarette smoke has been associated with persistent OME in some children.
4. A therapeutic trial of suitable antimicrobial agents (such as trimethoprim-sulfamethoxazole, amoxicillin, erythromycin-sulfisoxazole, cefaclor (Ernston and Anari 1985) or amoxicillin-clavulanate) may be prescribed in an attempt to eradicate viable middle ear bacteria or prevent emergence of bacteria into the middle ear from the nasopharynx which may play a role in the pathogenesis of persistent OME.
5. While decongestant-antihistamine combination drugs are ineffectual in hastening the resolution of persistent OME (Cantekin et al. 1983), a short course of prednisone or prednisolone, in concert with one of the anti-

microbial agents listed in the previous suggestion, may, in some children, promote middle ear drainage and allow reventilation of the middle ear cleft. The efficacy of corticosteroids for this indication is unproven, although the results of some clinical investigations support the use of such agents (Schwartz et al. 1980). It is the author's current belief that 50% of children with chronic OME (more than 12 weeks), will improve dramatically with prednisone 1 mg per kg body weight per day for three or four days, followed by an additional week of 10 mg per day. The maintenance dose for infants is approximately 50% of the daily loading dose. All children treated with prednisone are also treated with trimethoprim-sulfamethoxazole for two to four weeks.

PERSISTENT OME: REFERRAL TO AN OTOLARYNGOLOGIST

The decision about who needs otolaryngological referral, and when, is based on historical, objective, subjective, and financial considerations. Variables to be considered include the presence of major craniofacial malformations or sensorineural hearing loss; unilateral vs. bilateral persistent OME; proximity to summer; the financial circumstances of the parents; and distance from the otolaryngologist. Children with unilateral OME can be observed for at least six months, while children with bilateral OME can safely be managed over a period of three or four months. If possible, audiometric, linguistic, and tympanometric assessments should be performed before otolaryngological consultation. Usually, the otolaryngologist will suggest insertion of tympanostomy tubes after aspiration of the middle ear cleft.

Consultation with an otolaryngologist should be requested for:

1. Two or three episodes of acute otitis media in an otitis-prone child who had received sufonamide or amoxicillin chemoprophylaxis on an intermittent or continuous regimen.
2. Bilateral otitis media with effusion (with presumed or documented 25 dB or more hearing loss) persisting over a three- or four-month period.
   During the midsummer months many children with persistent OME will, by some unknown mechanism, establish drainage and reventilation of the middle ear cleft (Tos, Holm-Jensen, and Sorensen 1981). Tympanostomy tubes have been proven to protect the middle ears of many otitis-prone children against recurrent episodes of AOM. Tympanostomy tubes inserted in mid-August or early September usually remain in situ and patent during the fall and winter "otitis season," whereas tympanostomy tubes inserted in May or June will usually become obstructed or extruded before or during the next "otitis season." This may then necessitate a second surgical procedure during the following January, February, or March.
3. Unilateral otitis media with effusion monitored by physicians over a six- to eight-month period.

The primary concern about chronic OME is significant conductive hearing loss, which can hinder learning and speech development, although an otherwise normal child with unilateral chronic OME will usually compensate. In addition, while warm weather may promote middle ear drainage and ventilation, it happens on rare occasion that a child with unilateral chronic OME may experience obstruction to drainage of the middle ear because of a nasopharyngeal tumor, such as a rhabdomyosarcoma or lymphoma. Nasopharyngoscopy or a lateral cephalometric roentgenographic view of the nasopharynx may be requested when clinically indicated, particularly for adolescents with persistent OME.

4. Children with an underlying moderate or severe sensorineural hearing impairment or mental retardation, children with cleft palates, and those with significant craniofacial anomalies should be taken for otolaryngological consultation after two or three months of persistent bilateral OME.

ADENOIDECTOMY

An exceptionally well controlled study (Gates et al. 1987) comparing four treatment modalities clearly demonstrates that adenoidectomy in conjunction with tympanocentesis, with or without placement of tympanostomy tubes, gave better results (fewer months of recurrent OME during prolonged follow-up) than tympanostomy tube insertion without adenoidectomy.

TYMPANOSTOMY TUBES: PROBLEMS AND DECISIONS

Although unquestionably efficacious in the reventilation of the middle ear cleft, restoration of hearing, and prevention of recurrent middle ear infections, tympanostomy tubes are not problem-free. Recurrences of acute middle ear infection can be expected in 20 to 40% of otitis-prone children, and are easily recognized by the appearance of otorrhea through a patent tympanostomy tube. Intermittent otorrhea can be managed by the same strategies useful in the management of the otitis-prone child.

However, persistent otorrhea is more difficult to control because oral antimicrobial agents are often ineffectual against the *Pseudomonas* bacteria that usually infect the chronically draining middle ear. Intramuscular or intravenously administered aminoglycoside antibiotics, in combination with anti-*Pseudomonas* drugs such as Ticarcillin, are occasionally necessary for effective treatment (Bluestone et al. 1985) when simpler measures (such as aural debridement and topical otic antibiodics) fail. Ear plugs or similar mechanical barriers to water are often prescribed for children with tympanostomy tubes who swim; but may not be absolutely necessary.

References

Berman, S., and Gross, K. 1986 (Abstract). Medical management of chronic middle ear effusion: Results of a clinical trial of prednisone combined with trimethroprim-sulfamethoxazole. *American Journal of the Disabled Child* 140:317.

Biedel, C. W. 1978. Modification of recurrent otitis media by short term sulfonamide therapy. *American Journal of the Disabled Child* 132:681–683.

Bluestone, C. D., Carder, H. M., Coffey, J. D. Jr., Kenna, M. A., Pelton, S. I., McCracken, G. H. Jr., and Nelson, J. D. 1985. Management of the child with a chronic draining ear. *Pediatric Infectious Diseases* 4:607–612.

Cantekin, E. L., Mandel, E. M., Bluestone, C. D., Rockette, H. E., Paradise, J. L., Stool, S. E., Friar, T. J., and Rogers, K. D. 1983. Lack of efficacy of a decongestant—antihistamine combination for otitis media with effusion ("secretory" otitis media) in children. *New England Journal of Medicine* 308:297–301.

Chan, J. C. M., Logan, G. B., and McBean, J. B. 1967. Serous otitis media and allergy and other causes. *American Journal of the Disabled Child* 114:684–692.

Ernston, S., and Anari, M. 1985. Cefaclor in the treatment of otitis media with effusion. *Acta Otolaryngologica* (supp) 124:17–21.

Fiellau-Nikolajsen, M. 1983. Epidemiology of secretory otitis media: A descriptive cohort study. *Annals of Otology, Rhinology and Laryngology* 92:172–177.

Fria, T. J., Cantekin, E. I., and Eichler, J. A. 1985. Hearing acuity of children with otitis media with effusion. *Archives of Otolaryngology* 111:10–16.

Friel-Patti, S., Finitzo-Hieber, T., Conti, G., and Brown, C. K. 1982. Language delay in infants associated with middle ear disease and mild, fluctuating hearing impairment. *Pediatric Infectious Diseases* 2:104–109.

Gates, G. A., Avery, C. A., Prihodat, J., and Cooper, J. C. 1987. Effectiveness of adenoidectomy and tympanostomy tubes in the treatment of chronic otitis media with effusion. *New England Journal of Medicine* 317:1444–1451.

Groothius, J. R., Sell, S. H. W., Wright, P. F., Thompson, J. M., and Altemeier, W. A. 1979. Otitis media in infancy: Tympanometric findings. *Pediatrics* 63:435–442.

Howie, V. M., Ploussard, J. H., and Sloyer, J. 1975. The "otitis prone" condition. *American Journal of the Disabled Child* 129:676–678.

Hubbard, T. W., Paradise, J. L., McWilliams, B. J., Elster, B. A., and Taylor, F. H. 1985. Consequences of unremitting middle ear disease in early life: Otologic, audiologic, and developmental findings in children with cleft palate. *New England Journal of Medicine* 312:1529–1534.

Kraemer, J. J., Richardson, M. A., Weiss, N. S. et al. 1983. Risk factors for persistent middle ear effusions: Otitis media, catarrh, cigarette smoke exposure, and atopy. *Journal of the American Medical Association* 249:1022–1024.

Lampe, R. M., Weir, P. N. R., Spier, J., and Rhodes, M. F. 1985. Acoustic reflectometry in the detection of middle ear effusion. *Pediatrics* 76:75–78.

Liston, T. E., Foshee, W. S., and Pierson, W. D. 1983. Sulfisoxazole chemoprophylaxis for frequent otitis media. *Pediatrics* 71:524–530.

Mackin, M. L., and Jones, P. K. 1985. Oral dexamethasone for treatment of persistent middle ear effuison. *Pediatrics* 75:329–335.

Marks, N. J., Mills, R. P., and Shakien, O. H. 1983. Cotrimoxazole in the treatment of serous otitis media: A follow up report. *Journal of Laryngology and Otology.* 97:213–215.

Nelson, J. D. 1971. Prop the baby, not the bottle. *Journal of Pediatrics* 79:348–350.

Schwartz, R. H., Puglese, J., and Schwartz, D. M. 1980. Use of the short course of prednisone for treating middle ear effusion: A double-blind crossover study. *Annals of Otology, Rhinology and Laryngology* (supp 68) 89:296–300.

Schwartz, R. H., Stool, S. E., and Rodriguez, W. J. 1981. Acute otitis media: Toward a more precise definition. *Clinical Pediatrics* 20:549–554.

Schwartz, R. H., Puglise, J., and Rodriguez, W. J. 1982. Sulfamethoxazole chemoprophylaxis in the otitis-prone child: A randomized, double-blind, placebo-controlled, crossover study. *Archives of Diseases of Childhood* 57:590–593.

Schwartz, R. H., and Rodriguez, W. J. 1982. Trimethoprim-sulfamethoxazole treatment of persistent otitis media with effusion. *Pediatric Infectious Diseases* 1:333–335.

Schwartz, R. H., Rodriguez, W. J., and Grundfast, K. M. 1984. Duration of middle ear effusion after acute otitis media. *Pediatric Infectious Diseases* 3:204–207.

Schwartz, D. M., and Schwartz, R. H. 1986. Validity of acoustic reflectometry in detecting middle ear effusion. *Pediatrics* 79:739–742.

Senturia, B. H., Bluestone, C. D., Klein, J. O., and Rhodes, M. F. 1980. Report of the ad hoc committee on definition and classification of otitis media and otitis media with effusion. *Annals of Otology, Rhinology and Laryngology* 85 (Suppl 68) 3(4):223–227.

Shurin, P. A., Pelton, S. I., Donner, A., and Klein, J. O. 1979. Persistence of middle ear effusion after otitis media in children. *New England Journal of Medicine* 300:1121–1123.

Teele, D. W., Klein, J. O., and Rosner B. A. 1980. Epidemiology of otitis media in children. *Annals of Otology, Rhinology and Laryngology* 89 (supp 68):5–6.

Teele, D. W., Klein, J. O., and Rosner, B. A. 1983. The Greater Boston Otitis Media Study Group: Middle ear disease and the practice of pediatrics. *Journal of the American Medical Association* 249:1026–1029.

Teele, D. W., Klein, J. O., and Rosner, B. A. 1984. Otitis media with effusion during the first three years of life and development of speech and language. *Pediatrics* 74:282–287.

Tos, M., Holm-Jensen, S., and Sorensen, C. H. 1981. Changes in prevalence of secretory otitis media from summer to winter in 4-year old children. *American Journal of Otolaryngology* 2:234–237.

Woodhead, J. C., Milavetz, G., Dusdieker, L. B., Booth, B. M., and Wilmoth, R. N. 1986 (Abstract). Prednisone treatment of otitis media with effusion. *American Journal of the Disabled Child* 140:318.

Issues on Identification and Assessment

Chapter 8

Re-Evaluating Our Approach to Evaluation: Demographics are Changing—Are We?

Noel D. Matkin

Significant differences in the impact of an acquired hearing loss in adulthood versus a prelingual loss in childhood must be recognized. Traditional service delivery models are not appropriate when considering the pediatric population. It is well documented that the effects of hearing impairment in early childhood are pervasive in terms of normal cognitive, social-emotional, and speech-language development. Further, the adverse impact of having a child with a major developmental disability upon family dynamics is well documented (Moses 1985). As a consequence, habilitative and educational needs in many cases are complex, extensive, and long term. This is especially true of the relatively large number of youngsters with one or more developmental disability in addition to their hearing loss. There is also growing evidence that selected cases of severe and profound unilateral hearing impairment of early onset, as well as those losses associated with the early onset of recurrent otitis media, may have negative impact on speech-language development and subsequent academic achievement (Bess 1986; Teele, Klein, and Rosner 1984). To complicate matters, successful management of pediatric cases depends in large part upon the acceptance of professional recommendations and active cooperation of the child's parents. Yet in many clinical settings, parents still are not viewed as active participants in the evaluation process. Further, as recommendations are formulated, changing family structures—such as two-career couples and single parents—often are not considered. For these reasons, the evaluation of hearing-impaired children is most effective when undertaken as a team endeavor. Otherwise, as noted in the Rand Report (Brewer and Kakalik 1973), services, at best, become fragmented and, at worst, conflicting recommendations for management are made. Far too often, each specialist's effectiveness is limited because evaluation services are provided as specialty assessments in relatively isolated clinical settings, and then the findings from the evaluation are communicated to parents, clinicians, and educators in a professional lexicon which has limited meaning.

The purpose of this paper is to focus on several shortcomings in service delivery for young children and infants at risk for developmentally significant hearing impairments. As the population of young hearing-impaired children changes and becomes more complex, there is a pressing need for modification of the traditional approach to evaluation. In many instances pediatric evaluations are based on a medical rather than a developmental model. Also, the need to facilitate interdisciplinary communication is apparent as one reviews the current clinical and research literature. Therefore, recommendations for change, based upon both a consideration of current demographic studies and clinical experience, will be offered.

EARLY IDENTIFICATION

The key to successful habilitation of hearing-impaired children is early identification, evaluation, and intervention. Ideally, the detection of an educationally signficant hearing loss will be immediately followed by provision of comprehensive remedial services which are individualized, i.e., based on each child's profile of strengths and current limitations across the major developmental areas.

At present, the screening of infants at risk for hearing loss is focused on two groups: babies in a well-baby nursery whose histories include one or more risk factors, and newborns who begin life in an intensive care unit. According to Alberti et al. (1985) the prevalence of at-risk infants is 92% in the NICU and 8% in the well-baby nursery. In view of such prevalence figures, it is not surprising that Simmons (1980) reports the incidence of sensorineural hearing loss to be 19 per 1000 in the NICU and 3.5 per 1000 in the well-baby nursery. While the dual thrust in current neonatal screening merits support, evidence is accruing that suggests a significant number of cases will not be detected even if screening of these two groups of newborns is universally implemented.

Stein, Clark, and Kraus (1983) reported that nearly one-half of hearing-impaired infants cared for in a well-baby nursery would not have been detected through utilization of the current risk register. More recently, a survey of the parents of children with confirmed bilateral sensorineural hearing loss—entitled the "Never Too Young" project—was completed in Arizona (Elssman, Matkin, and Sabo 1986). Briefly, the data based on a sample of 159 youngsters indicate that 125 or 79% of the sample was considered to have a congenital impairment. Approximately one-half (52%) of the congenital cases had no known risk factor in the prenatal or perinatal history. In other words, 65 of 159 babies were not suspected to be at risk for hearing loss and thus were not referred for hearing screening during the neonatal period. Recall that the Joint Committee on Infant Hearing (1982) recommends that hearing screening optimally should be completed by three months of age but no later than six months of age.

These findings should not be surprising when one considers that babies with a hearing loss due to autosomal recessive inheritance will be healthy at birth and will not have a family history for childhood hearing loss. A second relatively large group of babies who obviously will escape early detection are those youngsters with a silent clinical infection due to one of the TORCH[1] syndrome factors. Both the Stein et al. (1983) study and the "Never Too Young" project suggest that late identification of many pediatric hearing losses, under the best of circumstances, will continue to be a major deterrant to optimal management. In Arizona, the median age of identification varied inversely with the degree of the hearing impairment. Those with a profound impairment were identified at 16 months of age, those with severe losses at 18 months, while those with moderate losses at 22 months. It was not unusual for mild losses to be undetected until age three. These findings do not differ significantly from those reported a decade ago by Malkin, Freeman, and Hastings (1976). Only one category of infants identified in Arizona had been identified early and had treatment initiated by six months of age, i.e., the two babies with bilateral atresia.

The development of genetic screening programs to detect carriers of a recessive gene for hearing loss, and routine screening of all newborns for a silent TORCH infection both are sorely needed if the current situation is to change. Since the implementation of neither screening program is anticipated in the near future, the burden for early detection and referral of many infants at risk for congenital hearing loss will continue to fall upon the shoulders of the primary care physician.

From 20 to 30% of developmentally significant bilateral sensorineural impairments are acquired after the newborn period (Elssmann, Matkin, and Sabo 1986). In Arizona, the hearing loss in 28 of 34 acquired cases was due to meningitis with the average age of onset being 15 months and with a range of 5 to 42 months. Obviously, ongoing screening will be needed to identify such acquired cases as early as possible.

According to a survey from the Robert Wood Johnson Foundation study in Colorado (Walker, Downs, and Northern 1985), the majority of pediatricians report that they do routinely screen for hearing loss. In 82% of the cases, the case history is used as the primary screening tool. Unfortunately, the Arizona study as well as a report by Shah, Chandler, and Dale (1978) indicate that in the

---

[1]TORCH is an acronym to summarize the major infections that may be acquired in utero including: T—toxoplasmosis; O—other, including syphilis; R—rubella; C—cytomegalovirus; and H—herpes simplex.

majority of cases, the possibility of a hearing loss is first raised by the parents. The child's physician initially questioned the youngster's hearing status in only 7.5% of the cases in the Shah et al. sample. Thus, the sensitivity of a routine pediatric case history as the primary tool for identifying hearing loss in young children must be questioned.

The need for improved instruction in medical schools, as well as a national continuing education thrust with pediatricians, with family and general practitioners, as well as with pediatric nurses, is evident. Results from the "Never Too Young" survey revealed that, on the average, an additional seven month's delay in identification of a bilateral sensorineural hearing loss occurred among high-risk infants when the physician did not refer on the basis of the parents' initial statement of concern. In other words, the sensitivity of the managing physician to parental concern does have a direct impact on early identification. According to the Canadian Report (Health Services Directorate Task Force Report 1984), delays in early diagnosis of hearing loss are most often linked to lack of awareness of the signs and symptoms of childhood hearing loss by health care professionals, refusal of physicians to consider parental observations as valid, and reluctance of physicians to arrange prompt referral for audiologic assessment.

Not only is there a pressing need to enhance the knowledge of primary care physicians about hearing loss in children but to develop screening procedures having good reliability and validity. Such screening procedures must be easily incorporated into a busy clinic practice if they are to gain widespread acceptance.

With respect to increased awareness, a 35-minute videotape with an instructional manual designed for either self-study or group instruction is available for continuing education through the University of Arizona Medical Center (Fischler, Matkin, and Behrend 1985). The essential steps in identification and comprehensive assessment are highlighted, and the tape concludes with five mothers reporting their experiences from the time the hearing loss was suspected until it was confirmed.

While it is easy to direct criticism toward physicians, their limited knowledge of pediatric hearing loss suggests that audiologists have not made a consistent and sustained effort to provide continuing education. Further, there does not appear to be a consensus among audiologists as to either the preferred methodology for office screening or the referral criteria to be used by physicians. The current projects funded by the Robert Wood Johnson Foundation may provide research-based procedures and materials that will be universally applicable. In the meantime, the information kit on early identification and management of hearing-impaired children prepared by the Canadian Task Force merits consideration. Guidelines for office screening and referral by physicians also have been recommended by Matkin (1984). The importance of considering not only aberrant auditory behavior but delays in expressive language development was stressed in this latter publication.

MINIMAL HEARING LOSS

Growing evidence indicates that so-called minimal hearing losses, including those associated with recurrent otitis media (ROM), unilateral sensorineural impairments, and bilateral sensorineural hearing losses of borderline normal to mild degree, may have adverse effects upon normal development in selected children (Bess 1985). Data are not readily available to determine whether such cases are growing in number or whether our rate of detection has improved. Nevertheless, as the full spectrum of children with significant hearing loss is discussed, it is important to consider those youngsters who in past decades would not have been considered at risk for developmental delays or academic difficulties.

With respect to hearing loss associated with early recurrent otitis media, it has become increasingly apparent, despite the methodological flaws in many of the studies, that selected children do in fact encounter significant speech-language delays and subsequent academic problems. Of particular interest are those children, reported by Klein (1986), who despite active medical management have the persistence of middle ear effusion for more than three months. Certainly, these youngsters, who number approximately 5% of the children with ROM, merit careful monitoring and evaluation. Unfortunately, none of the available otitis media studies has serial audiograms for the cases investigated. Thus, one is not certain as to the degree of the hearing impairment during episodes of otitis media, whether the loss was unilateral or bilateral, and, importantly, how long the hearing loss was present. Clinical experience with a variety of children having a history of otitis media and flat tympanograms has revealed that the impairment may range from 10 dB or less to as great as 35 to 40 dB HL. It is not reasonable, therefore, to talk about an average hearing loss of 27.6 dB as being typically associated with otitis media (Kokko 1974). Since the variance in degree of hearing loss associated with ROM is so great, mean or median numbers have little meaning when one attempts to identify specific children with developmentally significant delays. The current debate on the adverse effects of early otitis media will continue until longitudinal audiologic information for such cases is available to correlate with speech-language and academic findings.

With respect to unilateral impairments, the recent article by Bess and associates (1986) suggests that 35% of their sample had failed at least one grade in school and an additional 13% had needed special resource services. In other words, the traditional belief that individuals with unilateral hearing impairment encounter little, if any, difficulty may not be valid. As reported by Bess, the majority of children with significant unilateral hearing losses are not identified until age five or older. Thus, late identification and use of a failure-based model, rather than early identification and preventive intervention, appear to be characteristic of this population of youngsters. As we focus on refinement of early intervention and continuing education needs, unilateral sensorineural hearing loss is a topic that merits consideration.

Finally, growing evidence from a number of speech-language and academic surveys reveals that children with so-called minimal bilateral sensorineural hearing loss encounter substantial communication and school problems. Unfortunately, current research indicates that our first line of defense in intervention, i.e., fitting hearing aids and providing assistive listening devices in adverse classroom acoustic environments, is not a common practice. As reported by Karchmer and Kerwin (1977) in a national survey, only 56% of those youngsters who have hearing losses less than 45 dB in the better ear are fitted with wearable amplifying devices. A review of the demographic data reported by Shepard, Gorga, Davis, and Stelmachowicz (1981) suggests that the situation may be more dismal than the earlier study indicated. To explain, those youngsters surveyed in the Iowa public school system who had relatively normal hearing in the low test frequencies but a significant bilateral high frequency hearing loss were rarely fitted with amplifying devices. Yet, acoustic studies of speech perception clearly indicate that most of the intelligibility of a speech message is contained in the frequencies above 1000 Hz.

A study by Blair, Peterson, and Viehweg (1985) indicates that significant delays across a number of academic areas became evident in the first grade. Of greater concern is the fact that such delays increased in magnitude when achievement scores for fourth grade were compared with those from the first grade. Interestingly, only 14% of this sample was fitted with hearing aids. As services are refined for the broad spectrum of children with developmentally significant hearing impairments, the child with a minimal to mild bilateral sensorineural hearing loss should be given priority. Certainly, there is no group of children with mild developmental delay who respond more readily to early identification and intervention than such youngsters. The cost of providing ongoing support services at school age or of letting children repeat grades due to academic failure far exceeds the expense of a preschool intervention program so that full integration into the regular classroom becomes a feasible alternative.

One hopes that audiologists will not continue to use adult guidelines when making a decision about whether a child with minimal hearing loss is a candidate for a wearable amplification device and language intervention. Without detailed information about the child's speech and language development and, when appropriate, performance in the classroom, such youngsters may be denied the opportunity to develop optimal auditory function, the basis of verbal language competence (Matkin 1986).

PROGRESSIVE HEARING IMPAIRMENT

Sensorineural hearing losses associated with certain etiological factors, including congenital impairments from maternal rubella and acquired losses following meningitis, may progress over time (Pappas 1985; Kean et al. 1979). As noted by Pappas in 1985, a number of additional etiological factors are known to be associated with progressive sensorineural hearing loss; however, in a significant number of cases the etiology is idiopathic. Pappas suggests that progression of the impairment among children with sensorineural hearing loss may be characterized by irregularity. Significant periods of time in which the hearing impairment appears to be stable may be followed by an additional decrement of hearing loss which is usually bilateral but occasionally may be unilateral. Recent research with respect to cytomegalic virus (CMV), the etiological factor considered to be the most common cause of congenital exogenous hearing impairment, indicates that in a number of such cases the impairment does not progress over time (Dahle et al. 1979). Keep in mind that without routine screening of newborns, CMV, as the etiological factor underlying the hearing impairment, will remain obscure. Thus, at present it is not possible to identify many youngsters who are at high risk for progressive sensorineural hearing loss. A clinical report by Walton et al. in 1985 and a more recent article by Naulty, Weiss, and Herer (1986) indicate that progressive sensorineural hearing loss also is encountered in at least one third of the NICU survivors with a history of persistent fetal circulation.

When one considers the detailed list of etiological factors associated with progressive hearing loss, as well as recent reports on cytomegalic viral cases and persistent fetal circulation infants, the importance of systematic and ongoing audiologic monitoring of all children with sensorineural hearing loss cannot be overstressed. A schedule that has been found to work quite well in the University of Arizona clinics is that children with such losses are routinely scheduled for re-evaluation on a three-month basis until age three. Retesting every six months is then utilized until age six. Finally, school-age children are seen on an annual basis. Not only does such a rigorous schedule allow identification of progressive hearing loss, but additional benefits justify the time and effort required. Longitudinal monitoring also permits the identification of conductive hearing loss as an overlay to the sensorineural impairment, parental acceptance and adjustment to their child's hearing impairment, assessment of hearing aid function and, finally, modification of earmolds to maximize the benefit of powerful ear-level aids. In short, numerous factors justify a rigorous ongoing audiologic monitoring program with pediatric cases.

ADDITIONAL DEVELOPMENTAL DISABILITIES

Many children with sensorineural hearing impairment have developmental disabilities in addition to the hearing loss. Over a decade ago, Vernon (1969) and the Office of Demographic Studies (Rawlings and Gentile 1970) both highlighted the increasing prevalence of multiple handicaps among hearing-impaired children. In 1982, the Office of Demographic Studies again conducted a national survey relative to the prevalence of multiple handicaps among those hearing-impaired children being served in special programs (Karchmer 1985). While the sample included approximately 55,000 students in more than

6,000 schools across the United States, youngsters with mild hearing loss being educated in regular classrooms were not well represented in this data. Nevertheless, the important finding is that approximately 21% of the children sampled were reported to have one additional developmental disability while another 10% were reported to have two or more additional handicapping disabilities. Briefly, the O.D.S. data indicate that at least 30% of children with sensorineural hearing impairment will have one, or more, additional developmental disability. The four disabilities shown to be most frequently encountered in youngsters with sensorineural hearing loss are mental retardation (8%), specific learning disabilities (7.5%), emotional/behavioral problems (6%), and uncorrected visual problems (4.4%). These prevalence figures highlight the point made earlier when the need was stressed for adopting a developmental rather than a medical service model for such youngsters and their families.

Unfortunately, a review of the literature suggests that many evaluation and remedial programs assume that children being served will have only a hearing impairment. The continued use of such terms as "the deaf child" or "the hard-of-hearing child" suggest that we are serving a homogenous population. Yet growing evidence indicates that the current population of hearing-impaired children in the United States is hallmarked by its heterogeneity.

Unless a proactive developmental approach is used, many children with multiple handicaps will be provided integrated comprehensive services only after they have experienced failure. These youngsters should be identified as early as possible and then services should be individualized with careful consideration of the particular youngster's developmental profile. Such an integrated comprehensive approach suggests that service delivery for young hearing-impaired children must involve interactive teamwork, requiring effective communication among the various professionals serving the youngster and his or her family.

As stated in an earlier publication (Matkin 1985), five major deterrants consistently impair effective communication among professionals during service delivery and limit the effectiveness of teamwork in many settings. These deterrants include the trend in this country for increased speciality training as reflected by current accreditation standards and certification requirements. As a result, graduate students often complete an extensive curriculum almost exclusively focused on one specialty area. Such clinicians enter practice with advanced degrees but with little knowledge or appreciation of the broad scope of research in child development or of the competencies among allied professionals.

Second, various professionals who work with children having developmental disabilities often lack a common terminology. As a consequence, evaluations or oral reports often are fully meaningful only to a colleague in the same discipline, but not to other specialists who also are evaluating the child.

A third deterrant is that many graduate programs do not include either academic instruction or clinical experience in teamwork. Without such a background, territorial defensiveness is often apparent as professionals interact with co-workers from other disciplines. There have been a number of publications that address the need for training models in teamwork, one of the best being a book by Brill (1976).

A fourth problem area is that a professional pecking order exists among various pediatric specialists. Unfortunately, clinicians, who spend the least amount of time with the child and parents, often have the most clout when it comes to establishing a diagnosis and to setting priorities for recommendations. In sharp contrast, the teacher and the parents, who spend the most time with the child, often have minimal input to the evaluation team.

The fifth, and final, issue that often impairs effective teamwork is related to time. In a situation where there is a major effort to contain costs for professional services, the expense of assembling a team for a comprehensive evaluation must be a major consideration. For this reason, developmental screening must be implemented as a routine clinical procedure so that only those cases needing evaluation by a full array of specialists are referred.

Despite these five deterrants, a number of benefits obviously accrue if comprehensive multi-disciplinary evaluations are available at the point of identification. Only by identifying the full array of developmental disabilities at the outset can appropriate intervention be undertaken. As noted in the Rand report (Brewer and Kakalik 1973), there is evidence that more effective parent management results when parents are provided with unified and coordinated information rather than fragmented recommendations.

SUMMARY

As the population of young hearing-impaired children becomes more heterogenous, there is the need to re-evaluate our approach to evaluation. Late identification still characterizes far too many children with developmentally significant hearing impairments of early onset. Once such a child is identified, stringent protocols for ongoing audiologic monitoring must be implemented so that amplification systems and intervention plans can be appropriately modified, especially in those instances where the hearing impairment progresses. Ongoing research is needed to understand the specific impact of so-called minimal hearing losses to ensure the optimal management of these youngsters. Finally, interactive teamwork is a key to providing optimal services, especially for the relatively large number of children with multiple developmental disabilities, including hearing loss.

Many of the preceding comments and recommendations were made in 1976 during the Second Symposium on Childhood Deafness, yet a number of the same problems persist. Most of the shortcomings can be minimized if each of us will make a concerted effort to reevaluate our current approach to evaluation. Young hearing-impaired children and their families deserve such quality assurance.

REFERENCES

Alberti, P. W., Hyde, M. L., Riko, K., Corbin, H., and Fitzhardinge, P. M. 1985. Issues in early identification of hearing loss. *The Laryngoscope* 95(4):373–381.

Bess, F. H. 1985. The minimally hearing-impaired child. *Ear and Hearing* 6:43–47.

Bess, F. H. 1986. The unilateral sensorineural hearing-impaired child: A Final Comment. *Ear and Hearing* 7(1):52–54.

Blair, J. C., Peterson, M. E., and Viehweg, S. H. 1985. The effects of mild hearing loss on academic performance of young school-age children. *The Volta Review* 87(2):87–93.

Brewer, G., and Kakalik, J. 1973. *Improving Services to Handicapped Children* (R-1420, HEW). Santa Monica, CA: Rand Corporation.

Brill, N. 1976. *Teamwork: Working Together in the Human Services.* Philadelphia, PA: Lippincott.

Dahle, A. J., McCollister, F. P., Stagnos, S., Reynolds, D. W., and Hoffman, H. E. 1979. Progressive hearing impairment in children with congenital cytomegalovirus infection. *Journal of Speech and Hearing Disorders* 44(2):220–229.

Elssmann, S., Matkin, N. D., and Sabo, M. 1986. *Early Identification: Fact or fiction.* Manuscript in preparation.

Fischler, R. S., Matkin, N. D., and Behrend, S. H. 1985. *Case Studies in Child Development: Katie* [videocassette]. Tucson, AZ: Arizona Health Sciences Center.

Health Services Directorate Task Force Report. 1984. *Childhood Hearing Impairment.* Ottawa, Canada: Minister of National Health and Welfare.

Joint Committee on Infant Hearing. 1982. Joint Committee on Infant Hearing Position Statement. *Asha* 24(12):1017.

Karchmer, M. A., and Kerwin, L. A. 1977. *The Use of Hearing Aids by Hearing-impaired Students in the United States,* Washington, D.C.: Office of Demographic Studies, Gallaudet College.

Karchmer, M. A. 1985. A demographic perspective. *In* E. Cherow, N. D. Matkin, and R. J. Trybus (eds.). *Hearing-Impaired Children and Youth with Developmental Disabilities* (pp. 36–70). Washington, D.C.: Gallaudet College Press.

Keane, W. M., Postic, W. P., Rowe, L. D., and Konkle, D. F. 1979. Meningitis and hearing loss in children. *Archives of Otolaryngology* 105:39–44.

Klein, J. O. 1986. Risk factors for otitis media. *In* J. K. Kavanagh (ed.). *Otitis Media and Child Development.* Parkton, MD: York Press

Kokko, E. 1974. Chronic secretory otitis media in children: A clinical study. *Acta Otolaryngologica* (supp) 327:7–44.

Malkin, S. F., Freeman, R. D., and Hastings, J. O. 1976. Psychosocial problems of deaf children and their families: A comparative study. *Audiology, Hearing, and Education* 2:21–99.

Matkin, N. D. 1984. Early recognition and referral of hearing-impaired children. *Pediatrics in Review* 6(5):151–156.

Matkin, N. D. 1985. Effective communication: Interactive interdisciplinary teamwork. *In* E. Cherow, N. D. Matkin, and R. J. Trybus (eds.). *Hearing-Impaired Children and Youth with Developmental Disabilities* (pp. 71–81). Washington, D.C.: Gallaudet College Press.

Matkin, N. D. 1986. The role of hearing in language development. *In* J. K. Kavanagh (ed.). *Otitis Media and Child Development.* Parkton, MD: York Press.

Moses, K. L. 1985. Dynamic intervention with families. *In* E. Cherow, N. D. Matkin, and R. J. Trybus (eds.). *Hearing-Impaired Children and Youth with Developmental Disabilities* (pp. 82–98). Washington, D.C.: Gallaudet College Press.

Naulty, C. M., Weiss, I. P., and Herer, G. R. 1986. Progressive sensorineural hearing loss in survivors of persistent fetal circulation. *Ear and Hearing* 7(2):74–77.

Pappas, D. G. 1985. *Diagnosis and Treatment of Hearing Impairment in Children: A Clinical Manual.* San Diego, CA: College Hill Press.

Rawlings, B., and Gentile, A. 1970. *Additional Handicapping Conditions, Age at Onset of Hearing Loss, and Other Characteristics of Hearing-impaired Students. United States: 1968–1969.* (Series D, Number 3). Washington, D.C.: Office of Demographic Studies, Gallaudet College.

Shah, C. P., Chandler, D., and Dale, R. 1978. Delay in referral of children with impaired hearing. *Volta Review* 80:206–215.

Shepard, N. T., Gorga, M. P., Davis, J. M., and Stelmachowicz, P. G. 1981. Characteristics of hearing-impaired children in the public schools: Part I—Demographic data. *Journal of Speech and Hearing Disorders* 46:123–129.

Simmons, F. B. 1980. Patterns of deafness in newborns. *The Laryngoscope* 90:448–453.
Stein, L., Clark, S., and Kraus, N. 1983. The hearing-impaired infant: Patterns of identification and habilitation. *Ear and Hearing* 4(5):232–286.
Teele, D. W., Klein, J. W., Rosner, B. A., and the Greater Boston Otitis Media Study Group. 1984. Otitis media with effusion during the first three years of life and development of speech and language. *Pediatrics* 74(2):282–287.
Vernon, M. 1969. *Multiply handicapped deaf children.* Research Monograph, Council for Exceptional Children, Inc., 1–112.
Walker, D. D., Downs, M. P., and Northern, J. L. 1985. Report on the Colorado Robert Wood Johnson Foundation project/screening children for communication disorders. *The Rocky Mountain Journal of Communication Disorders* 1:5–7.
Walton, J. P., Dalzell, L. E., Hendricks-Munoz, K., and Merle, K. 1985, November. Incidence of sensorineural hearing loss in infants with persistent fetal circulation. Paper presented at the American Speech-Language and Hearing Association Annual Convention, Washington, D.C.

Chapter 9

Screening of High-Risk Infants Using Auditory Brainstem Response Audiometry

Bruce A. Weber

The Problem

No one can reasonably argue against the early identification and management of congenital hearing loss. Hearing is critical to normal speech and language development, which in turn is vital for most aspects of normal human development. Responsiveness to auditory input begins in utero and by three months after birth the full-term infant has begun to enter the readiness stage for language acquisition (Illingworth 1980). A significant hearing impairment at birth can produce a major disruption in language learning (Menyuk 1977) and produce irreversible deficits in the development of the central auditory pathways (Moore 1985). Even a mild hearing impairment has been implicated in delayed development of auditory skills (Quigley 1978). Early identification of a hearing loss followed by appropriate management minimizes the auditory deprivation which can interfere with speech/language learning and central nervous system (CNS) maturation. It must be stressed that early identification is of little or no value if there are not appropriate follow-up measures.

The prevalence of some degree of permanent sensorineural hearing loss in the intensive care nursery (ICN) population is around 10%. About 2–5% of the ICN babies will have a moderate to profound bilateral hearing loss requiring amplification and habilitation. (Dennis et al. 1984; Galambos, Hicks, and Wilson 1984; Sanders et al. 1985). Transient conductive hearing loss is much more widespread. Prevalence of middle-ear effusion in ICN population may be as high as 25–35%, especially in babies who are intubated longer than seven days (Stein, Ogdamar et al. 1983).

In 1982 the Joint Committee on Newborn Hearing made recommendations for the identification, diagnosis, and management of hearing loss in the young infant (1983). The following factors are included in the Committee's "High-Risk Register": family history of childhood hearing impairment, congenital perinatal infection (rubella, herpes, etc.), anatomic malformations of the head and neck, birth weight less than 1500 grams, bilirubin levels indicating the need for a transfusion, bacterial meningitis, and severe asphyxia (Gerkin 1984).

The earliest time for hearing screening, of course, is in the newborn nursery shortly after birth. At this time the babies are readily available for testing which permits screening before the babies scatter geographically. As Mahoney (1986) notes there is a general problem of how to efficiently, effectively, and economically screen all newborns at risk for hearing impairment at an early enough age to begin optimum habilitation. Such an undertaking cannot be carried out without some form of governmental coordination and support. As of January 1985 eight states (Connecticut, Texas, New Jersey, Massachusetts, Oklahoma, Georgia, California, and Florida) have a legislated mandate for neonatal screening, but it does not necessarily follow that adequate funding for implementation has also been provided. Only Utah, Colorado, Oklahoma, New Jersey, and Massachusetts in the United States, and British Columbia and Nova Scotia in Canada, have operational state-wide or province-wide high-risk hearing screening programs for newborns at this time. Active regional programs are found in Arkansas, Georgia, Florida, and Connecticut. It is evident that large scale neonatal hearing screening is just beginning. Since governmental bureaucracy moves slowly, each hospital and medical center should consider how it wishes to address the problem of early detection of hearing impairment.

PRINCIPLES OF SCREENING

Fria (1985) presents an excellent discussion of the principles of screening as they relate to newborn infants; only a brief consideration of this topic will be presented here. The goal of any screening test is to separate the impaired from the unimpaired. In auditory brainstem response (ABR) screening in the ICN, the purpose is to sort the babies into two groups: those who are continued to be viewed as at risk for a significant hearing loss and those for whom there is no longer major concern about hearing status. As a screening procedure, it is not the purpose of the ABR test to confirm that a hearing loss is present in a specific baby; this is the role of the follow-up testing.

For any screening test there are four possible outcomes; two desirable and two undesirable. On the positive side, a baby with a hearing loss can fail the test and a normal-hearing baby can pass the test. Conversely, on the negative side a hearing-impaired baby can pass the test and a normal-hearing baby can fail it. These outcomes are shown in figure 1. The probability that an impaired baby will fail the test (HIT) is called the test's sensitivity. The probability that a normal-hearing baby will pass the screening (CORRECT REJECTION) is called the test's specificity. The ideal screening tool would have perfect (100%) sen-

	HEARING LOSS	NORMAL
FAIL SCREEN	A 42	38 B
PASS SCREEN	3 C	317 D

Figure 1. Typical results of an ABR hearing screening program in the intensive care nursery.

sitivity and perfect specificity, but in practice this is seldom achieved with any screening procedure. The actual sensitivity and specificity of hearing screening can be determined by examining the relationships of the number of babies who fall in each of the four possible screening outcomes. Figure 1 gives an example of the results of ABR screening on 400 babies. Sensitivity is calculated by dividing the number of HITS (Box A) by the total number of babies who have a hearing impairment (Boxes A + C) and multiplying this value by 100. In this example in figure 1, the sensitivity is 93%. Specificity is calculated by dividing the number of normal-hearing babies who passed the ABR screening (Box D) and dividing this value by the total number of babies who have no hearing loss (Boxes B + D) and multiplying the result by 100. In the example, the specificity is 89%.

In conducting a screening program the tester has some control over the likelihood of the four different test outcomes and, in turn, the sensitivity and specificity of the screening. By making the screening criterion for passing the test more stringent (e.g., requiring a detectable response at 30 dB HL, rather than 40 dB HL) more babies will fail the test. This will increase the likelihood that a hearing-impaired baby will fail the screening, thus, sensitivity is raised. However, the more stringent screening criterion will also increase the likelihood that normal-hearing babies will fail the test, so specificity is reduced. It is also important to know that the number of overreferrals does not necessarily indicate that a screening test is inaccurate. Even if a screening test is performing effectively very high overreferral rates must be expected when the prevalence of an impairment is very low. It is beyond the scope of this chapter to discuss these principles of screening in detail. It is essential, however, that everyone involved in newborn hearing screening understands these principles and their practical implications. The reader is referred to Fria's (1985) thorough discussion of this topic.

Alternative Hearing Screening Procedures

Primary considerations in neonatal hearing screening are the effectiveness of the test procedure and the costs involved. It makes no sense to use an ineffective hearing screening technique just because it can be conducted cheaply. Likewise, a highly sensitive test procedure is of little value if it is too costly to implement. Anyone considering developing an ICN hearing screening program must evaluate critically the alternative available methods for testing the hearing of a neonate. A number of audiometric procedures have been used in ICN hearing screening. It is not the intent here to consider each technique fully, but rather to consider the strengths and weaknesses of ABR audiometry in relationship to alternative testing procedures. Certainly, no one should undertake an ABR screening program unless he or she is convinced that its advantages justify its added administration time and expense.

BEHAVIORAL OBSERVATION AUDIOMETRY (BOA)

As its name implies this technique relies on the detection of a behavioral response when a high intensity (e.g., 90 dBA) auditory stimulus is presented to the baby. Testing may be conducted using narrow-band stimuli centered at such frequencies as 500 Hz, 1000 Hz, and 2000 Hz. (Gerber and Dobkin 1984); or high pass filtered white noise, the "Nova Scotia spectrum," may be used (Gerber 1985). The high intensity stimulus is presented by a hand-held screener positioned approximately one inch from the baby's ear; the nature of the responses include cessation of activity, eye-widening, subtle changes in facial expression, crying, and gross startle responses. The determination of whether a response has occurred is highly subjective and is often difficult even for experienced clinicians. There is concern about the effectiveness of BOA screening. Using BOA, Plotnick and Leppler (1986) identified only two severely hearing-impaired babies among 356 newborns screened in the ICN. Assuming a very conservative 2% prevalence of significant sensorineural hearing loss in the ICN, at least three times as many hearing-impaired babies would be anticipated in the group tested. False negative rates of 40 to 86% have been reported for BOA (Alberti et al. 1983; Durieux-Smith and Jacobson 1985), which indicates that babies with a significant hearing loss are passing the behavioral screening and are thus lost to follow-up. Though there are still proponents of BOA for neonatal screening, it is no longer widely viewed as an effective screening procedure (Jacobson and Morehouse 1984).

CRIB-O-GRAM (COG)

This screening technique uses sensitive motion detectors positioned under the baby's crib mattress to detect changes to the test stimulus. A microprocessor determines when to present the high-intensity test stimulus (a 92 dB sound pressure level (SPL) band of noise centered at 3000 HZ) and measures changes in ongoing motor activity. The COG apparatus also indicates whether the baby has met the criteria for passing the hearing screening. Responses range from subtle changes in respiratory patterns to startle reflexes. The COG has a major advantage over many other test procedures because it is automated, thereby requiring little examiner time (McFarland, Simmons, and Jones 1980).

Because high stimulus intensities are needed to elicit a detectable behavioral response, COG, like BOA, may miss mild and moderate hearing losses. There is a major question about the sensitivity and specificity of the COG because the responses recorded from the newborns depend as much on their motor states as on their sensory abilities. Durieux-Smith et al. (1985) found that 32% of the babies tested with COG shifted from pass to fail, or vice versa, when they were retested within 48 hours.

Similar to COG, the Linco-Bennett Auditory Response Cradle (ARC) (Shepard 1983) uses an 85 dB SPL high pass noise stimulus and records cardiac and respiration changes, as well as such behavioral responses as startles and changes in bodily activity. ARC screening can be conducted in less time than with the COG, but possesses essentially the same advantages and limitations as are listed above for COG.

ACOUSTIC REFLEXES

Relatively little attention has been given to the use of acoustic reflex measures in the hearing screening of newborns. A primary reason for this is that only a small percentage of babies demonstrates a detectable contralateral reflex when a conventional 220 Hz probe tone is used (Himelfarb et al. 1978). Ipsilateral stimulation and a 660 Hz probe tone both appear to increase the number of babies who demonstrate a response. Even so, McMillan et al. (1985) were able to elicit reflexes in only 76% of the healthy full-term infants who were free of middle-ear problems. Sprague et al. (1985) were able to elicit a detectable acoustic reflex in 80% of full-term newborns with a 660 Hz probe tone and only 50% with a 220 Hz probe tone. The number of babies demonstrating a reflex should be even lower in the ICN where otitis media and neurological problems are much more common.

In acoustic reflex testing high intensity stimuli are used, and though the testing is brief and relatively simple to perform, reflex testing cannot be expected to identify mild or moderate hearing impairments even under the best testing conditions. Interpretation of reflex test results is also a problem. Further investigation in this area is certainly warranted, but it is unlikely that reflex measures will play a significant role in hearing screening in the ICN (Keith and Bench 1978).

AUDITORY BRAINSTEM RESPONSE (ABR)

The term Auditory Brainstem Response (ABR) is used in this discussion. In the pediatric and neonatology literature the term Brainstem Auditory Evoked Response (BAER) is more widely used. The two terms refer to the same response.

Schulman-Galambos and Galambos (1975) first reported the use of ABR Audiometry in the intensive-care nursery. Because it permits testing at low stimulus intensity levels, it is now generally considered to be the most sensitive test procedure and has been used by some as the standard by which the others are compared (Durieux-Smith and Jacobson 1985). Unlike the procedures discussed above, ABR audiometry utilizes a purely sensory response which is not altered by changes in arousal level.

The ABR does have two major limitations: 1) The raw acoustic click routinely used in neonatal screening contains frequencies predominately in the 2000 Hz–4000 Hz range, and hearing sensitivity for other frequencies is not evaluated. This will be discussed more fully later in this chapter. 2) The ABR reflects synchronous neural firing within the brainstem and is not a conscious response at the level of the cortex. It is important to remember that a normal ABR does not provide the same information about the auditory system as a normal behavioral response. Fortunately, for the vast majority of babies the ABR is a good estimator of overall hearing status, so when it is used with caution, reasonable statements about hearing can be made from ABR test results.

The real test of the value of an ABR screening program is its predictive validity, that is, its ability to detect hearing-impaired babies and separate them from the unimpaired. Such information has been scarce because it requires longitudinal data on babies tested in the ICN. Recently, Murray, Jarvel, and Watson (1985) examined the literature to determine how much we know about the predicitive validity of ABR ICN screening. Thirty-two studies (involving a total of 4,945 newborns) met the investigators criteria regarding follow-up. After examining the data from these studies, they concluded that, while there is adequate information on "HIT" and "FALSE ALARM" rates, data on "MISS" and "CORRECT REJECTION" rates are lacking. Therefore, it is not possible to determine accurately the predictive validity of ABR screening at this time. Murray et al. (1985), however, used signal detection theory to estimate the validity of ABR screening and concluded that ABR screening is "apparently neither very sensitive nor grossly insensitive." Considering the limitations of the alternative techniques, ABR audiometry is widely viewed as the best overall hearing screening procedure presently available (Cox 1984). As a result, the remainder of this chapter will be confined to a discussion of ABR screening in the ICN.

DEVELOPMENT OF AN ABR HEARING SCREENING PROGRAM

When an ABR hearing screening program is contemplated, certain questions must be asked during the planning phase. The resulting answers will determine if a screening program is feasible and, if so, what form it should take.

How will the costs of the ABR screening program be supported? Prior to the initiation of any ABR hearing screening program in the ICN it must be determined if the program has the necessary professional and administrative support. It is not difficult to get acknowledgement that early detection of hearing loss is important, but few hospitals will welcome the initiation of an ABR screening if it is likely to be a deficit operation. Most audiology programs in a medical setting are expected to be self-supporting or nearly so. Careful consideration should be given to the costs involved. Without some idea of how the costs of the screening program will be covered, it makes little sense to spend time dealing with the procedural aspects of ABR screening. Costs of the program include telephone and mail follow-up and the costs of retesting babies who fail the initial screening. Support for appropriate patient management, e.g., hearing aids, must also be considered.

The most logical source of financial support is through the fees charged to parents of babies who are tested. However, as a result of a nationwide prospective payment system (PPS) in 1983, billing for services within the ICN has changed dramatically in most hospitals in the United States. The PPS provides the hospital, prior to treatment, a set dollar amount based on the patient's diagnosis rather than retrospectively reimbursing for the actual services provided. Once the patient's diagnosis related group (DRG) has been determined, the hospital knows exactly how much it will receive for the treatment it provides (Shakno 1984). The system, devised originally for Medicare patients, has now been adopted by state and federal agencies which support certain babies in the ICN. A review of the babies who received ABR screening at Duke in 1985 showed that 36% were covered by a DRG system.

The PPS concept using DRGs was designed to motivate hospitals to limit patient services and thereby reduce costs. If costs are kept low, a hospital will make money on a DRG patient. Conversely, if expensive services are provided, the hospital will lose money because it will receive no additional money for these services. Therefore, hospitals now have an incentive to streamline services as much as possible. One way to accomplish this is through reduction in use of non-essential test procedures. As a result, the ICN medical staff is reluctant to order an expensive elective procedure such as ABR hearing screening. Because there is no way to bill for the costs of ABR screening for many babies in the ICN, it is clear that support for the hearing testing of these babies must to be obtained elsewhere.

At Duke the screening program has been fortunate in obtaining financial support from local Sertoma service clubs to cover the costs of testing those babies whose insurance will not pay ABR test fees. Other ICN screening programs have received support from the Lions Club (Ruth, Dey-Sigman, and Mills 1985). If there is sufficient support from the hospital administration and the medical staff, and the financial aspects of the screening seem manageable, then some more specific questions can be considered.

Which babies should be screened? The high-risk register developed by the Joint Committee on Newborn Hearing is often used as the basis for selecting the babies who should receive ABR hearing screening (Ruth, Dey-Sigman, and Mills 1985, and Gerkin 1984). However, not all specific risk factors are strong indicators of the likelihood of hearing loss (Cox, Hack, and Metz 1984). Duara et al. (1986) found that only low birth weight, immature gestational age, and extended stay in the hospital showed an independent correlation with permanent hearing loss by discriminant analysis. Babies who possess one or more of these risk factors are highly likely to spend at least part of their hospital stay in the ICN. In a retrospective study Pappas (1983) found that only 46% of children with a hearing loss would have been placed on the high-risk register. For these reasons we have chosen routinely to screen all the babies in the ICN rather than spending time reviewing medical records for risk factors. We believe that this approach is the most time-efficient way to screen babies who are at risk for hearing loss. Since only about 5% of newborns require placement in the ICN, restricting routine hearing screening to this ICN group markedly reduces the number of babies to be routinely tested.

It would be desirable to perform an ABR screening on all newborns, but practical considerations, such as time and cost, must be considered. Though we do not routinely screen full term nursery (FTN) babies, we do test them on request. Such selective screening of FTN babies is aimed at detecting the one or two non-ICN babies per 1000 who have a significant hearing impairment (Matkin 1984). If FTN babies are not routinely tested the staff of the full term nursery must be alerted to request ABR screening if they encounter a baby with a family history of hearing loss. This is the most frequently occurring risk factor for profound deafness in the general newborn population (Mahoney 1984) and should be readily picked up in the hospital intake interview. Defects of the head and neck also indicate the need for a hearing screening test.

Once the target group for routine hearing screening has been identified it is highly desirable to have a standing order for the testing of this group. As shown in figure 2, at Duke, ABR screening is one of the test procedures to be conducted prior to discharge on all ICN babies. With a standing order, professional time need not be spent contacting and talking to parents in order to obtain their approval. This is obviously desirable for practical reasons, but, equally as important, the standing order demonstrates that the nursery staff recognizes the value of the screening program. The standing order greatly facilitates the acceptance of the screening by new nursery personnel.

What ABR protocol should be used? The ABR test procedure is now widely used and has been well reported in the literature, so there is no need for a detailed discussion here. It is sufficient to say that two scalp electrodes are

DUKE UNIVERSITY MEDICAL CENTER

INTENSIVE CARE NURSERY
DISCHARGE CHECKLIST

Name

History #

D.O.B.

PROCEDURE		DATE ORDERED	DATE PERFORMED
Thyroid Screen	On Admission (1st. 48 hrs.)		
PKU	After 72 hr. Enteral Feeds		
Type and Screen	On Admission		
S.T.S.	On Admission		
Hgb Electrophoresis	On Admission for all Non-Caucasian Infants		
Head Circumference	On Admission		
Head Ultrasound	On day 5 for all Infants <1500 gms.		
Ophthamology Consult: Rule out Retinopathy of Prematurity	On day 28 for <1250 gms - all infants 1251-1500 gms-if O_2 re'cvd >1500 gms- 80% O_2 x 72 hr		
Brainstem Auditory Evoked Response	When Stable (Usually in unit 3)		
Infant Tracking			
FAMILY NOTIFIED OF PENDING TRANSFER/DISCHARGE			

DISCHARGING MD — SIGNATURE:

DISCHARGING RN — SIGNATURE:

Figure 2. ABR hearing screening as an integral part of the routine pre-discharge workup of every baby in the intensive care nursery.

attached to the baby's head (one off the fontanel close to the vertex or forehead and the other on the mastoid or earlobe). A ground electrode is placed on a convenient location such as the foot. Even though the tenderness of the neonate's skin does not permit hard scrubbing or the use of abrasive electrode gels, sufficiently low electrode impedance (below 10,000 ohms) can usually be obtained. Not infrequently, however, there are babies who demonstrate impedances greater than 20,000 ohms even though the skin was carefully prepared. Fortunately, it is often possible to carry out the ABR screening in spite of electrode impedances higher than desired (Eccard and Weber 1983).

The basic test protocol is the same as would be used in the testing of the hearing status of older children or adults. However, the scalp distribution of the neonates response is different from those of older children and adults. Contralateral recordings are not nearly as good as ipsilateral (Edwards, Durieux-Smith, and Pieton 1985), so there must be an electrode on the mastoid or earlobe of the stimulated ear. As mentioned above, an unfiltered click stimulus provides information only about hearing for frequencies between about 2000 Hz and 4000 Hz. This signal is chosen because its abrupt onset makes it most effective in producing a detectable response. Given the poor recording conditions in the ICN it is inadvisable to use more frequency specific stimuli (e.g., tone bursts) which are less effective in eliciting a response. There are preliminary reports that frequency specific information can be obtained from newborns using tone pip stimuli imbedded in band-reject noise (Hyde 1985). Further investigation is required to validate the frequency specificity of such stimuli and to determine if they significantly improve the information that can be obtained from a clinical hearing screening program.

Because the concern in ABR hearing screening is with the detection of a response, rather than obtaining maximum resolution of the component waves of the ABR, it is possible to reduce the low pass filter to 1500 Hz if excessive high frequency interference is a problem. It must be noted, however, that changing analog filter settings will influence the ABR latencies. The immature ABR from the neonate is quite cyclic in nature (figure 3). In the event that

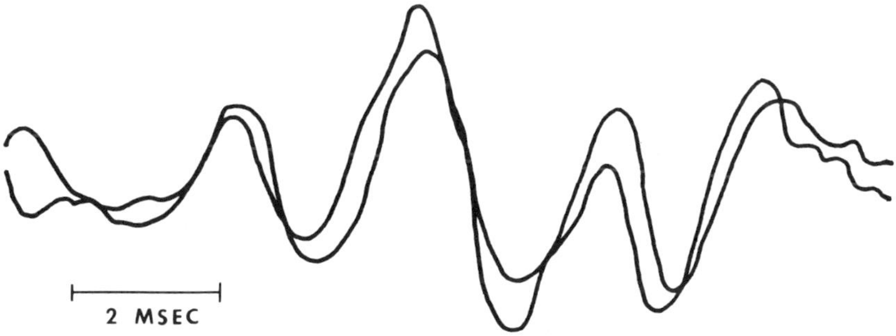

Figure 3. A typical ABR from a premature newborn in the intensive care nursery. Note the cyclic nature of the response which is similar to the artifact which can be produced by electrical interference.

electrical interference in the test environment matches the 300–400 Hz frequency of the ABR, chance time-locking of the signal averaging to this interference may produce a tracing which mimics an ABR. Controls (no stimulus runs) are important in all ABR testing and are essential in ICN screening. Increasing stimulus rate reduces testing time, but also reduces the quality of the resulting responses. A good compromise is a click rate of around 30–40/sec (keeping away from an even multiple of the ever present 60 Hz electrical interference and its harmonics). Cox (1984) recommends a somewhat slower rate of 21/sec.

What transducer should be used? The TDH-39 or TDH-49 earphones are frequently used for ABR testing. With the premature newborn, however, these two transducers are large and heavy and may create a collapsed ear canal (Hosford-Dunn et al. 1983). A small "walkman-style" earphone works well with the neonate. We have just begun using an insert earphone with good success. It is particularly valuable in maintaining a controlled level of stimulation to an active baby. Ruth, Dey-Sigman, and Mills (1985) also report good results with a similar insert sound delivery system. As will be discussed more fully below, a bone conduction oscillator is also useful in differentiating conductive from sensorineural hearing losses.

What should be the screening criterion? The screening criterion (the dividing line between passing and failing the test) will be dictated by the goal of the screening program. If the goal of the screening program is to detect unilateral, as well as bilateral hearing losses, it is obvious that both ears will need to be tested. However, if the purpose is to rule out a handicapping hearing loss which will significantly affect speech and language development, this can be accomplished by screening only the most accessible ear. It is obvious that a bilateral hearing impairment can be ruled out if the baby passes the hearing screening of one ear.

Because ABR screening is a costly and time-consuming procedure we have chosen to screen a single ear in our program at Duke. This does not imply that a unilateral hearing loss is without clinical significance. On the contrary it is well established that a unilateral hearing loss can create cognitive and academic problems in school-age children (Culbertson and Gilbert 1986). However, it was our decision that the additional expense of testing the second ear offsets the benefits. This decision was based on three factors: 1) A review of our retesting of ICN screening failures revealed a very small number of unilateral sensorineural hearing impairments. 2) Screening a single ear will, by chance, result in the testing of the affected ear in half of the babies with a unilateral hearing loss. 3) Even if a unilateral hearing loss is missed in the ABR hearing screening, the delay in its detection should not have a major impact on early speech and language development. Thus, we believe that this concession to practical considerations has not significantly reduced the clinical value of our ICN screening program.

It must be stressed again that the presence of an ABR at the screening intensity level only indicates that peripheral hearing is grossly intact for the high frequency portion of the speech range. Though it is reasonably safe to report that the baby has adequate peripheral hearing for speech and language development, it must be clear to all concerned that central auditory problems cannot be ruled out. Because it is not influenced by the auditory cortex, ABR audiometry cannot be viewed as the electrophysiologic equivalent of behavioral audiometry.

A screening criterion of 30 dB HL is recommended. This level is 30 dB above the behavioral threshold of normal listeners in a quiet (non-ICN) environment. As discussed earlier in this chapter, such a stringent screening criterion will increase the number of false positives and reduce the number of misses. Alberti et al. (1983) found that the failure rate at 30 dB is triple that at 40 dB. Because of the importance of early detection of a hearing loss it is preferable to reduce the likelihood of missing an impaired baby at the expense of more false positive results. However, there are times when the recording conditions do not permit the detection of an ABR at a 30 dB intensity level. Routinely, the testing conditions in the ICN are far from optimum. The auditory brainstem of the baby is immature and the test environment is electrically and acoustically noisy. The incubator, monitors, and infusion pumps generate 60 Hz interference (along with its high frequency harmonics) which can swamp and even mimic the small amplitude ABR. Acoustic noise in the ICN, if sufficiently high can also influence the ABR (Richmond, Konkle, and Potsik 1986). The absence of a response at 30 dB under these conditions would not be unexpected even from a baby with excellent hearing.

We find that we are encountering this problem more frequently than we did in the past. A major reason for this is the age and health status of the babies being screened. Because tertiary care ICNs may lose considerable money on each baby supported under a DRG system (described earlier in the chapter), the babies in the ICN tend to be transferred or discharged sooner than they were just a very few years ago. As a result, at Duke, for only about one baby in three is it possible to conduct ABR screening when the baby is near full term and in an open basinette. It is nursery policy to transfer the baby to a local hospital as soon as the baby is able to safely travel. Therefore, it is usually necessary to test babies when they are age 36–38 weeks, still in an incubator, and attached to monitors. These testing conditions are less than optimum and a response at 30 dB HL may not be detected.

If such conditions are encountered, retesting in the ICN at a later date is indicated. When this is impossible (e.g., if the baby is scheduled for immediate discharge) we have chosen to modify the screening criterion to pass a baby if he demonstrates a clear response at 45 dB and the most prominent ABR component wave has a latency that falls within normal limits on our clinic norms. The baby's Wave III and/or Wave V latencies are compared with norms for the appropriate conceptual age. Normal ABR latencies are used as an indication that the 45 dB stimulus was sufficiently above threshold so that grossly normal peripheral hearing can be inferred. It must be stressed that a response at 30 dB is the routine screening criterion and a response at 45 dB is accepted only when there are adverse recording conditions which cannot be corrected and when retesting is impossible. If reponse latency is used in this manner it is essential that the examiner have latency norms for different conceptual ages at 2 to 3 week intervals. Many sets of latency norms for premature infants have been reported in the literature (Weber 1982); however, each testing facility must establish its own set of norms using its specific equipment and testing protocol.

It can be argued that if a baby fails the screening test there is little reason to carry out testing at higher intensity levels, because the need for a retest has already been established. However, probing for approximate threshold is recommended for two reasons: 1) the baby may not return for retesting, so it is important to get as much information about hearing status as reasonably possible at the time of screening and 2) responsiveness at higher intensity levels provides information about the severity of the hearing loss and this information can be used to determine how to proceed in scheduling retesting. This topic will be discussed in some detail later in this chapter.

It must be decided whether the goal of the screening program is to identify all babies with a hearing loss (even a transient conductive hearing loss) or whether the target group consists of only those babies with a permanent sensorineural loss. If the purpose is the latter, some effort must be made to separate screening failures into two groups: babies with conductive problems and babies with permanent sensorineural hearing loss. Hooks and Weber (1984) have demonstrated the feasibility of recording ABRs from neonates using bone conducted (BC) click stimuli. We attempt to record BC responses from every baby who fails the air conduction screening. A comparison of air conduction and bone conduction responses helps differentiate babies with conductive (and often transient) hearing impairments from permanent sensorineural hearing losses. Though an ABR to a 30 dB bone conduction signal may actually be due to a normal cochlea in the non-test ear, the response does provide evidence of an intact sensorineural mechanism in at least one ear. This information is of value in determining appropriate management and follow-up. For example, if an external or middle ear problem is confirmed by a physician, an attempt will be made to retest the baby in the hospital after treatment. If AC and BC ABRs are in agreement, consistent with a sensorineural hearing loss, no retesting will be performed prior to discharge from the ICN. It must be cautioned that because of the larger mass of a bone conduction oscillator, the BC click has its maximum energy in lower frequencies than an AC click (Hooks and Weber 1984; Schwartz, Larson, and De Chicchis 1985). As a result, a baby with a markedly sloping high frequency sensorineural loss may demonstrate a better ABR to the BC click because of better low frequency hearing and would mistakenly be suspected as having a conductive hearing loss. To minimize the likelihood of this error, an otoscopic examination by an ICN physician is performed on every baby who shows better ABRs to bone conduction stimuli. If there is no evidence of a conductive hearing impairment, it is assumed that the baby has a significant sensorineural hearing loss.

Further limitations of bone conducted ABR testing are: 1) the maximum output is considerably less than for an earphone (Schwartz, Larson, and De Chicchis 1985) and 2) response latencies are markedly affected by oscillator placement (Yang, Rupert, and Moushegian 1986). It is of interest to note that Hooks and Weber (1984) found that normal-hearing newborns were somewhat more responsive to BC clicks than AC clicks. This may well be because the cochlear response mechanism is more mature for low frequencies than high frequencies (Wolf and Goldstein 1980).

When should the screening be performed? ABR screening should be carried out as close to discharge or transfer as possible. This will permit testing when the babies are as mature and healthy as possible. In our experience it is best for ABR screening to be conducted on a regular basis in order to keep up with the flow of babies through the ICN. However, there must be considerable flexibility because discharge plans often change with little forewarning and the ICN census fluctuates markedly. In our screening program we devote two half-days to regular testing and during these times we choose the babies to be tested based on their expected discharge date, other procedures scheduled, and whether they are sleeping quietly. Ideally we try to test all babies shortly after feeding when they are likely to be entering an extended period of sleep. As needed, an attempt will be made to perform screening at other times of the week if a baby is due for an unexpectedly early discharge.

Who should do the testing? Though ABR test equipment is expensive, the major expense involved in a neonatal screening program is the personnel needed to perform the testing, interpret the findings, and perform the necessary follow-up. One solution to high personnel costs is to use volunteers. Gerkin and Weyland (1985) report good success with the Infant Hearing Assessment Foundation (IHAF) which utilizes volunteers to perform testing with a semi-automated ABR screening device (the Synap I). The authors report no problems with volunteers betraying patient confidentiality or misleading parents or with objections from hospital personnel. Similar satisfactory use of IHAF volunteers has been reported by Duara et al. (1986). Gerkin and Weyland (1985), however, did encounter volunteers who were not comfortable with the test equipment or handling young babies, and volunteers who received time-consuming training and shortly thereafter ceased to participate in the program. Anyone who has relied on volunteer support is well aware that there is usually a core of dedicated individuals who are very reliable and who perform their tasks with a high level of skill and efficiency. Unfortunately, it is the rare volunteer program that does not spend time training individuals who are less reliable and committed. Success in the use of volunteers is influenced by many factors and it is impossible to make a general sweeping statement on the wisdom of using volunteers. It must be kept in mind, however, that a professional must be intimately involved in the screening program to interpret the test results, insure adequate volunteer training, serve as a liaison to the nursery, and monitor all aspects of the program. At Duke we have decided that our relatively small program (about 250 babies screened a year) can best be conducted without volunteer support.

The commonly used alternative to the use of volunteers is for an audiologist to conduct the testing and follow-up. Though this is a costly alternative, many believe that the level of expertise required to handle the babies properly, interact with the nursery staff, conduct the ABR screening and interpret the results cannot be entrusted to volunteers. There is little question that an audiologist is better able to respond appropriately to questions and interpret the test results for parents and the hospital staff. Hearing screening is also likely to be accepted more enthusiastically by the doctors and nurses in the ICN when they deal with a small number of professionals, rather than a larger and ever changing group of volunteers.

A much less frequently used alternative to the use of volunteers or audiologists is to employ a trained technician. In a hospital setting technicians perform a wide range of procedures such as X-ray, EEG, and EMG under the direction of a physician. Audiology has seldom followed this medical model. However, in ABR screening a technician, under the direction of an audiologist, may provide a reasonable alternative which falls between the uncertainty and uneveness of volunteer support and the very expensive use of an audiologist.

One way to get around the problem of who should administer the ABR screening is to have it conducted by the testing apparatus itself. A new automated ABR neonatal hearing screener has been introduced recently that requires no sophistication on the part of the examiner. The Algo-1 is a battery-operated ABR screener that weighs seven pounds and is about the size of a portable typewriter. After the recording electrodes are attached to the baby's scalp the screener will automatically begin presenting click stimuli at 35 dB HL if there is sufficiently low electrode impedance, and when ambient noise level and movement artifacts are within acceptable limits. The clicks are presented at a rate of 37/sec through a unique disposable circumaural earphone that has an adhesive surface for holding it firmly in place. Whenever the recording conditions are unsatisfactory, the click stimuli will be automatically interrupted until noise level and/or movement artifacts are reduced. The ALGO-1 compares the accumulated response in memory with a nine-point template of a neonatal ABR. When the likelihood of a response reaches a predetermined criterion level the test stimuli automatically cease and a display panel indicates that the baby has passed the hearing screening test. If the likelihood of response is not sufficiently high at the end of 15,000 sweeps, testing is halted and the display panel indicates that the baby should be referred for additional testing.

A primary advantage of the automated ABR screener is that it does not require an audiologist for administration and interpretation. Thus, cost per test should be less than for conventional ABR screening. However, it is likely that the busy ICN nurse will be expected to assume the additional responsibility of hearing screening and this may be met with some resistance.

The Algo-1 is fully automated and is very conservative. It will not begin a test run if ambient noise, electrical interference, or movement artifact exceed predetermined levels. When babies are restless or are on monitors in incubators the automated screener may not accept the recording conditions, even though conventional ABR screening may be successfully conducted under the same conditions. This automated ABR screener, therefore, is not without its limitations. On the positive side, it certainly has the automated characteristics of the Crib-O-Gram procedure without relying on high intensity stimulation or a motor response. At present there is little information on the clinical performance of the Algo-1. There is an encouraging report from its developers (Thornton, Sprague-Hermann, and Berrick 1985) and field testing is underway in several hospitals. Determination of its place in ICN screening programs must await the results of controlled testing by independent investigators.

Implementing The Screening Program

If the above questions have been adequately addressed and the decision is to proceed with an ABR hearing screening program, then the next step is to purchase equipment, if needed, and carry out inservice training for ICN nurses, neonatologists, and residents. One cannot plunge immediately into the screening of at-risk babies, so it is wise initially to conduct some testing in the full-term nursery. This will provide experience with newborns and will indicate the lowest intensity level that will elicit a detectable ABR under good recording conditions. However, it is one thing to test a term baby in an open bassinet and something else to enter the ICN and test a premature baby who is in an incubator and is attached to artifact-producing monitors and infusion pumps. Experience obtained in the full term nursery is very important, but cannot replace the need for several weeks of experience in the ICN before actual screening begins. During this "shakedown" period the suitability of the selected screening criterion can be evaluated. When the clinical phase of the screening program is initiated it is recommended that ABR latency data be gathered to start the development of latency norms for different conceptual ages. As these norms develop they will begin to be of value in determining if ABR latencies of individual babies are abnormally extended (Weber 1982).

The failure rate of most ICN ABR screening programs ranges from 11 to 19%. Of those babies who fail the screening, reports of false positive rates range from 0 to 96%, with most reports clustered around 30 to 50% (Fria 1985). If a baby passes the repeat hearing screening after failing the ABR screening in the ICN it is likely due to such factors as a self-resolved middle ear problem, increased maturation, improved neurological, and general health status, and better testing environment in the retesting site.

Because failure of the ABR hearing screening test does not confirm that a baby has a hearing loss, it is important that the failure is interpreted clearly in the baby's medical record and that this information is appropriately conveyed to the parent(s). Stein and Jabaley (1981) provide an excellent discussion of this very important topic. It is important that the parent(s) be told that a significant hearing loss cannot be ruled out by the screening test and that further testing is needed under more favorable test conditions. At that time it will be possible to determine if the baby's lack of responsiveness is due to a hearing loss or to other causes. It should be obvious that parents should never be told that their child has a hearing loss based on the failure on the ABR screening test in the ICN.

Because ICN ABR screening has a 30–50% false positive rate, some have argued against attempting to identify hearing-impaired infants while they are in the nursery (Downs 1982). Instead it is recommended that hearing screening be deferred until the babies can return as outpatients at a later date (such as four months of age). This has several advantages: increased likelihood of picking up adventitious or progressive hearing loss, less confounding factors such as illness and immaturity, avoidance of additional testing during a critical parent-child bonding period, and relative ease in scheduling the testing on an outpatient basis (Alberti et al. 1985). Though there are clearly arguments in favor of postponing initial hearing screening until after the infant has been discharged from the nursery, this writer still strongly supports screening in the ICN. High risk babies often come from unstable home environments. This greatly complicates follow-up of babies who fail the ICN screening test and underscores the importance of performing as much testing as possible prior to discharge. The difficulties experienced in getting ABR retests on the relatively few babies who fail the ICN screening has convinced us of the wisdom of testing babies prior to discharge. At least with our patient population, far too many babies would never receive an early hearing screening if it was conducted strictly on an outpatient basis.

RETESTING

The conventional approach to retesting of screening failures is to attempt to bring back each of these babies after a specified period of time. This approach assumes that all ICN failures have the same likelihood of a significant premanent hearing impairment. An alternative approach, which we utilize at Duke, is to divide the ICN failures into two groups: 1) those who demonstrate a normal ABR at 45 dB and who are suspected of having no more than a mild, possibly temporary, hearing loss; and 2) those who do not have a normal response at 45 dB and who are suspected of having a substantial hearing loss. For the latter group, we contact the parents(s) to arrange to bring the baby back at four or five months of age when he will have stabilized and matured and have a good chance of showing behavioral responses. There is sufficient reason for concern about the baby's hearing so that an all-out effort is made to make contact with the baby's caregiver to insure that follow-up testing is performed. In contrast, for the group of babies who failed the screening test, yet gave responses at 45 dB in the ABR screening, the family is contacted when the baby is three to four months conceptual age. This contact is initially by letter, with a follow-up by phone if at all possible. The letter contact provides the family with expected response behaviors and milestones for normal-hearing infants. The subsequent telephone contact is made to determine the parent's perception of the baby's responsiveness to sound. A repeat hearing test is always offered to the parent. However, if the parent has no concerns about hearing status and provides information which indicates that the baby is responding normally to sound, no retest is scheduled and the baby's name is removed from the list of infants being followed. Even if the family has no concerns about the baby's hearing status and is not interested in coming to the medical center for a follow-up hearing test, the family is always given information about how they can call to arrange for a hearing retest at any time if in the future they have concerns about the child's hearing. Such an approach to follow-up hearing testing is considered to be a reasonable compromise between the ideal and what is practical. It must be remembered that returning a baby for follow-up testing may cause the parents mental anguish and certainly it causes them to make time and financial commitments. In contrast with programs that routinely schedule follow-up hearing tests for all babies who fail the screening, this approach minimizes "no shows" in instances where the parents were never convinced that repeat hearing testing was necessary. It also reduces time spent retesting normal-hearing babies who had transient problems in the ICN. Our experience has been that parents who are in daily contact with a baby are good judges of whether their child has a significant hearing impairment at four or five months of age.

It can be argued that waiting until a hearing-impaired infant is four or five months of age before performing repeat hearing testing is needlessly delaying the habilitation process. However, in our center we require behavioral audiometric findings that are also compatible with a hearing loss before beginning management (such as the fitting of a hearing aid). A repeat ABR test shortly after discharge would be of value if the baby demonstrated normal hearing. However, if the baby again shows ABR results suggestive of a hearing loss, behavioral testing will still be needed. Since confidence in behavioral audiometry for very young infants is quite low, we have chosen to delay retesting of babies who fail the ICN screening until the babies reach the age of four or five months when a repeat ABR test and behavioral audiometry can be conducted on the same visit. Delaying follow-up testing until four or five months of age still permits appropriate habilitative procedures in time to maximize normal speech and language development and is within the six months age recommended by the Joint Committee on Infant Hearing (1983). It is also a marked improvement over the findings of Horton and Hanners (1977) who reported that only 11% of hearing-impaired infants receive some habilitation by six months of age. It is also markedly better than the Stein, Clark, and Kraus (1983) report of a median age of 18 months for hearing-impaired infants first enrolled in therapy.

Neurological Problems

By the very nature of the newborns who are transferred to the ICN, a high percentage have some form of temporary or permanent neurological problem.

When these disorders affect the brainstem they may alter the ABR and complicate interpretation of the test results. Thus, an abnormal or absent ABR may indicate a peripheral hearing loss or it may be the result of neural dyschrony as a result of a neurological problem in the brainstem. Often these two problems cannot be separated and incorrect interpretations may result (Stockard, Stockard, and Coen 1983). When the examiner suspects that a neurological problem is present, such as the presence of ABR Wave I and the absence of later waves, he or she should interpret the test results as they relate to a hearing impairment and should report the abnormal responses with the recommendation for further testing to clarify the nature of the problem. The view of the traditional audiologist's role relative to neurological disorders is: a) to be aware that they may contaminate the hearing test results, and b) to report possible indications of neurological dysfunction so that professionals trained in this area may take appropriate action.

In contrast, it can be argued that the value of ABR screening in the ICN population goes well beyond ruling out a significant hearing impairment. Because of the expense involved, it is not likely that many of the ICN babies will also recieve ABR testing to evaluate brainstem status. Rather than being a factor that contaminates hearing testing, some view the evaluation of auditory brainstem status as another aspect of the screening program. Kileny and Robertson (1985) used the ABR to screen asphyxiated newborns and concluded that its value was two-fold: it evaluated auditory sensitivity and was also sensitive to the sequelae of hypoxic encephalopathy. Though such dual screening clearly increases the value of the screening program, making decisions relative to brainstem status in a premature infant does not fall within the expertise of most audiologists. Such an expanded ABR screening program must not be undertaken unless the audiologist has considerable experience in this area and has a close working arrangement with the neonatologists and pediatric neurologists. However, if the examiner in a hearing screening program elects not to make statements about the baby's neurological status, he must have a good understanding of both audiological and neurological determinants of response abnormalities (Hecox 1985). Both peripheral and central factors influence the ABR and it is not possible to screen adequately for one without adequately understanding the other.

References

Alberti, P. W., Hyde, M. L., Riko, K., Corbin, H., and Abramovich, S. 1983. An Evaluation of BERA for hearing screening in high-risk neonates. *Laryngoscope* 93:1115–1121.

Alberti, P. W., Hyde, M. L., Riko, K., Corbin, H., and Fitzhardinge, P. M. 1985. Issues in early identification of hearing loss. *Laryngoscope* 95:373–381.

Cox, L. C. 1984. The current status of auditory brainstem response testing in neonatal populations. *Pediatric Research* 18:780–783.

Cox, L. C., Hack, M., and Metz, D. A. 1984. Auditory brainstem response abnormalities in the very low birthweight infant: Incidence and risk factors. *Ear and Hearing* 5:47–51.

Culbertson, J. L., and Gilbert, L. E. 1986. Children with unilateral sensorineural hearing loss: Cognitive, academic, and social development. *Ear and Hearing* 7:38–42.
Dennis, J. M., Sheldon, R., Toubas, P., and McCaffee, M. A. 1984. Identification of hearing loss in the neonatal intensive care unit population. *The American Journal of Otology* 5:201–205.
Downs, D. W. 1982. Auditory brainstem response testing in the intensive care unit: A cautious approach. *ASHA* 24:1009–10015.
Duara, S., Suter, C. M., Bessard, K. K., and Gutberlet, R. L. 1986. Neonatal screening with auditory brainstem responses: Results of follow-up audiometry and risk evaluation. *The Journal of Pediatrics* 108:276–281.
Durieux-Smith, A., and Jacobson, J. T. 1985. Comparison of auditory brainstem response and behavioral screening in neonates. *The Journal of Otolaryngology* 14:47–52.
Durieux-Smith, A., Picton, T., Edwards, C., Goodman, J. T., and MacMurray, B. 1985. The Crib-O-Gram in the NICU: An evaluation based on brain stem electric response audiometry. *Ear and Hearing,* 6:20–24.
Eccard, K. D., and Weber, B. A. 1983. Influence of electrode impedance on auditory brain stem response recordings in the intensive care nursery. *Ear and Hearing* 4:104–105.
Edwards, C. G., Durieux-Smith, A., and Picton, T. W. 1985. Neonatal auditory brain stem responses from ipsilateral and contralateral recording montages. *Ear and Hearing* 6:175–178.
Fria, T. J. 1985. Identification of congenital hearing loss with the auditory brainstem response. *In* J. T. Jacobson (ed.). *The Auditory Brainstem Response* (pp. 317–334). San Diego, CA: College-Hill Press.
Galambos, R., Hicks, G. E., and Wilson, M. J. 1984. The auditory brain stem response reliably predicts hearing loss in graduates of a tertiary intensive care nursery. *Ear and Hearing* 5:254–260.
Gerber, S. E., and Dobkin, M. S. 1984. The effect of noise bandwidth on the auditory arousal response of neonates. *Ear and Hearing* 5:195–198.
Gerber, S. E. 1985. Stimulus, response, and state variables in the testing of neonates. *Ear and Hearing* 6:15–19.
Gerkin, K. P. 1984. The high risk register for deafness. *ASHA* 26:17–23.
Gerkin, K. P., and Weyland, C. 1985. Infant hearing assessment foundation programs. *Hearing Instruments* 36:22–24.
Hecox, K. 1985. Neurologic applications of the auditory brainstem response to the pediatric age group. *In* J. T. Jacobson (ed.). *The Auditory Brainstem Response* (pp. 287–296). San Diego: College-Hill Press.
Himelfarb, M. Z., Shanon, E., Popelka, G. R., and Margolis, R. H. 1978. Acoustic reflex evaluation in neonates. *In* S. E. Gerber and G. T. Mencher (eds.). *Early Detection of Hearing Loss* (pp. 109–127). New York: Grune & Stratton.
Hooks, R. G., and Weber, B. A. 1984. Auditory brain stem responses of premature infants to bone-conducted stimuli: A feasibility study. *Ear and Hearing* 5:42–45.
Horton, K. B., and Hanners, B. A. 1977. Trends in educational programming: The early years of the hearing-impaired child, zero to three. *In* F. H. Bess (ed.). *Childhood Deafness* (pp. 313–320). New York: Grune and Stratton.
Hosford-Dunn, H., Runge, C. A., Hillel, A., and Johnson, S. J. 1983. Auditory brain stem response testing in infants with collapsed ear canals. *Ear and Hearing* 4:258–260.
Hyde, M. L. 1985. Frequency-specific BERA in infants. *The Journal of Otolaryngology* 14:19–27.
Illingworth, R. S. 1980. *The Development of the Infant and Young Child: Normal and Abnormal.* London: Churchill Livingston.
Jacobson, J. T., and Morehouse, C. R. 1984. A comparison of auditory brain stem response and behavioral screening in high risk and normal newborn infants. *Ear and Hearing* 5:247–253.
Joint Committee on Infant Hearing Screening Position Statement (1982). 1983. *Ear and Hearing* 4:3–4.
Keith, R. W., and Bench, R. J. 1978. Stapedial reflex in neonates. *Scandinavian Audiology* 7:187–191.
Kileny, P., and Robertson, C. M. T. 1985. Neurological aspects of infant hearing assessment. *The Journal of Otolaryngology* 14:34–39.
McFarland, W. H., Simmons, F. B., and Jones, F. R. 1980. An automated hearing screening technique for newborns. *Journal of Speech and Hearing Disorders* 45:495–503.
McMillan, P., Bennett, M. J., Marchant, C. D., and Shurin, P. A. 1985. Ipsilateral and contralateral acoustic reflexes in neonates. *Ear and Hearing* 6:320–324.

Mahoney, T. 1984. High-risk hearing screening of large general newborn populations. *Seminars in Hearing* 5:25–36.

Mahoney, T. M. 1986. Large-scale high-risk neonatal hearing screening. *In* E. T. Swigart (ed.). *Neonatal Hearing Screening* (pp. 123–141). San Diego: College-Hill Press.

Matkin, N. D. 1984. Early recognition and referral of hearing impaired children. *Pediatrics in Review* 6:151–156.

Menyuk, P. 1977. Effects of hearing loss on language acquisition in the babbling stage. *In* B. F. Jaffee (ed.). *Hearing Loss in Children* (pp. 621–629). Baltimore: University Park Press.

Moore, D. R. 1985. Postnatal development of the mammalian central auditory system and the neural consequences of auditory deprivation. *Acta Otolaryngologica Supplement 421*:19–30.

Murray, A. D., Javel, E., and Watson, C. S. 1985. Prognostic validity of auditory brainstem evoked response screening in newborn infants. *American Journal of Otolaryngology* 6:120–131.

Pappas, D. G. 1983. A study of the high-risk registry for sensorineural hearing impairment. *Otolaryngology—Head and Neck Surgery* 91:41–44.

Plotnick, C. H., and Leppler, J. G. 1986. Infant hearing assessment: A program for identification and habilitation within four months of age. *The Hearing Journal* 39:23–25.

Quigley, S. P. 1978. The effects of early hearing loss on normal language development. *In* F. N. Martin (ed.). *Pediatric Audiology* (pp. 35–63). Englewood Cliffs, NJ: Prentice-Hall.

Ruth, R. A., Dey-Sigman, S., and Mills, J. A. 1985. Neonatal ABR hearing screening. *The Hearing Journal* 38:39–45.

Richmond, K. H., Konkle, D. F., and Potsic, W. P. 1986. ABR screening of high-risk infants: Effects of ambient noise in the neonatal nursery. *Otolaryngology—Head and Neck Surgery* 94:552–560.

Sanders, R. A., Durieux-Smith, A., Hyde, M., Jacobson, J., Kileny, P., and Murnane, O. 1985. Incidence of hearing loss in high risk and intensive care nursery infants. *The Journal of Otolaryngology* 14:28–33.

Schulman-Galambos, C., and Galambos, R. 1975. Brain stem auditory-evoked responses in premature infants. *Journal of Speech and Hearing Research* 18:456–465.

Schwartz, D. M., Larson, V. D., and De Chicchis, A. R. 1985. Spectral characteristics of air and bone conduction transducers used to record the auditory brain stem response. *Ear and Hearing* 6:274–277.

Shakno, R. J. 1984. *Physician's Guide to DRGs*. Chicago: Pluribus Press.

Shepard, N. T. 1983. Newborn hearing screening using the Linco-Bennett Auditory Response Cradle: A pilot study. *Ear and Hearing* 4:5–10.

Sprague, B. H., Wiley, T. L., and Goldstein, R. 1985. Tympanometric and acoustic-reflex studies in neonates. *Journal of Speech and Hearing Research* 28:265–272.

Stein, L., Clark, S., and Kraus, N. 1983. The hearing-impaired infant: Patterns of identification and habilitation. *Ear and Hearing* 4:232–236.

Stein, L., Ozdamar, O., Kraus, N., and Paton, J. 1983. Follow-up of infants screened by auditory brainstem response in the neonatal intensive care unit. *The Journal of Pediatrics* 103:447–453.

Stein, L., and Jabaley, T. 1981. Early identification and parent counseling. *In* L. Stein, E. Mindel, and J. Jabaley (eds.). *Deafness and Mental Health,* (pp. 23–35). New York: Grune and Stratton.

Stockard, J. E., Stockard, J. J., and Coen, R. W. 1983. Auditory brain stem response variability in infants. *Ear and Hearing* 4:11–23.

Thornton, A. R., Sprague-Hermann, B., and Berrick, J. M. 1985. Automated neonatal hearing screening using the auditory brainstem response. *IX Biennial International Symposium of the International Electric Response Audiometry Study Group,* 25.

Weber, B. A. 1982. Comparison of auditory brain stem response latency norms for premature infants. *Ear and Hearing* 3:257–262.

Wolf, K. E., and Goldstein, R. 1980. Middle component AERs from neonates to low-level tonal stimuli. *Journal of Speech and Hearing Research* 23:185–201.

Yang, E. Y., Rupert, A. L., and Moushegian, G. 1986. Bone conduction auditory brainstem responses in human neonates and adults. *Abstracts of the Ninth Midwinter Research Meeting of the Association for Research in Otolaryngology,* 99–100.

Chapter 10

Behavioral Evaluation of Hearing-Impaired Children

Allan O. Diefendorf

Introduction

Over the past decade there has been an increasing emphasis on the potential effects of unilateral hearing losses, mild hearing losses, and high frequency hearing losses on the development of communication and academic skills. Thus, a growing significance has come to bear on the early identification of hearing loss among the childhood population.

Sensorineural hearing losses ranging from moderately severe to profound are no longer the primary target in pediatric assessment. In addition to screening for the generalized presence or absence of hearing loss, a comprehensive pediatric evaluation must include the accurate assessment of young children with varying degrees, different types, and different configurations of hearing loss.

Improved assessment procedures for infants and young children have meant greater precision in quantifying hearing losses at an early age. In order to help the reader develop more accurate and precise skills for measuring and interpreting young children's auditory behavior, this chapter examines the available assessment procedures.

Obviously, a reliable determination of a child's hearing sensitivity is only the first step in a comprehensive pediatric evaluation. Once the hearing loss has been described in terms of degree, type, and configuration, the focus should shift from the loss of sensitivity to the child's usable residual hearing.

Two General Approaches to Assessment

Behavioral assessment of auditory function is based on the observation of overt responses to controlled auditory signals. The two general approaches that have been employed clinically depend upon whether or not reinforcement is used.

Historical precedent has favored the approach without reinforcement. Here, although the response is active, the infant is viewed as being passively involved with his environment. A typical example would be the introduction of an acoustic stimulus into an adequate sound room where the infant is in a light sleep, or at least quiet, and the observation of behavioral changes (responses) that occur within a specified time following stimulus onset. The probability of a response is dependent on the state of the infant, the nature of the auditory stimulus, the definition of response, and background ambient noise levels. In the nonreinforced paradigm the stimulus elicits the response, which is then prone to habituation.

The second approach demonstrates that the behavioral assessment of infants can be accomplished through an operant conditioning paradigm. Applying the operant paradigm does not mean merely presenting an auditory stimulus, observing a response, and reinforcing that response. The stimulus does not "elicit" the response.

In the operant conditioning paradigm, the auditory stimulus is introduced as a contingency to indicate the time interval during which an appropriate response will have a consequence—that is, reinforcement. Subsequently, the response is strengthened by reinforcement. This approach recognizes a view of infants as active receptors of auditory information who, if given the chance, will interact with their auditory environment.

While assessment procedures without reinforcement can be implemented at birth (see figure 1), procedures using reinforcement cannot be implemented until the infant reaches approximately six months. The age factor highlights developmental differences; specifically, when normal developing children can consistently demonstrate a specifically defined motor response.

SENSITIVITY AND SPECIFICITY

The validity of any assessment procedure depends on its sensitivity, specificity, false positive rate, and false negative rate (see figure 2). The sensitivity of

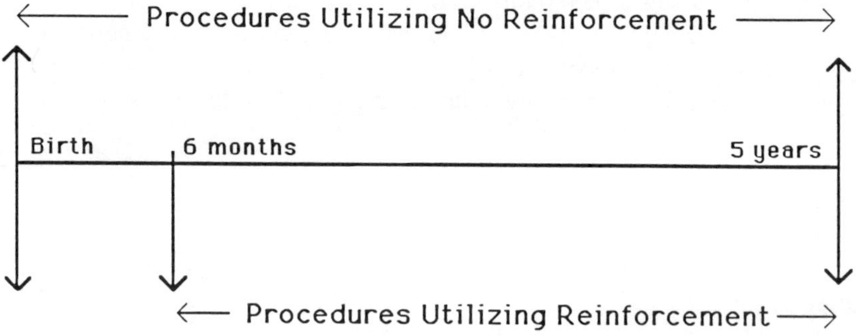

Figure 1. Schematic of the two behavioral approaches along an age continuum

POPULATION

	WITH HEARING LOSS	WITHOUT HEARING LOSS
POSITIVE TEST RESULTS	HAVE HEARING LOSS HAVE POSITIVE TEST = TRUE POSITIVES (TP)	NO HEARING LOSS HAVE POSITIVE RESULTS = FALSE POSITIVES (FP)
NEGATIVE TEST RESULTS	HAVE HEARING LOSS HAVE NEGATIVE TEST = FALSE NEGATIVES (FN)	NO HEARING LOSS HAVE NEGATIVE TEST = TRUE NEGATIVES (TN)

SENSITIVITY (in %)

$$\frac{TP}{TP + FN} \times 100$$

SPECIFICITY (in %)

$$\frac{TN}{TN + FP} \times 100$$

Figure 2. Evaluating the accuracy of an assessment procedure: sensitivity and specificity

a test is its accuracy in correctly identifying disordered individuals. Specificity establishes the test's accuracy in correctly identifying nondisordered individuals. It would be ideal if an assessment procedure was 100% accurate in its sensitivity and specificity; however, there is always an expected number of false-positive and false-negative identifications. All four of these conditions must be considered when evaluating the accuracy of an assessment procedure. The sensitivity of different assessment techniques used with young children should be an ongoing concern. Moreover, until a better understanding of auditory behavior and measurement in auditory assessment is found, the whole concept of assessment should be viewed as an ongoing process. Once a test's sensitivity and specificity are established, a more accurate interpretation of abnormal auditory behavior is possible.

Procedures Utilizing No Reinforcement

Although the primary focus of this chapter is behavioral assessment, the screening process must be considered as a prerequisite to assessment. Hence, screening techniques using behavioral responses will be considered briefly: neonatal screening and the high-risk alternative, and screening older children with Behavioral Observation Audiometry.

NEONATAL SCREENING

The desirability of early detection of hearing loss in infants has led to experimentation with several behavioral techniques in the newborn nursery: the Crib-O-Gram (Simmons and Russ 1974), the Auditory Response Cradle (Bennett 1975), and Behavioral Observation Audiometry (BOA) (Downs and Sterritt 1967). These techniques share certain similarities. Each introduces a high intensity, wide-band stimulus into a room where the infant is quiet or in a light sleep, and each involves monitoring or observing various overt responses from the infant.

Caution should guide interpretations drawn from these techniques—and from any behavioral assessments of hearing loss based on procedures without reinforcement. That is, judgments should not be elevated to a level of precision beyond that defined by the resolving power of our instrument. For example, the signal levels used in these approaches with newborns would, at best, identify only those infants with moderately-severe to profound hearing losses. Furthermore, intensive care nursery (ICN) babies may show further decreased responsiveness to external stimuli due to poor health and general weakness. Thus, there may be difficulty in coordinating a response in the ICN, where motor responses may be restricted.

Durieux-Smith et al. (1985) evaluated the Crib-O-Gram as a screening test for hearing loss in the ICN using the Auditory Brainstem Response (ABR) as the standard. With regard to false postives and false negatives, the results of this study indicated that approximately one-third of infants with ABR response levels of 30 dB nHL failed the Crib-O-Gram screening, while some of the infants with hearing losses that required medical or audiological management were not identified by the Crib-O-Gram. Sensitivity reached 100 percent when an ABR pass criterion of 50 dB HL was used. Furthermore, because of the high rate of failures, Durieux-Smith et al. suggested that the reliability of the Crib-O-Gram is better for infants of 38 weeks and older.

Feinmesser and Tell (1976) utilized Behavioral Observation Audiometry (BOA) in a neonatal hearing screening program and concluded that the procedure of observing motor responses of awake infants was not sensitive enough to detect deafness in neonates. That is, the high number of false positives and false negatives indicated that the procedures was inefficient and invalid.

If BOA is elected as a screening procedure for moderately severe to profound hearing loss, the research of Gerber (1985) should be considered. Specifically, Gerber suggests utilizing a fixed observational interval (2½ seconds) during which time only a specific behavior (eye movement and the movement of at least one limb) is an accepted response. The specific behavior must be observed by two independent observers or by one masked observer. The paradigm advocated by Gerber is referred to as the Arousal Response.

THE HIGH-RISK ALTERNATIVE

Concern about the efficiency of neonatal hearing screening programs using the BOA procedure (Ling et al. 1970) led to the formation of the Joint Committee on Infant Hearing Screening. In 1972, the committee recommended that infants at risk for hearing impairment be identified by means of five criteria, and suggested follow-up audiologic evaluation of these infants until accurate assessments of hearing could be made. Because acoustic testing of all newborn infants utilizing BOA can have a high incidence of false-positive and false-negative results, it was not universally recommended.

In 1982, the committee expanded and clarified the 1972 criteria (see table I). Further recommendations included screening the hearing of infants who manifest any feature on the list of risk criteria. Based on a retrospective study by Stein, Clark, and Kraus (1983), however, hearing screening procedures may need to be expanded in the newborn nursery, since 25 to 30% of their hearing-impaired children (N = 108) did not manifest any of the risk factors set forth in the 1982 position statement. Pappas (1983), in a similar study, determined that 54% of his sample (N = 109) would not have appeared among those infants with high-risk factors had the 1982 registry alone been used. Because of the limitations of BOA on newborn screening however, alternative electrophysiological measures should be considered (see chapters 7, 9, and 12 this volume).

The restrictions imposed by stimulus factors and response factors on the validity and reliability of behavioral procedures in the newborn nursery are clear: Suprathreshold stimulation is required to elicit reflexive responses, and the probability of obtaining a response is dependent on the nature of the stimulus (Hoversten and Moncur 1969; Thompson and Thompson 1972), the state of the child (Eisenberg 1969; Downs 1976), examiner bias (Weber 1969; Mencher, McCulloch, Derbyshire, and Dethlefs 1977;), and the ambient noise levels of the test environment. Even though BOA lacks precision in determining the ex-

Table I

1982 Joint Committee
Expanded High-Risk Criteria

1. Family history of childhood hearing impairment
2. Congenital perinatal infection (e.g., cytomegalovirus, rubella, herpes, toxoplasmosis, syphilis)
3. Anatomic malformations involving the head or neck (e.g., dysmorphic appearance including syndromal and nonsyndromal abnormalities, overt or submucous cleft palate, morphologic abnormalities of the pinna)
4. Birth weight <1500 g.
5. Hyperbilirubinemia at level exceeding indications for exchange transfusion
6. Bacterial meningitis, especially *Haemophilus influenzae*
7. Severe asphyxia which may include infants with Apgar scores of 0 to 3 or who fail to institute spontaneous respiration by 10 minutes and those with hypertonia persisting to 2 hours of age

act hearing status of a child, it is still an alternative for older children who are profoundly retarded or severely developmentally delayed, and for those youngsters who cannot be conditioned to procedures utilizing reinforcement. Hence, it is important to know the restrictions imposed by BOA on slightly older children.

SCREENING OLDER CHILDREN WITH BOA

Different investigators (Murphy 1961; Northern and Downs 1974), using similar behavioral approaches without reinforcement, have reported dissimilar threshold results for children of the same age. These disparities also are reported in the literature for speech thresholds. Furthermore, utilizing the BOA procedure, minimum response levels to different stimuli show improvement with increasing age (see table II). One interpretation of these data suggests that a developmental change in responses takes place during the first two years of life. Another interpretation—after comparing responses of infants of the same age utilizing the operant paradigm and appropriate reinforcement—suggests that the observed change in responses over time reflects the differences in methodology rather than marked changes in true sensitivity. The data reported in table II may be more accurately intepreted by suggesting that neurological maturation, response habituation found in BOA, and mean data extracted from groups of children, account for the change in response levels as a function of age.

A second restriction with BOA relates to the fact that thresholds (minimum

Table II

Response Levels as a Function of Signal and Age
From Northern and Downs (1978) (used with permission)

Age	Noisemakers (Approx. Spl)	Warbled Pure Tones (Re: Audiometric Zero)	Speech (Re: Audiometric Zero)
0–6 wk.	50–70 dB	78 dB (SD = 6 dB)	40–60 dB
6 wk.–4 mo.	50–60 dB	70 dB (SD = 10 dB)	47 dB (SD = 2 dB)
4–7 mo.	40–50 dB	51 dB (SD = 9 dB)	21 dB (SD = 8 dB)
7–9 mo.	30–40 dB	45 dB (SD = 15 dB)	15 dB (SD = 7 dB)
9–13 mo.	25–35 dB	38 dB (SD = 8 dB)	8 dB (SD = 7 dB)
13–16 mo.	25–30 dB	32 dB (SD = 10 dB)	5 dB (SD = 5 dB)
16–21 mo.	25 dB	25 dB (SD = 10 dB)	5 dB (SD = 1 dB)
21–24 mo.	25 dB	26 dB (SD = 10 dB)	3 dB (SD = 2 dB)

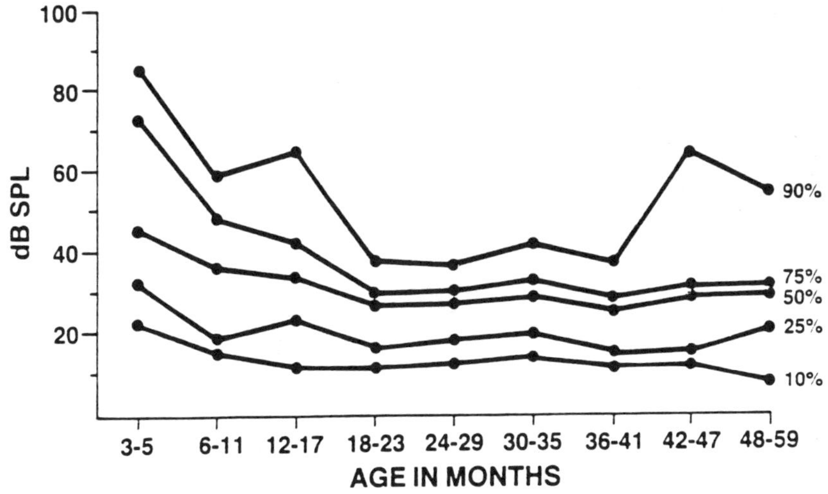

Figure 3. Intersubject variability in BOA as a function of age. From Thompson and Weber (1974)

response levels) show a wide range that qualify as normal. For example, Thompson and Weber (1974) looked at the intersubject variability among children ranging in age from three months to four years. They found a range of 24 dB on the low end (24 to 29-month-old children) to 65 dB at the high end (3- to 5-month-old children), for responses between the 10th and 90th percentiles (see figure 3).

A final restriction with the BOA approach is the need to select the auditory stimulus based on what is novel to the youngster, and not necessarily on what stimulus might be needed for assessment purposes. For example, if a high frequency stimulus is needed to rule out a high frequency hearing loss, this could pose a problem; a number of investigators (Hoversten and Moncur 1969; Thompson and Thompson 1972) have shown that high frequency signals are not effective with young children in a BOA procedure. Figure 4, from Thompson and Thompson, shows the percentage of response to five different stimuli across four different intensity levels. These data show clearly the interaction of different stimuli at different levels on responses observed from a BOA procedure.

PROCEDURES UTILIZING SYSTEMATIC REINFORCEMENT

OPERANT BEHAVIOR

In order to overcome the restrictions imposed by BOA, it is possible to approach the behavioral assessment of hearing in children through an operant

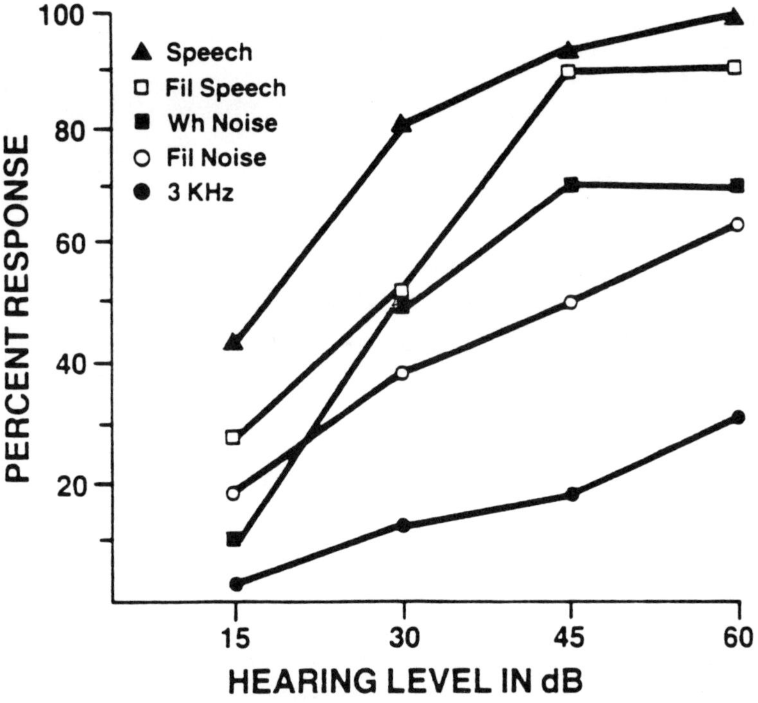

Figure 4. Percent response to five stimuli as a function of hearing level. Infants 7 to 12 months of age. From Thompson and Thompson (1972)

conditioning procedure; specifically, through an operant discrimination procedure. In an operant discrimination procedure, the stimulus is used to cue the child that a response will result in reinforcement. Operant behavior is increased by the application of positive reinforcement. Thus, it is possible to increase the rate of response if a positive reinforcer can be identified and used. Since audible signals of the type used in assessing auditory function are known to have little reinforcing value in children (Moore, Thompson, and Thompson 1975; Moore, Wilson, and Thompson 1977), it is best to use a test procedure in which the signal and reinforcer are separate and the signal serves only to cue the youngster that a correct response will result in reinforcement.

CONDITIONING TECHNIQUES

Even a brief review of the literature reveals that the following operant procedures used for auditory assessment have a relatively long history: the foundation for work on visual reinforcement audiometry (VRA) was laid by Suzuki and Ogiba in 1960, and the label VRA was coined in 1969 by Liden and Kankkunen; the concept of tangible reinforcement operant conditioning audiometry

(TROCA) was developed by Lloyd and his colleagues in 1968; and conditioned play audiometry is referenced in the literature by Barr in 1955.

This may suggest that these are "old" conditioning procedures, and new procedures need to be developed. Instead, what is needed to help redirect the focus of behavioral assessment is not another "new" test of hearing for young children, but rather a better understanding of existing principles of behavior and measurement in auditory assessment. In the decade ahead it will be the precision with which these "old" techniques are utilized that will serve to quantify hearing loss accurately in infants and young children.

VISUAL REINFORCEMENT AUDIOMETRY

VRA has emerged as a successful assessment procedure for infants and young children six months through two years of age (Moore, Wilson, Thompson 1977). In VRA, conditioned turns of the head toward a sound source (localization in a sound field and a conditioned behavior under earphones) are reinforced by an attractive three-dimensional animated toy (Moore, Thompson, and Thompson 1975). The success of VRA is certainly related to the fact that the response (head turn) and reinforcer (animated toy) are well suited to the developmental level of children between these ages.

The test-room arrangement used in the VRA procedure is shown in figure 5. The examiner in the control room has full view of the testing situation and activates the auditory stimulus and visual reinforcer. The test room is arranged with the parent and infant located behind a table in the center of the room. A loudspeaker is positioned at a 45° azimuth to the right or left of the infant's midline of vision. The visual reinforcer, housed in a dark plexiglass enclosure, is located at eye level. In order to maintain the infant's head in a midline position, a second examiner, seated at the infant's side, encourages the child to observe passively or play with colorful, nonnoisy toys. The auditory stimulus is not presented if the infant is looking at the assistant or loudspeaker, or is vocalizing, crying, or moving excessively.

Wilson, Moore, and Thompson (1976) investigated the auditory thresholds[1] of infants, utilizing the VRA procedure described in their ealier work (Moore et al. 1975; Moore et al. 1977). Ninety infants between 5 and 18 months of age were divided into groups of 15 according to age. Minimum response level, using a protocol of attenuating the signal 20 dB after each response and increasing it 10 dB after each failure to respond, was defined as the lowest presentation level at which the infant responded at least three times out of six presentations. Figure 6 presents the minimum response levels obtained by VRA and provides

[1] Since "auditory threshold" represents a minimum auditory response level dependent upon choice of psychophysical method and measurement step size, and therefore not one absolute level; and since auditory response levels may improve slightly with age due to attention and motivation, it may be more appropriate to use the term minimum level (MRL) (Matkin 1977) rather than auditory threshold.

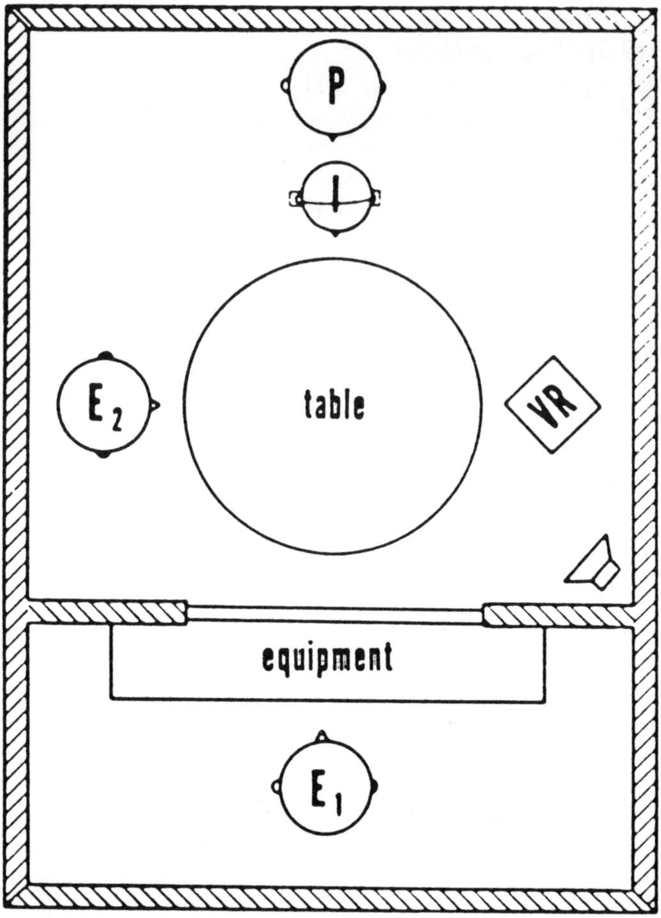

Figure 5. Test-Room arrangement. E1—Examiner, E2—Test-Room Examiner, P—Parent, I—Infant, VR—Visual Reinforcer

comparative data from BOA procedures (Thompson and Weber 1974). The VRA data indicates that the mean response levels improved slightly with age, ranging from about 30 dB SPL for 5-month-olds to about 20 dB SPL for 7- to 18-month-olds. For comparative purposes, the median threshold of 10 normal-hearing adults was 20 dB SPL under the same signal and measurement step conditions. The 10th and 90th percentile points were 20 and 40 dB SPL for 5-month-olds and 20 to 30 dB SPL for 6- through 18-month-olds.

In comparing the VRA MRLs to the BOA MRLs for the same ages, it is obvious that the difference favors the technique utilizing reinforcement. Even more important, for infants six months of age and older the range between the 10th and 90th percentile is reduced from the 45 to 50 dB reported on BOA to 10

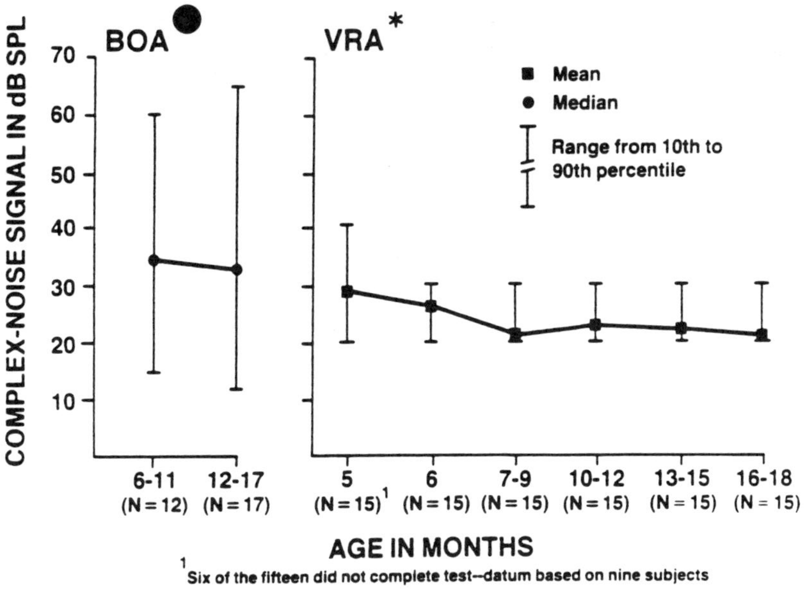

Figure 6. Auditory thresholds of infants as obtained by BOA and VRA methods. *From Wilson, Moore, and Thompson (1976) •From Thompson and Weber (1974)

dB for the VRA procedure used in this study. Certainly for the audiologist evaluating mild hearing losses, the substantially tighter dispersion data obtained with the operant conditioning paradigm would be desirable.

Auditory Assessment. Different studies (Wilson and Moore 1978; Goldman 1979; Diefendorf and Jennings 1983) using the protocol and precision suggested by Wilson and Moore have reported similar sound-field minimum response levels for VRA. In each report, minimum response levels are within a conservative definition of normal hearing (<20 dB HTL) and only slightly elevated from adult comparisons. These data support the accuracy of the VRA test procedures in correctly identifying normal hearing (good specificity). More important, however, is the indication from these data that the VRA test procedure yields a very tight grouping of MRLs for a normal population, thereby resulting in a wide range available for defining abnormal MRLs. Thus, VRA can meet the goals of identifying mild and moderate degrees of hearing loss, as well as hearing losses with varying configurations. As shown in figure 7, the test-retest reliability of VRA (using conditioned play audiometry as the standard) is excellent with children who demonstrate different degrees and configurations of hearing loss. These three clinical cases serve to support the sensitivity of the VRA test procedure.

Results of earphone assessment are also provided by Wilson and Moore. Earphone to pinna attachments in this study may have resulted in sound pressure leakage, thus causing elevated low-frequency MRLs; however, the results pro-

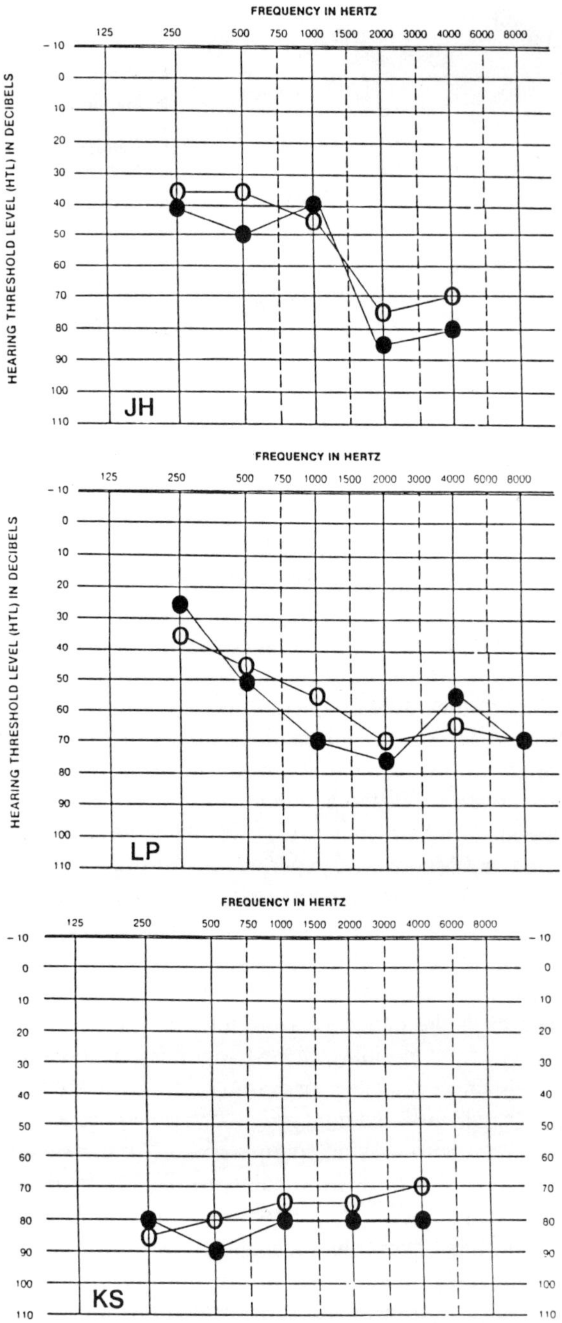

Figure 7. Longitudinal results of assessment. ●Visual Reinforcment Audiometry (VRA) and ○Conditioned Play Audiometry (CPA) (Sound field). VRA before 18 months CPA after four years

vide strong evidence supporting the use and success of earphone assessment with infants utilizing VRA. As a final note, with an appropriate headband arrangement (and cooperation from the youngster under test), bone conduction measurements can be made successfully using VRA.

TANGIBLE/VISUAL REINFORCEMENT OPERANT CONDITIONING AUDIOMETRY

The basic paradigm used in the TROCA/VROCA procedure involves a bar press response coupled with either tangible (e.g., cereal) or visual reinforcement. The procedure uses principles and terminology associated with operant conditioning; specifically, positive reinforcement for appropriate responses and a mild punishment (time out) for false responses. The child's behavior is conditioned until he learns to push a response button whenever a sound is detected. With most children, it has been found that a secondary social reinforcement enhances auditory stimulus-response control. The procedure is most effective with children between two and four years of age developmentally, but has also been shown to be effective with younger children, as well as many difficult-to-test persons including those with mental impairment. In addition, TROCA/VROCA can be used successfully as a fall-back procedure when preschoolers have lost interest in play audiometry and further audiometric information is necessary.

Auditory Assessment. The investigations of Fulton, Gorzycki, and Hull (1975) and of Wilson and Decker (1977) reported minimum response levels for young children utilizing the TROCA/VROCA procedures. Each of these investigations demonstrated that MRLs were tightly grouped and within normal ranges for their subjects, who ranged in age from 12 months to 2 years, suggesting good specificity with this procedure. Also significant is the general agreement that conditioning time, and therefore total testing time, is extended with the TROCA/VROCA procedure. Once a child is brought under auditory stimulus-response control however, testing moves quickly across different stimuli and back and forth between ears.

CONDITIONED PLAY AUDIOMETRY

Conditioned play audiometry is probably the most common procedure used in the assessment of young children. Through conditioning, the child learns to engage in some activity—putting rings on a peg, dropping or stacking blocks—each time he hears the signal. These activities are assumed to be interesting to the child and to reinforce his response. As Fulton (1978) asks, however, if the play activity is the reinforcement, what is the response? Conversely, if the play activity is the response, what is the reinforcement? Because conditioned play audiometry does not follow a strict model of auditory Stimulus → Response → Reinforcer, the procedure can lead to confusion for the youngster, which may result in noncontingent, random playing. In children for whom conditioned play audiometry is appropriate, separation of response from reinforcement, and adherence to the principles of the operant paradigm, may improve this procedure's validity and reliability.

Pediatric literature clearly suggests that conditioned play audiometry is widely accepted among clinicians who interact with young children; however, Barr (1955) tested 135 children between the ages of two and six years using this procedure, and found that the percentage of success was directly related to age. Furthermore, Thompson and Weber (1974) concluded that the rate of success in obtaining detailed information with conditioned play audiometry is limited for children under the age of 30 months.

Auditory Assessment. Experience with conditioned play audiometry indicates that reliable minimum response levels can be obtained when auditory stimulus-response control has been established and response criteria are maintained. Results from a clinical study (Diefendorf 1981) of 40 preschoolers, ages 30 to 48 months, revealed MRLs at a level of 10 dB or better. These findings were in close agreement with other four-year-old children (Gerwin and Glorig 1974) with deviations of less than 5 dB.

MAXIMIZING PRECISION IN VRA, TROCA, AND CONDITIONED PLAY AUDIOMETRY

SOUND-FIELD ASSESSMENT

Sound-field assessment is often the only alternative available to a clinician evaluating the pediatric patient. Warble tones and narrow bands of noise both appear to be in common clinical use; however, there remain many questions about the specific parameters of each of these signals. Wide-band stimuli have been good for maintaining uniform sound fields, but are not good stimuli for identifying frequency-specific hearing losses (Stephens and Rintelmann 1978), and adequate modulation rate of FM tones in sound fields for normal-hearing individuals may be inadequate for accurately assessing hearing-impaired individuals. In addition to questions concerning the choice and standards of stimuli used in sound-field assessment, there are other areas that must be addressed; namely, the patient's position relative to the loudspeaker, the physical environment, and calibration considerations.

In an excellent article by Walker, Dillon, and Byrne (1984), these concerns are addressed and subsequent recommendations are made. This report suggests that the limitations of certain types of stimuli may not apply when the stimuli have optimal characteristics. Furthermore, the authors state that if the recommendations and techniques described are utilized in sound-field assessment, it is possible to achieve the same degree of precision and reliability that is achieved in audiometric measurements made under earphones. Regardless of conditioning technique used, the challenge now rests with the clinician whenever sound-field assessment is considered for the pediatric patient.

TEST-ROOM EXAMINER

The role of the individual in the room with the parent and child is crucial to the success of the VRA, TROCA, and Conditioned Play Audiometry procedures. When only one examiner is available, a micro-processing computer can be used to control the activation and signal intensity of the auditory stimulus.

In VRA the test-room examiner has two primary responsibilities: entertaining the child at the midline position (facing forward) with colorful nonnoisy toys, and judging responses. If the youngster being tested shows too much interest in the colorful toys, the results may be either no response during a signal trial, or elevated minimum response levels. On the other hand, if the youngster being tested shows no interest or is bored with the colorful toys, false responses may occur regularly. The test-room examiner must have a continuum of toys available, and must be astute at judging when a toy change in either direction (more entertaining/less entertaining) may be necessary to maintain the child's midline position and optimum response state.

Since the test-room examiner is required to judge responses, it is possible that knowledge of signal trials versus control trials could result in tester bias in the VRA test procedure. The test-room examiner therefore wears headphones and can be alerted by a signal (tone or light) that an observation interval is occurring.

With a number of children it has been found that secondary social reinforcement enhances auditory stimulus-response control. Thus, in addition to teaching the youngster the conditioned response in the TROCA and Conditioned Play Audiometry procedures, the test-room examiner must also be skilled in providing social reinforcement at the appropriate time and interval.

CONDITIONING IN OPERANT PROCEDURES

There are currently no recommended test procedures for conducting VRA, TROCA, or Conditioned Play Audiometry; however, if one adheres to the philosophy that reliable measurements are a direct result of the test instrument and the development of auditory stimulus-response control through conditioning, then the interaction between the subject, the test procedure, and the examiner, in achieving precise results, is an important part of that process.

Thompson and Folsom (1984) compared the effects of two conditioning procedures in the use of VRA with one- and two-year-old children. One conditioning procedure used an initial stimulus presentation level (30 dB HL) and only two conditioning trials prior to MRL exploration. The second procedure used a 60 dB HL initial presentation level and five conditioning trials prior to MRL exploration. The data from the Thompson and Folsom study indicated no significant differences between the two conditioning procedures in regard to obtained MRLs or to the number of false-positive responses observed during control trials.

If a child fails to respond in VRA the examiner can quickly introduce hearing level increments until a spontaneous response is observed. It must also be recognized, however, that for some hearing-impaired children localization to a sound source may not be a realistic response task.

If there is reason to believe—based on case history information or initial testing trails—that a child may not adapt well to the VRA procedure, it would be clinically advantageous to consider a test strategy that begins at a relatively soft level, so that if habituation occurs after a few trials, the opportunity to observe spontaneous responses at a soft level is at least available. This rationale would support the use of the 30 dB conditioning level in cases where there is doubt about the VRA procedure.

When any operant procedure is used in a case of either known or suspected hearing loss in a child, it is likely that several paired conditioning trials (with a visual reinforcer; demonstrating the bar press response; or completing the motor activity) at suprathreshold levels will be required to condition the response prior to MRL exploration. Obviously, the auditory signal must be audible if conditioning is to be established.

FALSE-POSITIVE RESPONSES

False-positive responses are monitored by means of control trials. Both signal trials and control trials occur during the MRL exploration; the occurrence of either trial initiates an observation interval during which responses are judged. If a response occurs during a signal trial it is considered a correct detection; if, however, a response occurs during a control trial (that is, when no acoustic stimulus is presented) it is considered a false-positive response. Control trials are interspersed among actual stimulus trials on a random schedule. The presence or absence of false-positive responses during control trials allows the examiner to calculate the percentage of false-positive responses. The purpose of the control trial is to exclude data on any youngster who reaches a false response rate that would cast suspicion on his response data. This information is important in establishing response validity, which is the basis for examiner confidence in test results.

LOGIC CIRCUIT

The logic-control circuit in VRA and TROCA provides a strict definition of the response interval for both signal trials and control trials (monitoring false-positive responses). Initiation of the auditory test stimulus starts an adjustable timer which is used to define the observation (response) interval. A head turn or bar press response is judged to be a positive response only if it occurs during this interval—usually set at three to four seconds. If the infant responds correctly during this interval and a positive vote is rendered by the test-room assistant, the visual or tangible reinforcer is automatically activated. (In VRA the reinforcer is set for a pre-selected duration of usually two or three seconds.) If the examiner renders a vote after the four-second response interval has elasped, the visual or tangible reinforcer will not be activated. Since the response interval timer is automatically activated by the onset of stimulus presentation, and reinforcement is automatically controlled, the test procedure is made easier for the examiner, who can then devote full attention to the behavior of the youngster under test.

SUMMARY

In summary, the importance of adopting a developmental, age-appropriate approach to the measurement of hearing in young children through the utilization of a pediatric test battery cannot be overemphasized. When youngsters can be successfully conditioned for assessment, audiological information relative to peripheral and central auditory function (Diefendorf 1982) can be obtained. Furthermore, for the hearing-impaired youngster significant information can be obtained with respect to understanding how that child uses his residual hearing.

REFERENCES

Barr, B. 1955. Pure tone audiometry for pre-school children. *Acta Oto-Laryngologica Supplement* 121.

Bennet, M. J. 1975. The auditory response cradle: A device for the objective assessment of auditory state in the neonate. *Symposium Zoological Society London* 37:291–305.

Diefendorf, A. O. 1981. The effect of a pre-play period on play audiometry. Paper presented at the Tennessee Speech-Language-Hearing Association Annual Convention, Memphis.

Diefendorf, A. O., and Jennings, S. 1983. Stimulus response comparisons between visual reinforcement audiometry (VRA) and behavioral observation audiometry (BOA). Paper presented at the American Speech-Language-Hearing Association Annual Convention, Cincinnati.

Diefendorf, A. O., 1982. Update in pediatric hearing assessment. *Monographs in Contemporary Audiology* 3:1–21.

Downs, M. 1976. Early identification of hearing loss: Where are we? Where do we go from here? *In* G. Mencher (ed.). *Proceedings of the Nova Scotia Conference on Early Identification of Hearing Loss.* Basel: S. Karger.

Downs, M. P., and Sterritt, G. M. 1967. A guide to newborn and infant hearing screening programs. *Archives of Otolaryngology* 85:15–22.

Durieux-Smith, A., Picton, T., Edwards, C., Goodman, J. T., and MacMurray, B. 1985. The Crib-O-Gram in the NICU: An evaluation based on brain stem electric response audiometry. *Ear and Hearing* 6:20–24.

Eisenberg, R. B. 1969. Auditory behavior in the human neonate: Functional properties of sound and their ontogenetic implications. *International Audiology* 1:34–35.

Feinmesser, M., and Tell, L. 1976. Evaluation of methods for detecting hearing impairment in infancy and early childhood. *In* G. Mencher (ed.). *Proceedings of the Nova Scotia Conference on Early Identification of Hearing Loss.* Basel: S. Karger.

Fulton, R. T., Gorzycki, P. A., and Hull, W. L. 1975. Hearing assessment with young children. *Journal of Speech and Hearing Disorders* 40:397–404.

Fulton, R. T. 1978. Pure-tone tests of hearing—age one year through five years. *In* F. N. Martin (ed.). *Pediatric Audiology* (pp. 174–235). Englewood Cliffs, New Jersey: Prentice-Hall.

Gerber, S. E. 1985. Stimulus, response, and state variables in the testing of neonates. *Ear and Hearing* 6:15–19.

Glorig, A. 1974. Pure tone sweepcheck as an indicator of the pure tone threshold test. *In* K. S. Gerwin, and A. Glorig (eds.). *Detection of Hearing Loss and Ear Disease in Children* (pp. 149–151). Springfield, Illinois: Charles C Thomas.

Goldman, T. M. 1979. Response of infants of warble-tone signals presented in soundfield using visual reinforcement audiometry. Master's thesis, University of Cincinnati.

Hoversten, G., and Moncur, J. 1969. Stimuli and intensity factors in testing infants. *Journal of Speech and Hearing Research* 12:687–702.

Joint Committee on Infant Hearing Screening. 1972. Supplementary Statement on Infant Hearing Screening. *ASHA* 16:160.

Joint Committee on Infant Hearing Screening, 1982. Policy statement issued jointly by The Academy of Otolaryngology—Head and Neck, The Academy of Pediatrics, The American Nurses Association, and The American Speech-Language-Hearing Association.

Liden, G., and Kankkunen, A. 1969. Visual reinforcement audiometry. *Acta Otolaryngologica* 67:281–292.

Ling, D., Ling, A. H., and Doehring, O. G. 1970. Stimulus response and observer variables in the auditory screening of newborn infants. *Journal of Speech and Hearing Research* 13:9–18.

Lloyd, L. L., Spradlin, J. E., and Reid, M. J. 1968. An operant audiometric procedure for difficult-to-test patients. *Journal of Speech and Hearing Disorders* 33:236–245.

Matkin, N. D. 1977. Assessment of hearing sensitivity during the preschool years. *In* F. H. Bess (ed.). *Childhood Deafness, Assessment and Management* (pp. 127–134). New York: Grune and Stratton.

Mencher, G. T., McCulloch, B., Derbyshire, A. J., and Dethlefs, R. 1977. Observer bias as a factor in neonatal hearing screening. *Journal of Speech and Hearing Research* 20:27–34.

Moore, J. M., Thompson, G., and Thompson, M. 1975. Auditory localization of infants as a function of reinforcement conditions. *Journal of Speech and Hearing Disorders* 40:29–34.

Moore, J. M., Wilson, W. R., and Thompson, G. 1977. Visual reinforcement of head-turn responses in infants under 12 months of age. *Journal of Speech and Hearing Disorders* 42:328–334.

Murphy, K. P. 1961. Development of hearing in babies. *Hearing News* 29:9–11.

Northern, J. L., and Downs, M. P. 1974. *Hearing in Children.* The Williams and Wilkins Company: Baltimore.

Northern, J. L., and Downs, M. P. 1978. *Hearing in Children.* The Williams and Wilkins Company, Baltimore.

Pappas, D. G. 1983. A study of the High-Risk Registry for sensorineural hearing impairment. *Head and Neck Surgery* 91:41–44.

Simmons, F. B., and Russ, F. N. 1974. Automated newborn hearing screening, the Crib-O-Gram. *Archives of Otolaryngology* 100:1–7.

Stein, L., Clark, S., and Kraus, N. 1983. The hearing-impaired infant: Patterns of identification and habilitation. *Ear and Hearing* 4:232–236.

Stephens, M. M., and Rintelmann, W. F. 1978. The influence of audiometric configuration on pure-tone, warbled-tone and narrow-band noise thresholds of adults with sensorineural hearing losses. *Journal of American Auditory Society* 3:221–226.

Suzuki, T., and Ogiba, Y. 1960. A technique of pure-tone audiometry for children under three years of age: Conditioned orientation reflex (COR) audiometry. *Revue de Laryngologie, Otologie, Rhinologie* 81:33–45.

Suzuki, T., and Ogiba, Y. 1961. Conditioned orientation audiometry, *Archives of Otolaryngology* 74:192–198.

Thompson, M., and Thompson, G. 1972. Response of infants and young children as a function of auditory stimuli and test method. *Journal of Speech and Hearing Research* 15:699–707.

Thompson, G., and Weber, B. 1974. Responses of infants and young children to behavioral observations audiometry (BOA). *Journal of Speech Hearing and Disorders* 39:140–147.

Thompson, G., and Folsom, R. C. 1984. A comparison of two conditioning procedures in the use of visual reinforcement audiometry (VRA). *Journal of Speech and Hearing Disorders* 49:241–245.

Walker, G., Dillon, H., and Byrne, D. 1984. Sound field audiometry: Recommended stimuli and procedures. *Ear and Hearing* 5:13–21.

Weber, B. A. 1969. Validation of observer judgments in behavioral observation audiometry. *Journal of Speech and Hearing Disorders* 34:350–355.

Wilson, W. R., Moore, J. M., and Thompson, G. 1976. Sound-field auditory thresholds of infants utilizing visual reinforcement audiometry (VRA). Paper presented at The American Speech and Hearing Association Annual Convention, Houston, Texas.

Wilson, W. R., and Decker, N. T. 1977. Auditory Thresholds of Infants using Operant Audiometry with Tangible and/or Visual Reinforcement. Unpublished Research, University of Washington.

Wilson, W. R., and Moore, J. M. 1978. Pure-tone earphone thresholds of infants utilizing visual reinforcement audiometry (VRA). Paper presented at The American Speech-Language-Hearing Association Convention, San Francisco, California.

Chapter 11

Audiologic Application of Auditory Evoked Potentials in Children

Daniel M. Schwartz and *Jamie A. Costello**

In 1976 at the Second International Symposium on Childhood Deafness, Zerlin and Naunton (1976) described a technique for constructing an electrophysiologic audiogram based on whole nerve action potential responses recorded transtympanically. This invasive electrocochleographic procedure served as a last resort alternative to assessing the status of the auditory periphery in children with whom conventional behavioral pediatric test protocols were precluded. Transtympanic electrocochleography has never achieved widespread clinical use as an electrophysiologic test of hearing sensitivity.

In the decade to follow, our understanding of the neurophysiologic mechanisms that underlie auditory bioelectric potentials and their correlation to peripheral and central auditory pathophysiology has increased substantially. Much of what has been written about auditory evoked potentials in pediatrics has related principally to its application as an electrophysiologic correlate of behavioral audiometric threshold in the form of a latency-intensity function for wave V, and as an initial screening test for intensive-care unit newborns at risk for hearing loss.

The search for a reliable, valid, non-invasive bioelectric index of peripheral hearing sensitivity in the behaviorally untestable child has continued for more than two decades. Logically, the premise of electric response audiometry is to derive an approximate correlate to the behavioral pure-tone audiogram. Although the early, middle, and late auditory evoked potentials have each received research attention toward achieving this goal, the short-latency auditory brainstem response has enjoyed the most clinical success with very young and/or difficult-to-test children, and the slow vertex response the least. Unfor-

*At the time that this chapter was prepared Jamie A. Costello was affiliated with the Speech, Hearing and Neurosensory Center, San Diego Children's Hospital, San Diego, CA tunately, despite the observation that the endogenous slow vertex response permits a valid, frequency-specific electrophysiologic audiogram, its sensitivity to patient state of consciousness and arousal limits its use to the cooperative, unsedated older child.

This chapter focuses on the pediatric application of auditory evoked potentials to estimate hearing sensitivity. Although we have made liberal use of reference citation, we purposely avoided topographic descriptions of individual research studies. Rather, we opted for a laconic, sometimes philosophical overview of the subject.

THE CLICK EVOKED LATENCY-INTENSITY SERIES

CONDUCTIVE HEARING LOSS

The organized relationship between wave V latency of the auditory brainstem response (ABR), and stimulus intensity serves as the foundation for brainstem electric response audiometry, as exemplified in figure 1. This exponentially decaying response series, shown as a monotonically decreasing curve, represents a normative template against which individual patient data are compared. Hence, the discrepancy between the normal wave V threshold and the visual detection threshold of wave V for a given patient defines the estimated degree of peripheral sensitivity loss, while the slope of the function is used to infer (but is not diagnostic of) the peripheral site of lesion, as well as the audiometric contour.

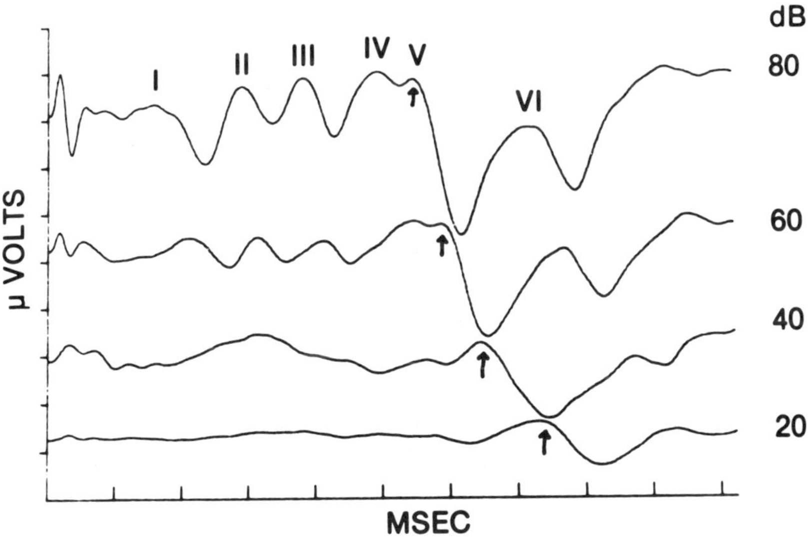

Figure 1. Example of a latency intensity function for wave V used to estimate hearing sensitivity loss.

There is general consensus that disorders affecting sound transmission through the external and/or middle ear result in a temporal prolongation of ABR waves I-V. The latency-intensity function is characterized by displacement to the right of and parallel to the corresponding normal template as illustrated in figure 2. Theoretically this displacement should be proportional to the attenuating characteristics of the specific middle ear disorder relative to the loss of energy reaching the oval window and approaching the cochlea.

Shown in figure 2 are two wave V latency-intensity functions for conductive hearing loss. In both instances the latency-intensity function is shifted to the right with a slope similar to the non-linear normal template and a wave V threshold approximately equivalent to the degree of sensitivity loss.

THE BONE CONDUCTED ABR: A WORD OF CAUTION

Despite the value for estimating degree and type of hearing loss from the air-conducted latency-intensity series, it has been considered at times advantageous also to record the ABR to bone-conducted stimuli. The discrepency between air and bone conduction estimates of hearing loss presumably represents the electrophysiological analog of an air-bone gap. This is particularly appealing when faced with the dilemma of assessing sensorineural reserve in a behaviorally untestable infant or child having an atretic or microtic external ear.

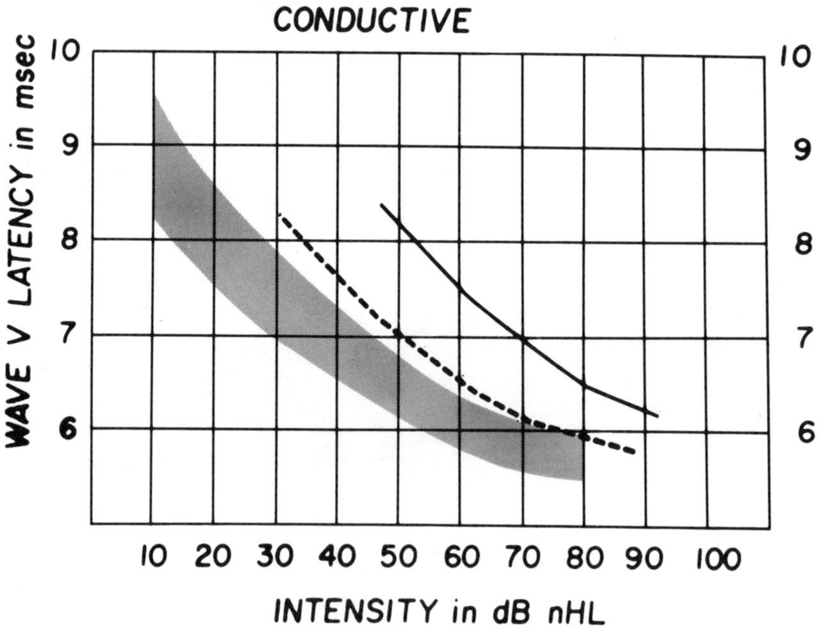

Figure 2. Example of a latency intensity function for two patients with conductive hearing loss. The shaded area represents a normal template.

Berlin (personal communication), for example, states quite dogmatically that the bone-conducted click-evoked ABR must be obtained on any child who presents with no recordable ABR by air conduction.

Given the limited data describing the spectral characteristics of brief transients transduced through standard audiometric bone-conduction oscillators, Schwartz, Larson, and De Chicchis (1981) investigated the differences in acoustic spectra across five air- and bone-conduction transducers commonly used in ABR measurement.

Figure 3, from Schwartz et al. 1981, depicts the output levels of two air- and three bone-conduction receivers when driven just below and at saturation by a 100 microsecond rectangular electrical pulse generated by a Nicolet CA 1000 evoked potential system.

Each of the bone vibrators showed its greatest concentration of energy in the 2000 Hz region with the Radioear B-70A providing the most output and the B-72 the least. For all three vibrators there was a precipitous decrease in output above and below 2000 Hz. Even at maximum, however, output never exceeded the equivalent of 35 dB HL. Moreover, when driven at high stimulus input levels there is considerable non-linear distortion at the resonance peak across vibrators.

Obviously, the consequence of the severely reduced output and distortion characteristics of these bone-conduction devices is that its use in click-evoked ABR testing is, at best, limited to those children whose cochlear reserve does not exceed much more than 30 dB. When used to evaluate those children who

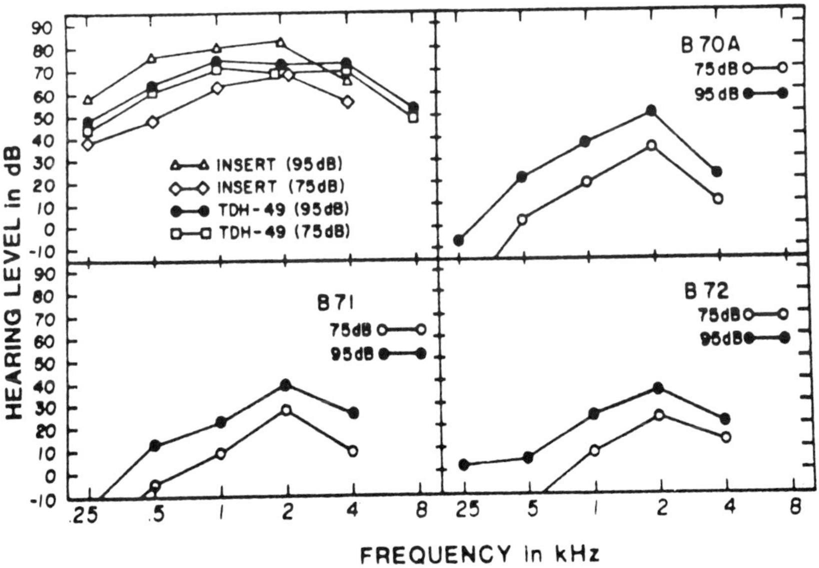

Figure 3. Acoustic spectra of three bone-conduction devices at input intensities of 75 and 95 dB (re: attenuator setting). (Taken from Schwartz, Larson and De Chicchis 1985.)

do not present with an air-conduction ABR as suggested by Berlin, however, the signal intensity needed to elicit a bone-conducted response will most likely drive the vibrator into saturation, thus confounding test measurement and interpretation.

SENSORINEURAL HEARING LOSS

The latency-intensity function for a flat and precipitous high frequency cochlear hearing loss is illustrated graphically in figure 4. The primary features are that the slope of the function increases immediately above the wave V threshold such that for mild-to-moderate steeply sloping sensorineural hearing loss, wave V latency is normal at high levels of stimulation followed by a rapid latency prolongation beyond normal limits as intensity decreases, often thought to be indicative of loudness recruitment. In contrast, that for the flat configuration shows a constant latency shift similar to the conductively impaired ear with a slope sometimes less than normal.

TOWARD PLACE SPECIFICITY

Although the click-evoked ABR has proven to be of unlimited value as a "quasi objective" estimate of type and degree of sensitivity loss, and in neu-

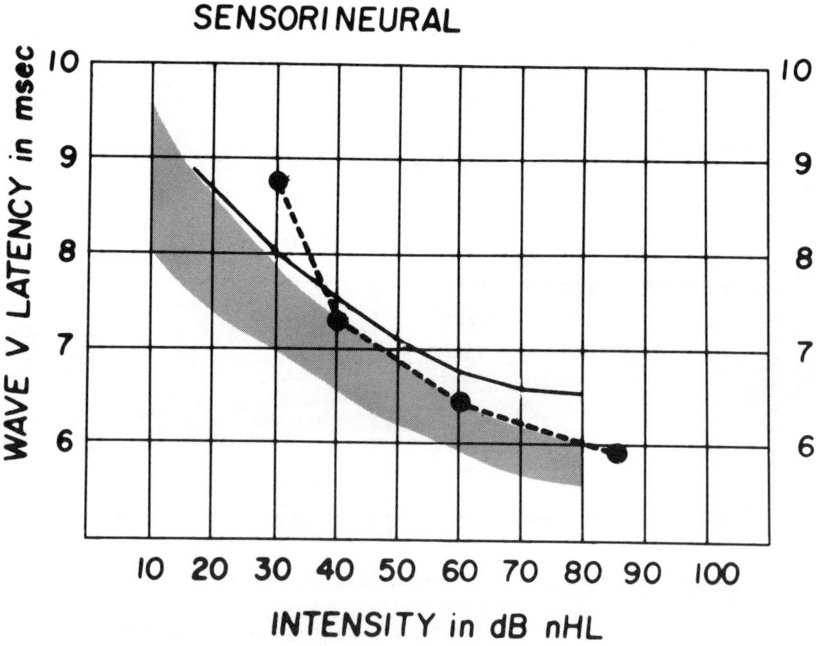

Figure 4. Example of a latency intensity function for an ear with sensorineural hearing loss.

rodiagnosis since the almost instantaneous rise-time assures highly synchronized neural excitation, there are several inherent problems associated with the use of a broad spectrum rectangular pulse for approximating an audiogram that deviates from a flat contour. In such cases, the degree of loss across one band of frequencies may differ substantially from that in a second band as is seen in low-frequency rising or high frequency sloping configurations. Clearly, this variable becomes critical when one is restricted to electric response audiometry for defining the hearing loss in otherwise behaviorally untestable children with the end goal being the development of an appropriate program of intervention. Indeed, the notion of fitting a hearing aid based on a test that does not quantify residual low frequency hearing or, in fact, that is insensitive to interfrequency threshold differences within the 1000–4000 Hz region, seems rather contrary to traditional or contemporary audiologic philosophy.

As a consequence of the lack-of-place specificity for click stimuli, there has been an increasing trend, and debate, as to the best approach for estimating more definitively the pure-tone audiogram. These strategies have included, but are not limited to, ABRs to tonal stimuli, notched-noise paradigms, and derived ABRs to clicks and tones in high-pass, narrow-band and wideband noise.

THE 500 Hz TONE PIP

In an effort to resolve the problem of frequency specificity, Davis and Hirsh 1976 attempted early on to determine if reliable wave V responses could be elicited to low- and high-frequency tone pips. Discouragingly, they concluded that responses to 500 Hz tone pips were difficult to identify and were most likely mediated near the cochlear apex. One year later, however, two Japanese studies (Suzuki, Hirai, and Horiuchi 1977; Suzuki and Horiuchi 1977) revealed that the influencing factor in eliciting a detectable ABR to low-frequency tone pips was the high-pass filter cut-off frequency. They reported that the high frequency cut-off selected for routine neurodiagnostic evaluation causes marked suppression of Wave V amplitude, particularly for a 500 Hz tone pip, when used for threshold estimation.

The latency of wave V in response to tone pips is influenced heavily by stimulus rise time, frequency, and intensity. As frequency decreases the wave V latency is prolonged relative to that of a higher frequency brief tone as depicted in figure 5. Of course, the magnitude of this shift is tied to the stimulus intensity whereby the latency delay between frequency conditions is magnified as intensity decreases.

MASKING PARADIGMS

In recent years, many modifications to the tone-pip paradigm have been explored as a means of restricting the spread of acoustic energy from a tone pip to a constrained place along the basilar membrane while still maintaining sufficient neural synchrony to evoke a morphologically organized ABR. This is par-

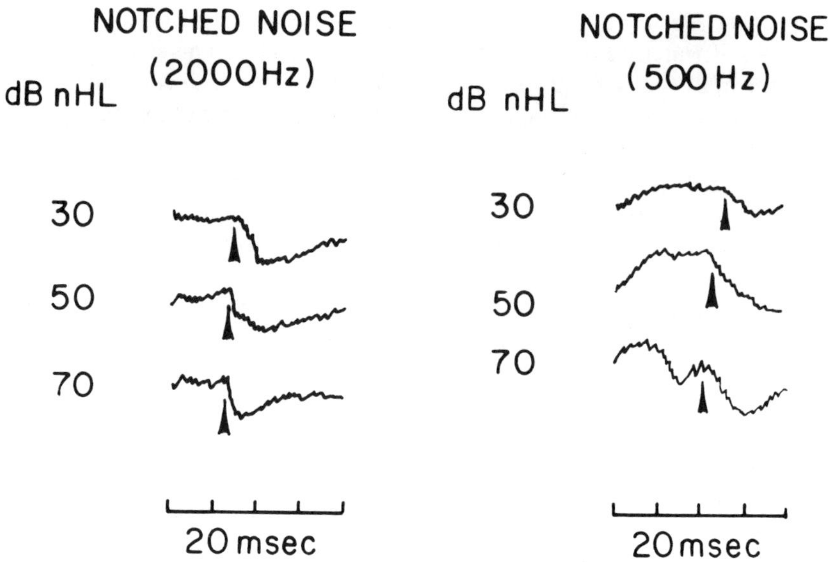

Figure 5. Auditory brainstem responses to 500 Hz and 2000 Hz tone pips. (Modified from Stappells et al. 1985).

ticularly important for low-frequency stimuli since the spatial distribution of cochlear excitation is so broad.

Notch filtering. One rather attractive method schematized in figure 6 is based on the "busy line" theory and incorporates a band reject filtering of a broad band masking noise imposing a notch within a nominally restricted frequency band with the test tone at its center. Figure 7 compares response characteristics of a 500 and 2000 Hz tone pip in notched noise as a function of stimulus intensity as described by Stappells et al. (1985). The responses have been artistically smoothed, but unaltered for presentation clarity. Observe that changes in frequency from high to low influences amplitude and latency of the response due, at least in part, to traveling wave mechanics.

The pleasing advantage of the band-reject or notched noise method over the more elaborate, albeit more place-specific, derived response technique is that it does not appear to lengthen overall test time significantly relative to the use of unmasked clicks; thus, it is a clinically feasible alternative to a broad spectrum click for estimating place-specific threshold in the otherwise untestable child.

THE DERIVED BAND MASKING TECHNIQUE

Based on early animal studies (Teas, Eldredge, and Davis 1962) designed to separate the click-evoked whole-nerve action potential into its component parts, a series of studies have applied special masking techniques in an attempt to reconstruct the audiogram (Elberling 1974; Don, Eggermont, and Brackmann 1979; Eggermont and Don 1982).

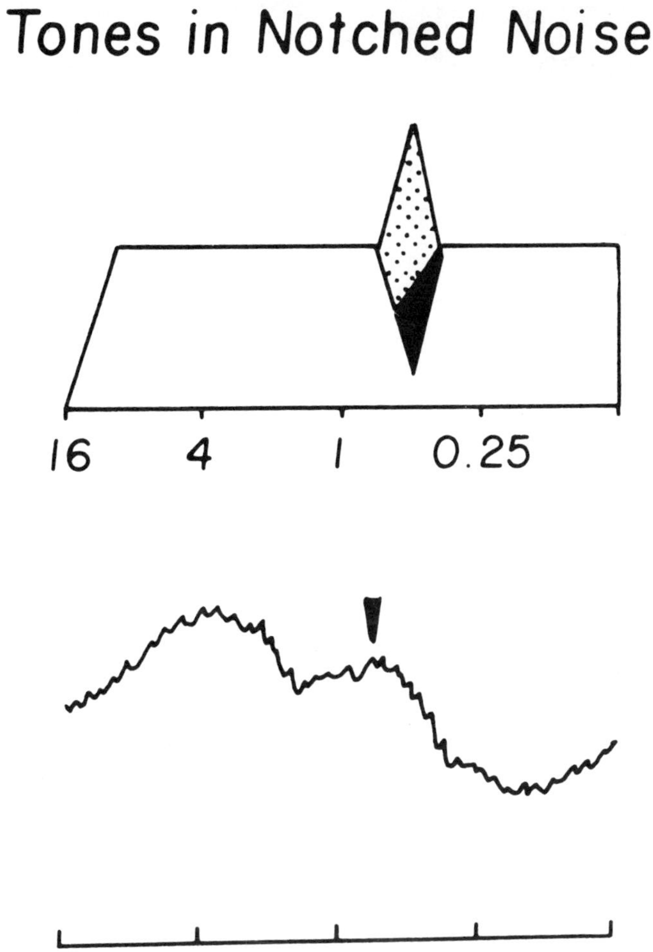

Figure 6. Schematic of the notched noise paradigm for place specificity of the ABR. Also shown is an examplary tracing for a 500 Hz tone in notched noise. (Modified from Stappells et al. 1985).

The derived band technique utilizes the simultaneous presentation of a broad-band click and a high-pass masker presented at the minimal masking level (MML) for an unfiltered broad spectrum noise and a 60 dB SL click. This signal-to-noise (S/N) ratio is then held constant as click intensity is decreased.

For the test procedure, a click-evoked ABR intensity series is developed in the presence of octave-spaced high pass maskers until a derived electrophysiological audiogram is reconstructed. To illustrate, the click-evoked ABR is recorded with a high-pass masker having a 2000 Hz cut-off frequency. Next, the procedure is repeated with a 1000 Hz cut-off thereby resulting in masked regions 1000 Hz and above. The two responses are subtracted via computer and this derived narrow band ABR is presumed to represent the contribu-

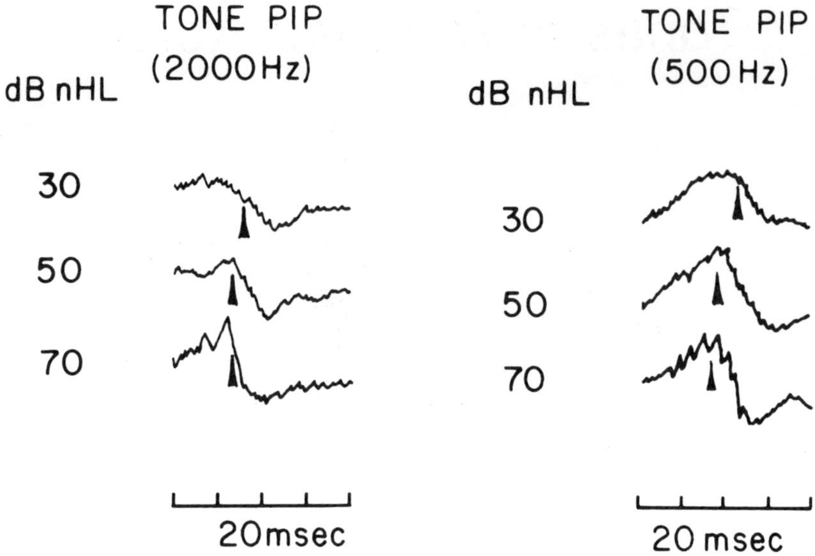

Figure 7. Example of auditory brainstem responses recorded to 500 Hz and 2000 Hz tone pips in notched noise. (From Stappells et al. 1985).

tion of the neural pathway initiated by the 1000–2000 Hz region of the basilar membrane.

To date, the derived response technique has been applied primarily to normal hearers with mixed success for estimation of low frequency threshold, and has not been replicated on sufficiently large patient populations with hearing loss to warrant universal clinical adoption (Laukli and Mair 1986). Furthermore, reconstruction of a derived response audiogram can take up to two hours of test time thereby necessitating prolonged sedation with young children. Moreover, the method is limited only to those evoked potential systems capable of performing computer subtraction.

In addition to stimulus modifications for developing a more frequency-specific wave V latency-intensity function, at least three additional auditory evoked potential tests have been proffered as permitting frequency-specific approximations of the pure-tone audiogram. These include 1) the middle latency response (MLR), 2) the slow negative response (SN-10), and, 3) the 40 Hz steady state potential.

MIDDLE LATENCY RESPONSES

Middle latency responses (MLR) represent a triphasic series of vertex positive scalp-evoked potentials occurring between 10 and 50 msec following the onset of an acoustic stimulus (see Kileny 1983 for an excellent review of the middle response). Salient to electric response audiometry, however, is that the MLRs of adults can be recorded rather easily in response to frequency-specific tone bursts, with MLR threshold agreeing quite favorably with the pure-tone audiogram. Clearly, this paradigm lends itself well to the derivation of an electrophysiologic audiogram in those cases in which the click-evoked ABR may be misleading.

Successful, stable and presumedly reliable MLRs were thought early on to have been recorded both from neonates and young infants (Mendel, Adkinson, and Harker 1977; Wolf and Goldstein 1980; McRandle, Smith, and Goldstein 1980). Recently, however, a series of investigations reported most compelling evidence to cast doubt on many of the earlier claims for the reliability and stability of MLR threshold recordings in young children (Scherg 1982; Kileny 1983; Suzuki, Hirabayashi, and Kobayashi 1984). Each of these investigators demonstrated rather convincingly that the MLR configuration depends on the characteristics of analog high-pass filtering. They went on to suggest that considerable waveform distortion is introduced by high-pass analog filtering, whereas low-pass filtering results can effect peak latency.

The end product of this finding, as portrayed in figure 8, is that the infant and adult MLRs differ significantly and that the earlier claims for similarity most likely represented the effect of analog filter distortions which, when accounted for, alter the infant MLR to the point of an absence or serious depression of the dominant Pa component so robust in the adult. In fact, there is some question as to whether the MLR is even present in young children; it may not mature into a clinically useful response until pubescence. Suzuki et al. have suggested that the pronounced effect of high-pass filtering in young children is most likely attributable to the observation that the dominant frequency component of the MLR in young children is more closely allied to 20 Hz rather than 30–50 Hz of their adult counterparts. At least for the present time, therefore, recording the MLR in infants and young children as an unbiased approximation of hearing threshold is indeed presumptive and tenous.

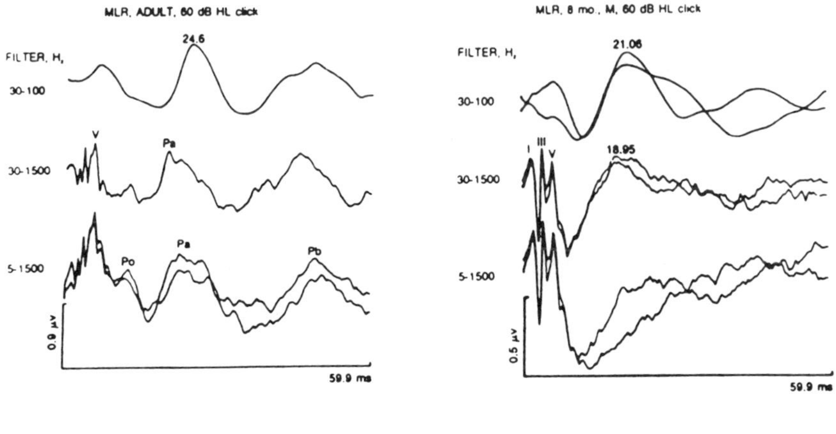

Figure 8. Comparison of adult and neonate middle latency response demonstrating the affect of analog filtering on response morphology.

In 1981 Galambos, Makeig, and Talmachoff excited the audiologic community with the description of an auditory steady-state response referred to as the 40 Hz event related potential (ERP). In their initial report, Galambos et al. demonstrated that when acoustic stimuli are presented at a rate of 40/sec, there occurs a superimposition of successive negative and positive peaks of the MLR such that each cycle of a sinusoidal response lasts approximately 25 msec. The result is an amplitude increase two–three times greater than the conventional MLR evoked at slow rates of stimulus presentation. From this, they went on to report that the 40 Hz ERP can be recorded quite robustly to low frequency (250–500) tonal stimuli, and more importantly, remains clearly visible at intensity levels approximating those of the behavioral threshold. This observation had such an immediate impact on audiology that one manufacturer quickly introduced a 40 Hz screening device, while others modified their respective averaging computers to permit response overlap.

Unfortunately, little attention was paid to see if the same phenomenon held true in those patients with whom the test was most applicable; that is the behaviorally untestable child. Recent studies, for example, have shown that the amplitude of the response and hence the response threshold, may be influenced by natural sleep, not to mention twilight sedation (Szyfter, Dauman, and deSauvage 1984; Brown and Shallop 1982; Jerger et al. 1986). Equally as important, however, is that the 40/sec rate at which maximum amplitude of this steady state potential occurs may not be the same for children and adults (Suzuki, Hirabayashi, and Kobayashi 1983).

Fifer, Jerger, and Null (1985) demonstrated most impressively that in contrast to the adult 40 Hz sinusoidal response, the neonate response achieves maximum amplitude at stimulation rates near 20/sec. as presented in figure 9. More recently, Stapells, Galambos, and Costello (unpublished data) reported that infants showed no consistent steady state response (SSR) amplitude peak, regardless of stimulation rate. In fact, at 1000 Hz, the 39/s SSR mean amplitude was only 43% of the adult.

Surely this is a disconcerting finding given the initial impetus toward refining this technique for electric response audiometry. Undoubtedly, considerably more research on this steady state response is needed before we can incorporate it comfortably into routine pediatric practice.

THE SN-10

The slow-negative potential SN-10 was first introduced by Davis and Hirsh (1979) following the two Japanese reports (Suzuki et al. 1977; Suzuki and Horiuchi 1977) on the influence of high-pass filtering on the wave V ABR to low-frequency (500 Hz) tone pips. Specifically, it was noted that the amplitude of wave V increased either with no high-pass filtering or when using a much lower (<50 Hz) and a steeper rejection rate than that typically employed in ABR testing. Davis and Hirsh (1979) followed suit and demonstrated a descending ver-

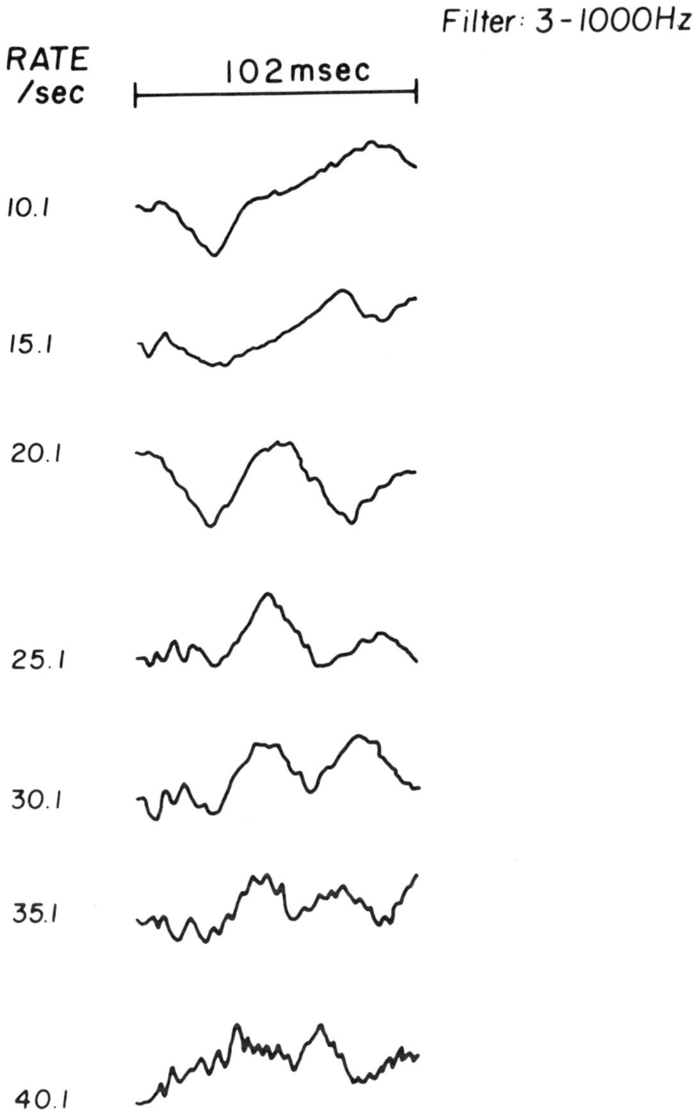

Figure 9. Example of the effect of click rate on the middle latency response of newborns. (From Fifer et al. 1985).

tex negative tail following wave V that is easily resolved when using appropriate wide and steep filter characteristics and, more importantly, that can be visualized at intensity levels close to the 500 Hz behavioral threshold.

Shown in figure 10 is the effect of high-pass filter cut-off frequency on the tone-elicited ABR as reported by Hyde (1985). At a cut-off of 0 Hz the ABR is characterized by a broad symmetrical wavelet. As the high-pass cut-off in-

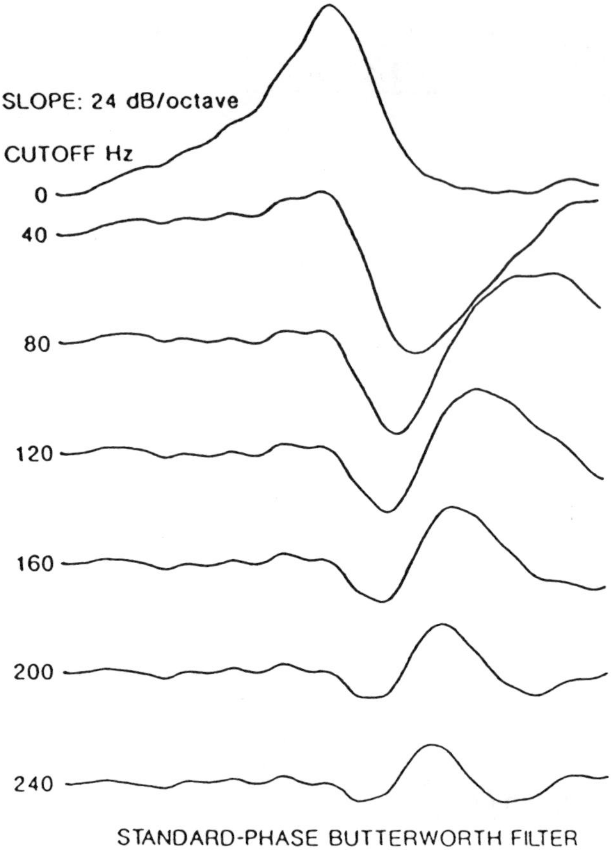

Figure 10. Effect of high-pass filter cut-off frequency on the tone-elicited ABR. (From Hyde 1985).

creases to 40 Hz as used by Davis and Hirsh (1979), there emerges an exaggerated negative slope to a depressed wave V most likely the result of phase distortion; this is the SN-10. Of course, continued increases in cut-off frequency influence further this entire wave complex. Like all other so-called frequency specific responses, the efficacy of SN-10 for frequency-specific audiometric mapping continues to be debated, but deserves additional exploration.

In their comparison of eight electric response audiometric techniques involving most of those mentioned herein, Stapells et al. (1985) found that the ABR to tones (2 msec rise-1 msec plateau-2 msec fall) in notched noise yielded the best approximation to behavioral thresholds at 500 and 2000–4000 Hz, respectively, followed next by ABR to unmasked tones. Simply stated then, the recommended stimulus for an audiologic ABR would be a 500 and 2000–4000 Hz tone in notched noise using a broad filter passband (e.g., 30–3000 Hz) at a rate somewhere near 40/sec. Again, while this approach offers no guarantees in all cases, it should reduce hearing loss estimation error by a sufficient amount to warrant its inclusion in the test battery, unless new conflicting data are reported.

ILLUSTRATIVE CASES

Armed with a review of the many ways that auditory evoked potentials can be used to estimate degree and type of sensitivity loss in those children with whom behavioral techniques are precluded or misleading, we present a select series of audiologically provocative pediatric material.

CASE #1

The first case is that of a nearly five year old cytomegalic child. The sequelae of this ubiquitous herpes virus include: intellectual and developmental impairment, neuromuscular disorder, systemic malformations, visual impairment secondary to chorioretinitis, and sensorineural hearing loss.

The child was first seen for auditory brainstem response testing at one year of age as a cross-check to the inconsistent responses in the moderate hearing loss range noted during sound-field behavioral testing.

The results, shown in figure 11 are represented by a clearly observable and repeatable wave V down to 75 dBnHL in the right and 55 dBnHL in the left, thereby suggesting probably no poorer than a severe and moderate sensorineural loss for the right and left ears, respectively. She was subsequently fitted with appropriate binaural amplification and enrolled in an auditory rehabilitiation program. The child has since been monitored annually via age appropriate behavioral audiometric techniques.

At the age of almost five years her sound-field responses at 1000 and 4000 Hz showed evidence of marked threshold shift to the severe hearing loss range. Repeat auditory brainstem responses, presented in figure 12, supported the onset of a progressive hearing loss wherein wave V threshold for the right ear was now at 80 dB, while that for the left was at 70 dBnHL representing a 15 dB threshold shift.

This case favors continued ABR monitoring as a complement to behavioral techniques that do not allow intra-aural separation of threshold responses in children at risk for acute progressive disseminating disease. By so doing, we are able to institute immediate management modifications relative to amplification needs and educational goals.

CASE #2

The second scenario presents a reverse image. This 23 month old female born with unconjugated, or indirect hyperbilirubinemia secondary to hemolytic disease was initially seen for ABR screening in the intensive-care nursery.

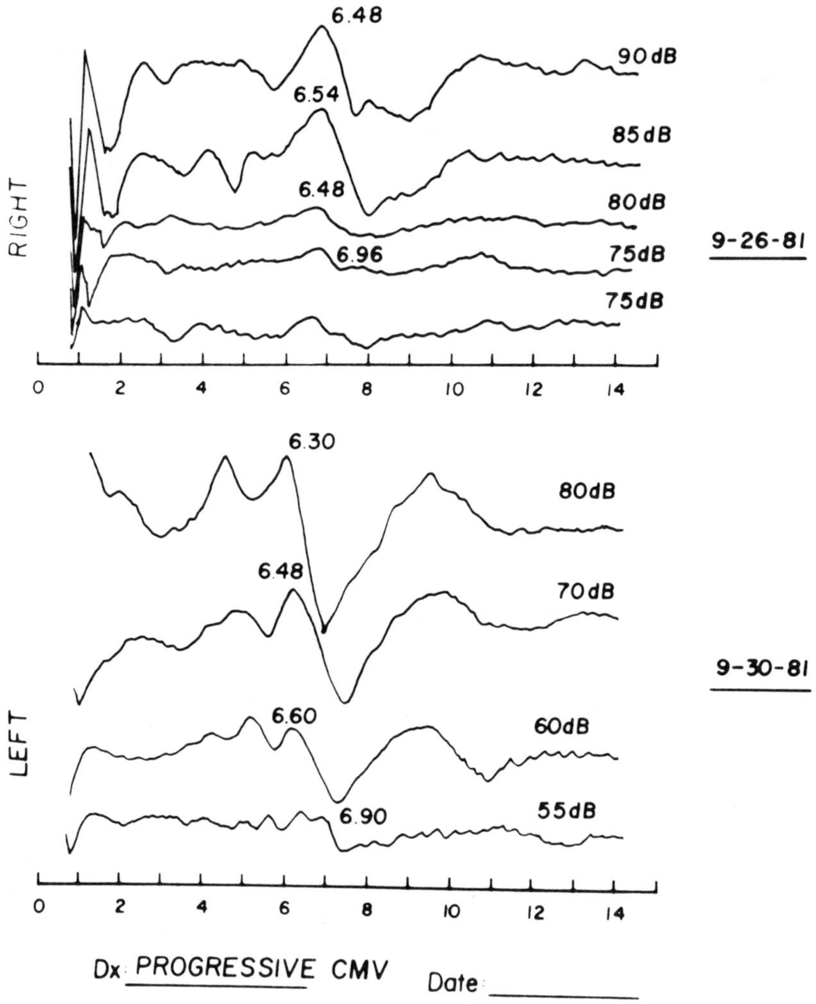

Figure 11. Auditory brainstem responses for a child with progressive CMV (Case #1).

The results shown in figure 13 depict essentially no visually detectable response, except perhaps a fragment of Wave I. A more detailed latency-intensity series at age three months (figure 14) demonstrated a visible, I, III, and V at 90 dBnHL in the left ear with wave V and consequently the I-V inter-peak interval abnormally prolonged. Wave V responses were apparent and replicated down to 75 dB on the left. On the right ear, however, only wave I continued to be observed through 90 dBnHL supporting that initially seen in the ICN and highlighting the combined peripheral and central effects so common in these children. These estimates of severe bilateral hearing loss continued to exist both in terms of ABR monitoring and as evidenced by an absence of acoustic responsi-

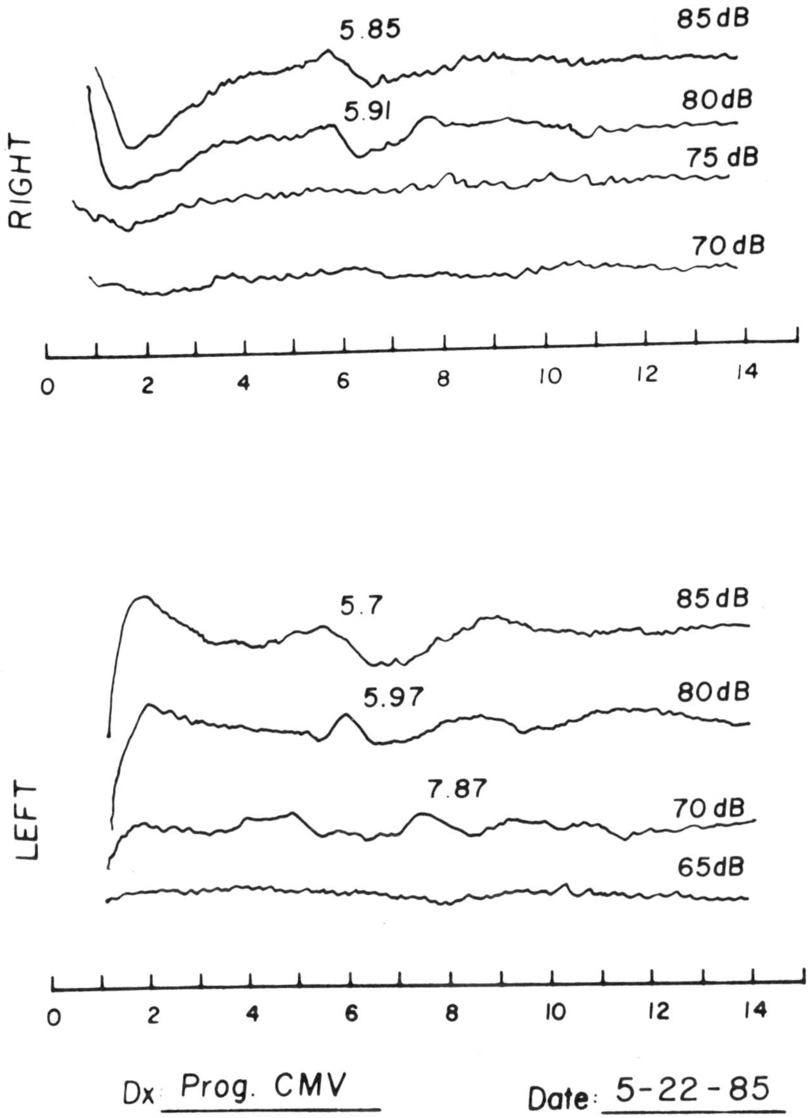

Figure 12. Repeat auditory brainstem responses for the child described in Case #1 illustrating the progressive nature of the disease.

vity to visual reinforcement strategies. Consequently, she was fitted with binaural amplification, and auditory rehabilitation therapy was initiated.

Represented in figure 15 is the most recent latency-intensity series for the right ear obtained to click stimuli on this child. Results for the left ear are equally as dramatic although the slope of the wave V function is slightly shifted to the right. As can be seen, at 80 dBnHL, waves I-V appear at normal, abso-

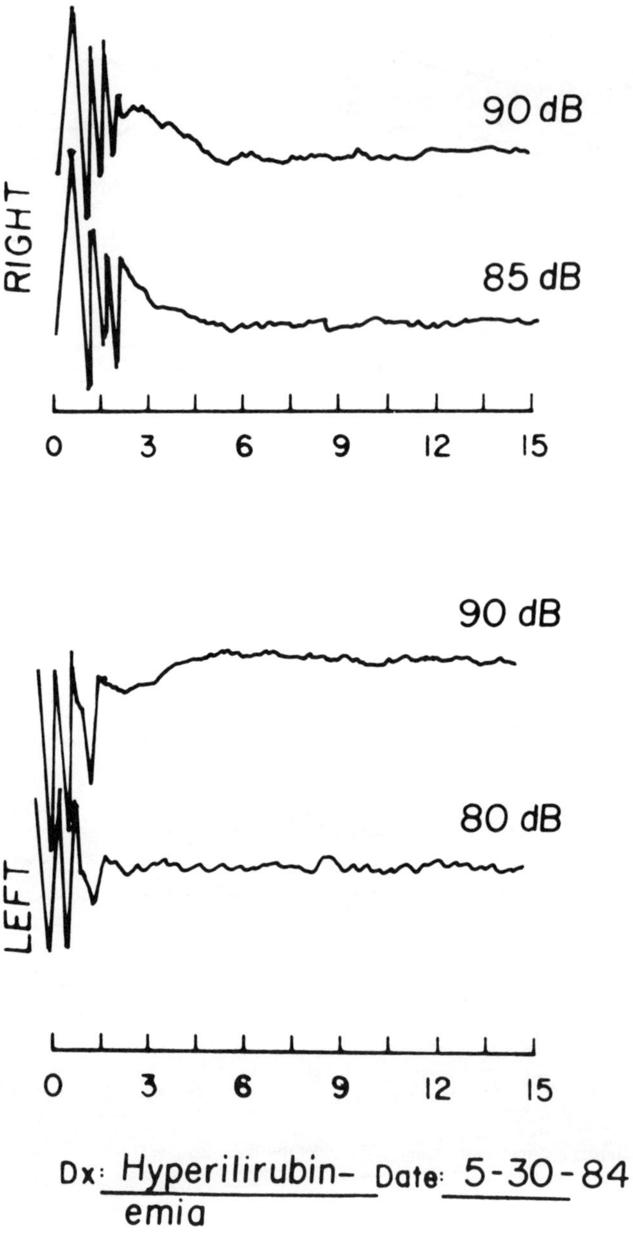

Figure 13. Initial auditory brainstem responses recorded in the neonatal nursery for a child born with hyperbilirubinemia. (Case #2).

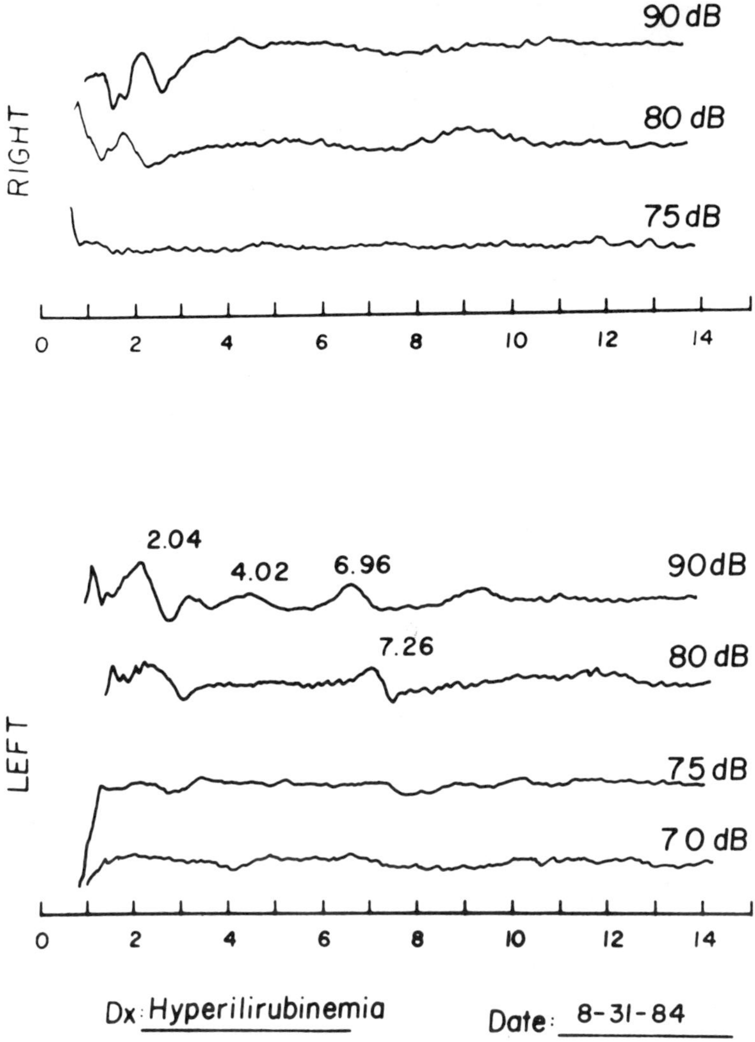

Figure 14. Latency-intensity series for Case #2 suggesting some slight improvement in hearing sensitivity.

lute, and interpeak latencies, although amplitudes are somewhat depressed. Of critical importance to the child's management, however, is that wave V threshold is now 20 dBnHL, bilaterally; an improvement of about 60 dB. Tone-pip thresholds were 30 dBnHL in the right and 35 dBnHL in the left. Obviously, the hearing aids have since been removed from the child and she continues to develop well.

This case again highlights the need for continuous evoked potential monitoring in high-risk children. We, and others (Dennis, J. M., personal communica-

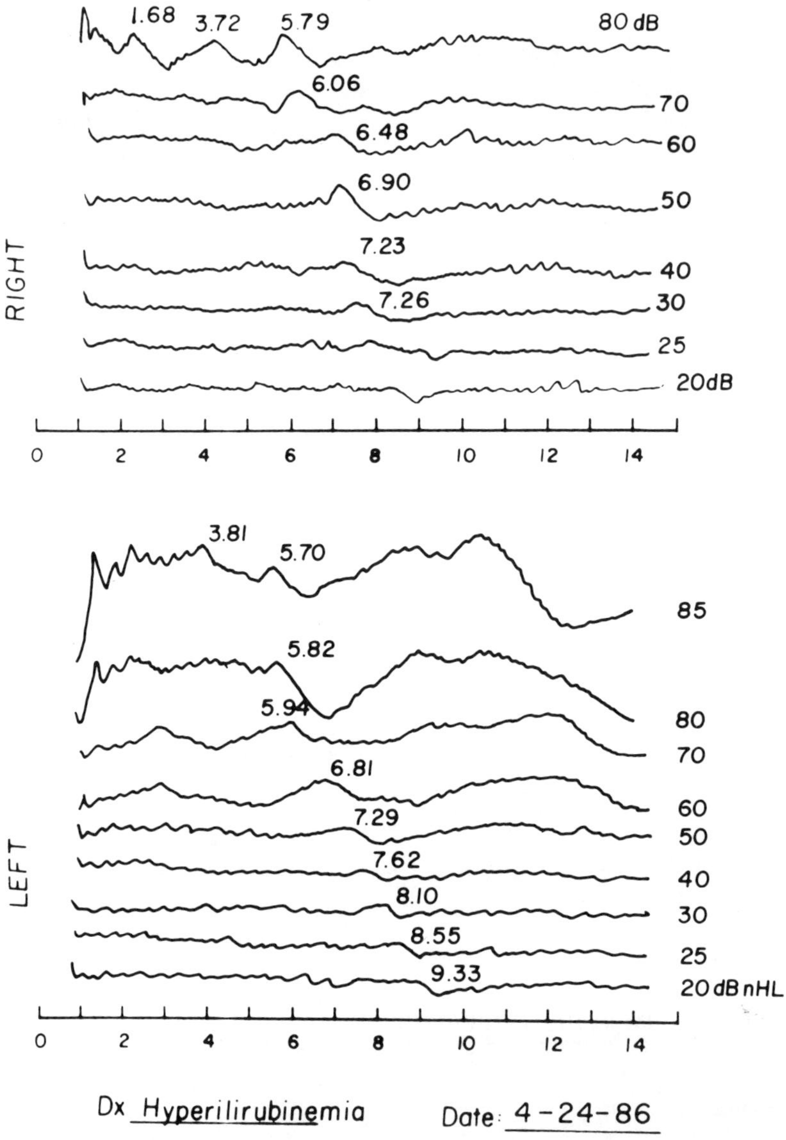

Figure 15. Latency-intensity series for Case #2 recorded two years following the initial ABR screening. Note the clear presence of wave V down to near normal limits, bilaterally.

tion), have seen several cases of improvement in auditory sensitivity over time in hyperbilirubinemic children. All too often, such children are lost to routine electrophysiological follow-up. Clearly, untimely management of this child could have led to amplification-induced hearing loss, thus compromising the child's future developmental course.

CASE #3

The final case represents a departure from the two previous ones. This was a two year old male who was first seen at age 21 months to substantiate behavioral sound field results consistent with moderate-to-severe-hearing loss in at least the better ear. The child presented with speech and language delay and maternal reports of unresponsitivity to sound.

Auditory brainstem responses shown in figure 16 revealed an observable wave V down to 75 dBnHL on the right, coupled with no response to left ear click stimulation. Right ear 1000 and 4000 Hz tone-pip thresholds were 80 dB and 70 dBnHL, respectively as illustrated in figure 17. Complimentary tympanometry showed evidence of increased stiffness in the absence of a pressure disturbance perhaps due to minor thickening of the tympanic membrane. The child was ultimately referred for otologic examination to insure against hearing aid contraindication at which time some streaking was observed on both drumheads along with some reduced mobility at pneumo-otoscopy. More obvious

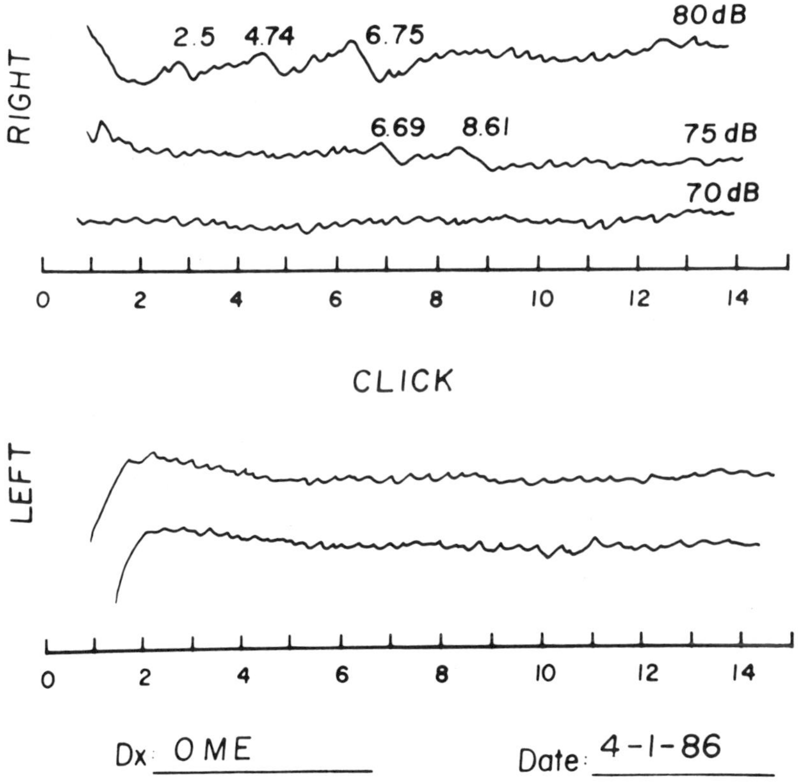

Figure 16. Initial ABR of a 21 month old child who presented with speech and language delay (Case #3).

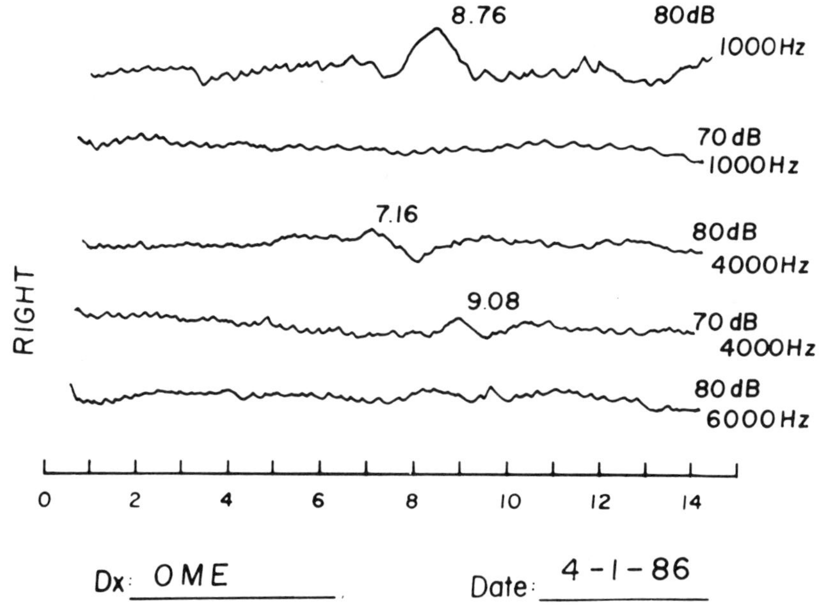

Figure 17. Auditory brainstem responses for Case #3 recorded to 1000 Hz and 4000 Hz tone pips.

was the presence of a mucoid nasal discharge bilaterally. The child was subsequently treated with amoxicillin prophylaxis for early otitis media. Although hearing-aid recommendation was provided, fitting was delayed in favor of repeat ABR evaluation to determine if the quiescent OME might not have affected the initial results. Recall that neither the immittance results nor pneumo-otoscopic exam were very impressive for OME.

The repeat click-evoked ABRs two months post antimicrobial therapy are presented in figure 18. Wave V threshold is now 50 dB on the left and 45 dBnHL on the right; certainly a dramatic decrease in threshold sensitivity, and moreover, a situation that may have led to inappropriate amplification selection had it not been for a very astute pediatric electrophysiologist and an equally aware pediatric otolaryngologist who had confidence in ABR.

These three cases serve to remind us of the exquisite value of sensory evoked potentials in pediatric audiologic diagnosis and monitoring. We are naturally convinced that the entire complement of evoked potentials represents the most powerful tool available to the audiologist today in determining the integrity of the peripheral and central auditory pathway.

Afterword

In this paper we have attempted to review at least some of the current thought on hearing loss estimation using auditory evoked potentials. It is evident that despite a flurry of research attempts to design a technique to estimate low frequency hearing, none has been very successful. In fact, one can even argue

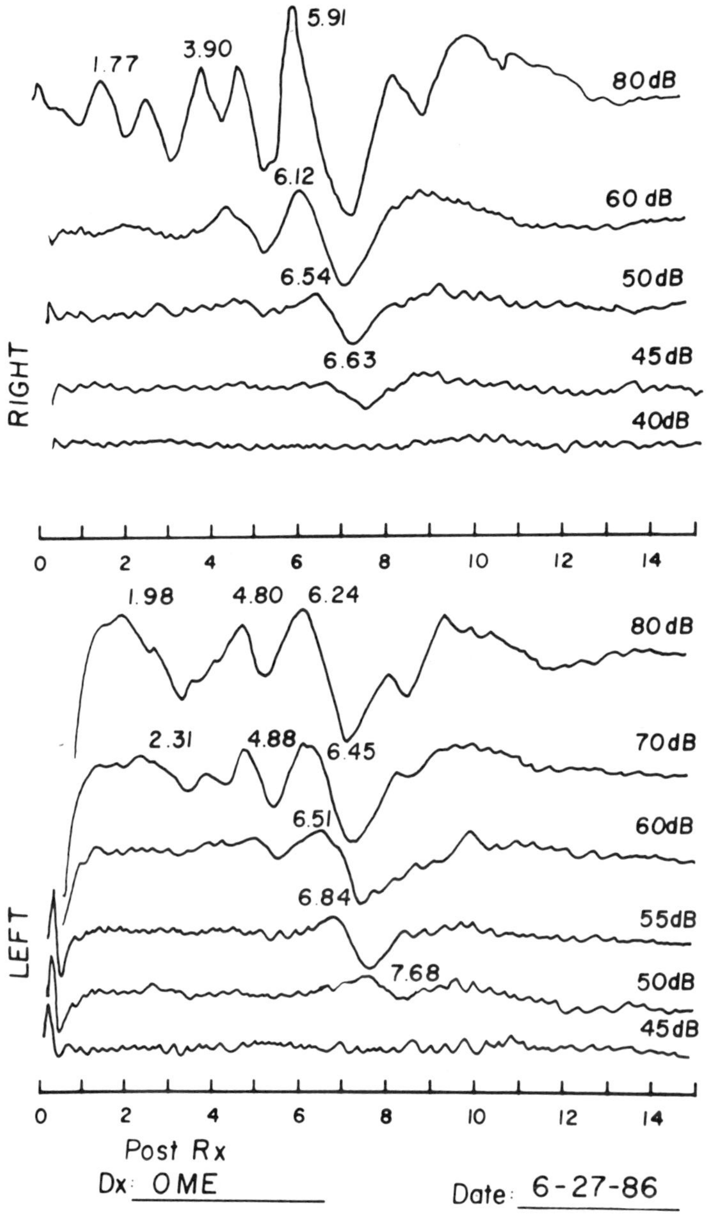

Figure 18. Auditory brainstem responses for Case #3 following treatment for otitis media with effusion.

against the need for any of these so-called place-specific procedures over the click evoked ABR in hearing loss estimation. We presume that the point prevalence of rising audiometric contour in children is quite low. Thus, is all of the research effort put forth in the search for a low-frequency predictor justified?

Will such information on this select group of children actually alter our habilitative management strategy? Conversely, in good hands the click evoked ABR does respectably well in estimating hearing loss in the frequency region critical to consonant recognition (i.e., 1000–4000 Hz). Not only is this frequency band important to speech understanding, but it is also given the most emphasis in the fitting of appropriate amplification.

With reference to amplification we add one final caveat. There has been some impetus over the past several years for employing ABR threshold strategies under conditions of amplification in an effort to derive an electrophysiological analog to functional gain. We have always maintained that this is a rather dubious technique since, to our knowledge, no hearing aid can respond rapidly enough to an onset transient without creating marked spectral splatter. The result from this, of course, will be measurable downward shift in the wave V latency-intensity function regardless of the frequency response characteristics of the amplifier, thus supporting the cochlear excitation pattern from base to apex. One could be easily led into a false sense of security by thinking that this single numerical value correlates to the gain-by-frequency function. This point was recently substantiated by Beauchaine et al. (1986) who showed that the aided wave V latency-intensity function was the same for a series of three electroacoustically heterogeneous hearing aids. Clearly, with recent advances in probe tube microphone technology for measuring the output spectrum of a hearing aid in-situ, even with young infants, there is no plausible reason to rely on a click-evoked ABR to determine functional gain, since it will neither identify nor quantify the gain that a hearing aid provides across individual frequencies.

Finally, while definitive knowledge of peripheral auditory system integrity is an indispensable prerequisite to formulating early and appropriate treatment and management of the hearing-impaired child, auditory evoked potentials can be equally contributive to evaluating the effects of the wide spectrum of neuropathologies that compromise a child's normal developmental course. Nonetheless, the neurodiagnostic and monitoring applications of these robust bioelectric events have not received the same degree of attention as they have with the adult population. Unfortunately, to review the wealth of clinical ABR material we have gathered on a host of these unique pediatric disorders is beyond the scope of this chapter.

References

Beauchaine, K. A., Gorga, M. P., Reiland, J. K., and Larson, L. 1986. Application of ABRs to the hearing-aid selection process: Preliminary data. *Journal of Speech and Hearing Research* 29:120–128.

Brown, D. D., and Shallop, J. K. 1982. A clinically useful 500 Hz response. *Nicolet Potentials* 1: 9–12.

Davis, H., and Hirsch, S. K. 1976. The audiometric utility of the brain stem response to low frequency sounds. *Audiology* 15:181–195.

Davis, H., and Hirsch, S. K. 1979. A slow brainstem response for low-frequency audiometry. *Audiology* 18:445–461.

Don, M., Eggermont, J. J., and Brackmann, D. E. 1979. Reconstruction of the audiogram using brain stem responses and high-pass noise masking. *Annals of Otolology, Rhinolology and Laryngology* 88:(Suppl. 57), 1.

Eggermont, J. J., and Don, M. 1982. Analysis of click-evoked brainstem auditory electric potentials using high-pass noise masking and its clinical application. *Annals of the New York Academy of Science* 338:471.

Elberling, C. 1974. Action potentials along the cochlear partition recorded from the ear canal in man. *Scandinavian Audiology* 3:13.

Fifer, R. C., Jerger, J. F., and Null, D. 1985. Low-frequency threshold prediction in neonates. *Asha* 27:81.

Galambos, R., Makeig, S., and Talmachoff, P. J. 1981. A 40-Hz auditory potential recorded from the human scalp. *Proceedings of the National Academy of Sciences of the United States of America* 78:263–264.

Hyde, M. 1985. Instrumentation and signal processing. *In* J. Jacobson (ed.). *The Auditory Brainstem Response*. San Diego: College Hill Press.

Jerger, J., Chmiel, R., Frost, J. D., and Coker, N. 1986. Effect of sleep on the auditory steady state evoked potential. *Ear and Hearing* 7:240–245.

Kileny, P. 1983. Auditory evoked middle-latency responses; Current issues. *Seminars in Hearing* 4:403–413.

Laukli, E., and Mair, I. W. S. 1986. Frequency specificity of the auditory brainstem responses: A derived study. *Scandinavian Audiology* 3:141–146.

McRandle, C., Smith, M., and Goldstein, R. 1974. Early averaged electroencephalic responses to clicks in neonates. *Annals of Otology, Rhinology and Laryngology* 83:695–702.

Mendel, M. I., Adkinson, C. D., and Harker, L. A. 1977. Middle components of the auditory evoked potentials in infants. *Annals of Otology, Rhinology and Laryngology* 86:293–299.

Sherg, M. 1982. Distortion of the middle latency auditory response produced by analog filtering. *Scandinavian Audiology* 11:57–60.

Schwartz, D. M., Larson, V., and De Chicchis, A. R. 1981. Spectral characteristics of air and bone transducers used to record the auditory brainstem response. *Ear and Hearing* 6:274–277.

Stappells, D. R., and Picton, T. W. 1981. Technical aspects of brainstem evoked potential audiometry using tones. *Ear and Hearing* 2:20–29.

Stappells, D. R., Picton, T. W., Perez-Abalo, M., Read, D., and Smith, A. 1985. Frequency specificity in EP audiometry. *In* J. Jacobson (ed.). *The Auditory Brainstem Response*. San Diego: College Hill Press.

Suzuki, T., Hirai, Y., and Horiuchi, K. 1977. Auditory brainstem responses to pure tone stimuli. *Scandinavian Audiology* 6:51–56.

Suzuki, T., and Horiuchi, K. 1977. Effect of high-pass filter on auditory brainstem responses to tone pips. *Scandinavian Audiology* 6:123–126.

Suzuki, T., Hirabayshi, M., and Kobayashi K. 1983. Auditory middle responses in young children. *British Journal of Audiology* 17:1–4.

Suzuki, T., Hirabayashi, M., and Kobayashi, K. 1984. Effects of analog and digital filtering on auditory middle latency responses in adults and young children. *Annals of Otology, Rhinology and Laryngology* 93:267–270.

Szyfter, W., Dauman, R., and de Sauvage, R. C. 1984. 40 Hz middle latency responses to low frequency tone pips in normally hearing adults. *The Journal of Otolaryngology* 13(5):275–280.

Teas, D. C., Eldredge, D. H., and Davis, H. 1962. Coclear responses to acoustic transients: and interpretation of whole-nerve action potentials. *Journal of the Acoustical Society of America* 34:1438.

Wolf, K. E., and Goldstein, R. 1980. Middle component AERs from neonates to low-level tonal stimuli. *Journal of Speech and Hearing Research* 23:185–201.

Zerlin, S. S., and Naunton, R. R. 1976. Electrocochleographic detection of hearing impairment. *In* F. H. Bess (ed.). *Childhood Deafness: Causation, Assessment & Management*. New York: Grune & Stratton, Inc.

Chapter 12

Recent Developments in Acoustic Immittance Measurements with Children

Jerry L. Northern

The use of acoustic immittance measurements in the auditory evaluation of children has improved dramatically the efficiency and accuracy of pediatric audiology. In fact, it is generally agreed that the hearing evaluation of any child is incomplete without acoustic immittance measurements. The applications of acoustic immittance measurements are broad enough to include hearing screening programs, diagnostic audiology work-ups, prediction of hearing sensitivity with acoustic reflex measurements, and management/monitoring of children with middle ear effusion.

The development of new immittance equipment reflects the widening market and increased demand for easy-to-use instruments. There are currently more than 20 commercially available immittance meters ranging from microprocessor-based clinical units with data storage capabilities to miniaturized hand-held screening devices. Although this increase in the number of instruments has led to automated and easy-to-use test equipment capable of recording an automatic tympanogram as well as measuring an ipsilateral acoustic reflex in a matter of seconds, the lack of agreement in manufacturing standards is readily apparent. Few if any validating studies exist for the majority of immittance meters currently available for clinical use (Schwartz 1986).

An important part of this growth of immittance audiometry is the increased awareness among primary care physicians, especially pediatricians and family practitioners, of its use in identifying middle ear effusion in children (Downs and Northern 1986). A 1984 Colorado statewide survey of 484 primary care physicians, who manage the health care of children younger than three years of age, found that 22% of these physicians owned tympanometers, including 39% of the responding pediatricians. In this Colorado survey, only 14% of the physicians reported using tympanometry at each well-child check, and the average number of times used per day was only 2.2. These numbers represent an obvious underuse of this important technique. In a similar study conducted in Tennessee, 33% of the primary care physicians surveyed, who see children under the age of 36 months, used tympanometry at each well-child visit (Bess and Kenworthy 1986).

The clinical utility of acoustic immittance measurements with children is well established and does not need additional discussion (Brooks 1982). Therefore, this chapter will focus on immittance applications that are undergoing development or refinement, as well as on immittance applications that may be considered controversial, including recent advances in immittance measurements in infants, the application of immittance measurements in predicting hearing sensitivity, acoustic reflectometry, and the role of immittance testing in mass screening programs.

Immittance Measurements In Infants

The use of immittance measurements in neonates and infants has had a stormy, albeit interesting, development (Northern 1981). Keith published the first reports of acoustic immittance tests in infants in 1973 and 1975. With an instrument using a 220-Hz probe tone, Keith evaluated 60 neonates whose ages ranged between 2½ hours and 151 hours, and found that although most of the neonates had normal tympanograms, he did note a number of tympanograms with a "*w*-shape," or bimodal peak pattern. He attempted to elicit acoustic reflexes with a 220-Hz probe tone in these newborns, but found that only 33% of the babies showed stapedial reflex responses. Ten percent of the infants did not have an acoustic reflex in either ear at the time of testing, but later were confirmed to have normal hearing responses. Keith and Bench (1978) reached an important conclusion: that tympanometry and acoustic reflex measurement must always be done together when testing neonates; ". . . to do less may result in the erroneous conclusion that tympanometry is neither accurate nor reliable in infants."

In an often cited publication by Paradise, Smith, and Bluestone (1976), results were reported that showed a high positive correlation of 86% between tympanometry and otoscopy in 280 children between 10 days and 5 years of age. Poor correlation, however, was noted between these two measures in infants less than 7 months of age. In fact, from 43 infants less than 7 months of age, nearly half had middle ear effusion confirmed by myringotomy; yet 24 of the 40 abnormal ears displayed normal tympanograms. It was then concluded that although tympanometry had much to offer in the diagnosis of middle ear effusion, the use of tympanometry in infants less than 7 months of age was not recommended. This guideline has been widely accepted as a matter of undisputed fact by most primary care physicians, who then generalize this finding to indicate that immittance measurements should not be conducted in neonates and young infants.

Subsequent studies have been conducted and published showing that tympanometry with acoustic reflex measurements can be used to determine the status of the infant middle ear with high validity and reliability. Schwartz and Schwartz (1978) report data showing that while a normal tympanogram cannot be considered evidence of a mobile tympanic membrane or effusion-free middle ear, the presence of an acoustic reflex with a normal tympanogram confirms normal middle ear status. Freyss et al. (1980) found that the presence of the acoustic reflex provided a higher sensitivity than tympanometry alone for separating normal dry middle ears from middle ears with fluid; however, as initially reported by Keith (1973), measurement of the acoustic reflex in infants is no simple task.

An intriguing finding concerning infant acoustic reflexes was reported by McCandless and Allred (1978), who showed that with a 220-Hz probe tone only 4% of 53 infants less than 48 hours of age demonstrated an acoustic reflex. But when the probe tone was increased to a frequency of 660 Hz, an astounding 89% of the same infants had an acoustic reflex. McCandless and Allred opened the door for subsequent research on immittance measurements in infants by suggesting that although a 220-Hz probe tone was superior for infant tympanometry tracings, the 660-Hz probe tone was clearly better for acoustic reflex evaluation.

In a series of studies of acoustic reflexes in infants, Bennett and Weatherby (1979, 1982; Weatherby and Bennett 1980) used a two-component variable probe-tone immittance meter to record contralateral acoustic reflexes in newborns. Their studies show that as the probe-tone frequency is raised, the prevalence of the reflex increases, while the threshold of the acoustic reflex decreases. With a maximum intensity of 96 dB sound pressure level (SPL), no reflexes were detected with a 220-Hz probe tone, whereas with probe tones above 800 Hz all newborns exhibited acoustic reflexes. Bennett (1984) pointed out that calibration of the contralateral earphone stimulus in infants is important because of the smaller volume of newborn ear canals, and that differences in sound-pressure levels between adults and infants under earphones can easily exceed 6 dB. Bennett confirms that the optimal probe-tone frequency for detecting acoustic reflexes in neonates is 1400 Hz. At low frequencies the reduced impedance of the tympanic membrane effectively shunts the higher impedance of the middle ear, and small impedance changes caused by the reflex contraction cannot be measured.

The interaction between developmental changes in the newborn tympanic membrane and the acoustics of the external ear canal help to clarify immittance results in infants. Several studies, including Vanhuyse, Creten, and Van Camp (1975), Margolis and Popelka (1977), and Himelfarb, Popelka, and Shannon (1979), have shown that the double-peaked tympanograms are related to interactions between the acoustic resistance and acoustic reactance components of acoustic impedance. If the resistance value is greater than the reactance value near ambient pressure, a double-peaked susceptance tympanogram occurs. The introduction of positive air pressure to make the ear canal act like a hard-wall cavity is suspect in infants, whose osseous portion of the external auditory meatus is not completely developed. This fact may be responsible for the oft-noted monotonically increasing tympanogram obtained from newborn ear canals, and the smoothed, or humped tympanograms which can be obtained from infants with middle ear effusion.

Recently, in a thorough study of tympanometry and acoustic reflexes in neonates, Sprague, Wiley, and Goldstein (1985) reported 80% observable reflexes with the 660-Hz probe tone, and 50% observable reflexes with a 220-Hz probe tone with ipsilateral and contralateral activating stimuli. Instead of a standard earphone cushion for the contralateral stimulus, these researchers used insert receivers and found lower acoustic reflex thresholds than previously reported in other studies. The characteristics of the neonatal acoustic reflex reported by Sprague et al. (1985) were similar to those seen in adults. Reflex magnitude increased with stimulus activator intensity level, but the slope of acoustic reflex growth varied from infant to infant. The actual magnitude of the infant acoustic reflex was smaller than generally noted in adults. Barajas et al. (1981) had previously found that ipsilateral neonatal reflexes were present to broadband noise with a 1000-Hz stimulus. No clear relations were observed between tympanometric patterns and acoustic reflex characteristics. Thus, the tympanogram alone was not sensitive enough to reflect the acoustic-admittance characteristics of the neonatal ear.

McMillan et al. (1985) investigated ipsilateral and contralateral acoustic reflexes in neonates with probe tones of 220 Hz and 660 Hz. Their results indicated that ipsilateral and contralateral reflexes to pure-tone activators occurred three times more frequently with a 660-Hz probe tone (76%) than with the 220-Hz probe tone (24%). The maximum detection rate of 76% occurred with 1000- and 2000-Hz ipsilateral activating stimuli and the 660-Hz probe tone.

Wright et al. (1985) followed 210 infants during the initial two years of life with routine pneumatic otoscopy and immittance at each physician encounter. Tympanometry proved to have high predictive value (86%) for confirming normal ears, but relatively poor predictive value (58%) for detecting abnormal ears. In general, the tympanometrically abnormal ear often appears normal during the otoscopic exam. The real problem is the determination of which procedure is really the criterion against which the other procedures should be compared. Otoscopy is most often accepted as the criterion test against which to compare other screening techniques, although it is well known that the accuracy of otosocopy is only as valid as the individual behind the otoscope (Paradise et al. 1976). Since otoscopy is so subjective, it can be argued that *immittance* should be the criterion procedure because of its objectivity and test-retest reliability. Generally speaking, otoscopy used as the criterion (as reported by Wright et al. 1985) produces higher sensitivity agreement, since fewer subjects "fail" otoscopy while many subjects may "fail" tympanometric screening (Northern and Downs 1984).

During the past decade researchers have systematically supported Margolis's (1978) description of infant immittance measurements as both "promising and perplexing." There is indeed ample reason to continue utilizing immittance techniques in infants; however, clinical interpretation must be based on a thorough understanding of the complex interaction between the anatomy and development of the infant ear canal and the acoustic characteristics of the immittance measuring instrument. It would appear that the ultimate clinical infant immittance meter is not yet commercially available, but the data base now seems substantial enough for equipment manufacturers to devise an easy-to-use, multi-frequency probe-tone device for tympanometric and acoustic reflex measurement in newborns.

Hearing Prediction With The Acoustic Reflex

An area of acoustic immittance application that has caught the interest of researchers is the attempt to predict hearing levels through elicitation of the acoustic reflex. Since the revolutionary report by Niemeyer and Sesterhenn (1974), who initially developed the technique of determining air-conduction hearing thresholds from stapedial reflex measurements with broadband noise and pure tones, scores of papers have been published with various refinements of the procedure. Although the implications of these techniques with children are most important, it is somewhat surprising that few publications have actually reported data from hearing-impaired youngsters.

The various procedures for predicting hearing are based on the fact that the acoustic reflex threshold for broadband noise is lower than the acoustic reflex threshold for pure tones, and that the difference in decibels between the two thresholds is related in linear fashion to the severity of sensorineural hearing impairment. The specific techniques have been divided into three general categories: Sensitivity Prediction with the Acoustic Reflex (SPAR), regression equations, and the bivariate plot system (Hall and Bleakney 1981). According to Hall (1980), the original optimism expressed for this objective estimation of hearing sensitivity through a clinically efficient procedure has been tempered because of inherent weaknesses that have come to light with each of the general prediction methods. The original Niemeyer and Sesterhenn equation and the Sensitivity Prediction (SPAR) technique of Jerger et al. (1974) are characterized by a sizable proportion of prediction errors in the 20 to 40% range; the regression equations often underestimate severe hearing loss; and the bivariate plot system simply categorizes patients as having either normal hearing or hearing loss greater than 30 dB HL. Thorough discussions of each of the prediction techniques and their underlying assumptions, as well as reviews of the data that identified various influencing factors of prediction accuracy, have been published (Popelka 1981 and Silman 1984).

The SPAR methods, regression equations, and bivariate plot systems all estimate hearing loss with accuracy rates in excess of 60%, but none of the techniques is able to predict invariably the presence of hearing loss without error (Hall and Bleakney 1981). Hearing loss prediction from the acoustic reflex is influenced by a number of variables which unfortunately are common in the evaluation of hearing in children. These variables include chronological age, minor middle ear abnormalities, and audiometric configuration of hearing loss. Studies by both Keith (1977) and Jerger et al. (1978) suggest that predictive accuracy of hearing levels through the acoustic reflex is more successful in children than in adults. The Jerger et al. study (1978), utilizing the SPAR procedure, predicted normal hearing in children with 100% accuracy, severe hearing loss with 85% accuracy, and moderate hearing loss with somewhat less accuracy at 54%. Using the acoustic reflex threshold for the broadband noise alone, Keith, in his 1977 study, was able to identify normal-hearing children with 87% accuracy, and children with hearing impairment with an astonishing 97% accuracy. Based on these data, Keith proposed a cutoff screening point of 85 dB SPL for the broadband acoustic reflex threshold, to be used as a simple screening measure to separate normal-hearing and hearing-impaired children.

One extremely beneficial application of the prediction of hearing loss through the acoustic reflex should be in the examination of difficult-to-test special populations such as the mentally retarded. Only two studies have reported data from retarded populations, and both studies were composed primarily of retarded adults (Niswander and Ruth 1977; Poole, Sheeley, and Hannah 1982). Both studies utilized the SPAR procedure and reported accuracy in predicting hearing levels to be somewhat less than 60%. Both studies concluded that the SPAR test is a useful addition to the audiologist's repertoire, particularly for retarded individuals who are difficult to test.

In reviewing the literature dealing with immittance measurements of the acoustic reflex to assess hearing levels, it must be noted that the studies are dominated by adult data, and few studies report data from children. Although Margolis et al. (1981) state that neonate acoustic reflex thresholds appear to stabilize to adult norms by two to four months of age, Silman et al. (1984) point out the need to collect normative data from a large pediatric sampling, in which the degree and configuration of hearing loss is unrestricted, in order to present an unbiased data base for this population.

An innovative application of acoustic reflex measurement was described recently by Jerger et al. (1986). Jerger et al. used standard immittance measurement techniques to demonstrate contralateral stapedial reflex contractions to intracochlear electrical stimulation in an adult cochlear implant recipient. Their results indicate that various electrode configurations of a multi-channel implant device may be evaluated with acoustic reflex measurements. This immittance application may be especially valuable with the preoperative and postoperative evaluation of potential implant candidates who are too young to make adequate physiological responses to cochlear implant settings.

ACOUSTIC REFLECTOMETRY

Recently a new device known as the acoustic otoscope has been introduced as a simple, noninvasive screening instrument for identifying the presence of middle ear fluid in children. Initially described by Teele and Teele (1984), the acoustic otoscope was designed to overcome the disadvantages of acoustic immittance measurement. That is to say, the acoustic otoscope requires no hermetic seal at the ear canal and is effective even when the child is crying or when the ear canal is partially obscured with cerumen.

The acoustic otoscope generates a 100-millisecond multifrequency sweep beween 2000 Hz and 4500 Hz at a sound pressure of 80 dB SPL. The pickup microphone measures the amplitude of the reflected probe tone from the plane of the tympanic membrane. The instrument works on quarter-wavelength theory, so that the reflected wave completely cancels the principle wave in the external ear canal at a distance of one-quarter wavelength from the tympanic membrane. Thus, the reflected sound is inversely proportional to the total sound; a greater reflection produces a reduced amplitude suggestive of middle ear effusion.

To conduct the test, the examiner simply "aims" the speculum of the acoustic otoscope into the child's ear canal and presses the activator button. The instrument is quickly repositioned until the highest level of reflectometry is noted on the LED vertical display. Interpreters of the reflectometry scale generally agree that readings of 0 to 2 represent a normal middle ear; readings of 3 to 4 represent possible middle ear effusion; and readings greater than 5 indicate the presence of middle ear fluid.

The early studies of Teele and Teele (1984) reported results from nearly 260 children examined with the acoustic otoscope. Their acoustic otoscope reflectivity sensitivity scores were 94% and 99% with specificity scores of 79% and 83%. These investigators concluded that acoustic reflectometry adds considerably to the screening tools currently available for identifying children with middle ear effusion.

Lampe et al. (1985) compared results from acoustic reflectometry with tympanocentesis or myringotomy in 75 patients between 6 months and 13 years of age. They found a highly significant relationship between ears with middle ear effusion and reflectivity values of 5 or greater, and ears with no middle ear effusion and reflectivity values of 4 or less. With a reflectivity reading of 5 or greater, the acoustic otoscope correctly identified nearly 87% of ears with middle ear effusion, and correctly identified 70% of ears without effusion based on a reading of 4 or less. These authors found the reflectometry technique to be a valuable adjunct to current diagnostic tools because it is objective, rapid, and reliable irrespective of age, crying, cerumen, or lack of cooperation from the child.

A less positive report on the reflectometer was published by Buhrer, Wall, and Schuster (1985), who evaluated 60 children with the acoustic reflectometer, pure tones, immittance, and otologic evaluation. They found reflectometry to be the least sensitive and least specific of the screening procedures. Their study differed from previous studies in that they used the acoustic otoscope in a general otologic clinic situation—not just for identifying the presence or absence of middle ear fluid. They also used a reflective fail value of 3 and considered this reading in conjunction with the length reading available on the acoustic otoscope. The ear canal length reading is described by the manufacturer, but is generally disregarded by clinicians; however, Buhrer et al. concluded that when the acoustic otoscope is used as intended, i.e., as a supplement to pneumatic otoscopy in the diagnosis of middle ear effusion, the test can be beneficial and can save clinical time. They suggest that the reflectometer performs best when (1) digital readings of 5 or greater are considered positive, (2) ear canal length readings are ignored, (3) it is used to confirm middle ear effusion, and (4) ears are clear of cerumen occlusions.

Kenworthy, Bess, and Wright, in a personal communication, discuss evaluating the acoustic otoscope in tests of children under 12 months of age, using smaller experimental tips of 6.25, 4.5, and 3.0 cm. Based on their initial evaluation of 36 ears from 22 children, agreement between otoscopic examinations and reflectometry results are approximately 60%, thereby leaving some question about the suitability of the experimental small tips for infants at this time.

A thorough evaluation of the acoustic otoscope in children was reported by Schwartz and Schwartz (1986) from a cohort of 511 ears of 256 children seen in a private practice pediatric office. The ages of the children ranged from 2 months to 14 years. Schwartz and Schwartz applied decision-making analyses and established Receiver Operating Characteristics (ROC) curves with a large sample of 160 children to illustrate the effects of various cut-off criteria on true- and false-positive rates for reflectometry and tympanometry. For example, consistent with the manufacturer's suggestion, the cutoff criterion of 5 provides a sensitivity of 88% and a specificity rate of 83%. They noted that the length measurement provided by the acoustic otoscope has no clinical usefulness. Schwartz and Schwartz concluded that the acoustic otoscope complements traditional methods for detecting middle ear fluid in otherwise asymptomatic children. They caution, however, that the acoustic otoscope should not be used as a technique to identify general pathologies of the ear.

SCREENING FOR MIDDLE EAR DISEASE

This topic has generated an overwhelming volume of literature, primarily initiated by a national conference held in Nashville during the summer of 1977, dealing with the use of immittance measurements in screening for middle ear disease in children. The Nashville conference resulted in a statement that ". . . the Task Force does *not* recommend the use of impedance measurements for universal [mass] screening on a routine basis for the detection of middle ear disorders in children of any age group" (Harford et al. 1979); however, the Nashville Task Force proceeded to generate a set of guidelines for those immittance screening programs already in existence, as well as to stimulate additional research to evaluate immittance testing as a screening method for infants and children.

Not long after publication of the Nashville guidelines, the American Speech-Language-Hearing Association (ASHA) generated their own set of Guidelines for Acoustic Immittance Screening of Middle-Ear Function (1979). The procedural considerations for both sets of recommendations are remarkably similar—utilizing tympanometry and the acoustic reflex to reach a "pass/fail" decision. Their primary difference centers on the outcome for children who fail the initial screening. The Nashville guidelines recommend a retest of all failures within four to six weeks, while the ASHA guidelines recommend immediate medical referral for all those children who have an abnormal middle ear pressure and an absent acoustic reflex.

Several investigators have undertaken mass screening projects with a goal of evaluating one or both sets of guidelines, but no clear advantages have emerged for either set of referral criteria (Wall et al. 1985); in fact, several studies found it necessary to alter referral criteria midstream in their data collection because of overreferral problems (Lucker 1980; Queen et al. 1981; Dermody, Curotta, and Mackie 1983; Roush and Tait 1985). These studies generally found overreferral of children to be based on the absence of the acoustic reflex accompanied by abnormal middle ear pressure. Bess and Kenworthy (1986) cite the work of Tos and Poulsen (1980) and Hallett (1982) to support the recommendation to retest following initial failure because their data indicate that many middle ear effusions will resolve spontaneously with no residual effects.

The efficacy of six different school screening programs for otitis media was reported recently by Wachtendorf et al. (1984) of San Antonio. These authors concluded that the use of the acoustic reflex as an indicator of middle ear disease in hearing screening programs results in low specificity and a high rate of false-positive results. Based on their study of six screening protocols, they recommend decreasing the rate of overreferrals by (1) not referring children on the basis of absent acoustic reflexes alone; (2) confirming a suspected hearing loss with audiometry; (3) rescreening all type C tympanograms at six weeks, and (4) referring only children with peak pressure $\leq$ -200 mm. H20 and hearing loss verified by audiometry. The Wachtendorf et al. article makes an interesting point: those who initiate mass screening programs must accept the responsibility of identifying real disease states rather than placing that burden on the physician and creating a financial burden for the family.

Robinson and Allen (1984) attempted to demonstrate potential racial differences in tympanometric results with 253 children from day-care centers in metropolitan Detroit. They based their study on the premise that ethnicity is a factor affecting the incidence of otitis media. Specifically, previous studies had shown that black children have a significantly lower incidence of otitis media than white children (Klein 1978; Griffith 1979; Schubert, Lassman, and LaBenz 1980). The purpose of their study was to provide data on middle ear dysfunction, as inferred from tympanometry, across and within black and white middle-class preschool children between 30 and 48 months of age.

The results of their carefully conducted research confirmed that black children have significantly less middle ear dysfunction, as indicated by failure of tympanometric screening, than do white children of the same age and social class. Robinson and Allen showed that both races show a higher risk for failure of tympanometry at younger ages, with black children approaching the failure rate of white children at less than two-and-a-half years; but quickly diverging failure rates appear with maturation up to four years of age. Black children showed a significant ($p < .05$) lower incidence of failure with tympanometry at 23% compared to 38% for white children. The authors cite evidence of differences between races in eustachian tube and mastoid anatomy (Doyle 1977; Lindeman and Shea 1980). Although the cause of these reported differences in middle ear dysfunction is not clear, the findings are important for planning school and community hearing screening programs.

In recent years several large-scale studies of immittance screening have been published, based on controlled interpretation of parameters and variables to determine effects of failure criteria, and these are worthy of careful study. Scandinavian studies by Fiellau-Nikolajsen (1983), as well as a Canadian screening study by FitzZaland and Zink (1984), have demonstrated that the following factors can be manipulated to achieve any desired result: sensitivity; specificity; predictive value of a positive test; optimal range of false positives; number of children referred for medical evaluation; and number of children retested by the screening program. Thus, the end result of any screening program can be tailored to coincide with the availability of treatment facilities in any given geographic area, by manipulating the algorithm used to determine medical referral from the results of the screening program.

The controversy regarding the role of immittance screening is closely tied to the issue of speech and language problems in children as sequela of middle ear effusions. These topics have been the central theme of two outstanding national workshops summarized by Bluestone et al. (1983, 1986) as special articles in *Pediatrics*. These two special articles are highly recommended resources for current, state-of-the-art information on the effects of otitis media on the child and for a synopsis of the controversies in screening for middle ear disease and hearing loss in children. The conclusions of Bluestone (1986) are germane to the present discussion: an untold number of children, in at least 24 states in this country, fail screening tests for asymptomatic otitis media with effusion and are referred for treatment despite the lack of (1) a clear definition of the target population to be identified, i.e., children at risk of developing functional/structural impairment secondary to otitis media; (2) meaningful guidelines for screening protocols based on the natural history of the disease (most episodes of otitis media with effusion resolve spontaneously in a few weeks or, at most, two or three months); and (3) information from controlled studies showing that the costs/risks of the various medical and surgical treatments do not exceed those of the disease.

As Bess and Kenworthy (1986) point out, there is no immediate resolution in sight to the impedance screening controversy. The issues set forth in a debate between Bess (1980) and Northern (1980) raise legitimate concerns both for and against the use of immittance in mass screening programs, and these questions will not be settled easily. There is still a need for comprehensive, well controlled research. It is now time for existing guidelines for immittance screening to be revised in light of the current field data.

CONCLUSIONS

To be sure, acoustic immittance measurements continue to be our most powerful and most clinically efficient pediatric auditory evaluation technique; however, there is still a significant need to conduct additional research among pediatric populations. Improvements in the technical aspects of immittance equipment, as well as continued test procedure refinements—including multifrequency probe-tone applications—will no doubt enhance future utilization of acoustic immittance measurements.

REFERENCES

American Speech-Language-Hearing Association. 1979. Guidelines for Acoustic Immittance Screening of Middle-Ear Function. *Asha* 21:283–288.

Barajas, J., Olaizola, M., Tapia, M., Alacron, J., and Alaminos, D. 1981. Audiometric study of the neonate: Impedance audiometry, behavioral responses and brain stem audiometry. *Audiology* 29:42–52.

Bennett, M., and Weatherby, L. 1979. Multiple probe frequency acoustic reflex measurements. *Scandinavian Audiology* 8:233–239.

Bennett, M., and Weatherby, L. 1982. Newborn acoustic reflexes to noise and pure-tone signals. *Journal of Speech and Hearing Research* 25:383–387.

Bennett, M. 1984. Impedance concepts relating to the acoustic reflex. *In* S. Silman (ed.). *The Acoustic Reflex: Basic Principles and Clinical Applications* (pp. 35–61).

Bess, F. 1980. Impedance screening for children: A need for more research. *Annals of Otology, Rhinology and Laryngology* 89(3) Supplement 68:228–232.

Bess, F., and Kenworthy, O. 1986. Current status of impedance screening in the United States. *In* C. Bluestone et al., Controversies in Screening for Middle Ear Disease and Hearing Loss in Children. *Pediatrics* 77(1):65.

Bluestone, C., Klein, J., Paradise, J., Eichenwald, H., Bess, F., Downs, M., Green, M., Berko-Gleason, J., Ventry, I., Gray, S., McWilliams, B., and Gates G. 1983. Workshop on effects of otitis media on the child. *Pediatrics* 71:4, 639–652.

Bluestone, C., Fria, T., Arjona, S., Casselbrant, M., Schwartz, D., Ruben, R., Gates, G., Downs, M., Northern, J., Jerger, J., Paradise, J., Bess, F., Kenworthy, O., and Rogus, K. 1986. Controversies in screening for middle ear disease and hearing loss in children. *Pediatrics* 77(1):57–70.

Brooks, D. 1982. Acoustic impedance studies on otitis media with effusion: A review. *International Journal of Pediatric Otorhinolaryngology* 4:89–94.

Buhrer, K., Wall, L., and Schuster, L. 1985. The acoustic reflectometer as a screening device: A comparison. *Ear and Hearing* 6(6):307–314.

Dermody, P., Curotta, J., and Mackie, K. 1983. Pass/fail criteria in screening for otitis media in children with learning disorders. *International Journal of Pediatric Otolaryngology* 6:151–162.

Downs, M., and Northern, J. 1986. Mass screening for otitis media: The audiologist's viewpoint. *In* C. Bluestone et al., Controversies in Screening for Middle Ear Disease and Hearing Loss in Children. *Pediatrics* 71(7):61.

Doyle, W. 1977. Functional anatomic description of Eustachian tube vector relationships in four ethnic populations: An osteologic study. Dissertation Abstracts International, 38:3891A.

Fiellau-Nikolajsen, M. 1983. Tympanometry and secretory otitis media: Observations on diagnosis, epidemiology, treatment and prevention in prospective cohort studies of three-year-old children. *Acta Otolaryngologica* Supplement 394.

FitzZaland, R., and Zink, G. 1984. A comparative study of hearing screening procedures. *Ear and Hearing* 5(4):205–210.

Freyss, G., Manac'h, Y., Narcy, P., and Toupet, M. 1980. Acoustic reflex as a predictor of middle ear effusion. *Annals of Otology, Rhinology and Laryngology* 89 (Suppl. 68):196–199.

Griffith, T. 1979. Epidemiology of otitis media—an inter-racial study. *Laryngoscope* 89:22–30.

Hall, J. 1980. Predicting hearing loss from the acoustic reflex. *In* J. Jerger and J. Northern (eds.). *Clinical Impedance Audiometry* (2nd Ed.). Acton, MA: American Electromedics Corp., Chapter 8.

Hall, J., and Bleakney, M. 1981. Hearing loss prediction by the acoustic reflex: Comparison of seven methods. *Ear and Hearing,* 2:156–164.

Hallett, C. 1982. The screening and epidemiology of middle ear disease in a population of primary school entrants. *The Journal of Laryngology and Otology* 96:899–914.

Harford, E., Bess, F., Bluestone, C., and Klein, J. (eds.). 1979. Recommendations from the Task Force on Impedance Screening for Children. *Impedance Screening for Middle Ear Disease in Children.* New York: Grune and Stratton, 3–7.

Himelfarb, M., Popelka, G., and Shanon, E. 1979. Tympanometry in normal infants. *Journal of Speech and Hearing Research* 22:179–191.

Jerger, J., Burney, P., Mauldin, L., and Crump, B. 1974. Predicting hearing loss from the acoustic reflex. *Journal of Speech and Hearing Disorders* 39:11–22.

Jerger, J., Hayes, D., Anthony, L., and Mauldin, L. 1978. Factors influencing prediction of hearing level from the acoustic reflex. *Monographs in Contemporary Audiology* 1(1):1–20.

Jerger, J., Fifer, R., Jenkins, H., and Mecklenburg, D. 1986. Stapedial reflex to electrical stimulation in a patient with cochlear implant. *Annals of Otology, Rhinology and Laryngology* 95:151–157.

Keith, R. 1973. Impedance audiometry with neonates. *Archives of Otolaryngology* 97:465–467.

Keith, R. 1975. Middle ear function in neonates. *Archives of Otolaryngology* 101:376–379.

Keith, R. 1977. An evaluation of predicting hearing loss from the acoustic reflex. *Archives of Otolaryngology* 103:419–423.

Keith, R., and Bench, R. 1978. Stapedial reflex in neonates. *Scandinavian Audiology* 7:187–191.

Kenworthy, O. T., Bess, F., and Wright, P. 1986. Personal Communcation.

Klein, J. 1978. Epidemiology of otitis media. *In* E. R. Harford, F. H. Bess, C. D. Bluestone, and J. O. Klein (eds.). *Impedance Screening for Middle Ear Disease in Children.* New York: Grune and Stratton.

Lampe, R., Weir, M., Spier, J., and Rhodes, M. 1985. Acoustic reflectometry in the detection of middle ear effusion. *Pediatrics* 76(1):75–78.

Lindeman, P., and Shea, J. 1980. Size of the mastoid air cell system in children with middle ear effusion. *Laryngoscope* 90:1840–1844.

Lucker, J. 1980. Application of pass-fail criteria to middle ear screening results. *Asha* 22:839–841.

Margolis, R. 1978. Tympanometry in infants: State-of-the-art. *In* E. Harford et al. (eds.). *Impedance Screening for Middle Ear Disease in Children.* New York: Grune and Stratton, 41–56.

Margolis, R., and Popelka, G. 1977. Interactions among tympanometric variables. *Journal of Speech and Hearing Research* 20:447–662.

Margolis, R., Popelka, G., Handler, S., and Himelfarb, M. 1981. The effect of age on acoustic-reflex thresholds in normal hearing subjects. *In* G. Popelka (ed.). *Hearing Assessment with the Acoustic Reflex.* New York: Grune and Stratton, 85–96.

McCandless, G., and Allred, P. 1978. Tympanometry and emergence of the acoustic reflex in infants. *In* E. Harford et al. (eds). *Impedance Screening for Middle Ear Disease in Children*. New York: Grune and Stratton, 56–67.

McMillin, P., Bennett, M., Marchant, C., and Shurin, P. 1985. Ipsilateral and contralateral acoustic reflexes in neonates. *Ear and Hearing* 6(6):320–324.

Niemeyer, W., and Sesterhenn, G. 1974. Calculating the hearing threshold from the stapedius reflex threshold for different sound stimuli. *Audiology* 13:421–427.

Niswander, P., and Ruth, R. 1977. Prediction of hearing sensitivity from acoustic reflexes in mentally retarded persons. *American Journal of Mental Deficiency* 81:474–481.

Northern, J. 1980. Impedance Screening: An integral part of hearing screening. *Annals of Otology, Rhinology and Laryngology* 89(3) Supplement 68:233–235.

Northern, J. 1981. Impedance measurements in infants. *In* G. Mencher and S. Gerber (eds.). *Early Management of Hearing Loss*. New York: Grune and Stratton, 131–149.

Northern, J., and Downs, M. 1984. *Hearing in Children* (3rd Edition). Baltimore: Williams and Wilkins.

Paradise, J., Smith, C., and Bluestone, C. 1976. Tympanometric detection of middle ear effusion in infants and young children. *Pediatrics* 58:198–206.

Pestalozza, G. 1984. Otitis media in newborn infants. *International Journal of Pediatric Otorhinolaryngology* 8:109–124.

Poole, P., Sheeley, E., and Hannah, J. 1982. Predicting hearing sensitivity and audiometric slope for mentally retarded persons. *Ear and Hearing* 3(2):77–82.

Popelka, G. (ed.). 1981. *Hearing Assessment with the Acoustic Reflex*. New York: Grune and Stratton.

Queen, S., Moses, F., Wood, S., Harryman, D., and Couty, C. 1981. The use of immittance screening by the Kansas City, MO Public School District. *Seminars in Speech, Language and Hearing* 2:119–122.

Robinson, D., and Allen, D. 1984. Racial differences in tympanometric results. *Journal of Speech and Hearing Disorders* 49:140–144.

Roush, J., and Tait, C. 1985. Pure-tone and acoustic immittance screening of pre-school aged children: An examination of referral criteria. *Ear and Hearing* 6(5):245–250.

Schubert, E., Lassman, F., and LaBenz, P. 1980. Hearing. *In* F. M. Lassman, R. O. Fisch, D. K. Vetter, and E. S. LaBenz (eds.). *Early Correlates of Speech, Language and Hearing*. Littleton, MA: PSG Publishing.

Schwartz, D. 1986. Current status of techniques for screening and diagnosis of middle ear disease in children. *In* C. Bluestone, et al., Controversies in Screening for Middle Ear Disease and Hearing Loss in Children. *Pediatrics* 77(1):59.

Schwartz, D. and Schwartz, R. 1978. A comparison of tympanometry and acoustic reflex measurements for detecting middle ear effusion in infants below seven months of age. *In* E. Harford, et al. (eds.). *Impedance Screening for Middle Ear Disese in Children*. New York: Grune and Stratton, 91–96.

Schwartz, D. and Schwartz, R. 1980. Tympanometric findings in young infants with middle ear effusion: Some further observations. *International Journal of Pediatric Otorhinolaryngology* 2:67–72.

Schwartz, D. and Schwartz, R. 1987. Validity of acoustic reflectometry in detecting middle ear effusion. *Pediatrics* 29(5):739–742.

Silman, S. (ed.). 1984. *The Acoustic Reflex: Basic Principles and Clinical Applications*. New York: Academic Press.

Silman, S., Silverman, C., Showers, T., and Gelfand, S. 1984. Effect of age on prediction of hearing loss with the bivariate-plotting procedure. *Journal of Speech and Hearing Research* 27:12–19.

Sprague, B., Wiley, T., and Goldstein, R. 1985. Tympanometric and acoustic-reflex studies in neonates. *Journal of Speech and Hearing Research* 28:265–272.

Teele, D., and Teele, J. 1984. Detection of middle ear effusion by acoustic reflectometry. *Journal of Pediatrics* 104:832–838.

Tos, M., and Poulsen, G. 1980. Screening tympanometry in infants and two-year old children. *Annals of Otology, Rhinology and Laryngology* 89 (Suppl. 68):217–222.

Vanhuyse, V., Creten, W., and Van Camp, K. 1975. On the W-notching of tympanograms. *Scandinavian Audiology* 4:45–50.

Wachtendorf, C., Lopez, L., Cooper, J., Hearne, E., and Gates, G. 1984. The efficacy of school screening for otitis media. *In* D. Lim et al. (eds.). *Recent Advances in Otitis Media with Effusion*. Toronto: B. C. Decker, Inc., 242–245.

Wall, L., Naples, G., Buhrer, K., and Capodanno, C. 1984. A survey of audiological services within the school system. *Asha* 27:31–34.

Weatherby, L., and Bennett, M. 1980. The neonatal acoustic reflex. *Scandinavian Audiology* 9:103–110.

Wright, P., McConnell, K., Thompson, J., Vaughn, W., and Sells, S. 1985. A longitudinal study of the detection of otitis media in the first two years of life. *International Journal of Pediatric Otorhinolaryngology* 10:245–252.

Chapter 13

Hearing Aid Selection and Evaluation with Young Children

Mark Ross and *Richard C. Seewald*

Despite the accelerated pace in technological improvements and an ever-burgeoning literature in recent years, the essential considerations and basic goals in fitting hearing aids to young children have not changed. We take the view that the genesis of a hearing-impaired child's communication, educational, and psycho-social problems is the hearing loss itself, and that the most effective means of precluding or diminishing these problems is to provide early and appropriate amplification.

The consequences of a hearing loss are visible—often dramatic—and it is these visible consequences that usually engage our most sustained efforts. What is less apparent is the efficiency of an amplification device in giving children an optimum representation of speech signals consistent with their hearing loss. This goal will be the general focus of this chapter, beginning with a brief review of the rationale for early amplification; followed by specific procedures designed to select an appropriate amplification device; and ending with some comments on current hearing aid issues pertaining to young hearing-impaired children. The scope of the chapter does not permit an extensive exploration of general habilitative concerns. It should be explicitly understood, however, that hearing aids cannot be selected in an habilitative vacuum, and that the ultimate success of our efforts will depend as much on parental involvement, follow-up procedures, and educational decisions as upon the selection of specific electroacoustic parameters.

Rationale for Early Amplification

A mark of progress in the field has been the general acceptance of the need for early amplification. While there is little direct evidence available supporting this belief, we are able to make compelling inferential judgments from basic research dealing with auditory sensory deprivation and early language development.

Auditory sensory deprivation studies in rats and chicks have examined the physiological effects and structural changes in the brain stem auditory nuclei due to sound deprivation and/or excised peripheral auditory structures. The results of the early studies (Tees 1967a, 1967b), in which deprived animals were unable to resolve differences in sound patterns, particularly those embodying time differentiations, have been extended and essentially corroborated by later ones. Early sound deprivation has been shown to increase the latency of auditory neural responses by a factor of 2 to 3 (Clopton and Silverman 1978). Webster and Webster (1977, 1979) found incomplete maturation of most brain stem auditory neurons after both postnatal auditory deprivation and an experimentally produced conductive loss. Feng and Rogowski (1980) examined the effects of both monaural and binaural deprivation and demonstrated that an imbalance in sensory experience caused asymmetrical dendritic growth on one side. Silverman and Clopton (1977) and Clopton and Silverman (1977) also showed abnormal binaural interaction effects after monaural deprivation. Webster (1983) and Evans, Webster, and Cullen (1983) reported pathological changes in auditory brain stem structures after ablation or deprivation. The evidence demonstrating physiological and/or pathological changes in the auditory systems of animals appears conclusive.

We do not know the degree to which these findings apply to children. We can be fairly confident that the period of deprivation would have to be longer in children than in experimental animals (which generally varies from a few days after birth to 90 days) in order for irreversible structural and physiological changes to take place. Given the findings with animal research, we do not know what the behavioral correlates in human beings would be. It should be safe to assume—erring on the side of caution—that similar deprivation effects may occur in human beings, and that the longer the deprivation period, the more pronounced these effects will be. Conceptually, we view auditory sensory deprivation effects in humans as a movable ceiling: the longer we delay in fitting children with appropriate amplification, the lower their auditory potential. We believe, however, that *some* benefit can be obtained from amplification, no matter when amplification is begun.

These considerations apply mainly to severely and profoundly hearing-impaired children—those who would not experience auditory sensations without amplification. It is our firm conviction that one major reason for the limited benefit of amplification obtained by many children is that they suffer from the irreversible effects of auditory sensory deprivation. These are the children who appear to demonstrate tolerance problems, who are acutely aware of an "alien presence" in their ears, and whose attention has to be consciously drawn to sounds in order for them to "listen." The other major reasons for this limited benefit—including a low and inconsistent speech-to-noise ratio and the absence of full parental involvement in the process of habilitation—while crucial, do not appear to reduce the auditory potential ceiling in the same manner as does sensory deprivation.

Insofar as early language and speech development is concerned, there is no longer any doubt about the significance of the early years. The young child has an awesome capacity for organizing language input into a complex, rapidly evolving oral language system. In the absence of an adequate auditory channel, the child would evolve a visually oriented system. The point is that the hearing-impaired child possesses the same biological capacity for developing language as does a normal-hearing child. This facility is apparently an outgrowth of the rapid development of the central nervous system in the early years (Lennenberg 1967). It is at this time that children demonstrate the greatest facility for acquiring new behavior, of which language and speech is one subset. Fry (1978) is but one of the many psycholinguists who have affirmed the necessity of early diagnosis and treatment, so that sensory inputs can be available during the early years. For the great majority of hearing-impaired children likely to be seen by audiologists, the most effective sensory input would be appropriately amplified sound, which clearly appears to be better adapted than any possible substitute to take full advantage of this favorable developmental period (Fry 1978).

Selection Procedures

PRESELECTION CONSIDERATIONS

Hearing aids often must be selected for a child before a complete measurement of thresholds in each ear can be obtained. To preclude deprivation effects, and to take advantage of the early readiness period for language development, we must nevertheless proceed even if we only have approximate information. We cannot support the practices of previous years, where hearing aids would not be fitted on a child until complete bilateral thresholds were obtained. Hearing selection for children, then, must be viewed as an ongoing process; as more accurate and detailed audiometric information is obtained, modifications can be made in the specific electroacoustic recommendations.

The hearing aid(s) recommended for a young child must therefore incorporate sufficient electroacoustic flexibility so that desired modifications can be made easily. At a minimum, the aid(s) must permit a range of output and frequency response changes. Furthermore, for all ear-level hearing aids, we recommend the inclusion of directional microphones. An impressive amount of research support has been accumulated in favor of directional microphones over omnidirectional microphones (Hawkins and Yacullo 1984). Unfortunately, the hearing aid test boxes available in the average clinic do not permit measurement of the characteristics of directional microphones. Judging from the frequency with which specific aids vary from their nominal specifications, we can assume that the nominal directional characteristics of a microphone will also vary frequently from the specifications. Still, the advantages are sufficiently compelling to warrant more general recommendations of hearing aids with directional microphones.

Hearing aids recommended for young children should include provision for direct audio-input from an FM system, as well as a powerful inductance coil with an acceptable frequency response. Unlike directional microphones, the characteristics of inductance coils can be measured fairly simply with an inexpensive addition to a hearing aid test box. The children we see at a very early age in a clinic are shortly going to be enrolled in an educational program. They must be prepared to use a personal FM system in such a program, without resorting to standard FM system receivers (which ordinarily limit the high-frequency range), or to purchasing new hearing aids.

In our judgment, the use of a body-worn binaural arrangement, *for the profoundly hearing-impaired child,* should not be precluded for cosmetic reasons. A body aid will ordinarily provide more gain before feedback (Matkin 1984) and, because of the body baffle effect, will ordinarily demonstrate more low-frequency functional gain than a postauricular aid. Specifically, for children who may be considered candidates for a cochlear implant procedure, we would suggest the supervised use of a powerful body aid prior to the implantation. For the majority of children we see, however, behind-the-ear instruments are still the most desirable option.

Finally, the choice of a specific type of earmold should be considered a vital component of the entire process. The earmold should be a full shell-type fitting with thick-walled tubing. For the infant, it may not be possible to include desirable acoustic modifications in the mold because of size limitations, but the need for these should be continually assessed as the child grows and more information about the child's responses are obtained.

In a later section we shall discuss the provision of binaural hearing aids in some detail. Suffice to say now that we consider the routine recommendations of binaural hearing aids as the norm, to be modified as information develops which demonstrates that the child does worse (not the same!) with binaural than with monaural amplification.

ELECTROACOUSTIC SELECTION

The electroacoustic goal of our selection procedures is to deliver an amplified speech signal to the child that maximizes residual hearing across frequency. The theoretical basis for this goal is derived from the concept of the Articulation Index (AI) which, while initially developed for normal-hearing individuals (Boothroyd 1978), also has been applied to the hearing impaired with moderate success (Dugal, Braida, and Durlach 1978; Pavlovic 1984; Kamm, Dirks, and Bell 1985; Studebaker, Pavlovic, and Sherbecoe 1985). Briefly, what the AI does is evaluate the contributions to speech intelligibility of weighted bands of audible (above threshold or a noise floor) speech across frequency. Another such predictive scheme, termed the Speech Transmission Index (STI), takes into consideration reverberation effects—which the AI does not—and has been combined with the AI for improved prediction of speech intelligibility (Humes, Boney, and Ahlstrom 1985). Both of these schemes require an excellent speech-to-noise (or speech-to-threshold) ratio across frequency to achieve maximum speech intelligibility. This has always been our intention with hearing-impaired children, even without the impressive theoretical rationale. The problem has been, and still is, how to choose the electroacoustic characteristics to achieve this goal. We have devised a selection and evaluation procedure in which the goal is explicity addressed, if not conclusively solved.

In the following pages, we shall describe the general outline of the procedure. In the interests of clinical efficiency it was written as a computer program, although it may be applied without a computer. Only an abbreviated version of the program will be described here; we have presented it elsewhere in greater detail (Seewald and Ross 1988). Because the amount of audiometric information available for a young child typically is limited, the program is based on only unaided and aided thresholds. One basic requirement is an electroacoustic measurement system. Even though the responses obtained in a 2-cm^3 coupler differ markedly from real-ear measures, the standard coupler responses in conjunction with functional gain nevertheless are quite useful in the evaluation stage of the procedure.

The recent emergence of computerized probe-tube microphone systems promises to simplify the entire measurement process (Berlin 1985; Libby 1985). In addition to eliminating the known problems associated with 2-cm^3 coupler and real-ear performance differences, probe-tube systems—as a purely physical measurement—require only passive cooperation from the child and avoid a variety of difficulties associated with more conventional psychoacoustic tests (Hawkins et al. 1985). At present, however, relatively few centers have probe-tube systems available (Seewald, Whitehead, and Golardi 1986). Their advent, moreover, will not in itself change the procedure; it will just reduce some assumptions and simplify measurement.

It is necessary to discuss two other introductory points before going into the details of the procedure. The first point deals with the necessity of selecting an appropriate speech spectrum. Our procedure and a number of others require the inclusion of a specific speech spectrum in order to determine the recommended functional gain (Skinner et al. 1982; Byrne 1981, 1982; Byrne and Murray 1985). The long-term average speech spectrum has been shown to vary as a function of talker age, gender, distance, vocal effort, and measurement factors (Byrne 1977; Levitt 1982). Presently, among selection procedures that depend upon a specific speech spectrum level for determining results, there are no agreed upon levels. For example, of the six such procedures we reviewed (Gengel et al. 1971; Shapiro 1976; Pascoe 1978; Byrne 1978; Berger 1976; Cox 1983), none employed the same values in defining the speech spectrum. It should be recognized, however, that any set of values chosen can only approximately represent the variation in speech spectrum that a child will encounter in everyday life. We have chosen to use the levels presented by Cox (1983); with an overall SPL of 70 dB, the one-third octave values are among the highest reported in the literature (see table I). Our reasoning for selecting this specturm was based on the close proximity of parents and young children during caretaking activities.

The second point concerns the calibration of the sound field and the stimuli used to measure aided and unaided sound-field thresholds. A comprehensive review of the issues related to sound-field measurements can be found in Walker et al. (1984). In accordance with their recommendations, we are employing 5% frequency modulated (warble) tones. The sound pressure level (SPL) reference levels were selected to conform to those recommended by Morgan et al. (1979). These reference levels, at 45-degree azimuth, have been demonstrated to coincide well with the American National Standards Institute (ANSI) 1969 standard reference levels for pure-tone stimuli presented via earphones. In our program, we present results in SPL and/or a hearing threshold level (HTL) format. The measurements are made in HTL, and the conversion values are stored in the computer program. Speech spectrum and hearing aid characteristics are generally reported in SPL values; we believe that an SPL format is preferable to HTL, particularly for clarity in plotting suprathreshold responses.

SETTING TARGET FREQUENCY RESPONSE

The first step is to measure the child's unaided sound-field thresholds across frequency, however it can best be done. We are well aware of the difficulty in measuring individual ear thresholds for the young child; this is one of the reasons we stress the necessity of continued audiometric follow-up with modifications made as needed. For our example we shall use the sound-field audiometric results shown in figure 1.

These threshold values are entered into the computer in dB HTL. The conversions for HTL to SPL have already been stored in memory. With a properly calibrated sound field, conversions also can be hand calculated, but this is far more time consuming. The unaided sound-field thresholds for our case example, converted to dB SPL, are presented in figure 2. Also shown in this figure is the average speech spectrum, which is stored in the computer memory. We

Table I

The Long-term Average Speech Spectrum in dB SPL (after Cox 1983).

Frequency in Hertz								
250	500	750	1000	1500	2000	3000	4000	6000
60	66.5	62.5*	55	57*	57*	51*	49	47

*Interpolated

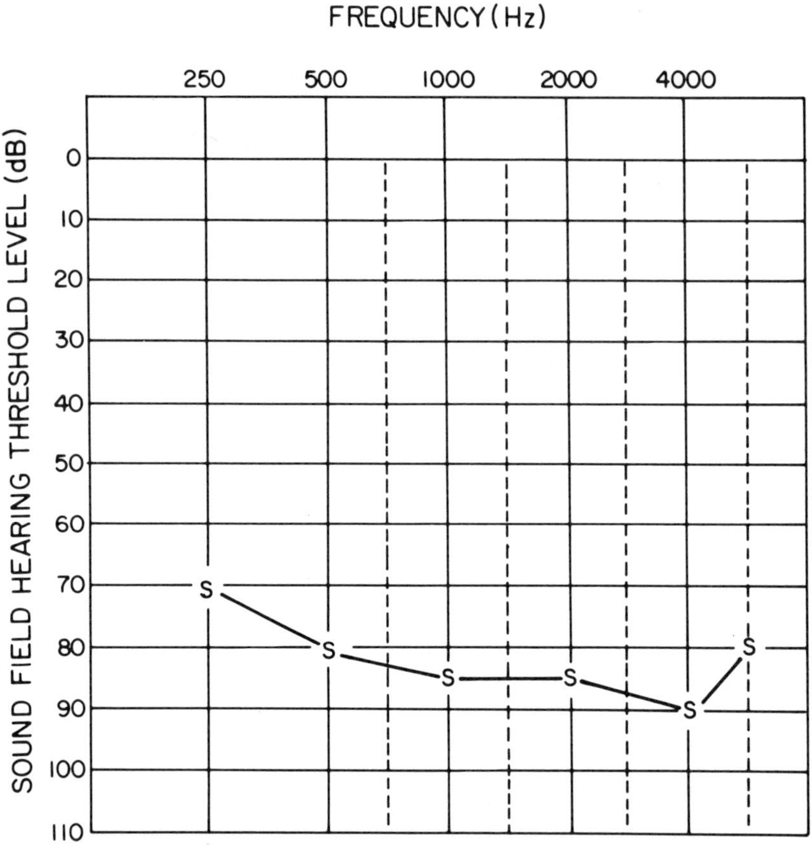

Figure 1. Unaided sound-field audiogram of case example.

should bear in mind that this is an *average* speech spectrum; within any frequency region, the intensity of speech fluctuations is approximately 30 dB, 12 dB above and 18 dB below the average values.

The selection of the target frequency response is made on the basis of the information supplied in figure 3. The abscissa displays the unaided sound-field thresholds, while the ordinate contains the desired sensation levels for the five frequency regions shown on the graph. Using the audiogram in figure 1 as an example, we can see that at 250 Hz, a 9 dB sensation level is the target. For the frequencies 500, 1000, 2000, 4000, and 6000 Hz, the target sensation levels are, respectively, 13, 10, 16, 11, and 12 dB. To simplify this presentation, we have omitted 750, 1500, and 3000 Hz; we strongly recommend, however, that whenever possible the thresholds for these frequencies also should be obtained. These functions are incorporated in the computer program. When the unaided thresholds are entered, the computations for the desired sensation level of speech by frequency region are made automatically by the computer.

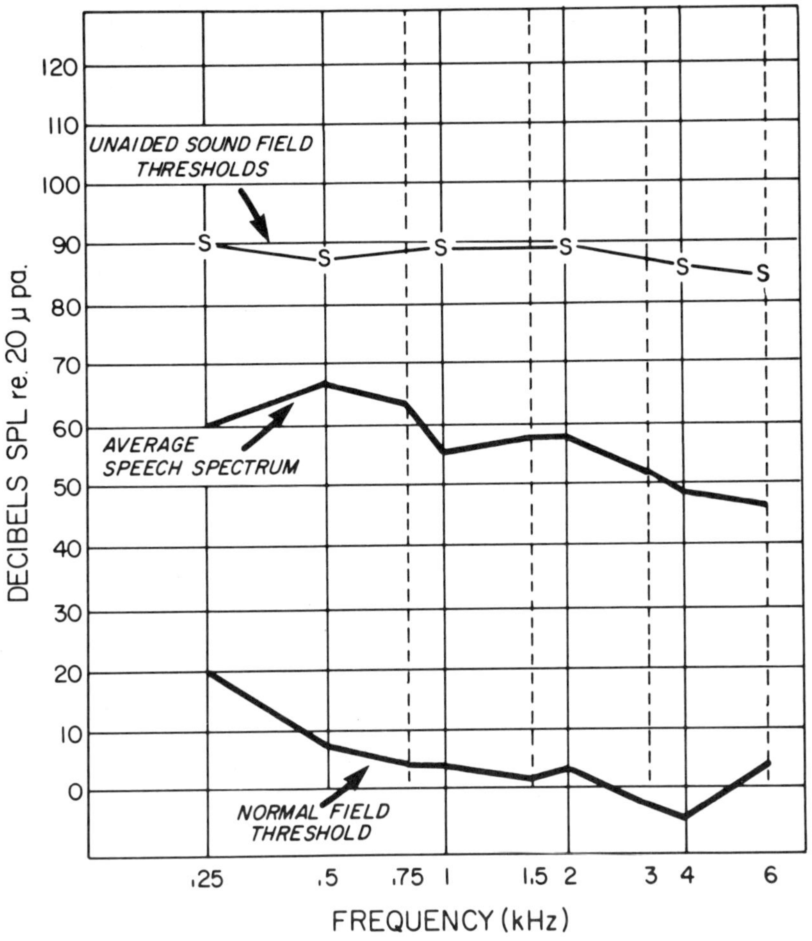

Figure 2. Unaided sound-field audiogram of case example on SPL scale. An average speech spectrum and average normal-hearing curve in dB SPL also are shown.

These desired sensation levels of the amplified speech spectrum were chosen to ensure audibility of the speech signal across the entire frequency spectrum. The sensation levels decrease as the degree of loss increases, with, however, a target of some audibility regardless of degree of loss. The different frequencies are given different weights in an attempt to reflect their relative contributions to speech intelligibility. We also want to ensure that there is sufficient "head room" between the amplified speech output and the saturation level of the hearing aid (to be discussed below) to reduce instances of saturation, keeping in mind the 12 dB peaks of speech above the value of the average speech output.

While we are trying to provide the audibility of as much of the speech spectrum as we can, we are particularly concerned that we do not overemphasize the

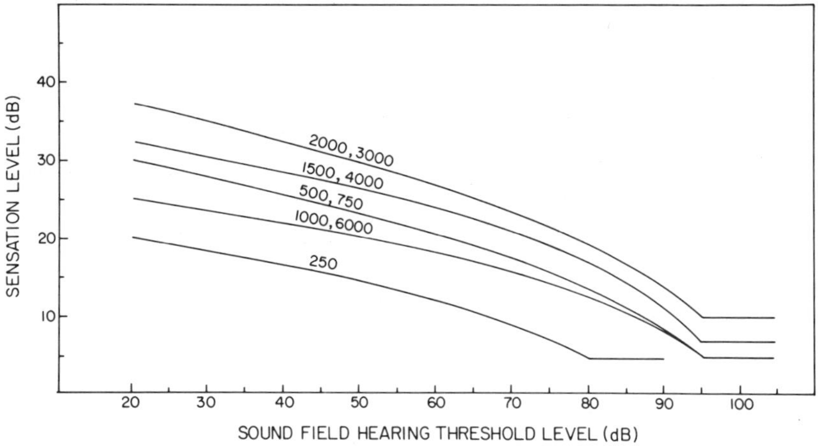

Figure 3. Desired sensation levels of amplified speech in dB as a function of hearing threshold level and frequency.

low frequencies in conformance with current clinical practices derived from the studies of Danaher, Osberger, and Pickett (1973) and Danaher and Pickett (1975). At the same time, however, some recent research suggests that we may have overreacted in our attempts to avoid an upward spread of masking by low frequency energy. In a recent, careful study by Punch and Beck (1986), an increase in low-frequency response was shown to be related to a positive judgment in perceived speech quality in quiet and noise, with an increase in syllabic recognition in quiet and no detrimental effects in noise. There is, therefore, sufficient disagreement about this point for us to compromise in our recommended sensation levels for the low frequencies by ensuring their audibility without overemphasizing them.

We also are concerned about providing sufficient audibility of the high frequencies so that the acoustic signature of crucial consonants can be detected by the child. We know that much of the energy of voiceless phonemes, particularly /s/, /f/, and the unvoiced /th/, falls about 4000 Hz (Levitt 1978). The /s/ phoneme, for example, conveys more morphological information than any other phoneme in the English language (e.g., past tense, plurals, third person present) as well as syntactic information (contractions such as it's and let's). Provided a child has sufficient residual hearing to detect the high frequency energy, it makes no sense to filter it out with an inadequate electroacoustic system. It is much more economical and effective to permit children to employ their biological capacities to *learn* language naturally rather than imposing artificially structured methods to *teach* them the same information.

In figure 4, the target amplified speech signal is shown as the dotted curve above the unaided sound-field thresholds. The numbers on the right side of the lines represent the desired sensation levels. The numbers on the left side of the line indicate the amount of functional gain necessary to achieve the desired

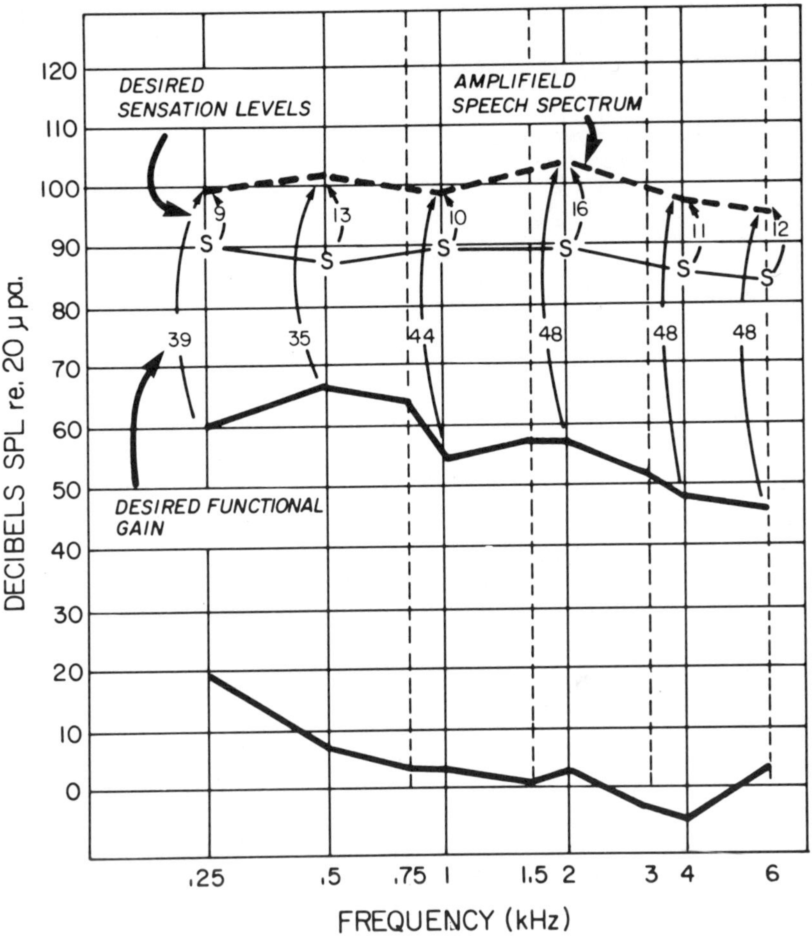

Figure 4. Target-amplified speech levels plotted above unaided sound-field thresholds. Numbers to the right of each frequency indicate desired sensation levels. Numbers to the left indicate amount of functional gain required to achieve the desired result of amplification.

result of the amplification, i.e., the difference between the target outputs and the speech spectrum.

In figure 5, the target-aided sound-field thresholds are shown. The differences between the unaided and aided sound-field thresholds are based on the target functional gain measures derived from the previous step. Clinicians accustomed to judging the suitability of a hearing aid on the basis of how close the aided thresholds approximate the normal thresholds may conclude that too little functional gain is being provided for this child. It should be noted, however, that audibility is obtained for all regions of the speech spectrum for an average input signal. Furthermore, functional gain can be increased simply by rotating the gain control. Our main concern is to develop a target frequency response that can be preserved, as gain or the input signal increases.

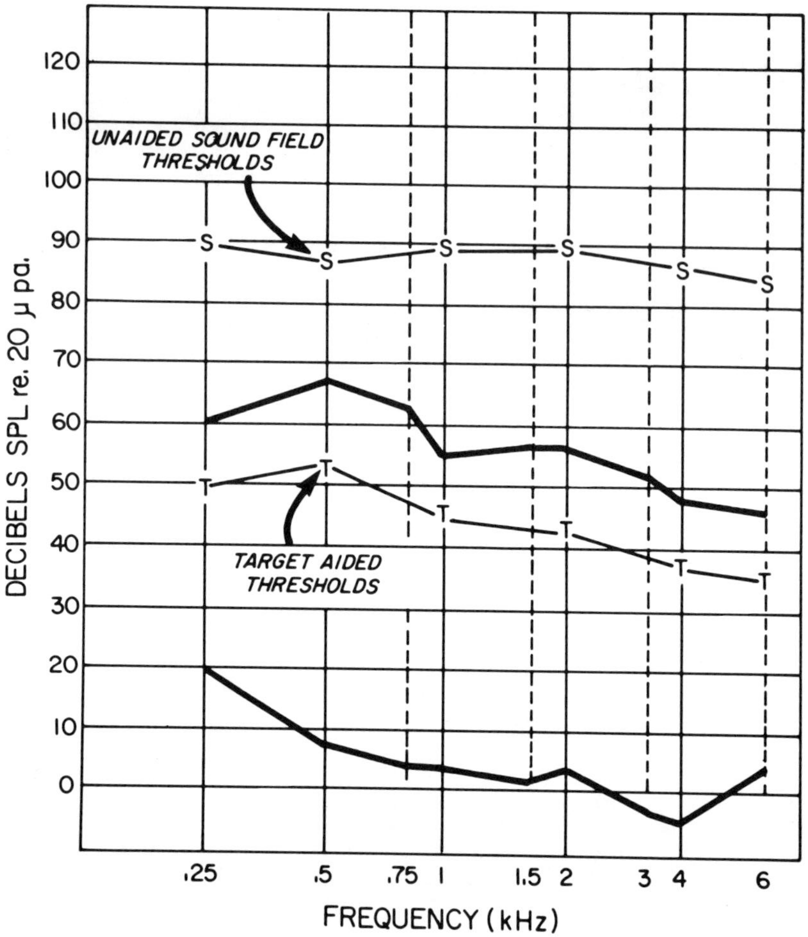

Figure 5. Required functional gain values from figure 4 plotted as target-aided sound-field thresholds.

Up to this point, the only actual measurements made were the unaided sound-field thresholds. When these are entered into the computer, it generates the target-aided thresholds based on the information stored in the program (speech spectrum, HTL to SPL conversion, and the target sensation levels). The information is printed in hard copy by the computer system. In the next step, the actual aided thresholds are compared to the target thresholds.

MODIFYING THE FREQUENCY RESPONSE

On the basis of unaided results, the clinician preselects a specific hearing aid/earmold combination with gain, frequency response, and output characteristics that generally appear appropriate for the child. We suggest that full ANSI curves be run on the hearing aid test box, prior to the aided measurements, although only the frequency response is required in this step. Monaural aided thresholds are then measured under the same conditions as the unaided thresholds. The actual aided sound-field thresholds in the example we have been using can be seen in figure 6.

In this figure, the divergence between our target and the actual measured thresholds is apparent. We are concerned not with the absolute levels, but with the shape of the curve. If, in this example, the same shape was obtained, but displaced upward or downward, then we would have met our goal. We would only have to rotate the gain control to achieve the aided thresholds we desire. In

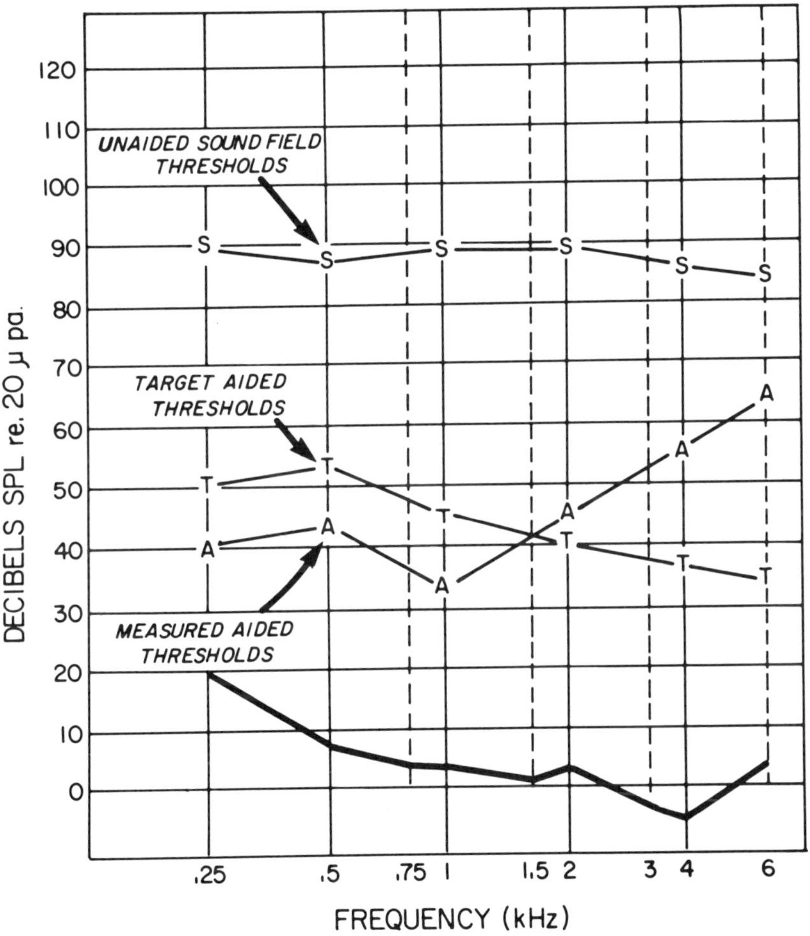

Figure 6. Comparison of measured sound-field thresholds and target-aided sound-field thresholds.

this example, however, there is a lack of congruence between the target and the actual thresholds, with too much gain in the lower frequencies and too little in the higher frequencies. By using the coupler frequency response curve obtained previously, we can make and observe modifications in the frequency response without having to test and retest the child. This is demonstrated in table II.

The first row in the table gives the coupler gain by frequency of the hearing aid first tried on the child. In the second row, the differences between the target functional gain as shown in figures 4 and 5 and the actual functional gain across frequency are shown. These are subtracted and/or added to the measured coupler gain to give the desired coupler gain, as shown in the third row. We are assuming that if the target frequency response can be obtained in the coupler, it would be reflected in the aided sound-field thresholds to achieve the target functional gain.

The task of the audiologist is to make changes in the frequency response characteristics of the hearing aid to achieve the target frequency response. If this is not possible with the first hearing aid tried on the child, then other aids may be selected by consulting manufacturer's specifications. This is a more economical and efficient method than repeated sound-field testing for modifying and/or selecting an appropriate frequency response for a child. By using the child's own aided functional gain measures as the base, this method has the advantage of reflecting the real-ear (hearing aid plus earmold) characteristics of a specific hearing aid.

While we would like to think that this method would result in functional gain measures precisely as "prescribed," we doubt that we would be so fortunate. Divergences will occur. Each audiologist working with a particular child will have to determine the extent of acceptable deviations. We suggest that differences of more than 10 dB at any frequency be considered unacceptable, with the added proviso that these differences not be in opposite directions at adjacent frequencies. Above all, however, it is necessary to ensure that the functional gain measures restore some audibility to a speech spectrum input, insofar as this is possible and not counterproductive (by developing feedback, for example).

Table II

Illustration of How the Difference Between the Actual and Desired Functional Gain Can Be Applied to the Coupler Frequency Response to Determine the Desired Coupler Frequency Response.

	Frequency in Hertz					
	250	500	1000	2000	4000	6000
Measured Coupler Gain	50	54	58	48	38	25
Desired/Functional Gain Difference	−11	−10	−11	3	18	28
Desired Coupler Gain	39	44	47	51	56	53

SETTING OUTPUT CHARACTERISTICS

We have discussed the rationale and procedures for determining appropriate function gain values across frequency. Our methods are grounded in solid theoretical constructions (the Articulation Index), while the several steps (unaided and aided sound-field measures) are straightforward and well within the capabilities of a young child. We are not so fortunate when it comes to determining an appropriate saturation sound pressure level (SSPL) across frequency.

The current procedures for determining the desired $SSPL_{90}$ setting of a hearing aid for adults is based on some measure of their Loudness Discomfort Levels (LDL). If any concept can be said to be well accepted in audiology, it is that the $SSPL_{90}$ must not exceed the LDL if the hearing aid fitting is to be satisfactory. Besides the variables inherent in a behavioral measure, the problem has been to relate LDL judgments made with earphones to the $SSPL_{90}$ of a hearing aid determined in a 2-cm^3 coupler. A simple but elegant method was described by Dillon et al. (1984), in which the output of an audiometer led to a receiver mounted in a behind the ear (BTE) case, with the client wearing a personal earmold. The LDL measures could then be referenced directly to the measures made in a coupler. Other researchers have described a similar method, employing a button-type receiver rather than one mounted in a BTE case (Hawkins 1980; Cox 1981). Young children, however, are unable to make the necessary LDL judgments, and this method cannot be used with them.

Attempts also have been made to determine if the LDL could be predicted from threshold measures. While general relationships have been established, the amount of individual variability from the general function is too great for predictive purposes for a specific person (Dillon et al. 1984; Byrne and Murray 1985). An additional complication is the fact that the LDL appears to be frequency dependent; that is, the LDL varies across frequency in an individualized fashion. In the past, we have used acoustic reflex measures as an approximate way of determining LDL, and have set the $SSPL_{90}$ accordingly (Ross and Tommassetti 1980). This clinical practice was not supported in a study that directly evaluated the relationship between the LDL and the acoustic reflex (Greenfield et al. 1985).

Since we cannot measure the LDL with young children, and since neither threshold nor acoustic reflex thresholds are sufficiently predictive, our decision on the appropriate output setting of the hearing aid must be based on other factors. On the one hand, we must try to ensure a sufficient range between the amplified speech output and the $SSPL_{90}$ of the hearing aid, while on the other, the $SSPL_{90}$ must not be so high as to produce discomfort or possibly dangerous sound levels (this point will be explored in more detail in a later section). In regard to discomfort, if a child is fitted with amplification at an early age, and if the earmolds fit and are seated properly, then in our opinion discomfort should be rare. Instances where it does occur may reflect structural changes in the auditory system secondary to delayed onset of amplification, although currently there is no direct proof for this assumption. Indirectly, we can recall cases where the children of congenitally deaf adults, fitted early with hearing aids, made successful adjustments to amplification; while their parents, with *similar* losses, could not tolerate sounds 5 to 10 dB above their thresholds.

At present, the state of the art in hearing aids does not permit controlling the maximum output by frequency. This is not to say that the $SSPL_{90}$ of every hearing aid is always flat across frequency; a frequency-dependent compression circuit will show variations at the maximum output. These variations are built into the hearing aid circuitry and are not susceptible to clinical modifications (with the exception of shutting off the compression circuit or increasing or decreasing the output). We must therefore select an overall limiting level; our decision is shown in figure 7, which shows the relationship between the target amplified speech spectrum output and the recommended maximum amount of sound pressure to be delivered to a child's ear. The amplified speech level is on the abscissa and the range above the amplified speech output is located on the ordinate. This function is stored in the computer program. Since the amplified speech output varies across frequency (but only slightly in this example), the recommended output also may vary as a function of frequency. For example, if the target output were 100 dB, the computer would select an output 20 dB above this, at 120 dB. As can be noted, the range decreases as the amplified speech output increases. The results of the computation are shown in figure 8.

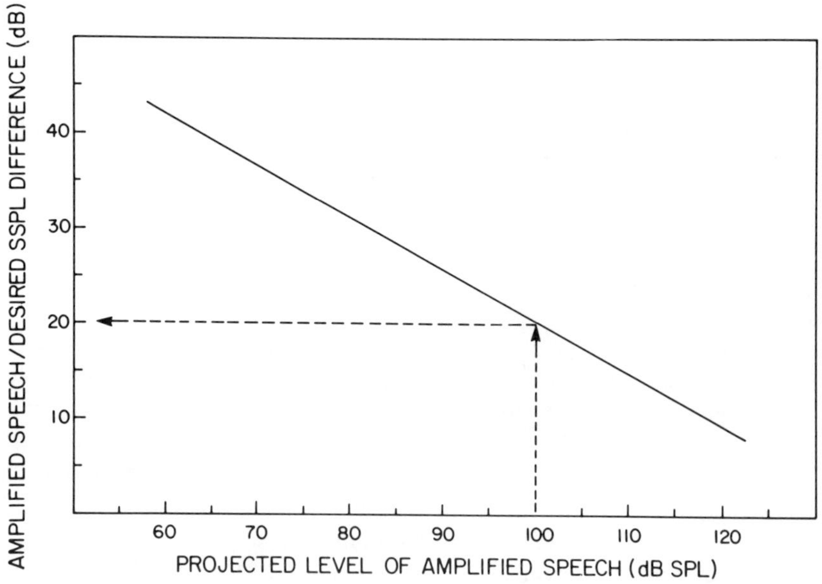

Figure 7. The linear function for the relationship between the projected level of amplified speech and the difference, in dB, between the projected amplified speech level and the desired real-ear SSPL. The dotted line shows that for a 100 dB amplified speech level, a value of 20 dB above this should be selected as the target SSPL (or 120 dB).

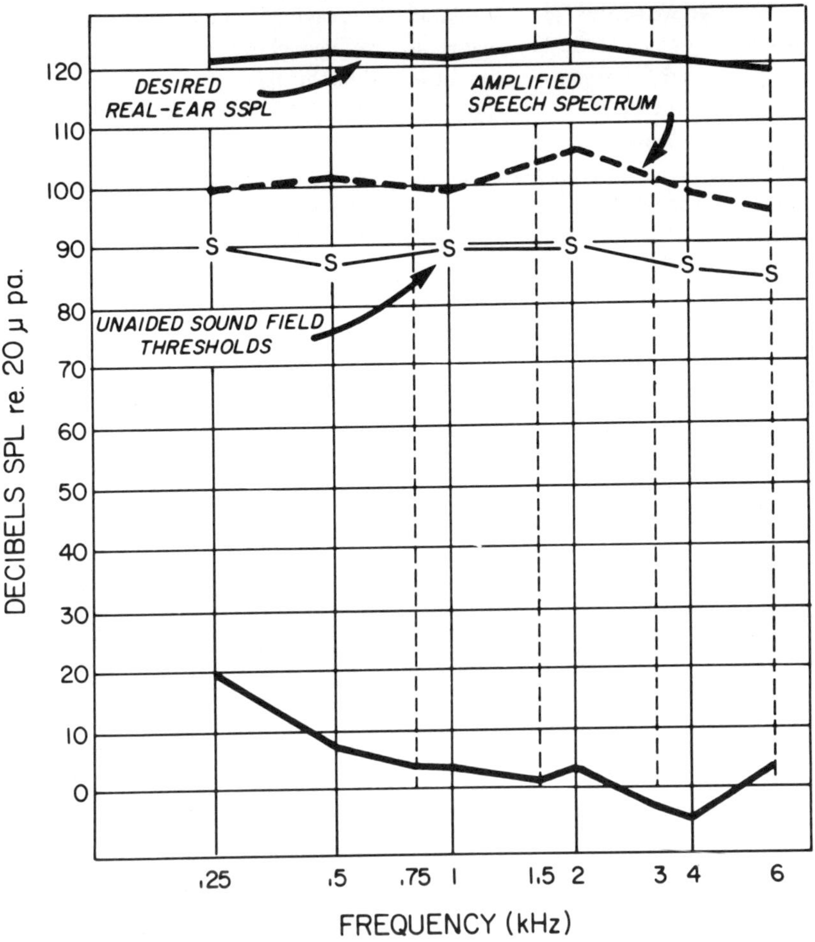

Figure 8. The desired real-ear SSPLs shown in relation to the target amplified speech spectrum and the unaided sound-field thresholds.

In our example, the recommended real-ear SSPL varies only slightly as a function of frequency. The nature of the program provides for a fairly flat output regardless of moderate variations in the amplified speech spectrum input. In order to achieve this real-ear SPL, the variation between real-ear and coupler measures have to be considered, since the $SSPL_{90}$ of a hearing aid is ordinarily defined in a 2-cm^3 coupler. What is necessary, then is to determine a coupler $SSPL_{90}$ which will produce the desired real-ear SSPL. For young children who have very small ear canals, the SPL generated in the ear canal by a hearing aid can be expected to be greater than that occurring in a 2-cm^3 coupler (Harford et al. 1983; Nelson-Barlow et al. 1985). The coupler-to-real-ear comparisons obtained by Nelson-Barlow et al. with young children reveal a mean deviation between the two measures of as much as 10 dB at some frequencies.

Although we recognize the limitations in applying average correction factors in selecting electroacoustic dimensions, we have chosen to apply the corrections reported by Nelson-Barlow et al. (1985) in lieu of a more supportable approach at the present time. The application of this approach is illustrated in table III. The average amount by which the coupler underestimates real-ear sound pressures is subtracted from the desired real-ear measures given by our program. The result is the target HA-2 coupler-defined $SSPL_{90}$ values. In other words, when these values are achieved in the coupler, they should produce the desired real-ear SPL outputs across frequency.

As can be seen the target $SSPL_{90}$ varies across frequency. We are unable to modify in any controlled fashion the frequency response of this output curve. Compromises will have to be made. If we set the output to coincide with the lowest value, then potentially significant acoustic information at other frequencies will be omitted. If we set the output at the highest value, we may be exceeding the child's tolerance level (which cannot be reliably measured with a young child). Our choice is to split the difference, provided we do not exceed the lowest value by more than 5 to 6 dB.

Because we are unable to measure directly the LDL of young children, selecting the proper $SSPL_{90}$ is the weakest link of the procedure. In addition to this approach—the most supportable because it is based on direct measurements of real-ear/coupler differences—there are several other possibilities that are attractive purely on an a priori basis.

Some of the newer versions of the computerized probe-tube microphone systems have the capacity to deliver to the ear either a speech spectrum signal or a controlled input on a frequency-by-frequency basis (as shown in table I). If these signals were delivered to a child wearing the aid with the selected frequency response, we should observe a real-ear SPL similar to that predicted in figure 4. By increasing the input across frequency by the amount given in figure 7 (or the difference between the target amplified speech spectrum and the desired real-ear SSPL given in figure 8), the resulting output should be quite close to the top curve in figure 8. The hearing aid then can be removed from the child and tested on a hearing aid test box, with the same inputs across frequency as in the previous step. The resulting SPLs appearing in the coupler should define the required $SSPL_{90}$ of the hearing aid. It is then necessary only to adjust the

Table III

Method for Arriving at the Desired $SSPL_{90}$ Coupler Values by Subtracting the Real-ear to HA2 Coupler Differences (Nelson-Barlow et al. 1985) From the Desired Real-ear SPL.

	Frequency in Hertz					
	250	500	1000	2000	4000	6000
Desired Real-Ear SPL	121	122	121	124	120	119
Correction	–	−2	−2	−10	−6	–
Desired HA2 Coupler $SSPL_{90}$	121	120	119	114	114	119

output to this level, using the internal controls of the hearing aid (again, realizing that some compromise will be necessary because of our inability to control the frequency response curve at the maximum output).

The other possibility is based on employing the differences between the obtained target functional frequency response and that observed in the coupler subsequent to this measurement. While the input levels used to measure these two different frequency responses are different, given a hearing aid functioning on the linear portion of its range, the relative differences between the two should reflect the real-ear/coupler differences for a particular child. These corrections can then be applied to the desired real-ear output curve, in the method demonstrated in table 3, to obtain the coupler sound pressures which should define the required $SSPL_{90}$ of the hearing aid. While both of these possibilities are purely speculative at present, they can easily be examined in a clinical research project. If either proves feasible, it would preclude the necessity of using average real-ear/coupler differences to arrive at the required $SSPL_{90}$ for an individual child.

Recurring Issues Of HearingAid Amplification For Young Children

SPEECH-TO-NOISE RATIO

Much of the effort we expend to ensure an optimum electroacoustic pattern (and certainly all of our theoretical speculation) is wasted in many of the acoustic environments that hearing-impaired children find themselves in. This may be difficult for someone with perfectly normal hearing to appreciate. Noise and reverberation levels that have only a mild effect on the speech recognition ability of a normal-hearing person will have a much more pronounced effect on someone with impaired hearing (Carhart and Tillman 1970; Finitzo-Hieber and Tillman 1978; Dirks et al. 1982). If that person is a congenitally hearing-impaired child, whose task is not just the *recognition* of language but its *development,* then competing acoustic stimuli will severely limit our best electroacoustic intentions. Of all the factors crucial to the auditory recognition of speech, and thus to a natural development of speech and language for the hearing-impaired child, the extent of the signal-to-noise (S/N) ratio is probably the most important.

In a chapter devoted to the electroacoustic selection of hearing aids for young children, it may seem odd to state categorically that this factor is secondary to ensuring a high S/N ratio. It should serve as a reminder of the statement we made earlier: The selection of hearing aids for young children cannot be made in an habilitative vacuum. An S/N ratio of +6 dB, and reverberation times of .7 or .9 seconds, will not seriously interfere with the speech comprehension of a normal-hearing child; a hearing-impaired child, on the other hand, requires an

S/N ratio in excess of 20 dB with minimal reverberation if his residual hearing is to be fully realized. The most effective way to accomplish this is simply to reduce the distance between the source and the child, either physically or with an FM system. This point cannot be overemphasized; audiologists dealing with young children (or with any hearing-impaired person, for that matter) must understand the deleterious effects of poor acoustical conditions and be sensitized to the need to ensure highly positive signal-to-noise ratios for hearing-impaired children.

BINAURAL HEARING AIDS FOR YOUNG CHILDREN

While the question of binaural hearing aids for young children is part of the larger issue of the binaural/monaural debate generally, it takes on unique aspects with children. At the time we must fit hearing aids to young children, we often do not have accurate threshold information for the two ears. We have suggested proceeding with approximate information in the selection of electroacoustic parameters, and, in spite of uncertainty about the relative thresholds in the two ears, we suggest proceeding also with binaural amplification. We view binaural hearing as the normal condition, to be contravened only when it can be demonstrated that a child functions more poorly with two hearing aids than with one. And even in such cases, for the older child we would recommend an organized auditory training program applied to the poorer ear to determine if after some period the ear was capable of contributing to the total auditory experience.

It is not our intention here to review studies on monaural versus binaural amplification; there is a wealth of data on this topic in the literature (e.g., Hawkins and Yacullo 1984; Nabelek and Robinson 1982). Our major concern is about delay, and relates to the possible effects of monaural amplification on eventual binaural functioning. In animal studies of auditory sensory deprivation, monaural deprivation has been found to produce structural changes in the auditory brainstem (Clopton and Silverman 1977; Silverman and Clopton 1977; Feng and Rosowski 1980; Evans, Webster, and Cullen 1983; Webster 1983). Physiologically, what these studies show are abnormalities in the ipsilateral suppression of contralateral activities at binaural synaptic junctions, as well as longer latencies to click stimuli from the contralateral nondeprived side at the level of the inferior colliculus. The animal research is extensive and in agreement: Monaural sound deprivation produces deviations in function and structure. The question is the degree to which these findings apply to human beings.

In a study that evaluated localization ability of several groups of children as a function of when binaural aids were obtained, Beggs and Foreman (1980) found that if a second aid was used prior to age four, localization ability was retained. Children who did not receive second aids until eight years of age stood little chance of developing localization ability. Sebkova and Bamford (1981a) found that training improved the ability of binaural hearing aid users to perceive speech in noise and to separate speech from noise source. This was not found to be true for a monaural group. In the second study, they showed significant relationships between the ability to localize a signal and binaural advantage in speech perception (Sebkova and Bamford 1981b).

What these studies suggest is that localization ability is related to early binaural exposure, that experience with binaural amplification can improve with training for a hearing-impaired group, and that the ability to localize is reflected in improved speech intelligibility scores. There is evidence, too, that long-term monaural amplification with adults will diminish their ability to discriminate speech in the deprived ear (Silman, Gelfand, and Silverman 1984). If this occurs in adults with early experience with two-ear listening, the effects of early and long-term monaural deprivation on congenitally hearing-impaired children can only be more profound (and consistent with the animal research reviewed above). Quite clearly we are dealing with a time-limited function, and children are not experimental animals; while the research and debate continues, they must receive the benefit of any clinical doubt. Too late, in this regard, is too likely to be too little.

EFFECT UPON RESIDUAL HEARING OF HEARING AID AMPLIFICATION

As with binaural versus monaural hearing aids, the possible effects upon residual hearing of hearing aid amplication is a perennial clinical issue in audiology. There are numerous case reports that this concern is warranted; one of us (M.R.) reported such an example over 20 years ago (Ross and Truex 1965). The results of large-scale studies completed in the last 10 years have shown that this event may occur, but is relatively rare.

The only prospective study we are aware of was completed by Markides in 1976. He used four groups of children, with 30 in each of the first three groups and 10 in the last group. In the first two groups, the children used aids with different maximum power outputs (MPOs), the third group did not use aids at all, and the fourth group used moderate-power binaural aids. After three years of testing, at six-month intervals, he concluded that there was no evidence of any threshold shift in the aided ears. Among the children he could find to follow up several years later, there was still no evidence of threshold shifts in the aided ears (Markides and Aryee 1980). Podoshin et al. (1984), in a retrospective study, examined 114 patients who had worn aids for at least eight years; no group evidence of deterioration in hearing sensitivity in the aided ear relative to the unaided ear occurred, although this was a possibility in several individual cases. Similar findings were reported by Reilly et al. (1981), who specifically examined cases of progressive loss. Of the 45 children with histories of progressive loss, the hearing aid could be implicated as a causative factor in only five cases. In a recent paper, Simmons (1986) reported that a number of these cases could well be due to perilymphatic fistulas.

According to Macrae (1985), approximately four cases in a thousand will show evidence of permanent threshold shifts (PTS) attributable to hearing aid usage, although instances of temporary threshold shifts are much more common. In his study, Macrae examined the relationship between temporary threshold shifts (TTS) and PTS, and concluded that individual susceptibility is too great for predictive purposes. The most complete report on the possible damage to hearing due to overamplification was contributed by Humes and Bess (1981). In their tutorial, they developed the relationships between the time that potentially damaging levels of amplified sound are experienced and possible permanent threshold shifts occur. The greater the hearing loss, the longer the individual can experience intense sounds before any additional shifts are noted.

We are not in favor of taking unnecessary risks in potentially further damaging a hearing-impaired child's residual hearing. We are also not in favor of an exaggerated concern which deprives children of speech sensation levels at the time they need it most. In response to the fear of overamplification, there appear to be as many children underfitted now as were previously overfitted. The children's residual hearing does them no good at the frequencies at which the amplified speech spectrum is below their thresholds. In the early years in particular, the children have to *hear*; without hearing there is no natural development of speech and language skills.

In a properly conducted aural habilitation program, we can have it both ways. We can fit children with hearing aids that provide an appropriate audible sensation of speech signals, and we can monitor their hearing frequently to detect possible instances of threshold shifts. After the initial fitting with amplification, the children should be tested at monthly intervals if possible, depending upon age, until accurate thresholds have been determined. The hearing thresholds of most of the children we see are going to be stable. For those for whom it appears that bilateral shifts are taking place (since we assume binaural amplification), remedial measures can be taken. Is there a medical condition underlying the shift? This should be ruled out. What are the real-ear sound pressure levels? Do they exceed our prescribed limits? A probe-tube microphone would be helpful here. Perhaps the $SSPL_{90}$ should be reduced. Is the child wearing a compression hearing aid with a too-low threshold of compression? If so, during pauses in speech, low-level background sounds will be maximally amplified. What happens when one aid is withdrawn? Is there recovery in thresholds in that ear? What we don't do is withdraw all amplification, except temporarily for testing purposes.

Concluding Remarks

In the first paragraph of this chapter, we stated that the considerations and goals in selecting hearing aids for young children have not changed over the years. We have presented no new information in this chapter, just some procedures to help us realize our goals and some personal comments on our clinical philosophy. Our clinical results have not kept pace with technological developments; too many children who should function as hard-of-hearing individuals are functionally deaf. Hearing aids are not the only issue, though clearly they are vital. No other therapeutic measure directly confronts the genesis of the child's communication and educational problems, the hearing loss itself. Management models that do not make provision for intensive and continued audiological involvement will not work. The audiologist has to see himself as an educator, with amplified sound his primary tool. And just as teachers continually review their results, so must the audiologist. It may not be the most glamorous activity an audiologist can engage in, but no others that we can think of pay such rewarding dividends.

References

Beggs, W. D., and Foreman, D. L. 1980. Sound localization and early binaural experience in the deaf. *British Journal of Audiology* 14:41–48.

Berger, K. W. 1976. Prescription of hearing aids: A rationale. *Journal of the American Audiology Society* 2:71–78.

Berlin, C. I. 1985. I.D. and management of hearing-impaired infants and neonates. *Hearing Instruments* 36:43–45.

Boothroyd, A. 1978. Speech perception and sensorineural hearing loss. *In* M. Ross and T. G. Giolas (eds.). *Auditory Management of Hearing-Impaired Children.* Baltimore: University Park Press.

Byrne D. 1977. The speech spectrum—some aspects of its significance for hearing aid selection and evaluaton. *British Journal of Audiology* 11:40–46

Byrne D. 1978. Selection of hearing aids for severely deaf children. *British Journal of Audiology* 12:9–22

Byrne D. 1981. Selective amplication: Some psychoacoustic considerations. *In* F. H. Bess, B. A. Freeman, and J. S. Sinclair (eds.). *Amplification in Education* (pp. 260–285). Washington, D.C.: A. G. Bell Association.

Byrne D. 1982. Theoretical approaches for hearing aid selection. *In* G. A. Studebaker, and F. H. Bess (eds.). *The Vanderbilt Hearing Aid Report* (pp. 175–179). Upper Darby, Pa.: Monographs in Contemporary Audiology.

Byrne D., and Murray, N. 1985. Relationships of HTL's, MCL, LDL's and psychoacoustic tuning curves to the optimal frequency responses characteristics of hearing aids. *The Australian Journal of Audiology* 7:7–16.

Carhart, R., and Tillman, T. W. 1970. Interaction of competing speech signals with hearing loss. *Archives of Otolaryngology* 91:273–279.

Clopton, B., and Silverman, M. 1977. Plasticity of binaural interaction. II: Critical period and changes in midline response. *Journal of Neurophysiology* 40:1275–1280.

Clopton, B., and Silverman, M. 1978. Changes in latency and duration of neural responding following developmental auditory deprivation. *Experimental Brain Research* 32:39–47.

Cox, R. M. 1981. Using LDL's to establish hearing aid limiting levels. *Hearing Instruments* 32:16–20.

Cox, R. M. 1981. Using ULCL measures to find frequency/gain and $SSPL_{90}$. *Hearing Instruments* 34:17–21.

Danaher, E. M., Osberger, M. J., and Pickett, J. M. 1973. Discrimination of formant frequency transitions in synthetic vowels. *Journal of Speech and Hearing Research* 16:439–451.

Danaher, E. M., and Pickett, J. M. 1975. Some masking effects produced by low frequency vowel formants in persons with sensorineural hearing loss. *Journal of Speech and Hearing Research* 18:261–271.

Dillon, H., Chew, R., and Deans, M. 1984. Loudness discomfort levels measurements and their implications for the design and fitting of hearing aids. *The Australian Journal of Audiology* 6:73–80.

Dirks, D. D., Morgan, D. E., and Dubno, J. R. 1982. A procedure for quantifying the effects of noise on speech recognition. *Journal of Speech and Hearing Disorders* 47:114–122.

Dugal, R. L., Braida, L. D., and Durlach, N. I. 1978. Implications of previous research for the selection of frequency-gain characteristics. *In* G. A. Studebaker and I. Hochberg (eds.). *Acoustical Factors Affecting Hearing Aid Performance.* Baltimore: University Park Press.

Evans, W., Webster, D., and Cullen, J. 1983. Auditory brainstem responses in neonatally sound deprived CBA/J mice. *Hearing Research* 10:269–277.

Feng, A., and Rogowski, B. 1980. Effects of monaural and binaural occlusion on the morphology of neurons in the medial superior olivary nucleus of the rat. *Brain Research* 189:530–534.

Finitzo-Hieber, T., and Tillman, T. W. 1978. Room acoustics effects on monosyllabic word discrimination ability for normal and hearing-impaired children. *Journal of Speech and Hearing Research* 21:440–458.

Fry, D. 1978. The role and primacy of the auditory channel in speech and language development. *In* M. Ross and T. G. Giolas (eds.). *Auditory Management of Hearing-Impaired Children.* Baltimore: University Park Press.

Gengel, R. W., Pascoe, D., and Shore, I. 1971. A frequency-response procedure for evaluating and selecting hearing aids for severely hearing-impaired children. *Journal of Speech and Hearing Disorders* 36:341–353.

Greenfield, D. G., Wiley, T. L., and Block, M. G. 1985. Acoustic-reflex dynamics and the loudness-discomfort level. *Journal of Speech and Hearing Disorders* 50:14–20.

Harford, E. H., Leijon, A., and Liden, G. 1983. A simplified real ear technique for verifying the maximum output of a hearing aid. *Ear and Hearing* 4:130–136.

Hawkins, D. B. 1980. Loudness discomfort levels: A clinical procedure for hearing aid evaluations. *Journal of Speech and Hearing Disorders* 45:3–15.

Hawkins, D. B., and Yacullo, W. S. 1984. Signal-to-noise advantage of binaural hearing aids and directional microphones under different levels of reverberation. *Journal of Speech and Hearing Disorders* 49:278–286.

Hawkins, D. B., Montgomery, A. A., Prosek, R. A., Walden, B. A., and Demorest, M. E. 1985. Examination of two issues concerning functional gain measurements. Paper presented at the convention of the American Speech-Language-Hearing Association, Washington, D.C.

Humes, L. E., and Bess, F. H. 1981. On the potential deterioration in hearing due to hearing aid use. *Journal of Speech and Hearing Research* 24:3–15.

Humes, L. E., Boney, S., and Ahlstrom, C. 1985. Comparison of two schemes for predicting speech recognition performance in normals. Paper presented at American Speech-Language-Hearing Association Convention, Washington, D.C.

Kamm, C. A., Dirks, D. D., and Bell, T. S. 1985. Speech recognition and the articulation index for normal and hearing-impaired listeners. *Journal of the Acoustical Society American* 77:281-288.

Lenneberg, E. H. 1967. *Biological Foundations of Language.* New York: John Wiley & Sons.

Levitt, H. 1982. Speech discrimination ability in the hearing impaired: Spectrum considerations. *In* G. A. Studebaker and F. H. Bess (eds.). *The Vanderbilt Hearing Aid Report,* (pp. 32–43). Upper Darby, Pa.: Monographs in Contemporary Audiology.

Libby, E. R. 1985. State-of-the-art of hearing aid selection procedures. *Hearing Instruments* 36:30–38, 62.

Macrae, J. 1985. Temporary and permanent threshold shift associated with hearing aid use. *The Australian Journal of Audiology* 7:45–54.

Markides, A. 1976. The effect of hearing aid use on the user's residual hearing. *Scandinavian Audiology* 5:205–210.

Markides, A., and Aryee, D. T. 1980. The effect of hearing aid use on the user's residual hearing. II: A follow-up study. *Scandinavian Audiology* 9:55–80.

Matkin, N. D. 1984. Wearable amplification: A litany of persisting problems. *In* J. Jerger (ed.). *Pediatric Audiology* (pp. 125–145). San Diego: College-Hill Press.

Morgan, D. E., Dirks, D. C., and Bower, D. R. 1979. Suggested thresholds sound pressure levels for frequency modulated (warble) tones in the sound field. *Journal of Speech and Hearing Disorders* 44:37–54.

Nabelek, A. K., and Robinson, P. K. 1982. Monaural and binaural speech perception in reverberation for listeners of various ages. *Journal of the Acoustical Society America* 71:1242–1248.

Nelson-Barlow, N. L., Auslander, M. C., Rines, D., and Stelmachowicz, P. G. 1985. Probe-microphone measures in hearing-impaired children and adults. Paper presented at the Convention of the American Speech-Language-Hearing Association, Washington, D.C.
Pascoe, D. P. 1978. An approach to hearing aid selection. *Wearing Instruments* 29:12–36.
Pavlovic, C. V. 1984. Use of the articulation index for assessing residual auditory function in listeners with sensorineural hearing impairment. *Journal of the Acoustical Society America* 75:1253–1258.
Podoshin, L., Kremer, M., Fradis, M., and Feiglin, H. 1984. Effect of hearing aids on hearing. *Laryngoscope* 94:113–117.
Punch, J. L., and Beck, L. B. 1986. Hearing aids and aural rehabilitation: Relative effects of low-frequency amplification on syllable recognition and speech quality. *Ear and Hearing* 7:57–62.
Reilly, K. M., Owens, E., Uken, D., McClatchie, A. C., and Clarke, R. 1981. Progressive hearing loss in children: Hearing aids and other factors. *Journal of Speech and Hearing Disorders* 46:328–334.
Ross, M., and Tommassetti, C. 1980. Hearing aid selection for pre-verbal hearing-impaired children. *In* M. C. Pollack (ed.). *Amplification for the Hearing Impaired.* (2nd Edition). New York: Grune and Stratton.
Ross, M., and Truex, E. H. 1965. Protecting residual hearing in hearing aid users. *Archives of Otolaryngology* 82:615–617.
Sebkova, J., and Bamford, J. M. 1981a. Evaluation of binaural hearing aids in children using localization and speech intelligibility tasks. *British Journal of Audiology* 15:126–132.
Sebkova, J., and Bamford, J. M. 1981b. Some effects of training and experience for children using one and two hearing aids. *British Journal of Audiology* 15:133–141.
Seewald, R. C., and Ross, M. 1988. Amplification for young hearing-impaired children. In M.C. Pollack (ed.). *Amplification for the Hearing Impaired.* (3rd Edition). New York: Grune and Stratton.
Seewald, R. C., Whitehead, G., and Golardi, S. 1986. Survey of hearing aid selection and evaluation procedures with young children. Paper presented at the Conference of the Canadian Speech-Language-Hearing Association. Winnipeg.
Silman, S., Gelfand, S. A., and Silverman, C. A. 1984. Late-onset auditory deprivation: Effects of monaural versus binaural hearing aids. *Journal of the Acoustical Society America* 76:1357–1362.
Simmons, B. 1986. Perilymphatic fistulas. Convention of the Alexander Graham Bell Association for the Deaf, Chicago.
Shapiro, I. 1976. Hearing aid fitting by prescription. *Audiology* 15:163–173.
Silverman, M., and Clopton, B. 1977. Plasticity of binaural interaction. I: Effect of early auditory deprivation. *Journal of Neurophysiology* 40:1266–1274.
Skinner, M. W., Pascoe, D. P., Miller, D. P., and Popelka, G. R. 1982. Measurements to determine the optimal placement of speech energy within the listener's auditory area: A basis for selecting amplification characteristics. *In* G. A. Studebaker, and F. H. Bess (eds.). *The Vanderbilt Hearing Aid Report:* (pp 161–196). Upper Darby, Pa.: Monographs in Contemporary Audiology.
Studebaker, G. A., Pavlovic, C. V., and Sherbecoe, R. L. 1985. Method for predicting speech discrimination of the hearing-impaired: Validation. Paper presented at American Speech-Language-Hearing Association Convention, Washington, D.C.
Tees, R. 1967a. The effects of early auditory restriction in the rat on adult duration discrimination. *Journal of Auditory Research* 7:195–207.
Tees, R. 1976b. Effects on early auditory restriction in the rat on adult pattern discrimniation. *Journal of Comparative Physiological Psychology* 63:389–393.
Walker, G., Dillon, H., and Byrne, D. 1984. Soundfield audiometry: Recommended stimuli and procedures. *Ear and Hearing* 5:13–21.
Webster, D., and Webster, M. 1977. Neonatal sound deprivation affects brain stem auditory nuclei. *Archives of Otolaryngology* 103:392–396.
Webster, D., and Webster, M. 1979. Effects of neonatal conductive hearing loss on brain stem auditory nuclei. *Annals of Otology, Rhinology and Laryngology* 88:684–688.
Webster, D. 1983. A critical period during postnatal auditory development of mice. *International Journal of Pediatric Otorhinolaryngology* 6:107–118.

Chapter 14

Communication/Language Assessment of the Hearing-Impaired Child

Richard R. Kretschmer, Jr. and *Laura W. Kretschmer*

In this age of educational accountability, the evaluation process has assumed an important role in both general and special education. Taxpayers expect their schools to report yearly improvement in reading or math scores for all students relative to national standards, while special education has legislated Individual Education Plans (IEPs) that require routine evaluation of pupil progress in areas from self-care to speech-sound production. Education of the hearing impaired certainly has not escaped evaluation pressures, especially in the areas of interpersonal communication and literacy. And, as we are all aware, significant deficits in English-language performance in these areas continue to characterize both deaf and hard-of-hearing students at all levels of the educational system, regardless of communication mode (Geers, Moog, and Shick 1984; Quigley and Paul 1986).

In a recent symposium on the last 20 years of language learning and teaching in the field of deafness, we reflected on the evidence that language test results of deaf children from 1965 to 1985 had not changed substantially even though our understanding of the normal language learning process and of the roles and functions of language in social communication had improved dramatically over that same period (Kretschmer and Kretschmer 1986). We wish to suggest that this new understanding of language learning and of its social communication functions *must* be incorporated into the evaluation process, as well as into our attitudes about the abilities of hearing-impaired children and youth.

We believe that one's view of language and its role in communication influences one's evaluation processes, as well as the way the products of evaluation are used in teaching. By the same token, teaching experiences, whether successful or otherwise, dispose one toward certain evaluation techniques.

To explain further, let us consider briefly how we define language and its role in social communication. From that perspective, we will consider recommendations for language/communication evaluation.

Description of Language

Language can be defined as a set of systematic rules, mutually agreed upon by a speech community, to designate experience and facilitate social interaction. From this definition, we can derive four basic aspects of language: discourse, semantics, syntax, and phonology (Clark and Clark 1977). The ordering of these components was deliberate, for it is clear from current research with English-speaking adults and children, that it is the discourse component that in large part determines semantic expression. Semantic need usually determines syntactic use, and it is the desired syntactic forms that determine phonological use at any given moment in the conversation. In other words, decisions about discourse and meanings to be expressed in discourse shape the syntactic constructions used. Since phonological considerations are beyond the scope of this presentation, we will focus instead on the discourse, semantic, and syntactic components of language. Keep in mind that learning to use these aspects of communication is driven by social motivation, which is particularly powerful in the early language development years.

Aspects of Discourse

Discourse governs how a conversation proceeds as individuals interact with one another. Semantic aspects relate to meaning; semantic rules in English outline how words may be joined to form larger units of meaning. Syntax, on the other hand, refers to the rules of sentence formation; syntactic selections are the means by which we order semantic units to facilitate the exchange of meaning in communication.

From the research literature and from observation, it is clear that each culture has certain constraints (or rules) that determine how people conduct social communication, particularly conversations (Wardhaugh 1985). American English, of course, has conventions which native speakers understand, and to which they adhere more or less—conventions that allow English speakers to predict how conversations will normally evolve. Without implicit knowledge of these conventions, the expectations of speakers and listeners of English conversations will be unmet; the smooth flow of a conversation can be impaired.

Briefly, to emphasize the critical nature of context in social communication, a few aspects of English conversation will be reviewed. We initiate conversations by engaging in opening sequences (Schegloff 1972; Williams 1976). One usually doesn't begin to converse until he has determined whether the other party wants to talk. These opening sequences are ritualistic and highly dependent on who the speaker is, on where the conversation is taking place, and on the specific reasons for the interchange (Wardhaugh 1985). One probably initiates conversations with an administrative supervisor in quite a different way than when conversing with a friend. Initiating conversation at a cocktail party is quite different from accomplishing the same task at a formal business meeting. If we intend to have an argument with our spouse, conversational initiation is different from trying to cajole our spouse into a six-week holiday in Europe. The purposes of any opening sequence are: (1) to establish "psychological" contact with the other person, and (2) to set the tone for the conversation itself.

To digress briefly, it can be shown that English has conventions not only for initiating conversations, but for terminating them as well (Schegloff and Sacks 1973). Once a speaker feels that he has said all he wishes to he can signal verbally (and nonverbally) to his communication partner that he wishes to terminate the interaction. This is referred to as a pre-closing and involves statements such as: "My, I didn't know it was so late" or "I have to pick up my kids from school." His communication partner would normally agree to terminate the conversation, by initiating the closing sequence. Like opening sequences, closing sequences are highly ritualized. Their extent and composition depend on the relation to the communication partner, the communication situation, and the purpose for interacting in the first place.

Once opening conventions are successfully negotiated, then communication partners normally embark upon the next task, that of choosing a topic (Wardhaugh 1985). As part of having an English conversation, the participants must agree implicitly on initial topics. The first topic is usually introduced through a conversational bid, such as: "Last summer, I went on this fabulous trip to Wales." At this point, one's communication partner can either accept this bid by saying: "Did you visit Aberystwyth?" or reject it by saying: "That's nice. By the way, did you hear about Mary and John?" This negotiating process continues until mutual agreement is reached, or until one partner acquiesces. Acts of choosing a topic occur throughout any conversation, either explicitly or implicitly. It is possible for speakers to introduce new topics into conversations by making a clean break between the previous dialogue and the new topic. For instance, one speaker might say: "I know we have been talking about Mary and her problems, but did you know that Mrs. Johnson decided not to move after all?" In fact, most new topics are introduced by association with other topics (Brinton and Fujiki 1984). For instance, a conversation could begin with an exchange about the relative merits of types of tea, then drift into an exchange on planning a trip to China, and finally end with an exchange on the merits of a newly discovered Chinese restaurant. What is important about these changes in topical direction is that the conversational partners should be able to recognize that changes are occurring; topics should not be changed so frequently as to make the conversation incoherent to all involved.

Once a topic has been decided on, the phase of information exchange should occur. The tone of a particular informational exchange sequence is set by the person who initiated the topic in the first place. Information exchange is shaped by three dimensions: cohesiveness, purpose, and text knowledge. These three dimensions interact to hold conversations together.

To explicate further, when speakers embark upon information exchange sequences, it is critical that each speaker's contribution is linked to the general topic while simultaneously showing awareness of the contributions of the other communication partners (Wardhaugh 1985). This awareness should exist at two levels, namely, the content being conveyed and the communication intention of the previous utterance. For instance, if a child produces a statement that is a prediction, then the next statement should respond not only to the content contained in the sentence, but also to the fact that a prediction was made. To ignore both shows a serious lack of involvement on the part of the listener. We would submit that these conversational intents have certain English syntactic structures strongly linked to them. For instance, when one wishes to make a prediction in English, it is very frequently accomplished using an internal state complement construction (I think he will fly away).

To exemplify these points, a short conversation between two pre-teen girls on the subject of pandas is presented in table I. Each contribution is on the topic of panda bears, but each utterance also recognizes previously generated utterances. In all cases, the children are responding not only to the content of the previous utterances, but also to their communicative intents. For instance, in sentence 2, Lauren says "Really" in response to Wanda's comment about seeing pandas, and uses the demonstrative pronoun [that] to represent the entire event, "seeing the panda bear in the Washington National Zoo" Wanda recognizes Lauren's comment through the use of "yeah," and extends the conversation by making the additional comment about what was fun about the event. In sentence 7, Wanda responds adroitly to Lauren's request for confirmation and then adds new information about how the national zoo is providing bamboo. In order for cohesion to work, each communication partner should be able to understand what has been said and what is intended by particular statements and then formulate responses that are appropriate and cohesive.

Central to the notion of conversational cohesion is the concept of monitoring old and new information (Clark and Haviland 1977). In order for a contribution to be cohesive, it must designate, in some way, the previous (old) information

Table I: Conversation between Wanda (W) and Lauren (L) on Pandas

W:	I was in Washington, D.C., and I saw the pandas in the national zoo.
L:	Really. That must have been fun. They're so cute and cuddly-looking.
W:	Yeah, they were both outside, so you got a good look at them.
L:	What were they doing?
W:	Well, Ling-Ling was walking around and eating stuff, while the other one was just sitting there looking grumpy.
L:	I think they just eat bamboo or something, don't they?
W:	Yeah, and the zoo has to grow it special for them. It's all around the place with signs that say it's being grown for the pandas.

to which one is linking. Once this has been done, the speaker normally adds new information. Facile communication partners rarely, if ever, merely add old information; each contribution usually carries new information as well. In some cases, the new information is conveyed through intonational patterns, which might indicate that the speaker either agrees with what has been said, or is contradicting previous information. The discourse function of certain semantic/ syntactic forms in English is to signal the presence of old and/or new information. For instance, pronouns are used normally only as old information markers. The determiner *the* tends to be an old information marker, while the determiner *a* is generally a new information marker. These syntactic forms could be said to have meaning only as they function within a conversational context. If we try to evaluate knowledge about such forms through isolated sentences, we may grossly underestimate or overestimate a hearing-impaired child's knowledge of English.

In addition to cohesion, information exchange sequences are dominated by the purpose of the speaker in undertaking a discussion of the topic. For instance, a speaker might undertake a topic in order to entertain; to tell a story; to explain a phenomenon; to describe an object; to convey personal feelings and/or emotions; to persuade; to challenge; or to tease a communication partner (Lindfors 1980). Once a topic is introduced, how the information exchange proceeds depends entirely upon the purpose of the speaker. Of course, his communication partner may not accept his purpose, or may attempt to subvert it. In order to achieve the latter goal, the communication partner must still be able to recognize what purpose is being attempted so as to frame his own responses accordingly.

Each information exchange purpose carries its own text organization, which is conveyed by the use of certain conventions. For instance, when telling a story in American English, the task of the narrator is to arrange the tale in chronological order, so that it is apparent how one event proceeds out of another event (Kemper 1984). This requires the narrator to provide physical and/or motivational links between the story events. Equally notable about these text organization conventions is that each has associated with it certain preferred linguistic structures (Halliday and Hasan 1976). For instance, when telling a story, *and* is used frequently, as are temporal words. If the story involves people conversing with one another, there is considerable use of indirect discourse. If the speaker engages in explanation, he is very likely to use many syntactic coordinators such as *because, but,* and *so*. Recounting personal feelings requires the frequent use of internal state verbs such as *want,* along with infinitive clauses. As suggested previously, syntactic forms are not used randomly, but rather are strongly linked to the speaker's purpose in conversing and to the text organization imposed on the conversation.

Finally, even though one's primary aim is clear communication, interpersonal conversations are still subject to ambiguity, as is any kind of communication. Even conversational partners from the same family have been known to misunderstand or to lose track of the topic entirely. Because English conversations are ruled by the "on track" principle, a variety of linguistic strategies for conversational repair have evolved (Jefferson 1972). These repair strategies enable the confused conversational partner to ascertain or verify topics, to clarify comments, to indicate communication purpose, or to encourage clearer oral production in order to hear what has been said. In English, repair sequences generally require the use of certain linguistic structures such as question-forms, embedded adjectives, and relative clauses. For example, table II presents a repair sequence between two teenage boys. As can be seen, the sequence was initiated by a question, and the response involved the use of both adjectives and relative clauses.

SEMANTIC/SYNTACTIC ASPECTS

Having briefly considered some aspects of English discourse, we turn to a consideration of the semantic/syntactic system. We accept that to be efficient communicators hearing-impaired children must use and understand the semantic/syntactic conventions of English. We further accept that some evaluation/assessment of that knowledge and ability must be made. We contend, however, that, as with learning when and how to have meaningful conversations, learning semantic/syntactic conventions occurs best while children are engaged in those same meaningful conversations. Thus, we would argue that when assessing semantic/syntactic knowledge, one must construct conversational environments where their use is natural. Further, in evaluation of syntax, we must consider assessing not only use of language forms per se, but also whether a child knows when to use those forms for effective communication.

The semantic and syntactic systems of English are so interwoven, that it is almost impossible to discuss them separately. Although individual words have meaning, it is the combination of words that gives meaning to sentences. The meaning of a sentence is not the summed meanings of individual words, but the product of the interaction between the primary lexical items in that sentence. As a consequence, the semantic system of English cannot be defined satisfactorily by its lexicon, but rather requires consideration of the types and number of meaning relations possible. These relations are called propositions. Each proposition contains a verbal unit—usually a verb, an adjective, or a preposi-

Table II: Conversation between Ben (B) and Jeremy (J)

B:	. . . so I was walking down the street and who did I see but that fox, Susie Watkins.
J:	Who's she?
B:	You know her.
J:	No, I don't.
B:	Well, she's that red-headed chick who lives in Greenfield, in the big white house next to Aaron.
J:	Oh, her. The one who drove me crazy in math class.
B:	Yeah, her. Well, I saw her yesterday and I go, "How about a date?" and she goes, "Yes!"

tion—and each verbal unit has associated with it a prerequisite number of arguments—usually nouns and/or adverbs. Thus, the verbal unit *in* carries with it two arguments: the entity that is *in,* and the place where the entity is. The verbal unit *put* carries three arguments: the entity who puts, the entity that is put, and the place where it is put.

We can encode propositions into single propositional sentences or we can combine and express them in multi-propositional sentences. A single propositional sentence in English normally occurs in a basic sentence frame. For instance, the verbal argument *hit* normally is organized into the basic frame N + V + N. Depending upon the immediate intent of the conversation, a modality may be attached to this basic frame; that is, we might decide to make a statement, ask a question, or give a command. If we decide to give a command, then the basic frame is modified in the following way: V + N. In addition, the speaker considers the immediate discourse requirements of his utterance, a consideration that determines the types of additional syntactic information to be included in the basic frame. For instance, if we wish to make a statement about a past event, then we need to use past tense, and if this past event includes an object that has already been introduced into the conversation, then we need to use the determiner *the* rather than *a*. These latter aspects of syntactic formation are called modulations. Modulation use is tied to the immediate discourse needs of the speaker.

In English, it is also possible to join propositions in single-sentence frames. There are three primary means by which this is achieved; namely, coordination, complementation, and relativization. Coordination involves the joining of two or more propositions into a single relationship; the intended relationship normally is signalled through the use of a connector such as *and, because, if,* or *whenever.* Complementation is the use of one proposition as the argument of another proposition. For instance, in the sentence, "I wanted to go," we have the main proposition, *I want something.* What is wanted is the event, *I go.* This is an example of a infinitive clause where the event, *I go,* acts as one of the arguments for the proposition, *I want something.* The form of complementation used is dependent on the semantic intentions of the speaker with regard to the information to be conveyed. For instance, if the speaker wishes to convey that someone asked a yes-no question, he will use a yes-no question, indirect discourse form, e.g., "He asked if he could go." On the other hand, if he wishes to convey the notion that the person is giving an order, he will use an indirect discourse–direct imperative form, e.g., "He told her to go." The third process for relating propositions is relativization, or the attachment of a proposition to an argument in another proposition for purposes of clarification. Thus, in the sentence, "I want the red ball," the proposition, *ball red,* has been attached to the argument, *ball,* in the proposition, *I want ball,* in order to clarify which ball is wanted. As stated previously, use of these more complex processes is dictated by the discourse purpose(s) of the speaker, namely, his intention when introducing certain topics.

Evaluation Procedures with the Hearing Impaired

From the reports of Heider and Heider in the 1940s to more recent summaries (Quigley and Paul 1986), evaluation of written, oral, signed, speechread, or auditory reception abilities of hearing-impaired persons has stressed their limitations in using English. Such evaluations have used tests developed on normal-hearing children, tests developed for exclusive use with hearing-impaired children, or tests that have been standardized on both normal-hearing and hearing-impaired populations. A variety of evaluation techniques has been used. Most prominent have been procedures that use acting-out techniques, elicited imitation, picture identification, grammatical judgments, and sentence completion tasks. Each of these techniques carries with it certain problems, which have been detailed elsewhere (Kretschmer and Kretschmer 1978; Darley 1979) and will not be reported here. These techniques all have in common a focus on evaluating syntactic or lexical item knowledge apart from the natural context of social communication. That is, these tests stress the evaluation of language out of context, in part, so the argument goes, to reduce ambiguity for the deaf child—that is, to ensure that the deaf child really *knows* something apart from context. In fact, the argument might be taken to its logical conclusion, namely, "Don't give the deaf child context; it only confuses him." Can you imagine how fluent those of us who are not deaf would be if we had to learn all of English discourse's semantic/syntactic conventions out of context? It is precisely what the deaf child does not need. Give him more context; evaluate him *in* context in order to understand the range of his communication assets and liabilities. Understanding language functions means knowing how and when to fit a particular syntactic form into an extended conversation so that conversation will work. It is not simply understanding and/or using a particular form to complete a noncommunicative sentence, to repeat exactly what someone else has said, or to do a picture discription.

Consider this specific example. Hearing-impaired children often are tested for their comprehension of adjectives by showing them a picture and then requesting that the child "show me the boy with blue eyes." If the child is able to accomplish one or more tasks such as this, he may be credited with having an age-appropriate knowledge of English adjectives. A brief consideration of the role of adjectives in a running conversation points out the weakness of such an approach. When there is potential ambiguity and one says "I saw the boy with blue eyes," it is normally assumed by listener and speaker that the adjective *blue* is required to differentiate this boy from others present. If a hearing-impaired child uses the adjective *blue* in this way and there are only boys with blue eyes present, then he doesn't really understand how English adjectives function in conversation. If the only observation about adjective knowledge is taken from this type of "test," regardless of the number of items tested, then the evaluator's understanding of a particular hearing-impaired student's language abilities is primitive at best. If you must, select those formal (standardized) tests that are at least powerful enough to tell you where to take the X-ray, to drill the well—or whatever other analogy you prefer.

To overcome the limitations of individual formal tests, many persons have advocated the use of a test battery in the evaluation of communication/language abilities of hearing-impaired children. Such an approach—which yields a profile of strengths and weaknesses in areas such as reception and expression of syntax, reception and expression of vocabulary, and so on—should also be treated cautiously. Each part of the test battery is, at best, a screening procedure for a certain limited aspect of language performance. When all the "tests" are shown in profile, that profile is thought to completely characterize a particular child. In fact, the profile characterizes only how that child responded at that point to the social event of repeated, intensive but decontextualized, test administration. We will say more about the social nature of test situations shortly.

Why are we so concerned about the exclusive use of formal tests? It is our contention that the evaluation procedures adopted by an educational program and/or an individual teacher, speech/language therapist, or school psychologist, are generally a reflection of how they believe language is learned, how it functions, or how it should be taught. In turn, the program and/or teacher uses these evaluation procedures to judge the success of their efforts to "teach" language. In short, focus on out of context test results seems to narrow the view of the consumer with regard to the abilities and/or needs of the deaf child.

We would argue that there can, and indeed must be, a judicious combination of theoretically sound formal tests along with examination of the conversational uses of language. We insist that hearing-impaired children must be evaluated on their knowledge of discourse conventions such as opening and ending conversations; choice of topic abilities; exchange of information; demonstration of cohesion skills; use of language for a variety of purposes; and knowledge of text organization, as well as whatever evaluation of specific semantic/syntactic forms are of interest. Even the latter evaluation should be tied to an examination of language in use rather than to tests conducted exclusively in isolation. The analysis of discourse abilities of hearing-impaired children can best be accomplished through examination of naturally occurring conversations. Specific semantic/syntactic use can be evaluated, when necessary, by some formal tests, but this can be done just as productively by developing communication problems that can best be solved through the use of particular linguistic forms. The former discourse evaluation will give insight into what the hearing-impaired child knows about conversations and about communicating, while the latter testing allows one to evaluate, when necessary, whether a child can use specific language forms to accomplish specific conversational goals.

CONCERNS ABOUT CONVERSATIONAL/INFORMAL ASSESSMENT

Before proceeding, we wish to address certain criticisms that have been leveled against the use of conversational evaluation. First, it has been argued by some that examining naturalistic conversation samples does not assess so-called reception or comprehension of language, only its production. This objection may be true if the emphasis is placed on analysis of the child's sentences apart from his contribution to the conversation itself. If a hearing-impaired child does not comprehend communication, it will quickly be apparent when he does not provide meaningful contributions to the interaction. If the child's contributions are examined in the context of the conversation and with regard to their discourse appropriateness, then both comprehension and production of language are being assessed.

Second, it is argued, unfortunately, that conversational analysis is unrealistic because teachers of the hearing impaired do not have sufficient knowledge of English and its discourse functions to analyze conversation. Given the fact that communication/language problems have long been recognized as one of the primary problems of hearing-impaired persons, it seems unacceptable to us to argue that teachers of the hearing impaired lack the knowledge to understand and assess all aspects of communication. If they do indeed lack knowledge of how to analyze English conversations, then it certainly must be said that they lack the primary information that enables them to be teachers of the hearing impaired. If there is substance to this argument, then the teacher-education programs for the hearing impaired must examine their curricula, and schools and programs for the hearing impaired must assess their in-service efforts. As educators, we must not abdicate our role as language experts. There is certainly enough work to go around when it comes to the issue of assessing and improving the communication abilities of hearing-impaired children.

Third, a corollary to the second objection, is the idea that even if teachers can accomplish conversational analysis, such procedures are too time consuming and take time from teaching. If one believes that assessment is independent of teaching rather than a necessary prerequisite, then this argument might hold weight; however, it is our contention that assessment is both a prerequisite to teaching and an ongoing component of instruction. If a teacher or program understands: (1) that meaningful use of language for communication is an integral part of education of the hearing impaired, and (2) that language grows from communication, then time for assessment ceases to be a problem. Evaluation time is simply built into the teaching process and occurs continually as the basis for measuring communication maturity.

Fourth, it has been suggested that use of conversational assessment makes it impossible to quantify "language age" or progress in language development. It could be argued, in return, that quantification, in and of itself, is not a valid goal with respect to assessing communication/language use. We seldom weigh the amount of communication of facile speakers, but we are certainly aware of the *effects* of that communication in everyday life. Still, granting the present concern for numerical accountability, it is possible to quantify any behavior you wish. Counting behaviors is the basis of any criterion-referenced testing procedure. One doesn't need a specific test in order to quantify language behaviors. For instance, listing number of appropriate versus inappropriate uses of if-clauses in situations requiring their use can be just as valid as giving the hearing-impaired child a standardized test that measures ability to identify if-clauses or complete sentences with such clauses.

Finally, it has been suggested that the use of formal language tests is more objective than the evaluation of natural conversations. In the formal test situation, the chances of evaluator bias are presumed to be reduced. Recent studies on intelligence and psychological testing have suggested just the opposite (Erickson 1981; McDermott and Hood 1982). Formal test situations are social encounters that develop over time, just as surely as informal conversations. The pacing, the types of examiner repetitions, the use of intonational patterns and nonverbal cues, and the biases of those persons who are administering the tests, are as important to formal testing situations as they are to any other social encounters. The perception of objectivity in any test situation varies in direct relation to one's social role in that assessment situation.

We reiterate that we do not question the requirement that hearing-impaired children must undergo standardized testing of the achievement or intelligence variety, in the same way that each of us has been forced to clear those obstacles. We do argue, however, that standardized or formal language tests alone do not offer a more objective basis for assessing communication than do informal procedures. Thus, why not employ informal procedures that are relevant to the interpersonal and classroom communication needs of each hearing-impaired child?

Recommendations for Assessment

Having discussed the need to evaluate language in its broadest context, namely, conversation, the question arises as to how evaluation could proceed. For school or program placement, we support the use of formal tests for which a sound psychometric and theoretical basis can be shown. A comprehensive evaluation procedure such as the one most recently suggested by Moeller, Osberger, Quinn, and Johnson (1986), which provides a useful variety of information rather than a single score to characterize language functioning, seems a step in the right direction. Once a child has been placed in a program, however, it is vital that more naturalistic data be obtained for purposes of planning his educational experience.

We do not advocate obtaining a pre-set number of utterances or interactions but rather suggest that children be observed in a variety of contexts to see how they adapt their language use across communication opportunities.

Specifically, we would suggest that each child be observed in interaction with several communication partners on the same topic, and with the same communication partner on a variety of topics. We would also suggest that children be placed in contexts where they: (*a*) narrate stories, (*b*) explain events, (*c*) describe events, (*d*) attempt to persuade others to perform tasks that they don't want to perform, and (*e*) negotiate roles and tasks, as in play situations. Along with this, children should be encouraged to write narrative, expository, and descriptive materials, on topics of their own choosing, addressed to various communication partners. The quality of what is written to the teacher may be quite different from that written to a best friend or one's mother. These tasks could be standardized for a particular school, based on its curriculum, with guidelines on how these samples would be derived.

Since evaluation should occur in a communication context, it is important that interpersonal communication efforts be videotaped. For instance, it is not possible to determine whether a child has responded to an indirect command unless we see the actions he performs when given the command. It is also important that the teacher provide field notes that put any videotaped segments into perspective. We recognize that not all programs have readily available videotape equipment; it is also possible to use field notes exclusively, or in combination with audiotape, when the child uses intelligible oral communication almost exclusively. Use of this latter technique, however, not only eliminates nonverbal information as well as the full communication context, but cannot be employed when the child's mode of communication is primarily visual.

We feel that there should be twice-yearly evaluations. These evaluations should be formalized with appropriate transcripts and interpretations. The most time-consuming aspect of conversation evaluation, of course, is the recording and transcribing of communication exchanges. Because of this difficulty, it may be time for school programs to consider employing language experts whose primary task it is to codify data that can be shared with classroom teachers and other professional staff. Because evaluation is ongoing, we also feel that there should be strategies for continually recording children's utterances and/or writings, but obviously these efforts need not to be as extensive as the beginning and end-of-the-year evaluations.

ANALYZING CONVERSATIONAL EXCHANGES

Once these data have been collected, they need to be analyzed. Analysis can occur on two levels, at the macro or conversation level and at the micro or sentence level. Conversational analysis should be focused at least on the ability of children to initiate and terminate conversations; to introduce and track topics; to generate and respond to clarification requests; to produce contributions that are cohesive; and to generate discourse organizations that reflect a variety of purposes.

Analysis at the micro or sentence level should consider at least four questions: (*a*) Was the form used appropriate to the context; that is, did it convey the function intended at that moment in the conversation? (*b*) Was the form used to encode semantic notions as they would normally occur in English? (*c*) Was the form produced a syntactically complete one? and (*d*) Were there forms the child did not use at all, that, if present, would facilitate his solving the communication problem he was facing? Often we attend to what the child is not producing well and do not consider areas where further growth is important. The answers to both macro- and micro-level questions need to be considered in relation to what we know about the normal development of language in children. Are the communication/linguistic behaviors exhibited by a particular child consistent with data on children learning English, or are there idiosyncratic developments? If the latter seems to be the case, then it is possible that this child is on the road to developing a linguistic system other than English. Information on communication/language development in normal children is growing at such an enormous rate that it is not reasonable for every teacher to keep abreast of it. This suggests another role that a specialist in language development might fill in school programs. The specialist could be expected to obtain information on the development of particular discourse aspects or linguistic structures and then provide this information to teachers to aid them in planning language/communication experiences.

Again at the micro or sentence level, attention should be given to knowledge of the following syntactic issues: (*a*) basic frames, (*b*) modalities, (*c*) modulations, and (*d*) complex forms including coordination, complementation, and relativization. From the language development literature, we learn that children normally master basic frames and modalities, then they develop modulations and complex operations (coordination first, then complementation, and finally relativization). Examination of dozens of language curricula for the deaf has shown us that most persons working with hearing-impaired children focus attention on modulations and delay assessing (or even teaching) complexity until the students are well into school, often even into high school. We would argue that this may be misplaced energy. Assessment and instructional focus should initially be placed on children's use of complexity rather than modulation. Although both normally develop simultaneously when children learn English, we would argue that a hearing-impaired speaker shows more linguistic maturity if he can express complex relationships despite syntactic "errors," as compared to producing only simple, albeit syntactically correct sentences, i.e., modulations.

At the micro or sentence level, specific evaluation might be accomplished by placing the child in communication situations where use of particular forms becomes critical because those forms normally encode certain linguistic functions. For instance, in play situations, one of the primary goals of communication is to negotiate roles (Kuczaj and Daly 1979). One of the common linguistic forms children use to negotiate these roles is if-clauses. Children often say, "If you be mommy, I'll be daddy," or "If you use the hose, be careful not to knock down the house." By putting a child in a situation where he has to negotiate certain aspects of play, his use and mastery of if-clauses within a naturalistic context could be assessed. Thus, when considering the evaluation of specific linguistic structures, one must first ask, under what conditions would such forms be generated? Use those conditions as a means of obtaining data about children's ability to generate language. Since each syntactic form is used for different functions in conversation, one cannot develop a single test that will work for each form. Instead, a different test may be required for each linguistic form being assessed, or for constellations of forms that fulfill essentially the same function within conversation. For instance, deVilliers and deVilliers (1986) have developed contextual referential communication tasks for use with deaf children that examine specification—a conversational function that normally entails the use of adjectives, *with* prepositional phrases, or relative clauses.

To organize communication evaluations, we think that school programs might assemble teams of teachers to work together in the evaluation process. Each teacher would be expected to bring information on his students to meetings where group discussion and group decision-making can occur. In this way, analysis of the macro-conversational and micro-sentence levels can be facilitated and verified. The evaluation team could also develop the specific situations through which particular linguistic forms can be evaluated. It is important that such teams have access to specialized personnel, such as a language development specialist, as well as the curricula committees for their schools, so that comprehensive assessment and programming decisions can be made.

The use of naturalistic evaluation has changed our own views of the communication/linguistic abilities of hearing-impaired children in some very positive ways. By considering what deaf children *know* about communication instead of simply what they don't know, the examiner is in for numerous surprises. A few years ago, we wouldn't have predicted that a 13-month-old deaf child would be able to switch communication styles according to which parent she was with (Blennerhassett 1984), or that a 2 ½-year-old deaf child with very limited oral communication could be expected to use the same utterances to respond differently to her mother's verbal teasing, to school language requests, or to homework routines (Plapinger 1985). Assessment of language knowledge by formal tests missed a pre-teen boy's sophisticated awareness of how conversations work outside of school. For instance, this young man used the utterance, "What's your problem?" to challenge his brother, to encourage his sister to seek new information, to end conflicts, and to initiate conversations. Without examining his interactions with others, we might have settled for the conclusion that there was much he couldn't do (Metzger 1985).

The Link Between Evaluation and Teaching

The power of evaluation procedures is shown, in large part, once that evaluation has been completed. We have stressed our belief that information about the maturity and immaturity of the communication/language system of a hearing-impaired child must be applicable to educational programming. We have argued that an assessment procedure that examines communication interactions can, and indeed must, be translated into an educational context. Schools are responsible for transmitting certain formal knowledge. Schools for the hearing impaired must simultaneously teach functional use of language as well. This latter goal is not impossible if the professional staff recognizes that content/knowledge can be taught *via* naturalistic communication exchange. Specifically, teaching in programs for the hearing impaired need not (indeed must not) be exclusively via lectures. What should be tried is construction of experiences that emphasize natural conversation while simultaneously developing aspects of knowledge. For instance, information about personal health care, such as regular visits to the doctor or dentist, can be provided by playing out the first visit to a dentist's office. Contemporary social issues can be explored as children obtain information about Martin Luther King, Jr., in order to reenact debates between Dr. King and other important people in his life. Any of these activities can be organized so that certain types of conversational and linguistic experience are emphasized. If discourse practice is needed in using a series of related comments, and if semantic/syntactic practice is needed for the target *and* for other simple conjoining, Martin Luther King might explain his experiences in Selma, Alabama to his wife Coretta, a format that encourages practice at both the conversational (macro-) and sentence (micro-) level. Using assessment information in this way requires planning and effort that is quite different from relying on teacher's textbook guides, or a universal language curriculum. Surely it is time we expected this sort of creative teaching from those who work with deaf children, since our traditional methods have not had a noticeable impact on the communication and/or literacy levels of a majority of deaf students.

There are, of course, many hearing-impaired children in the mainstream, an environment where the amount of formal language teaching or "therapy" is often confined to contact with an itinerant teacher or language therapist for one-half hour per day or week. Even in these cases, it is possible for the teacher/therapist to develop small communication problems that are best solved through the use of specific linguistic/communication acts. For instance, children can be given tasks that require them to express their desires, wishes, or intentions, such as telling another child what he/she hopes to do on a trip to Colorado. Focus on intentions will naturally provide practice in the use of simple infinitives, as the most efficient for English encoding.

Summary

In conclusion, language should be assessed for educational purposes in the communication context. Exclusive use of assessment procedures that emphasize out of context, noncommunicative responses, are, in our opinion, not providing the full range of information required to understand or to describe the abilities of deaf children. In our thinking, communication-based assessment procedures need to evaluate children engaged in natural conversations on a variety of topics, with a variety of communication partners, and for a variety of purposes. Micro-sentence level evaluation of specific semantic/syntactic forms should also be done in conversational context, taking into consideration not only semantic/syntactic accuracy, but also conversational appropriateness. In the evaluation of specific forms, one should identify what the child is doing well, what problems he/she is demonstrating, and any conspicuous absences. We urge teachers to use the evaluation data to devise learning experiences that recognize the extent of the child's communication abilities along with the curricular goals and normal language development literature. Emphasis should be on developing general notions of communication, in addition to any specific practice in using linguistic principles to solve communication problems. We urge that assessment of English-language knowledge be more than a testing exercise for hearing-impaired children. It should constitute the beginning of a process that allows the deaf child access to mature social interactions with any person in his society.

REFERENCES

Blennerhassett, L. 1984. Communicative styles of a 13-month-old hearing-impaired child and her parents. *Volta Review* 86:217–228.

Brinton, B., and Fujiki, M. 1984. Development of topic manipulation skills in discourse. *Journal of Speech and Hearing Research* 27:350–358.

Clark, H., and Clark, E. 1977. *Psychology and Language*. New York: Harcourt Brace Jovanich.

Clark, H., and Haviland, S. 1977. Comprehension and the given-new contract. *In* R. Freedle (ed.). *Discourse Production and Comprehension* (pp. 1–40). Norwood, NJ: Ablex.

Darley, F. (ed.). 1979. *Evaluation of Appraisal Techniques in Speech and Language Pathology*. Reading, MA: Addison-Wesley Publishing Company.

deVilliers, P., and deVilliers, J. 1986. Assessing expressive language by eliciting production in pragmatically appropriate settings. Paper presented at the International Convention of the Alexander Graham Bell Association for the Deaf, Chicago, IL.

Erickson, F. 1981. Timing and context in everyday discourse: Implications for the study of referential and social meaning. *In* W. Dickson (ed.). *Children's Oral Communication Skills* (pp. 241–269). New York: Academic Press.

Geers, A., Moog, J., and Shick, B. 1984. Acquisition of spoken and signed English by profoundly deaf children. *Journal of Speech and Hearing Disorders* 49:378–388.

Halliday, M., and Hasan, R. 1976. *Cohesion in English*. London: Longman.

Jefferson, G. 1972. Side sequences. *In* D. Sudow (ed.). *Studies in Social Interaction* (pp. 294–338). New York: Free Press.

Kemper, S. 1984. The development of narrative skills: Explanations and entertainments. *In* S. Kuczaj (ed.). *Discourse Development: Progress in Cognitive Development Research* (pp. 99–124). New York: Springer-Verlag.

Kretschmer, R., and Kretschmer, L. 1978. *Language Development and Intervention with the Hearing Impaired*. Baltimore, MD: University Park Press.

Kretschmer, R., and Kretschmer, L. 1986. Language in perspective. *In* D. Luterman (ed.). *Deafness in Perspective* (pp. 131–166). San Diego, CA: College-Hill Press.

Kuczaj, S., and Daly, M. 1979. The development of hypothetical reference in the speech of young children. *Journal of Child Language* 6:563–579.

Lindfors, J. 1980. *Children's Language and Learning*. Englewood Cliffs, NJ: Prentice-Hall.

McDermott, R., and Hood, L. 1982. Institutionalized psychology and the ethnography of schooling. *In* P. Gilmore and A. Glatthorn (eds.). *Children In and Out of School* (pp. 232–249). Washington, DC: Center for Applied Linguistics.

Metzger, H. 1985. *"What's Your Problem?" The Role of Questioning in the Social Interactions of a Hearing Impaired Preadolescent.* Unpublished Doctoral Dissertation, University of Cincinnati.

Moeller, M., Osberger, M., Quinn, M., and Johnson, D. 1986. Assessment of the communication skills of hearing-impaired children. Paper presented at the International Convention of the Alexander Graham Bell Association, Chicago, IL.

Plapinger, D. 1985. *Context: Its Effect on the Interaction Between a Hearing Mother and her Hearing-Impaired Child.* Unpublished Doctoral Dissertation, University of Cincinnati.

Quigley, S., and Paul, P. 1986. A perspective on academic achievement. *In* D. Luterman (ed.). *Deafness in Perspective* (pp. 55–86). San Diego, CA: College-Hill Press.

Schegloff, E. 1972. Sequencing in conversational openings. *In* J. Gumperz and D. Hymes (eds.). *Directions in Sociolinguistics: The Ethnography of Communication* (pp. 346–380). New York: Holt, Rinehart, and Winston.

Schegloff, E., and Sacks, H. 1973. Opening up closings. *Semiotica* 8:289–327.

Wardhaugh, R. 1985. *How Conversation Works.* Oxford, England: Basil Blackwell.

Williams, M. 1976. Presenting oneself in talk: The disclosure of occupation. *In* P. Harre (ed.). *Life Sentences: Aspects of the Social Role of Language* (pp. 145–162). London: John Wiley.

Chapter 15

Maturational Considerations in the Neuroauditory Evaluation of Children

Frank E. Musiek and *Karen M. Gollegly*

INTRODUCTION

An understanding of maturational effects is essential for the optimal diagnosis and management of children with auditory deficits. This is particularly important when the clinician is presented with apparent problems related to auditory reception, processing, and response systems. An awareness of the influence of maturation has become more critical because new hearing assessment procedures often probe the integrity of neural auditory mechanisms. We now know that brain functions related to hearing require more time to mature than peripheral auditory functions (Romand 1983). Therefore, hearing tests that are heavily dependent on neural function must be interpreted in the context of neuromaturational factors. Neuromaturation, or the lack of it, may explain discrepant test results in certain clinical instances. Knowledge of confounding maturational effects can help the clinician select the most appropriate audiological test(s) for a given child. The correct evaluation of the stage of audiological development for a particular child may also enhance management and habilitative strategies.

Although most audiological tests for children are influenced by maturation, this paper will focus primarily on selected neuroauditory test procedures. There are several reasons for this emphasis. One is that most of these tests are relatively new or experimental, and little is generally known about the maturational effects. In addition, these procedures tap various brain functions that may demonstrate long-term maturational effects. Therefore, maturation may remain a factor in evaluation for an extended period. Finally, the "neuroauditory" test results may allow insight, at least on a theoretical basis, into the mechanisms of maturation in the auditory system.

We will discuss the effects of maturation on the auditory brainstem response (ABR), middle latency response (MLR), the 'late responses' (i.e., N_1, P_2, P_3), and on dichotic listening. Though a variety of other audiological tests could be used to evaluate maturational effects, the selected measures reflect changes at various levels of the auditory system. Some mechanisms underlying neuroauditory maturation will also be discussed.

Auditory Brainstem Response (ABR)

The auditory brainstem response (ABR) is a commonly employed electrophysiological measure of peripheral hearing sensitivity and neurological status. As initially reported by Jewett and Williston in 1971, ABR provides a far-field recording of synchronous electrical activity in the auditory nerve and brainstem pathway in response to auditory stimulation. The ABR is characterized by five to seven waveforms in the first 10 msec following the presentation of a series of clicks or tone pip stimuli. Recordings are typically made with a referent electrode at the ear lobe or mastoid and an active site at the high forehead or vertex. Responses from the auditory nerve and brainstem are computer averaged and selectively filtered. Measures of absolute and interwave latencies, interaural latency differences, and amplitude ratios are commonly used to evaluate both hearing sensitivity and central nervous system function (Jacobson 1985; Hall 1983). However, these characteristics, as well as others, vary greatly as a function of age, with significant changes noted in the first three years of life.

MATURATIONAL VARIABLES IN THE ABR

Prior to 30 weeks gestational age, a repeatable ABR may or may not be recorded, with the variability seemingly related to both the intensity of the signal and the infant's general status (Starr et al. 1977). At 30 to 32 weeks gestational age, a waveform characterized by Waves I, III, and V is commonly noted. By three to four months of age (52 to 56 weeks gestation), Waves II and IV have emerged as well (Jacobson, Morehouse, and Johnson 1982; Krumholz et al. 1985; Salamy 1984).

ABR wave latency is a function of the age of the infant (figure 1). It is commonly recognized that Wave I attains adult latency values by three months of age, whereas Waves III and V continue to change until two to three years of age, reflecting the caudorostral development pattern (Cox 1985; Salamy et al. 1980). As a result of this progression, the interwave intervals will change as well. The I–V interval, commonly referred to as central conduction time, does not reach adult values until almost three years of age (figure 2) (Salamy 1984).

Some of the difficulty in obtaining repeatable latency measures is related to the inherent variablity in infant ABR recordings. Although the ABR does become more stable near term, the immature system provides a less synchronous response to the auditory stimuli when compared with adults. However, interestingly, within-subject tracings are fairly repeatable (Salamy 1984).

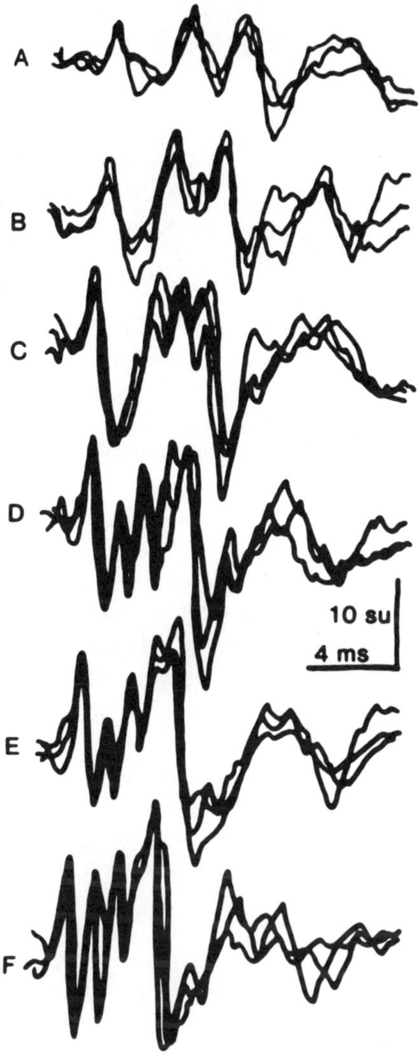

Figure 1. Maturational changes for the ABR. Changes can be seen in latency, amplitude, and morphology. Each ABR tracing represents a different infant or child at the following ages: A) 32 weeks conceptional age; B) 35 weeks conceptional age; C) full term; D) 3 months; E) 1 year; F) 3 years. (From Salamy 1984, with permission.)

Several additional factors are less commonly assessed but also reflect the ongoing maturation of the auditory system. The amplitude of the component waves and the resultant V/I amplitude ratio is one such measure. Contrary to the adult form in which Wave V is the largest wave, Waves I and III are equal to or slightly larger than Wave V in the neonate. Subsequently the V/I amplitude ratio is small. All waves increase in amplitude until approximately two to four

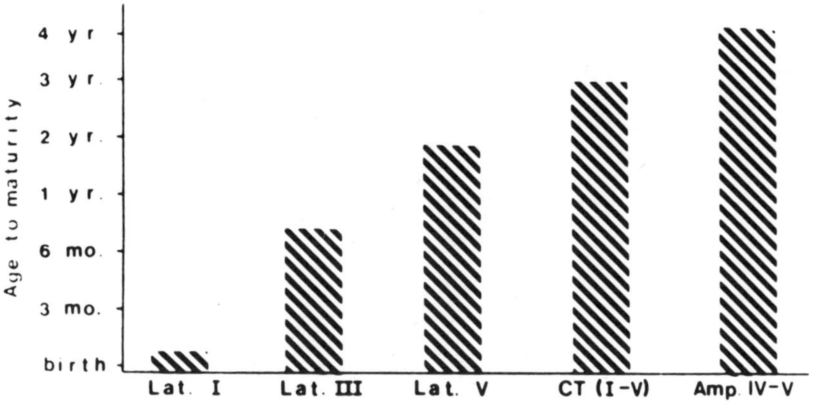

Figure 2. Maturation of selected ABR indices, from left to right: latencies of waves I, III, V, central transmission time (CT, I–V), amplitude of IV-V waves. (From Salamy 1984, with permission).

years of age with Wave V exhibiting the greatest growth (Cox 1985; Salamy 1984). Salamy (1984) relates that Waves I and V follow a similar growth pattern, reaching peak amplitude at two to four years, while Wave III reaches its peak at three years of age. Therefore, the V/I amplitude ratio increases during this period as well, reaching a plateau between two and four years of age. It is important to be cognizant of this difference in amplitude ratios when using this index as a measure of neural integrity.

The rate of stimulation is a factor affecting both neonatal and adult waveforms. Adults demonstrate an approximately 0.1 msec increase in Wave V latency each time the rate is increased by a factor of ten (Don, Allen, and Starr 1977). A similar function is seen in children. However, some studies have revealed absence of the ABR at rates above 40 clicks/sec prior to 30 weeks gestational age as well as markedly larger shifts in latency in preterm and term infants (Despland and Galambos 1980; Salamy 1984). In addition, a marked change in the response was noted for six- to seven-week-old infants at rates above 67 clicks/sec (Fujikawa and Weber 1977). In contrast, Salamy (1984) noted no significant change from normal at rates up to 100 clicks/sec for infants approximately this age. Though there is obvious disagreement about rate effects for "older" infants, it is clear that newborns and preterm infants reveal greater latency shifts than adults. These findings suggest that rate-affected changes may not reflect the neural refractory period alone but possibly adaptation and other neural mechanisms that vary from infant to infant.

A final additional measure of maturation reflected in the ABR is the comparison of the ipsilateral and contralateral responses. Adult tracings reveal an absence of Wave I in the contralateral response and differentiation of the Wave IV-V complex (Prasher and Gibson 1980). These differences are thought to reflect the contribution of different neural fibers in the ipsilateral versus contralateral conditions. Salamy, Eldredge, and Wakely (1985) reviewed developmental changes in the contralateral response in preterm and term infants. Their study revealed absence of a contralateral response in infants younger than 33 weeks post-conception. At 34 weeks, a highly variable response emerged, although Wave V was consistently later and Wave III consistently earlier than the ipsilateral response. In addition, the contralateral response was smaller in ampitude. Interestingly, when preterm infants were tested at term and compared with full-term infants, these significant differences in latency and amplitude persisted. This finding suggests some delay in neuromaturation in premature infants, even when they have reached term equivalence.

The above observations were made for preterm infants classified as "healthy." However, studies suggest that the previously discussed maturational changes in the ABR will vary between "normal" and "high-risk" infants. In particular, Salamy (1984) reports changes in ABR latencies and amplitudes between "normal" infants and "high-risk" infants. Although the latency pattern for high-risk infants generally parallels that of normal infants, wave amplitudes vary in a somewhat irregular manner. This information is important in effectively employing the ABR with the pediatric population.

Middle Latency Evoked Response (MLR)

The MLR, first described by Geisler, Frishkopf, and Rosenblith in 1958, is a series of evoked responses occurring after the ABR and up to 80–90 msec post stimulus. There are three negative (N_a, N_b, N_c) and three positive (P_a, P_b, P_c) waves that can be observed, but generally only the first two negative (N_a, N_b) and the first two positive (P_a, P_b) waves are used clinically or for investigative purposes (Musiek et al. 1984). The MLR can be elicited using clicks or tone pips generally presented at a rate of about 10/sec. This evoked response can be recorded using the same electrode montage as the ABR or a variety of other electrode arrangements (Musiek et al. 1984).

ASSESSMENT OF CHILDREN AND FILTER EFFECTS

Several reports indicated that MLRs could be obtained from infants and that these responses were similar to MLRs obtained from adults (McRandle, Smith, and Goldstein 1974; Mendel, Adkinson, and Harker 1977; Wolf and Goldstein 1978). Therefore, it appeared that there were no maturational influences on the MLR. In retrospect, this seems illogical in that the ABR demonstrates maturational effects and therefore the MLR, which probably is generated by higher auditory structures, should require longer to mature. This issue was addressed by Scherg (1982) and Suzuki, Hirabayashi, and Kobayashi (1983). Scherg demonstrated that narrow filtering with steep rejection slopes distorted the MLR waveform. This distortion was thought to be related to the "ringing" of the filters or a phase shifting resulting in the MLR waveform being smoother and more sinusoidal. Suzuki, Hirabayashi, and Kobayashi showed that when the filter settings were not as restricted as in the earlier studies (McRandle, Smith, and Goldstein 1974; Mendel, Adkinson, and Harker 1977; Wolf and Goldstein 1978), MLRs from infants and children were not similar to adults. It appeared that MLRs for infants and young children had a greater latency, were more variable, and had poorer waveform definition than for adults. These findings have been verified by subsequent reports (Kileny 1983; Sprague and Thornton 1982).

MATURATIONAL VARIABLES IN THE MLR

As can be observed in figure 3, the MLRs obtained with wide filter bands (i.e., 20–3000 Hz) reflect age specific changes despite individual variability with regard to wave presence, latency, and morphology. Several cases have been described where the latency of the P_a wave is considerably greater in the normal young child than in the adult (Kileny, 1983; Suzuki, Hirabayashi, and Kobayashi 1983). However, no extensive studies of age effects on the latency of MLR waves have been published. There is some preliminary data indicating that at 10–12 years of age MLR latencies are similar to those of adults (personal communication, Aaron Thornton 1982).

Perhaps one of the most extensive studies which has strong implications for maturational effects on the MLR is that of Kraus et al. (1985). This study reported the effect of age on the presence of the N_a and P_a waves of the MLR. Approximately 20% of the infants under one year of age did have a P_a response, while about 65% demonstrated an N_a wave. The presence of the MLR waves increased with age to nearly 100% at 10–12 years for both the N_a and P_a waves. Interesting recent work by Fifer (1985) and Jerger et al. (1987) suggests that the presence/absence of the MLR in infants may be related to the rate of stimulation with waveforms present at very slow rates (1–2/second) and absent at faster rates (5–10/second). This age-related trend in MLR wave presence implicates brain maturation effects.

Clinically, it is important to realize that, at this time, the absence of MLR in young children or infants is not necessarily an indication of abnormality (i.e., a hearing deficit). If the MLR waveform is present in the young child or infant it can be used to gain frequency specific information. If the MLR is absent in the older child (>10 years) or adult, one should consider the possibility of CNS involvement or delayed maturation (Kraus et al. 1982. Musiek et al. 1984).

LONG LATENCY POTENTIALS

The long latency potentials that we will discuss will be limited to the N_1, P_2, and P_3. These waves occur at approximately 100 (N_1), 200 (P_2), and 300 (P_3) msec post stimulus and are considerably larger (3.0–20.0 microvolts) than ei-

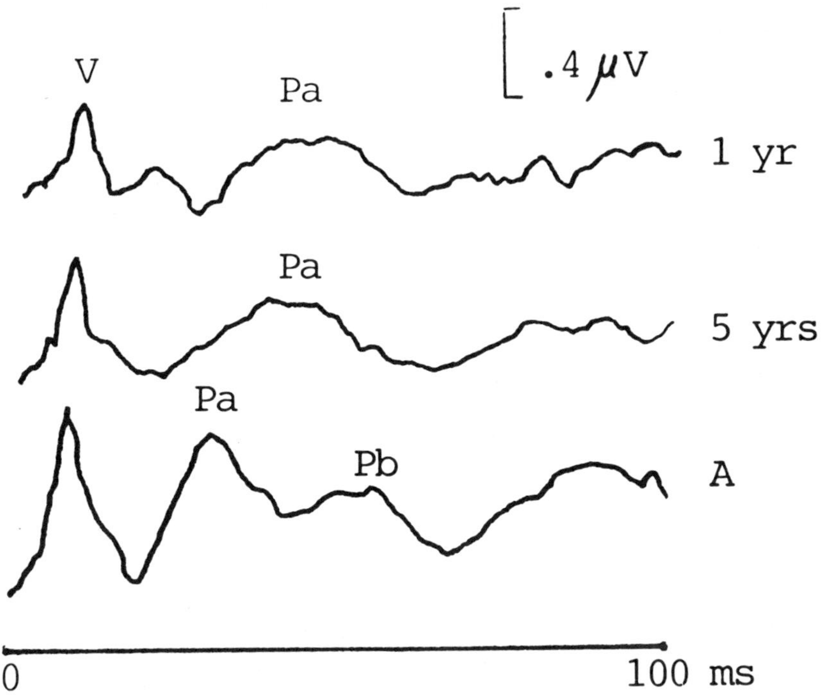

Figure 3. Middle latency responses (MLR) from 1 and 5 year old children and an adult. The latency, morphology, and amplitudes of the waveform change with age. (V = ABR Wave V, Filtering = 20–3000 Hz.) (Adapted from Suzuki et al. 1983.)

ther the ABR or MLR (Picton et al. 1977). The N_1 and P_2 waves are considered exogenous potentials; the P_3 is endogenous. Simply stated, exogenous potentials are elicited in response to externally generated environmental events while the endogenous potentials are related to internally generated events (Squires and Hecox 1983).

These later potentials can be generated by acoustic stimuli that may take the form of clicks, tone bursts, or short speech segments. The late components of the auditory evoked response may be recorded by electrodes placed at various scalp locations; however, optimal responses are usually obtained at or near the vertex (i.e., C_z, C_3, C_4, P_z) (Courchesne 1978).

The N_1 and P_2 can be obtained with the subject in a passive condition, that is, by simply listening to acoustic stimuli. However, the P_3 requires active processing on the part of the subject. For example, the conventional P_3 paradigm is to have the subject listen to frequent and rare stimuli. These stimuli are acoustically different with the rare stimuli occurring only 15–20% of the time. The subject is instructed to attend to and to count the number of rare stimuli heard for set trials. The process of identifying and counting the rare stimuli evokes the P_3. (See Polich and Starr 1983 for review.)

MATURATION OF THE N_1, P_2, AND P_3

As with the MLR, many of the questions regarding maturation effects on the long latency responses have yet to be answered. However, it is generally agreed that complete maturation of the later components requires many years with some components not stabilizing until adolescence or later (Polich and Starr 1983; Goldstein, 1973; Goodin et al. 1978; Ohlrich et al. 1978; Finley et al. 1985; Polich, Howard, and Starr 1985). Though there are definite maturational trends noted on group data, individual variance is great (Ellingson et al. 1974; Callaway and Halliday 1973). This variability, however, decreases as age increases (Callaway and Halliday 1973). Though latency and amplitude are the most common indices for measuring maturational effects, wave morphology, incidence of response, and threshold measures may also be used.

N_1, P_2 MATURATION

Though there is general agreement that maturation for N_1 and P_2 requires several years, it is difficult to find data that quantifies the age for complete maturation. In general statements, Goldstein (1973) and Polich, Howard, and Starr (1985) relate that the late potentials mature at approximately 8 to 10 years of age. These statements are consistent with data on a small pediatric population aged 6–15 years (Goodin et al. 1978 and with comments by Mendel 1985).

Perhaps one of the most systematic longitudinal studies on the N_1, P_2 with regard to maturation was performed by Ohlrich et al. (1978). These investigators tested 16 normal children biweekly from the age of two weeks to about three years. The stimuli were one msec clicks presented every 2.5 seconds at 108 dB SPL while the infants were asleep. The results indicated a mean reduction in P_2 latency of 70–80 msec from two weeks to three years of age. The mean N_1 change over approximately three years was not as dramatic (about a 10 msec latency reduction) (figure 4). These results are similar to a cross-sectional study on 130 children of the same age conducted by Barnet et al. (1975). These two studies also depicted an increase in the amplitude for P_2 (P_2–N_2) during the first three years of life.

Unusual maturational effects on the late potentials have been shown using speech stimuli (Kurtzberg, Stone, and Vaughn 1986). These researchers demonstrated marked changes in the morphology and latency for normal infants ranging from a few days to two years of age. The speech stimulus was "da" presented at 85 dB SPL with recordings from the midline and lateral locations on the head. Morphological changes with increasing age included increased amplitude and definition of a positive peak at approximately 120 msec poststimulus onset. A second positive peak at about 300 msec poststimulus onset reached maximum amplitude at three to six months of age, then decreased drastically in amplitude for a midline recording. Recordings from the electrodes over the temporal areas maintained both positive peaks with defini-

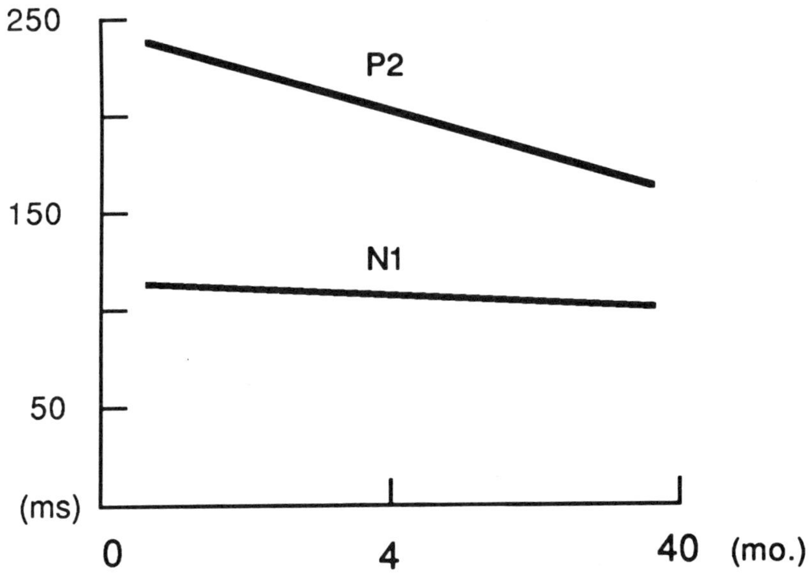

Figure 4. Regression lines indicating mean latencies of N_1 and P_2 acquired longitudinally from 16 infants. (Y axis = latency in milliseconds, X axis = age of infants in months.) (Adapted from Ohlrich et al. 1978, with permission from publisher.)

tion of both peaks improving through two years of age. Latencies of both positive waves decreased with increasing age for midline and lateral recordings.

It is clear from these studies that maturation has a marked effect on latency and amplitude of the N_1–P_2 complex through three years of age. However, little data is available for the late exogenous potentials (N_1, P_2, N_2) with regard to age effects for older children.

P_3 MATURATION

Since the conventional P_3 paradigm requires a rather sophisticated response, data on very young children is essentially unavailable. Therefore, maturational trends are limited to the child five years old and older. Goodin et al. (1978) tested seven normal children aged 6 to 15 years and found a systematic decrease in latency of P_3 with increasing age. The P_3 latency decreased at a rate of 18.4 msec per year for this group of children. Though not as striking, P_3 amplitude increased with increasing age.

Studies subsequent to Goodin's revealed similar findings. Polich, Howard, and Starr (1985) as well as Courchesne (1978) used larger numbers of children but again found the shortest P_3 latency to occur in the early to mid teen-age years (figure 5). Courchesne (1978) has shown changes in waveform morphology and amplitude for P_3 records from children 5 to 16 years of age. He has also shown that the recording site of the P_3 can affect morphology. Although matu-

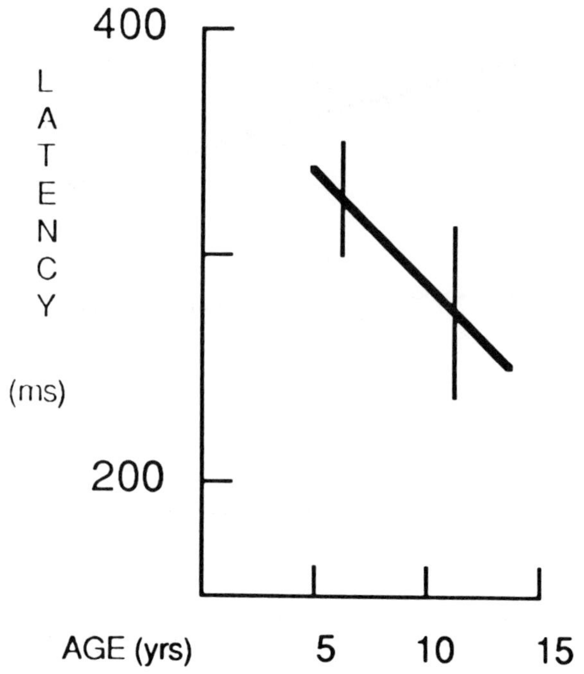

Figure 5. Mean latencies of the P-300 (P3a) as a function of age. (Interpolated from Polich et al. 1985, with permission.)

rational effects are seen at various recording sites, some sites yield different maturational trends. Because of inter-subject variability, especially in the early years, it is difficult to quantify maturational effects on the P_3. However, there is no doubt that children under 10 years of age have a much different P_3 than young adults (figure 6).

Dichotic Listening and Maturation

There are many psychophysical auditory tests that manifest maturational effects. However, in keeping with the neuroauditory theme of this paper, we have elected to profile a test procedure commonly associated with auditory cortical function—dichotically presented speech. General review of the literature and specific articles by Keith (1984) and Keith et al. (1985) indicate two extreme types of dichotic speech tasks. There are heavily linguistically loaded dichotic speech stimuli such as sentences, and there are those with minimal linguistic content such as nonsense syllables (e.g., consonant-vowels, "ba" and "da"). In between these two extreme examples are dichotic stimuli such as numbers or words which are moderately linguistically based. The reason that we mention light and heavily linguistically loaded dichotic speech stimuli is that maturational effects appear quite different for each.

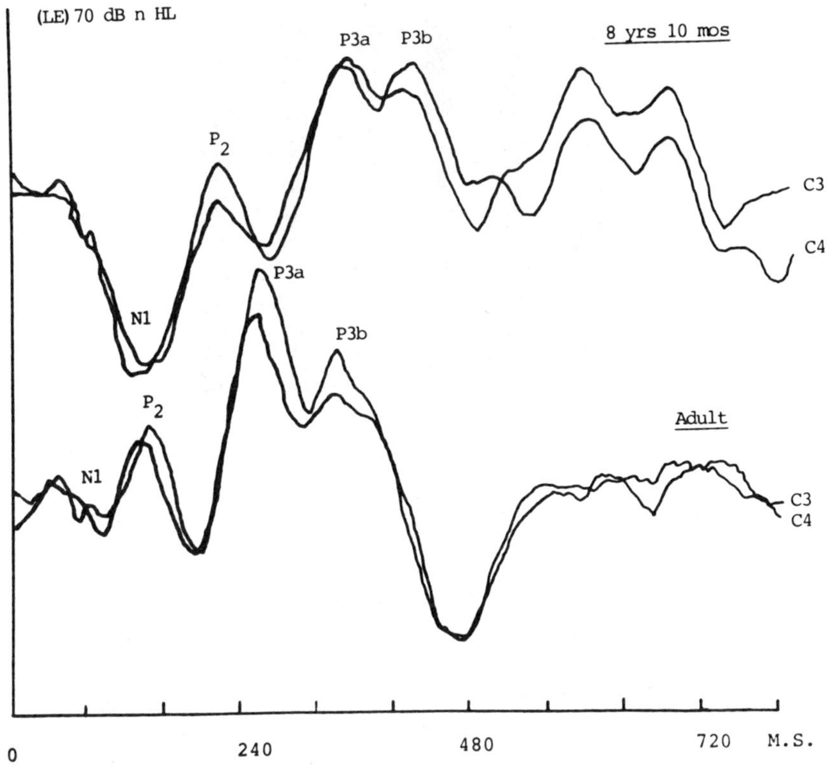

Figure 6. Examples of auditory evoked late potentials from an 8-year-old child and young adult. These were obtained using a P-300 paradigm with the stimuli presented to the left ear and recording taken at C-3 and C-4 positions on the scalp. These examples show clear differences in latencies in comparing a child and an adult.

In studies of normal children aged 5 to 13 years, a right ear advantage (REA) is observed to be relatively constant throughout this age range (Berlin, Tawfik, and Katbamno 1973; Obrzut et al. 1981). However, the number of double correct responses (i.e., both left and right ears correct) showed a definite increase with age (Berlin et al. 1973). This increase in bilaterally correct responses was thought to be related to an increased capacity of the brain to process two-channel stimuli.

Unlike the results obtained on consonant-vowels (CVs), dichotic sentences show definite laterality changes with age. It appears that with these stimuli young children show poor left-ear performance which improves with age (Willeford 1985; Keith 1984). The right ear scores are essentially as good at 5 years as they are at 10 years of age (figure 7). There are some relatively sound theoretical bases for the differing maturational effects on CVs and sentences. The CVs, which have a minimal linguistic load, may be processed somewhat equally in the two hemispheres and at a lower level than the sentences (Keith 1984; Porter and Berlin 1975). In contrast with the CVs, the dichotic sentences

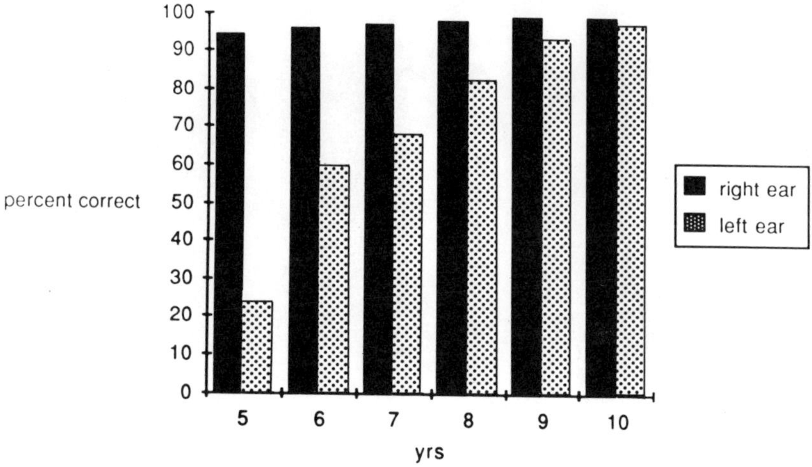

Figure 7. Left and right ear mean scores for the competing-sentences test by age. Based on the data from Willeford 1985 (with permission) and the authors. (N = > 40 for ages 7, 8, 9, and 10 years; N = > 25 for ages 5 and 6.)

seem to invoke considerable demand on the language-dominant hemisphere. The poorer left-ear scores in younger children may be attributed to the inability of the corpus callosum to transfer adequately a complex neural message from the right hemisphere to the intricate, language-dominant areas of the left hemisphere. The right-ear scores remain high because there is a direct neural route to the left hemisphere without crossing the corpus callosum (Keith 1984; Musiek, Kibbe, and Baran 1984; Musiek, Gollegly, and Baran 1984). As the child becomes older, the transcallosal auditory transfer between hemispheres matures and left-ear scores improve.

Of special interest is the case of a learning-disabled child (figure 8). It appears that after a lag in maturation this child's dichotic processing skills "catch up" by age 11. At nine this child shows left-ear scores far below the norm, but by age 11, scores became normal for both ears. In this particular case, not only did dichotic left-ear scores improve but so did the child's academic performance. This maturational trend in learning-disabled children is not limited to this case but has been observed in a number of subjects (Musiek, Gollegly, and Baran 1984; Musiek, Gollegly, and Ross 1985) (figure 9). Although the maturational ranges of various neuroauditory tests can only be estimated, it is important to realize the profound effect that maturation has on measures of auditory function.

UNDERLYING MECHANISMS OF NEUROAUDITORY MATURATION

We have given an overview of electrophysiological and behavioral correlates to maturation of the higher auditory system. Basic to the appreciation and un-

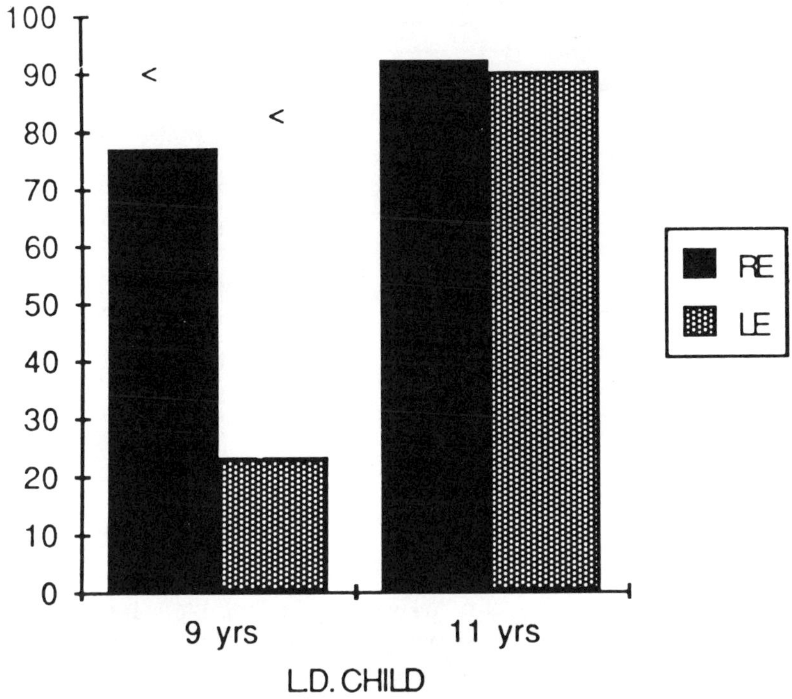

Figure 8. Results on the competing-sentences test from the same child at 9 and 11 years of age. At 9 years a severe left ear deficit is shown; at 11 years performance improves to normal bilaterally. (< = cut off norms for 9 years).

derstanding of these maturational changes in auditory function are age-dependent morphological alterations of the brain. Therefore, in this segment of the paper we will briefly discuss some of the main post-natal maturational changes in brain structure that may influence auditory electrophysiological and behavioral characteristics.

Though there are a variety of changes in the central auditory system postnatally (see Jacobson 1970, and Romand 1983 for reviews), due to the scope of this paper we will discuss only three main morphological factors. The first and most prominent is myelination, for which maturational cycles are quite well defined. The second and third mechanisms, dendritic branching and synaptogenesis, are interrelated, and for ease of communication will be discussed together.

MYELINATION

Simply stated, myelin is the white matter of the nervous system. Myelin, as it develops, covers the axons and facilitates the speed at which an impulse travels. In the brain some axons have little myelin; others are heavily myelinated; and

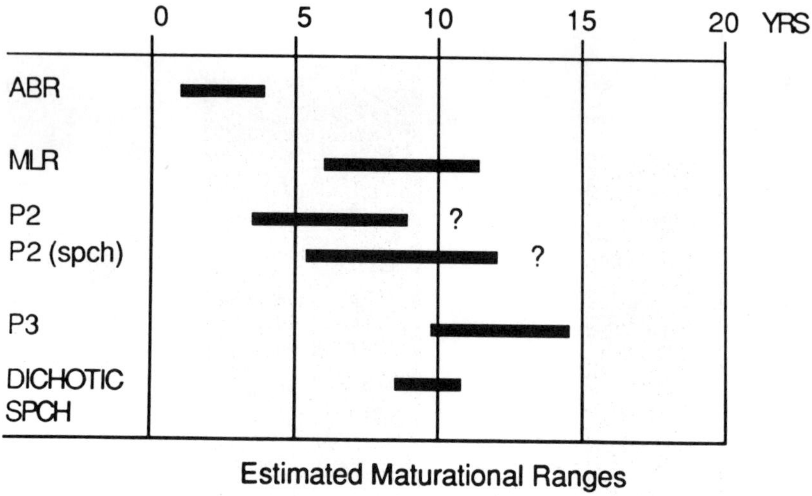

Figure 9. Authors' estimated age ranges for maturation of various audiological tests.

some are unmyelinated. The rate of myelination in the human (and animal) brain varies from region to region (Yakovlev and LeCours 1967). It appears that myelination is completed for brainstem structures before the first year of age. However, myelination may not be completed for the corpus callosum until age 10 or adolescence (Yakovlev and LeCours, 1967; Salamy 1978) (figure 10). Various intra- and intercortical connections (auditory association and language areas) may not be completely myelinated until years after myelination of the corpus callosum is complete (Yakovlev and LeCours 1967).

There is abundant evidence that suggests that myelin influences the latencies of various evoked potentials. Moreover, it appears that decrements observed in ABR interwave latencies with increasing age are related to increased myelination (Salamy 1984). These statements are supported by several studies. Shah and Salamy (1980) studied the cerebroside concentration in the rat brainstem over a 50-day post-natal period. Cerebroside is a lipid found only in myelin and can be measured to indicate the amount of myelin present in a given structure. A decrease in the II–V interwave latency was noted as cerebroside levels increased. Amochaev et al. (1979) reduced myelin density in the rat by triethyltin intoxication, and noted a significant increase in the ABR interwaves. After the drug was discontinued, ABR latencies returned to normal. Finally, studies on the quaking mouse (an animal suffering from a genetic disease in which myelin is not produced) implicate myelin as a major factor in neural transmission time. ABR interwaves are dramatically increased in quaking mice when compared with a control group (figure 11). Similar delays are also seen in the auditory long-latency potentials for these animals (personal communication, Alan Salamy 1986). There is also a general relationship between the age at which the corpus callosum and interhemispheric myelin mature and the age at which optimal responses may be recorded for the middle and late potentials.

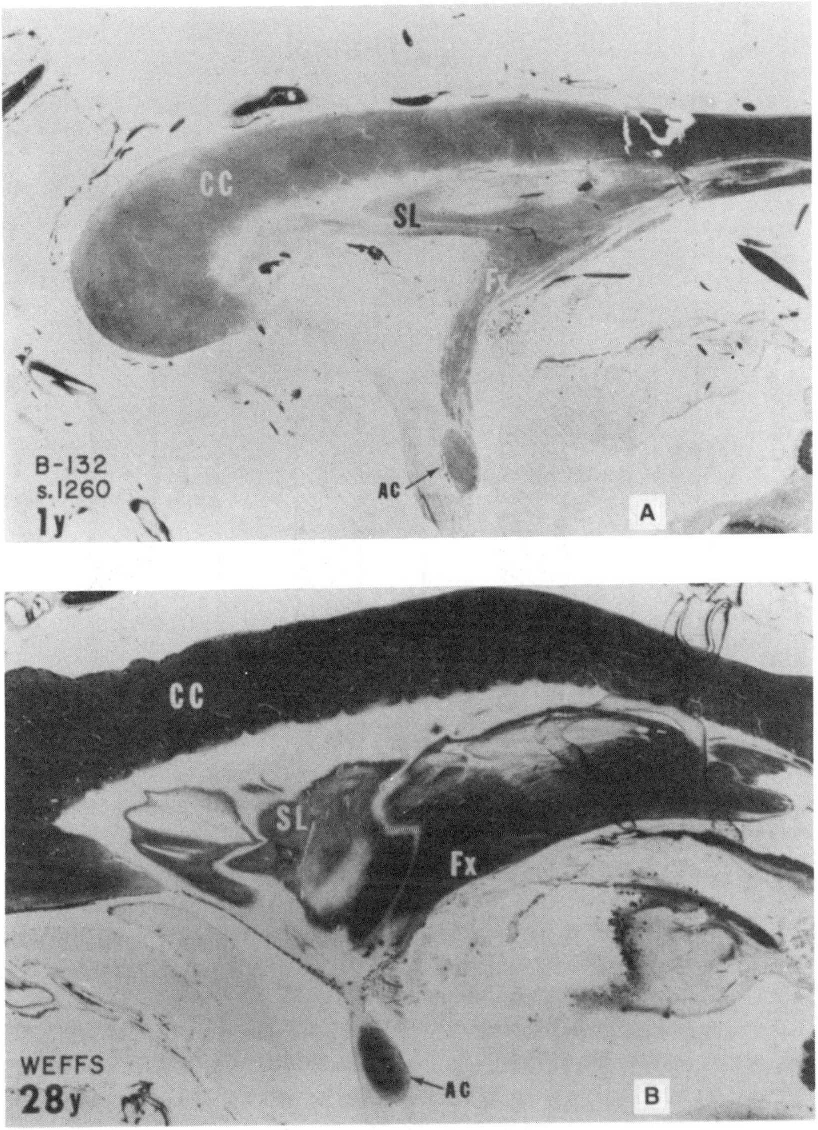

Figure 10. Corpus callosum of an infant (A) and adult (B). The Loyez method of staining has been used yielding a dark color for dense myelination and a light color for lack of myelination. As can be seen there are dramatic differences in myelin concentrations in the two examples. (From Yakovlev and LeCours 1967, with permission.)

Myelination of the corpus callosum may play an important role in the maturation of dichotic listening performance for heavily loaded linguistic stimuli (Musiek, Gollegly, and Baran 1984). As stated earlier, marked left-ear deficits are noted for young children (five years of age) but the left ear recovers by age 10. Incomplete or delayed myelination may prevent adequate transfer of com-

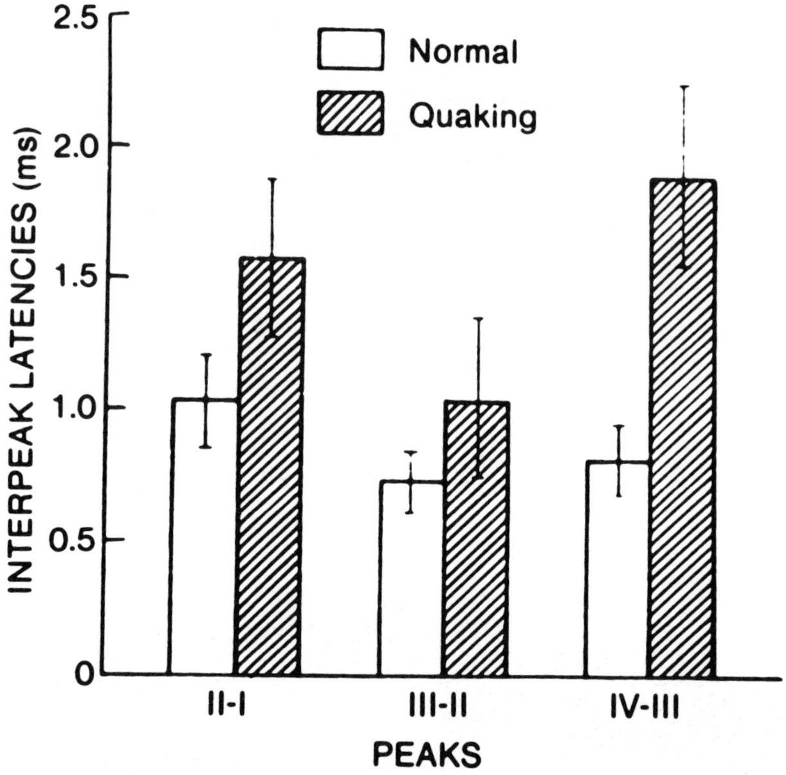

Figure 11. Interpeak ABR latencies for "normal" and "quaking" mice. (From Shah and Salamy 1980, with permission.)

plex linguistic stimuli from the right to left hemisphere in young children. These results mimic those of split-brain patients implicating poor interhemispheric transfer. As the child becomes older, myelination is completed, allowing better transfer and connection to the speech hemisphere; therefore, little deficit is observed in the left ear.

Interestingly, children reach adult levels of performance on dichotic sentence tasks at approximately 10 years of age, which is also approximately when corpus callosum myelination is completed. The left ear deficits (below-age matched norms) in the learning disabled child discussed earlier, makes one suspect a possible "lag" in myelination of the corpus callosum (Musiek, Gollegly, and Ross 1985).

DENDRITIC BRANCHING/SYNAPTOGENESIS

There are three parts to a neuron: the cell body (soma), axon, and dendrites. The dendrites are tapered cytoplasmic connections that have synaptic connections with other neurons. Dendritic branching or arborization is one of the main

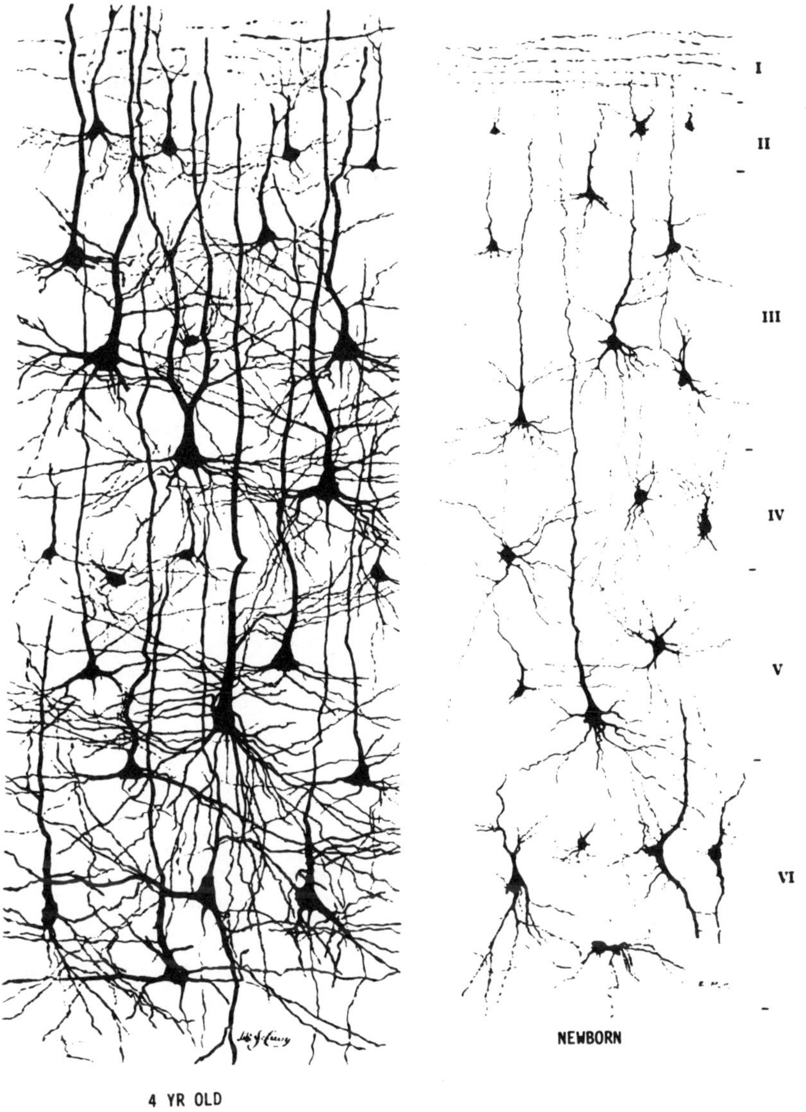

Figure 12. Cortical tissue taken from the superior temporal plane of the temporal lobe (Golgi-Cox stain) revealing dendritic branching density for a 4-year-old (left) and a newborn (right). (From Conel 1939, 1963, with permission.)

maturational processes of the neuron. During the first year of life, each cortical neuron, primarily through dendritic branching, establishes connections with about 10,000 other neurons (Crelin 1973). This increase in dendritic branching may continue, to some extent, for several years (Conel 1939, 1963) (figure 12). However, it is difficult to determine at what age arborization reaches its asymptote because it is greatly affected by environmental influences that increase with age (personal communication, Marin Padilla 1986).

Thus, dendritic branching provides an anatomical basis for additional synapses and therefore the integration, processing, and transfer of more information. However, dendritic branching in itself is of little functional value if the branches do not connect with other neurons. This connection takes place by axodendritic synapses. Some require functional validation for their normal maturation or even survival (Jacobson 1970); if dendritic branches do not connect, they may die; if they connect and synapse but the synapse is not used, they may become non-functional. Lack of use resulting from sensory deprivation reduces dendritic branching and synaptogenisis (Jacobson 1970).

Though there are many factors that contribute to the maturation of an auditory response, be it behavioral or physiological, myelination and dendritic branching are of prime importance. By our brief description of these basic phenomena one can realize the obvious relationship to CNS maturation as measured by audiological means. The understanding of both clinical and basic mechanisms of auditory maturation should help in defining the normal, as well as the abnormally developing, auditory system in children. This in turn should enhance our effectiveness in diagnostic and habilitative endeavors.

REFERENCES

Amochaev, A., Johnson, R., Salamy, A., and Shah, S. 1979. Brainstem and myelin changes in triethyltin-induced edema in young adult rats. *Experimental Neurology* 66:629–635.

Barnet, A., Ohlrich, E., Weiss, I., and Shanks, B. 1975. Auditory evoked potentials during sleep in normal children from ten days to three years of age. *Electroencephalography and Clinical Neurophysiology* 39:29–41.

Berlin, C., Hughes, L., Lowe-Bell, S., and Berlin, H. 1973. Dichotic right ear advantage in children 5 to 13. *Cortex* 9:393–401.

Callaway, E., and Halliday, R. 1973. Evoked potential variability: Effects of age, amplitude and methods of measurement. *Electroencephalography and Clinical Neurophysiology* 34:125–133.

Conel, J. 1939. *Postnatal Development of the Human Cerebral Cortex* (Vol. 1). Cambridge, MA: Harvard University Press.

Conel, J. 1963. *Postnatal Development of the Human Cerebral Cortex* (Vol. 7). Cambridge, MA: Harvard University Press.

Courchesne, E. 1978. Neurophysiological correlates of cognitive development: Changes in long-latency event-related potentials from childhood to adulthood. *Electroencephalography and Clinical Neurophysiology* 45:468–482.

Cox, L. C. 1985. Infant assessment: Developmental and age related considerations. *In* J. Jacobson (ed.). *The Auditory Brainstem Response*. San Diego: College Hill Press.

Crelin, E. 1973. *Functional Anatomy of the Newborn* (pp. 22–24). New Haven: Yale University Press.

Despland, P., and Galambos, R. 1980. The ABR is a useful diagnostic tool in the intensive care nursery. Pediatric Research 14:154–158.

Don, M., Allen, A., and Starr, A. 1977. Effect of click rate on the latency of auditory brainstem responses in humans. *Annals of Otology, Rhinology, & Otolaryngology* 86:186–195.

Ellingson, R., Danahy, T., Nelson, B., and Lathrop, G. 1974. Variability of auditory evoked potentials in human newborns. *Electroencephalography and Clinical Neurophysiology* 36:155–162.

Fifer, R. 1985. The MLR and SSEP in neonates. Doctoral dissertation. Baylor College of Medicine.

Finley, W., Faux, S., Hutcheson, J., and Amstutz, L. 1985. Long-latency even-related potentials in the evaluation of cognitive function in children. *Neurology* 35:323–327.

Fujikawa, S., and Weber, B. 1977. Effects of increased stimulus rate on brainstem electric response (BER) audiometry as a function of age. *Journal of the American Audiology Society* 3(3):147–150.

Geisler, C., Frishkopf, L., and Rosenblith, W. 1958. Extracranial responses to acoustic clicks in man. *Science* 128:1210–1211.

Goldstein, R. 1973. Electroencephalic audiometry. *In* J. Jerger (ed.). *Modern Developments in Audiology* (pp. 407–433). New York: Academic Press.

Goodin, D., Squires, K., and Starr, A. 1978. Long latency event-related components of the auditory evoked potential in dementia. *Brain* 101:635–648.

Goodin, D., Squires, K., Henderson, B., and Starr. A. 1978. Age related variations in evoked potentials to auditory stimuli in normal human subjects. *Electroencephalography and Clinical Neurophysiology* 44:447–458.

Hall, J. 1983. Auditory brainstem response audiometry. *In* J. Jerger (ed.). *Hearing Disorders in Adults: Current Trends*. San Diego: College Hill Press.

Jacobson, M. 1970. *Developmental Neurobiology*. New York: Holt, Reinhart & Winston.

Jacobson, J. (ed.). 1985. *The Auditory Brainstem Response*. San Diego: College Hill Press.

Jacobson, J., Morehouse, C. R., and Johnson, J. 1982. Strategies for infant auditory brainstem response assessment. *Ear and Hearing* 3(5):263–269.

Jerger, J., Chmiel, R., Glaze, D., and Frost, J. 1987. Rate and filter dependence of the middle-latency response in infants. *Audiology* 26:269–283.

Jewett, D., and Williston, J. 1971. Auditory-evoked far fields averaged from the scalp of humans. *Brain* 94:618–696.

Keith, R. 1984. Dichotic listening in children. *In* D. Beasley (ed.). *Audition in Children*. San Diego: College Hill Press.

Keith, R., Tawfik, S., and Katbamno, B. 1985. Performance of adults on directed listening tasks using a dichotic CV test. *Ear and Hearing* 6:270–273.

Kileny, P. 1983. Auditory evoked middle latency responses: Current issues. *Seminars in Hearing* 4:403–414.

Kraus, N., Ozdamar, O., Hier, D., and Stein, L. 1982. Auditory middle latency responses (MLRs) in patients with cortical lesions. *Electroencephalography and Clinical Neurophysiology* 54:275–287.

Kraus, N., Smith, D., Reed, N., Stein, L., and Cartee, C. 1985. Auditory middle latency responses in children: Effects of age and diagnostic category. *Electroencephalography and Clinical Neurophysiology* 62:343–351.

Krumholz, A., Felix, J., Goldstein, P., and McKenzie, E. 1985. Maturation of the brain-stem auditory evoked potential in premature infants. *Electoencephalography and Clinical Neurophysiology* 62:124–134.

Kurtzberg, D., Stone, C., and Vaughn, H. 1986. Cortical responses to speech sounds in the infant. *In* R. Cracco, and I. Bodis-Wollner (eds.). *Frontiers of Clinical Neuroscience-Evoked Potentials*. Baltimore: Williams & Wilkins.

McRandle, C., Smith, M., and Goldstein, R. 1974. Early averaged electroencephalic responses to clicks in neonates. *Annals of Otology, Rhinology, and Laryngology* 83:695–702.

Mendel, M. 1985. Middle and late auditory evoked potentials. *In* J. Katz (ed.). *Handbook of Clinical Audiology*. Baltimore: Williams and Wilkins.

Mendel, M., Adkinson, C., and Harker, L. 1977. Middle components of the auditory evoked potentials in infants. *Annals of Otology, Rhinology, and Laryngology* 86:293–299.

Musiek, F. E., Kibbe, K., and Baran, J. 1984. Neuroaudiological results from split-brain patients. *Seminars in Hearing*, 5(3):219–229.

Musiek, F. E., Gollegly, K., and Baran, J. 1984. Myelination of the corpus callosum and auditory processing problems in children: Theoretical and clinical correlates. *Seminars in Hearing* 5(3):231–241.

Musiek, F., Geurkink, N., Weider, D., and Donnelly, K. 1984. Past, present, and future applications of the auditory middle latency response (MLR). *Laryngoscope* 94:1545–1552.

Musiek, F., Gollegly, K., and Ross, M. 1985. Deficits in children with learning disabilities. *Journal of Childhood Communication Disorders* 9(1):43–63.

Obrzut, J., Hynd, G., Obrzut, A., and Pirozzolo, F. 1981. Effects of directed attention on cerebral asymmetry in normal and listening-disabled children. *Developmental Psychology* 17:118–125.

Ohlrich, E., Barnet, A., Weiss, I., and Shanks, B. 1978. Auditory evoked potential development in early childhood: A longitudinal study. *Electroencephalography and Clinical Neurophysiology* 44:411–432.

Picton, T., Woods, D., Baribeau-Braun, J., and Healey, T. 1977. Evoked potential audiometry. *Journal of Otolaryngology* 6:90–119.

Polich, J., Howard, L., and Starr, A. 1985. Effects of age on the P-300 component of the event related potential from auditory stimuli: Peak definition, variation, and measurement. *Journal of Gerontology* 40:721–726.

Polich, J., and Starr, A. (1983). Middle, late, and long latency auditory evoked potentials. *In* E. Moore (ed.). *Bases of Auditory Brainstem Evoked Responses*. New York: Grune & Stratton.

Porter, R., and Berling, C. 1975. On interpreting developmental change in the dichotic right ear advantage. *Brain and Language* 2:186–200.

Prasher, P., and Gibson, W. 1980. Brainstem auditory evoked potentials: Significant latency differences between ipsilateral and contralateral stimulation. *Electroencephalography and Clinical Neurophysiology* 50:240–241.

Romand, R. (ed.). 1983. *Development of Auditory and Vestibular Systems*. New York: Academic Press.

Salamy, A. 1978. Commissural transmission: Maturational changes in humans. *Science* 200:1409–1410.

Salamy, A. 1984. Maturation of the auditory brainstem response from birth through early childhood. *Journal of Clinical Neurophysiology* 1(3):293–329.

Salamy, A., Eldredge, L., and Wakely, A. 1985. Maturation of contralateral brain-stem responses in preterm infants. *Electroencephalography and Clinical Neurophysiology* 62:117–123.

Salamy, A., Mendelson, T., Tooley, W., and Chaplin, E. 1980. Differential development of brainstem potentials in healthy and high-risk infants. *Science* 210:553–555.

Scherg, M. 1982. Distortion of the middle latency auditory response produced by analog filtering. *Scandanavian Audiology* 11:57–60.

Shah, S., and Salamy, A. 1980. Brainstem auditory potentials in myelin deficient mice. *Neuroscience* 5:2321–2323.

Sprague, B., and Thornton, A. 1982. Clinical utility and limitations of middle-latency auditory evoked potentials. *Proceedings of the ASHA Convention,* Toronto, Canada, November, 1982.

Squires, K., and Hecox, K. 1983. Electrophysiological evaluation of higher level auditory processing. *Seminars in Hearing* 4:415–432.

Starr, A., Amile, R., Martin, W., and Sanders, S. 1977. Development of auditory function in newborn infants revealed by auditory brainstem potentials. *Pediatrics* 60:831–839.

Suzuki, T., Hirabayashi, M., and Kobayashi, K. 1983. Auditory middle responses in young children. *British Journal of Audiology* 17:5–9.

Willeford, J. 1985. Assessment of Central Auditory Disorders in Children. *In* M. Pinheiro and F. Musiek (eds.). *Assessment of Central Auditory Dysfunction: Foundations and Clinical Correlates*. Baltimore: Williams & Wilkins.

Wolf, K., and Goldstein, R. 1978. Middle component averaged electroencephalic responses to tonal stimuli for normal neonates. *Archives of Otolaryngology* 104:508–518.

Yakovlev, P., and LeCours, A. 1967. Myelogenetic cycles of regional maturation of the brain. *In* A. Minkowski (ed.). *Regional Development of the Brain in Early Life*. Philadelphia: F. A. Davis.

Issues on Management

Chapter 16

Options in Classroom Amplification Systems

David B. Hawkins

The decisions regarding the type of amplification system that a child should wear in a classroom have become increasingly complex in the last five to ten years. In the past there were only two options, a hearing aid or a large self-contained body-worn FM system. Today the options are numerous. Hearing aids can be coupled to various types of FM systems in a number of ways. Knowledge of these different arrangements is important to all clinical audiologists since many decisions regarding a child's classroom amplification arrangement must be made at the time of the hearing-aid selection. For instance, it may be important for the hearing aid to have a telecoil, direct audio input, or, ideally, both of these capabilities. The type of switching options on the hearing aid must be chosen so that the hearing aid will interface in the best possible way with the FM system. Audiologists should be familiar with the type of systems available, the electroacoustic properties and how to assess them, the behavioral results that can be expected, and the guidelines for when to consider the use of FM systems. This chapter will discuss some of these issues.

Signal-to-Noise Ratio: The Crucial Parameter

Performance with any amplification system is probably most directly related to the signal-to-noise ratio (S/N) delivered to the user's ear. A 5 dB change in S/N ratio could have a far greater effect on performance than a dramatic change in frequency response. Each of the classroom amplification options should be viewed in terms of its ability to provide the best possible S/N ratio.

In evaluating the S/N ratio that is provided by each system, the noise term should be thought of as the additive effect of both background noise and reverberation. To illustrate the effects of reverberation in a simple way, figure 1 shows a spectrogram of the same sentence spoken in a sound booth and in a room with a reverberation time of .5 s. The presence of reverberation causes elongation of vowels, smearing of transitions, and virtual elimination of silent gaps. When reverberation is present, a more positive S/N ratio is necessary to maintain the same level of performance. Figure 2 shows data from a study by Hawkins and Yacullo (1984) in which the effect of reverberation was quantified in S/N ratio terms. As the reverberation time was increased from .3 to .6 s, the hearing-impaired subjects required a 4 dB improvement in the environmental S/N ratio in order to maintain performance at the same level. From .6 to 1.2 s, a 9 dB change was necessary, and from .3 to 1.2 s, and 11.5 dB improvement was required. These data stress the clear need to consider the reverberation time in the selection of classrooms and make all possible changes to lower the values.

The environmental S/N ratio that is necessary to produce best performance by hearing-impaired children has not been studied extensively. Figure 3 shows the results from the only studies that have measured speech recognition in noise

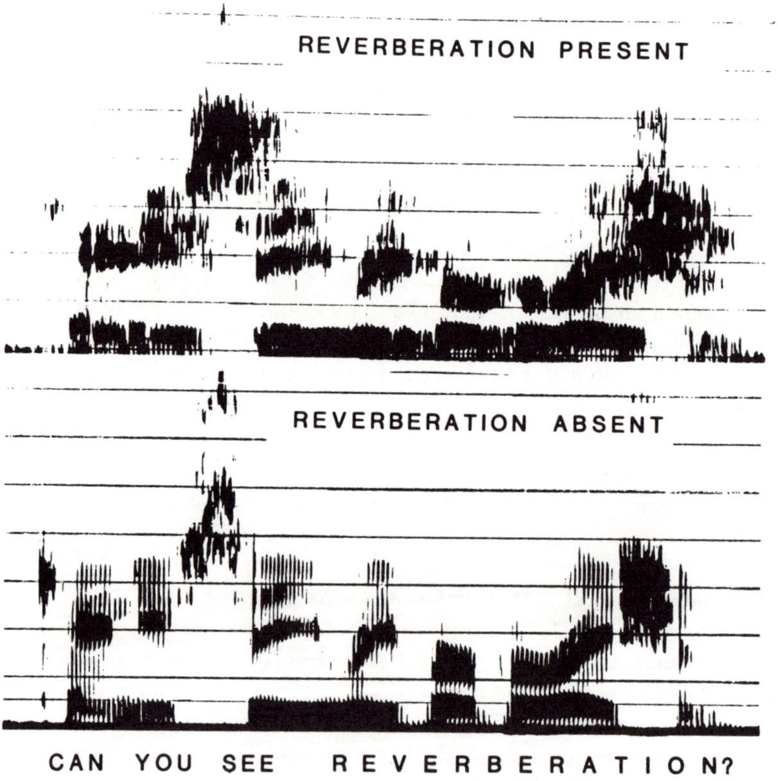

Figure 1. A sound spectrogram of the sentence "Can you see reverberation" spoken in a sound booth and a room with a reverberation time of .5 s. (Reprinted from Hawkins, D., *Audiological Acoustics*, 1985. Used with permission.)

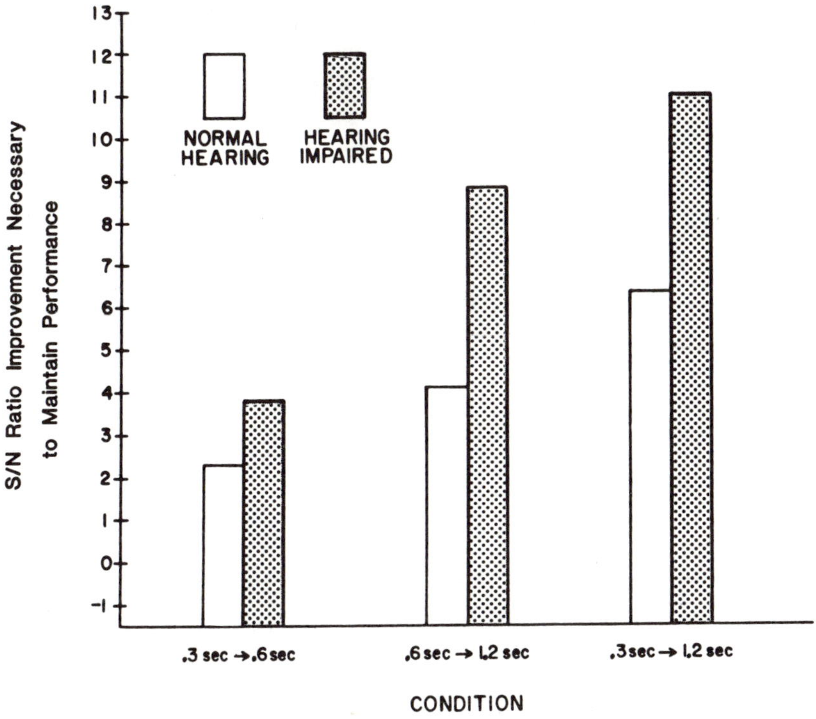

Figure 2. The S/N change necessary to maintain performance at a 50% correct level as the reverberation time is increased from .3 to .6 s, .6 to 1.2 s, and .3 to 1.2 s. (Data adapted from Hawkins and Yacullo 1984.)

and reverberation with hearing-impaired children. Averaging across studies and paying particular attention to the Finitzo-Hieber and Tillman (1978) data, it appears that a +15 to +20 dB S/N ratio is necessary for optimum performance at these moderate reverberation times. The values in the literature concerning the actual S/N ratios present in regular classrooms are disturbing. S/N ratios ranging from −6 to +15 dB have been reported, making even the best classroom marginally acceptable for the hearing-impaired child. These values should be kept in mind when making decisions regarding the necessity of special auditory equipment.

The advantage of the FM system in improving the S/N ratio lies exclusively in the distance from the speaker's mouth to the microphone that delivers the sound to the child's ear. With an FM system, the input to a child's ear originates approximately 15 cm (6 inches) from the mouth. Figure 4 shows the long-term average speech spectrum at the FM microphone. These data are from a study by Pearsons, Bennett, and Fidell (1977) and have been modified by correction factors given by the authors to provide the spectrum at the FM microphone. Notice that the overall level is 84 dB sound pressure level (SPL), approximately 20 dB higher than the level at 2 m, which is 65 dB SPL. Assuming that the noise level

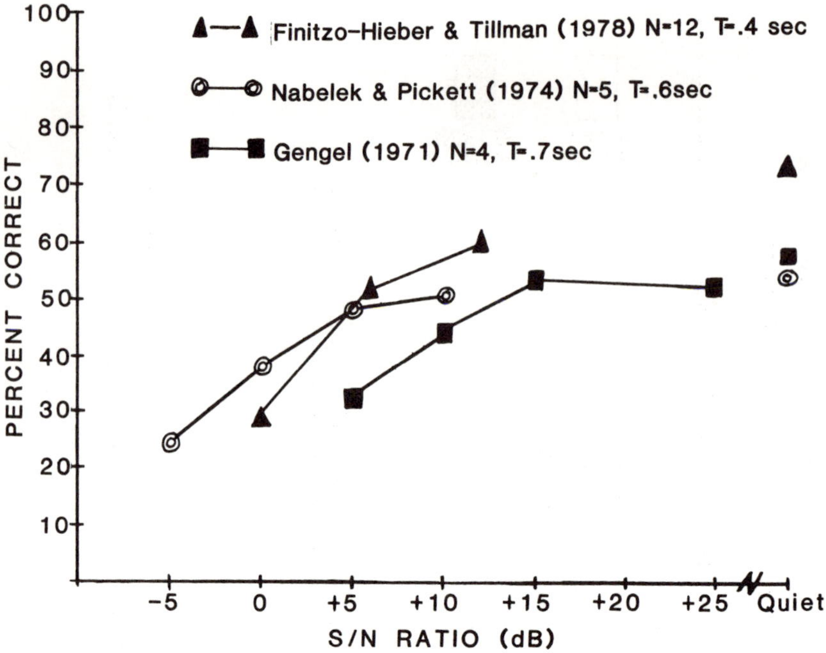

Figure 3. Results from three studies showing word recognition scores for children in the presence of noise and reverberation.

is the same at the two positions, by moving the input location from the front row of a classroom (2 m) to the FM microphone location around the teacher's neck (15 cm), the S/N ratio will be improved by 19 dB. In addition to this S/N improvement, the effect of reverberation is dramatically reduced because the microphone is in such close proximity to the source.

Options in Classroom Amplification

The first decision that must be made is whether individual hearing aids will be worn alone or whether an FM system is justified. If the choice is to use individual hearing aids, the two most important considerations impinging upon the S/N ratio issue are monaural versus binaural and omnidirectional versus directional microphones. Madison and Hawkins (1983), Hawkins and Yacullo (1984), and Hawkins (1984) have demonstrated that the most advantageous arrangement is binaural-directional. The improvement in S/N ratio in a reverberant room afforded by binaural aids is 1–3 dB and by directional microphones is 2–4 dB. When these two features are combined, a 3–7 dB improvement in S/N ratio can be achieved as compared to the traditional monaural-omnidirectional fitting. In the absence of any clear contraindication, bin-

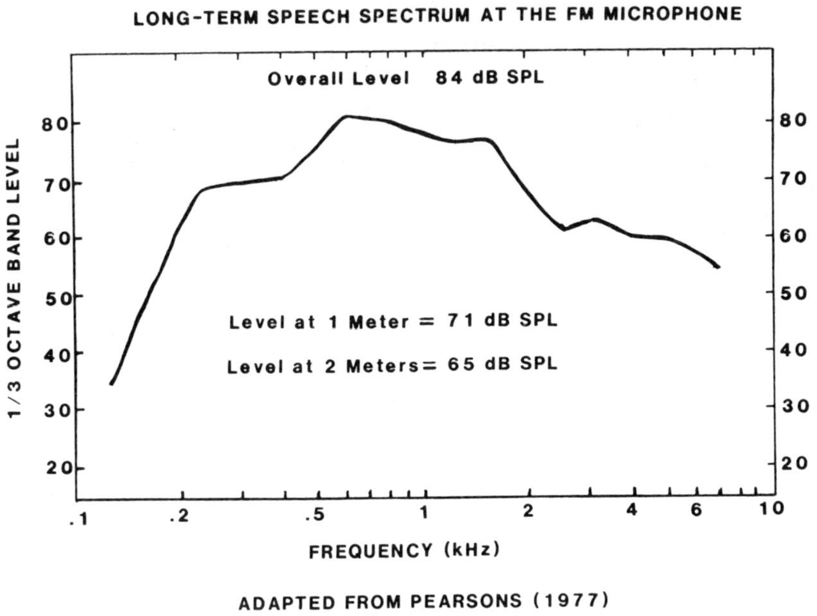

Figure 4. The long-term average spectrum of speech at the FM microphone location. (Data adapted from Pearsons, Bennett, and Fidell 1977.)

aural-directional should be the fitting of choice if S/N ratio concerns are dominant.

If the decision is made that an FM system is necessary or desirable, there are a number of options to consider. A diagram of the currently available options is shown in figure 5. The most popular system at present is probably still the self-contained FM system which replaces the hearing aid. Next in popularity is probably the neck loop (NL) arrangement, followed by direct input (DI), and silhouette inductor (SI). The trend in recent years has been for more of the personal FM systems (those attached to the hearing aid via NL, DI, and SI) to be used, especially with older hearing-impaired children. This is consistent with an increased awareness of the variety of assistive listening devices that are available.

ELECTROACOUSTIC CHARACTERISTICS OF PERSONAL FM SYSTEMS

Due to the increasing popularity of the personal FM system, it is necessary to examine how the electroacoustic characteristics of the hearing aid are altered when it is coupled to the FM system via NL, DI, and SI. First, however, there is the larger issue of how to assess electroacoustic characteristics of FM systems in general. The use of standard hearing aid measurements, such as ANSI S3.22

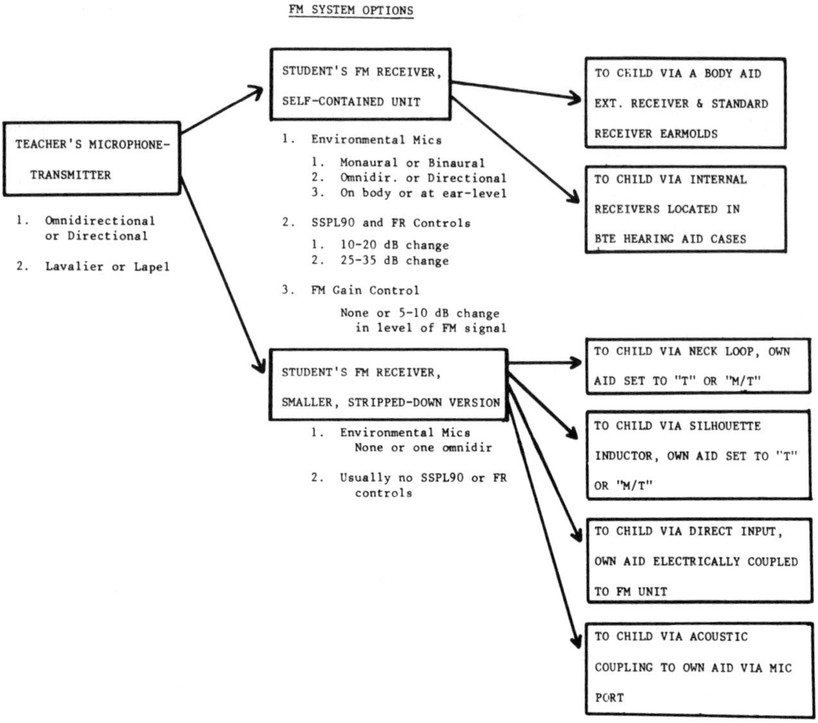

Figure 5. Diagram of the options available in FM system arrangements.

1982, may not be appropriate, as input levels of 50 and 60 dB SPL are used for determination of gain, frequency response, harmonic distortion, and internal noise. While these input levels may be appropriate for hearing aids, the input levels to the FM system are 20 dB higher, as mentioned earlier. Higher input levels, e.g., 70–80 dB SPL, may be required. Since most FM systems utilize a compression limiting system, it may also be more appropriate to use a broadband signal rather than sweep-frequency tone signals. The issue concerning use of a noise signal is a complicated one and is now being considered by the American National Standards Institute (ANSI) standards committee for hearing aid measurements.

A preliminary approach to measuring personal FM systems was outlined by Hawkins and Schum (1985). They used input levels of 60–65 dB SPL when measuring the hearing aid alone, and 80–85 dB SPL when measuring through the FM system attached to the hearing aid. The hearing aid volume control wheel remained at reference test gain position for both measurements, and in the FM measurements the FM receiver volume control wheel was adjusted such that with an 80 dB SPL input at 1000 Hz the output was the same as the hearing aid alone with a 60 dB SPL input. Using this approach, they evaluated the performance of four hearing aids attached to two FM systems via the three coupling methods. The following statements summarize their data:

1. When matched at 1000 Hz, the frequency response of the hearing aid attached to the FM system was typically different from that of the hearing aid measured alone.
2. The magnitude of the frequency response differences varied from minimal (2–3 dB) to substantial (20–25 dB).
3. The degree to which the original hearing-aid frequency response was preserved was not clearly different among the three coupling methods.
4. With the exception of the SI, harmonic distortion and internal noise was not greater for the personal FM system than the hearing aid alone.
5. The FM receiver volume control wheel taper curves varied dramatically (see figure 6 for an example) depending upon the coupling method, FM system, and hearing aid, with some combinations producing highly undesirable results.

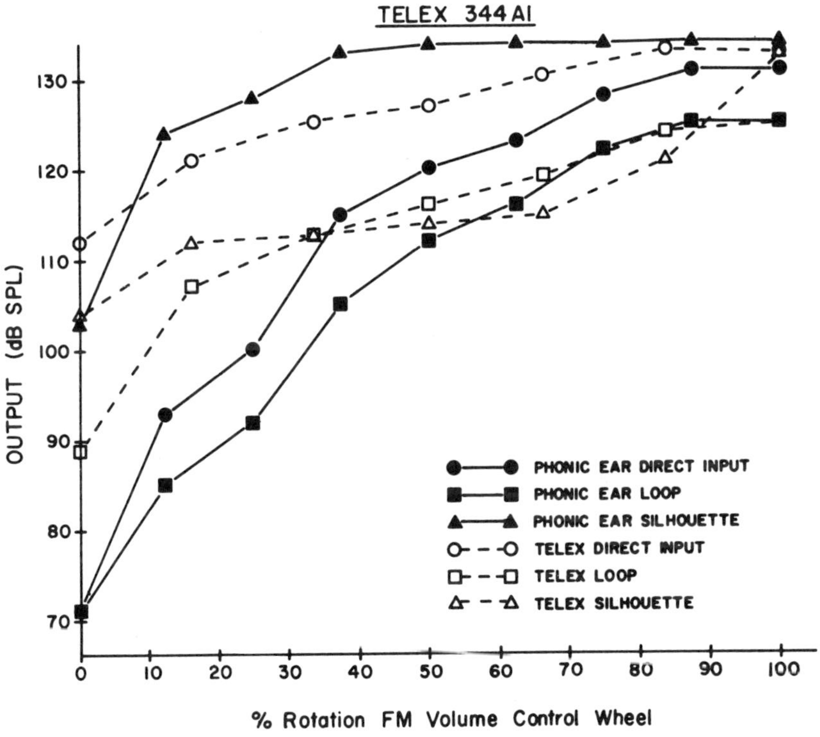

Figure 6. FM receiver volume control wheel taper curves for a hearing aid connected to two FM systems via DI, NL, and SI. (From Hawkins, D., and Schum, D. *Journal of Speech and Hearing Disorders* 1985. 50:132–141. Copyright 1985 by American Speech-Language-Hearing Association. Used with permission).

6. The input-output functions of some linear hearing aids were significantly altered when connected to an FM system having input compression (see figure 7 for an example).
7. Minor changes in the coupling between the SI and hearing aid can produce substantial changes in the system's output.
8. A teacher's directional FM microphone can improve the classroom S/N ratio by 4–7 dB.

In summary, the electroacoustic characteristics of a hearing aid can be altered in some minor and possibly major ways by connecting it to an FM system. Audiologists would be wise to assess these effects on a hearing aid test box before dispensing personal FM systems.

An alternative to assessing the FM-hearing aid combination with a test box is to use ear canal probe tube measurements. An example of a procedure described by Hawkins (1987) is shown in figure 8. First the output of the hearing aid alone is measured in the ear canal with a 60 dB SPL input signal and adjusted to be appropriate. The hearing aid is then coupled to the FM system, with the FM microphone clipped next to the compression microphone of the probe tube assembly. This location allows for a flat input across frequency to be

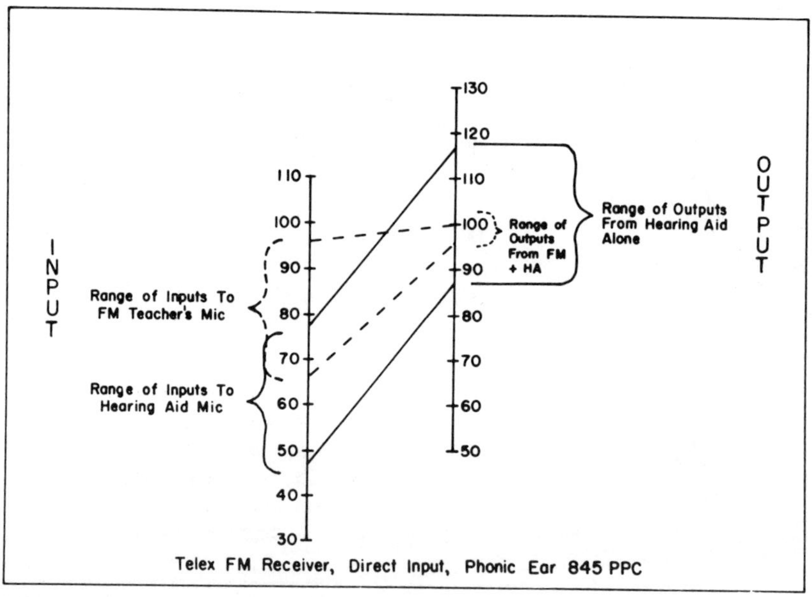

Figure 7. Input-output functions at 2000 Hz for a hearing aid alone and when connected via DI to an FM receiver. The solid lines connect the range of inputs to a hearing aid microphone to the outputs from the hearing aid alone. The dashed lines connect the range of inputs to the FM microphone to the outputs from the hearing aid when it is connected to the FM receiver via DI. The FM receiver volume control wheel was adjusted such that the output at 1000 Hz with an input of 84 dB SPL was equal to the hearing aid output alone with a 60 dB SPL input. (From Hawkins, D., and Schum, D. *Journal of Speech and Hearing Disorders* 1985. 50:132–141. Copyright 1985 by American Speech-Language-Hearing Association. Used with permission).

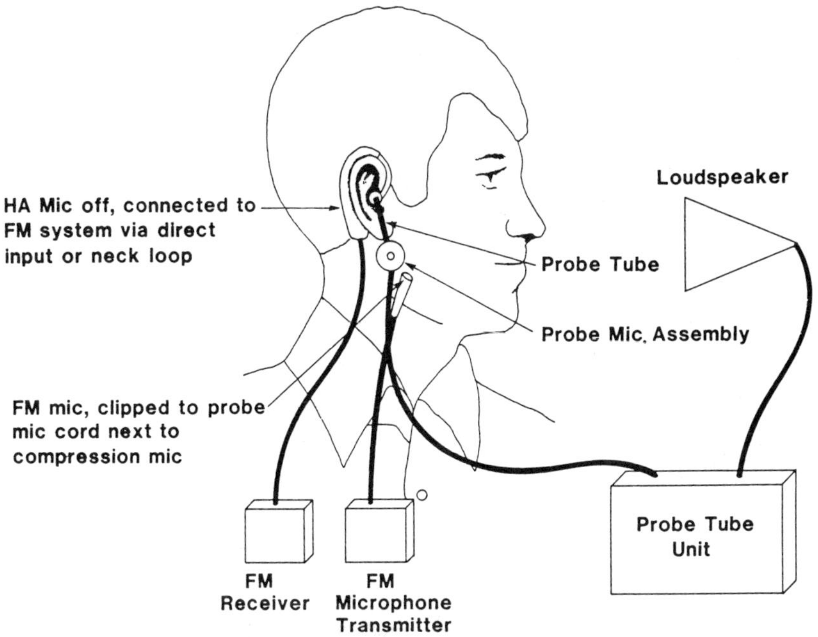

Figure 8. Arrangements to measure the real-ear response of an FM system attached to a hearing aid. The compression microphone in the probe microphone assembly serves to keep the sound pressure level constant at the FM microphone. (From Hawkins, D., *Ear and Hearing*, 1987, 8, 301–303. Used with permission.)

delivered to the FM microphone. The input level is increased to 80 dB SPL, the hearing aid microphone is turned off to allow for an FM only measurement, and the SPL in the ear canal is measured for a flat 80 dB SPL input to the FM system. The FM receiver volume control wheel can then be adjusted to produce the desired output level in the ear canal, perhaps matching the output of the hearing aid alone if that is desired. An example of measurements made with this procedure are shown in figure 9. The top curve shows the output in the ear canal of the hearing aid alone with a 60 dB SPL input. With the hearing aid volume control wheel remaining in the same position, the FM system with a neck loop was added and the FM volume control wheel adjusted so that, with a 80 dB SPL input, the output at 1000 Hz was the same as the hearing aid alone. The middle curve shows the resulting frequency response that was obtained. There is some decrease in the high-frequency response with the neck loop. The bottom curve shows similar measurements when the hearing aid was connected to the FM system via direct audio input. Notice that a further decrease in the high-frequency response resulted. This reduction in high-frequency gain could be compensated for by increasing the FM volume control wheel, but the response in the low and middle frequencies would then also be increased and be greater than the hearing aid alone. These data serve to make two important points: as mentioned earlier, differences can occur when the hearing aid is con-

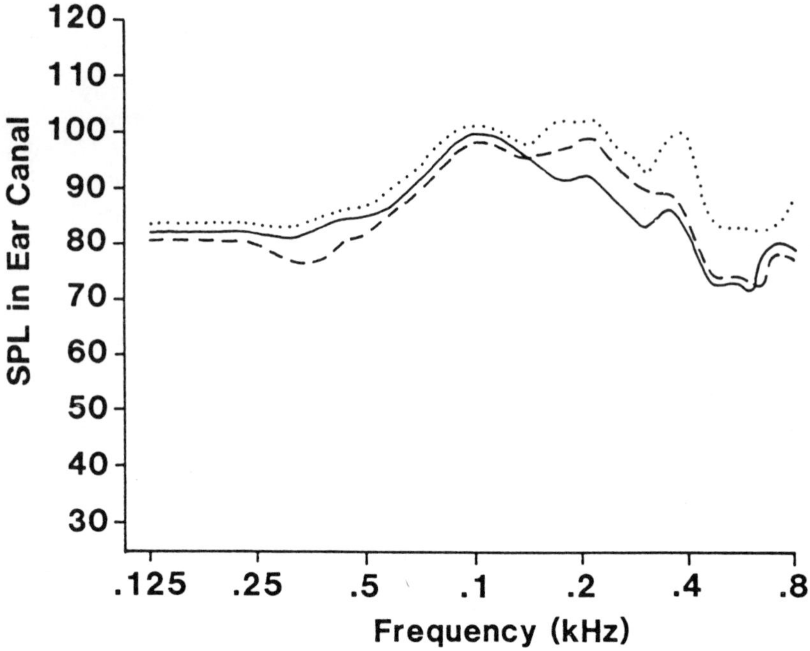

Figure 9. Output sound pressure levels in the ear canal for three measurement conditions utilizing the technique shown in figure 8. The dotted line is the output of the hearing aid alone. The dashed line is the output with the hearing aid coupled to an FM system via a neck loop and the solid line represents a connection via direct input. The FM receiver volume control wheel was adjusted such that the output at 1000 Hz was the same as with the hearing aid alone. (From Hawkins, D., *Ear and Hearing*, 1987, 8, 301–303. Used with permission.)

nected to an FM system, and these differences can be rapidly assessed as actual output levels in the ear canal with a real-ear probe tube system and maintain more appropriate input levels for the two measurements (60 dB SPL for the hearing aid and 80 dB SPL for the FM-hearing aid combination).

BEHAVIORAL RESULTS WITH FM SYSTEMS AND HEARING AIDS

A recent study by Hawkins (1984) used a group of moderately hearing-impaired children to compare a variety of amplification options on a speech recognition in noise task in a classroom environment. Four hearing-aid arrangements (monaural-omnidirectional, monaural-directional, binaural-omnidirectional, and binaural-directional), and seven personal FM systems were evaluated using an adaptive paradigm to determine the S/N ratio necessary for 50% correct performance. The important findings were the following: (1) among the hearing aids, best performance was obtained with binaural-directional and worst performance was obtained with monaural-omnidirectional; (2) the S/N ratio advantage of FM only (environmental microphone turned off) over hearing aids was 16–20 dB; (3) activation of the environmental microphones caused a major reduction in the FM advantage over hearing aids; (4) performance was not significantly different for the three coupling methods (DI, NL, or SI), but subjects complained about the signal strength variability with the SI; and (5) a directional FM system microphone improved the S/N ratio by 3 dB over an omnidirectional version.

In addition to the adaptive conditions, word recognition scores were obtained with hearing aids and an FM system (DI) at two environmental S/N ratios—+6 and +15 dB. The FM system provided a significant advantage at both S/N ratios, but the magnitude of the advantage decreased markedly as the S/N ratio improved. If the FM systems had been compared to the hearing aids at a +20 dB S/N ratio at this reverberation (.6 s), it is likely that equivalent performance would have been obtained. If, however, the reverberation time had been longer or the child had been seated further from the speaker (a 2 m location was used in this study), the FM advantage would increase and probably still be significant at +20 dB S/N ratio. In other words, the magnitude of the FM advantage is directly dependent upon the acoustic conditions in the classroom and the child's location relative to the teacher. In a quiet classroom with a reasonably short reverberation time (less than .5 sec) and a minimal child-to-teacher distance, the FM system will offer little, if any, advantage over a hearing aid or aids. When any of these factors (noise, reverberation, or distance) are altered in an adverse way, the FM advantage increases. Under the worst conditions of high noise, long reverberation, and substantial teacher-to-child distance, the improvement that an FM system offers is enormous.

SUMMARY AND CONCLUSIONS

Based on the available literature and this writer's opinions, the following recommendations are offered for classroom amplification systems:

1. Before making decisions regarding the type of amplification system, do whatever is possible to reduce the teacher-to-child distance, classroom noise level, and reverberation time.
2. After treatment of the room, if the reverberation time is less than .5 s and the S/N ratio at the child's ear is greater than +15 dB, there is no compelling reason to use an FM System. An FM system will still improve the S/N ratio and certainly will not be harmful, but whether performance will significantly improve is open to question. The preferred hearing-aid arrangement, barring contraindications, would be binaural with directional microphones.
3. If the reverberation time is greater than .5 s or the S/N at the child's ear is less than +15 dB, there is reason to consider an FM system for improving the S/N ratio and reducing the detrimental effects of reverberation.

4. If an FM system is chosen, consider the following:
   a. Use of a directional teacher's microphone.
   b. If the child has an appropriate hearing aid or aids and it is feasible within the specific educational setting, use a personal FM system; if not, use a self-contained system.
   c. If a personal FM system is to be used, consider the following:
      (1) If the child has strong cosmetic concerns, use a neck loop. Be sure the hearing aid's T-coil has sufficient strength.
      (2) If the child has no strong cosmetic concerns, use direct audio input.
      (3) Use a silhouette inductor only if it is known to work well with the specific FM system and hearing aid.
      (4) Carefully choose the switching options on the hearing aid(s). An appropriate switch contains positions for Hearing Aid Only, FM Only, and FM plus Hearing Aid Microphone. An ideal hearing aid for the personal FM system and assistive device use would have both a telecoil and direct audio input capability and be equipped with a five-position switch for Hearing Aid Only, FM Only Via the Telecoil, FM Only Via Direct Audio Input, FM Via Telecoil Plus the Hearing Aid Microphone Open, and FM Via Direct Audio Input Plus the Hearing Aid Microphone Open. This arrangement is currently offered by one manufacturer as a special order. Regardless of the specific arrangement, be sure that the hearing aid microphone can be turned off while the FM signal is being received.
      (5) If it is possible and there are no contraindications, connect the FM receiver to binaural hearing aids with directional microphones.
   d. Use the environmental microphone only when necessary. If the environment is noisy and the microphone is necessary, consider reducing the gain in the microphone circuit relative to the level of the FM signal.
   e. Check the total system on a hearing aid test box or preferably with a real-ear probe microphone system and listen to it yourself before dispensing it to a child.

REFERENCES

Finitzo-Hieber, T., and Tillman, T. 1978. Room acoustics effects on monosyllabic word discrimination ability for normal and hearing-impaired children. *Journal of Speech and Hearing Research* 21:440–458.

Gengel, R. 1971. Acceptable signal-to-noise ratios for aided speech discrimination by the hearing impaired. *Journal of Auditory Research* 11:219–222.

Hawkins, D. 1984. Comparisons of speech recognition in noise by mildly-to-moderately hearing-impaired children using hearing aids and FM systems. *Journal of Speech and Hearing Disorders* 49:409–418.

Hawkins, D. 1985. Methods of improving speech recognition in the presence of noise and reverberation. *Audiological Acoustics* 24:124–142.

Hawkins, D. 1987. A clinical method for assessing FM system performance with ear canal probe tube measurements. *Ear and Hearing* 8:301–303.

Hawkins, D., and Schum, D. 1985. Some effects of FM-system coupling on hearing aid characteristics. *Journal of Speech and Hearing Disorders* 50:132–141.

Hawkins, D., and Yacullo, W. 1984. The signal-to-noise ratio advantage of binaural hearing aids and directional microphones under different levels of reverberation. *Journal of Speech and Hearing Disorders* 49:278–286.

Madison, T., and Hawkins, D. 1983. The signal-to-noise advantage of directional microphones. *Hearing Instruments* 34, 18, and 49.

Nabelek, A., and Pickett, J. 1974. Monaural and binaural speech perception through hearing aids under noise and reverberation with normal and hearing-impaired listeners. *Journal of Speech and Hearing Research* 17:724–739.

Pearsons, K., Bennett, R., and Fidell, S. 1977. Speech levels in various noise environments. EPA Document 600/1-77-025, 1–70.

Chapter 17

Classroom Acoustics for Hearing-Impaired Children

Wayne O. Olsen

Introduction

Thirty years ago the special needs for control of noise and reverberation in classrooms for hearing-impaired children were pointed out by John and Thomas (1957). Research findings since then have demonstrated repeatedly the necessity for reduced noise levels and relatively short reverberation times for settings in which hearing-impaired children are expected to hear and understand speech (e.g., Finitzo-Hieber and Tillman 1978; Gelfand and Hochberg 1976; Hawkins and Yacullo 1984; Nabelek and Mason 1981; Nabelek and Pickett 1974a,b). Yet studies of classrooms in which hearing-impaired youngsters are expected to hear and understand speech, and to learn language structure, new concepts, and information critical to their academic success and ultimately to their vocational endeavors, generally have revealed conditions that are far too noisy, and often too reverberant (Bess, Sinclair, and Riggs 1984; Crum and Matkin 1976; Finitzo-Hieber 1981). The intent of this chapter is to review findings of some of the work dealing with noise and reverberation in classrooms, and to make some suggestions to improve those conditions.

"Acceptable" vs. Observed Noise Levels

Various relatively stringent criteria for noise levels in classrooms for hearing-impaired students have been suggested. Gengel (1971) recommended that noise levels in such classrooms should not exceed 30 dBA (A weighting scale on sound level meters) or the Noise Criteria (NC) 20 curve of Beranek (1954). (See figure 1.) He based this recommendation on his observations that the speech recognition performance of hearing-impaired college students remained relatively constant at +30 and +15 dB signal-to-noise ratios, but deteriorated at poorer signal-to-noise levels. Further, the students commented that listening

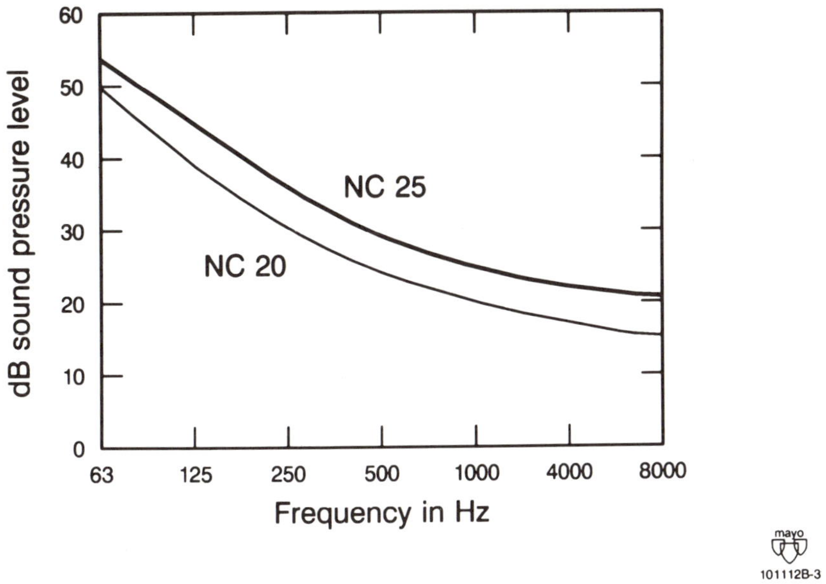

Figure 1. NC 25 and 20 curves of Beranek (1954) suggested by Niemoeller (1968) and Gengel (1971) as maximum noise levels in classrooms for hearing-impaired children.

was relatively effortless at the higher signal-to-noise ratios, but listening at signal-to-noise ratios less than +10 dB required so much effort that they would prefer to rely on speech reading and manual communication rather than use their hearing aids. On this basis Gengel recommended that ambient classroom noise levels should not exceed 30 dBA, or the NC 20 curve, in order to maintain signal-to-noise ratios of 20 dB or better.

Somewhat less stringent criteria for ambient noise have been suggested by Niemoeller (1968) and by Fourcin et al. (1980). Niemoeller's recommendation is that the NC 25 curve of Beranek be applied to classrooms for hearing-impaired youngsters. (See figure 1.) The recommendation of Fourcin et al. (1980) for British schools is more lenient, allowing noise levels up to 35 dBA in teaching areas of classrooms for hearing-impaired students. Scandinavian standards for classrooms for hearing-impaired children are more rigorous, allowing only noise levels of 25 dBA (Borrild 1978). In Sweden, the recommendations are that the noise levels not exceed 30 dB sound pressure level (SPL) in the octave bands from 125 to 1000 Hz, 25 dB SPL for the 2000 Hz octave band, and 20 dB SPL for the octave band centered at 4000 Hz.

Unfortunately, classrooms in the United States that meet any of the above criteria are the exception rather than the rule. In their study of 11 classrooms for hearing-impaired youngsters Crum and Matkin (1976) found only one with noise levels below the NC 30 curve. Finitzo-Hieber (1981) reported noise levels of 35–38 dBA in unoccupied self-contained classrooms for hearing-impaired youngsters. When 5 children and 1 teacher were active in the same area, the levels were 40–45 dBA. Noise levels in traditional classrooms evaluated in the same way were 42–44 dBA unoccupied, 58–60 dBA when 25 students and 1 teacher were present. Measurements for a carpeted classroom for hearing-impaired children in a mainstream environment were 36–39 dBA when unoccupied, 55–62 dBA with 15 students and 2 teachers in the room.

Similar noise levels were reported recently by Bess, Sinclair, and Riggs (1984). Their measurements of 19 classrooms for hearing-impaired children located in six schools revealed median noise levels of 41 dBA unoccupied, 56 dBA with students and teachers present. The ranges across the 19 rooms were 28 to 50 dBA empty, 48–66 dBA when occupied.

The median one-third octave noise levels for these 19 classrooms also are of interest. (See figure 2.) Note that noise levels for the unoccupied and occupied conditions were similar through 200 Hz, 40–50 dB SPL. Median levels dropped gradually to 30 dB SPL at 400 Hz, about 24 dB SPL at 1600 Hz, and approximately 12 dB SPL at 5000 Hz when the classrooms were empty, but remained at 40 dB SPL or higher through 1600 Hz and then decreased gradually to 30 dB SPL at 5000 Hz when the classrooms were occupied.

These levels can be converted to octave band levels and compared to the NC curves in figure 1 by adding 5 dB to the levels in figure 2 at the octave frequencies common to both graphs. Note that the octave band levels for the NC 25 curve in figure 1 is at 47 dB SPL at 125 Hz, decreases about 8 dB per octave through 500 Hz, then drops to 27 dB SPL at 1000 Hz, 24 dB SPL at 2000 Hz, and 22 dB SPL at 4000 Hz. If 5 dB were added at these levels for the unoccupied condition in figure 2, the resultant levels would exceed the NC 25 levels slightly at all octave bands except 4000 Hz.

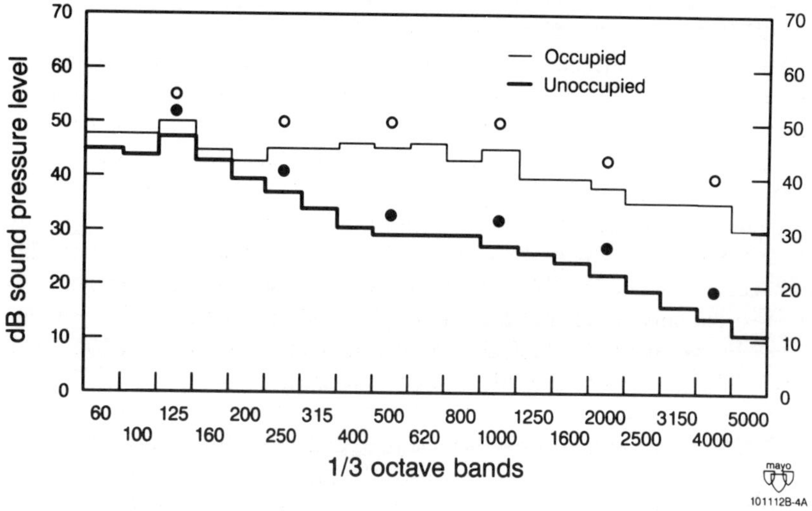

Figure 2. Median noise levels observed by Bess, Sinclair, and Riggs (1984) in 19 classrooms for hearing-impaired youngsters. Lines indicate one-third octave band levels, circles suggest one-octave band levels at indicated frequencies.

NOISE SOURCES AND THEIR "CONTROL"

External noises are those generated outside the building itself according to the classification system of John and Thomas (1957). Obvious sources are busy highways or streets, highway or street intersections, railroads, and airports. Noise problems associated with ground or air traffic are controlled best by careful selection of the school site. As noted by Fourcin et al. (1980) careful site selection is the most effective and economical means for controlling external noise problems. Construction to limit penetration of such noises into the classrooms of existing structures is costly and is never as successful, nor as easily achieved, as by good site selection.

If changes in the area around a school occur resulting in unacceptably high external noise levels, some steps can be taken to decrease their intrusion into the classroom. Solid walls of dense construction are preferable to a number of doors or large window areas. A 6-inch dense concrete wall has an average noise reduction index of 47 dB across the frequency region of 100 to 3200 Hz, whereas the noise reduction index of 32 oz glass used in windows is 22 dB (Fourcin et al. 1980). Use of heavier glass or of different weights of glass in the glass panes of double windows with the panes not directly parallel to one another can improve the sound insulation of windows. Obviously all sound attenuation is lost if windows are open or poorly installed. Virtually all sound attenuation in any construction is lost with even a small crack or opening in an otherwise well constructed wall or window.

Similarly, doors of high mass per unit area, well fitted and tightly sealed in the door frame must be used if entrance of external noise is to be reduced. If possible, doors should be located on the side of the building away from the noise source.

Landscaping can be used to diminish the intrusion of external noise into the school building. Grass-covered earthen banks and/or solid walls constructed between the source of the noise and the building can help deflect and reflect unwanted sound away from the school area. Planting thick growths of trees between the offending noise source and the school can be used to break up sound waves enroute to the classroom (Berendt, Corliss, and Ojalvo 1976).

The arrangement of space within the school building can assist in decreasing the interjection of unwanted external noise into classroom areas. A gymnasium or storage room might be located between the offending noise source and classrooms.

Noise generated within the school building but outside a given classroom is called internal noise by John and Thomas (1957). The choice of location of the classroom within the school building is vitally important. Clearly, areas immediately adjacent to the gymnasium, metal or woodworking shops, music rooms, etc., or next to mechanical equipment providing heat, air circulation, or air conditioning are not choice locations for any classrooms, and certainly not classrooms for hearing-impaired children. Unfortunately, classrooms for hearing-impaired youngsters are often located in just such areas (Crum and Matkin

1976). Space near noisy areas is better suited for storage rooms. Construction of such storage rooms places distance and additional walls between noisy activity or noisy mechanical equipment and the classroom.

Classrooms for hearing-impaired youngsters should not be located next to the main exit to the playground or at the junction of busy corridors within the building. Further, corridor areas in the vicinity of classrooms for hearing-impaired children can be quieted considerably by carpeting the floor and covering the ceiling with acoustic tile (Niemoeller 1968).

Doors leading into the classroom must fit the door frame snugly and the door frame should be lined with felt and rubber to ensure a tight seal. Obviously all sound isolation of a well-fitted, tightly sealed door is lost if there is an open ventilating duct in the door.

Partitions between classrooms and between classrooms and corridors must be fully contiguous between the floor and solid ceiling above. Walls extending just to a suspended false ceiling covering overhead ducts, pipes, and wiring provide excellent transmission paths for sound from room to room. Openings or cracks around ceiling ducts, pipes, etc. must be avoided. Even a small crack or opening in an otherwise satisfactory floor-to-ceiling wall negates the sound attenuating capacity of the construction.

The sound attenuating characteristics of a specific construction are based on sound transmission loss measured for 16 frequency bands between 125 and 4000 Hz. A single value derived from such measurements is used to give the construction material a sound transmission class (STC) rating (Berendt et al. 1976). For example, conventional wall construction, consisting of 2X4 studdings with 5/8 inch gypsum wallboard nailed to both sides, has an STC rating of 35. Loud speech is audible and intelligible through such walls. If two layers of 5/8 inch gypsum board are nailed to both sides of the 2X4 studdings, the STC rating is increased to 40. Loud speech is still audible through such wall construction (Berendt et al. 1976). Placing absorptive insulation material between the studdings can improve the sound attenuation of such walls somewhat (John and Thomas 1957). Use of 3 inch glass-fiber blanket material between 3 and 5/8 inch metal studdings with two layers of 5/8 inch gypsum wallboard on both sides attains an STC rating of 55. A shout is essentially inaudible through such walls (Berendt et al. 1976).

Temporary thin partitions, folding doors, sliding doors, etc. are not acceptable partitions between rooms or rooms and corridors. Not only are such "walls" of insufficient weight to serve as good insulators against sound transmission through them, but cracks at floor and ceiling levels and at joints allow direct paths of travel for the sound from room to room or from corridor to room.

Air circulation ducts create another sound path between rooms. Ducts can be lined with acoustical material and fitted with noise traps to avoid "cross talk" and noise transmission from room to room. Further, air circulation ducts should be large enough to allow air exchange at low velocity with a minimum of turbulence. Air turbulence in ducts also can be decreased with smooth joints and long radius turns rather than sharp corners and transitions in the paths of air flow. Flexible joints or sleeves at junctions and rubber supports should be used to diminish transmission of mechanical sounds and structure-borne sounds through the ductwork (Berendt et al. 1976).

Other structure-borne sounds created by the impact of one solid material against a solid surface of the structure itself should be diminished as much as possible. Vibrations generated by such impact are transmitted via paths provided by continuous rigid construction. Discontinuities in the material, with bridges between sections being of materials different from that of the sections themselves, interrupt transmission of structure-borne sounds. Pads underneath supporting beams also reduce structure-borne sounds (John and Thomas 1957). Although usually it is not feasible to modify existing buildings to provide discontinuities in floors etc., it should be a design consideration in construction of new school buildings.

Noise originating within the classroom itself was labeled "classroom noise" by John and Thomas (1957). Unavoidably, normal classroom activities result in generation of some noise, but efforts should be made to reduce the level of the necessary noise. Hard surfaced floors do little to mute noises. One of the best means of reducing noise within the classroom is by carpeting the floor. Carpeting softens the sounds of footsteps, sliding chairs and tables or objects dropping to the floor. If the use of carpeting is rejected for some reason, the legs of tables and chairs should have rubber or felt tips, and teachers and students should be encouraged to wear soft-soled shoes (John and Thomas 1957; Ross 1972).

Permanent, rather than temporary or mobile chalkboards, should be used in the classroom. Mobile chalkboards are noisier than permanently mounted chalkboards and therefore should be avoided (John and Thomas 1957). Permanently installed chalkboards might be backed with a soft material to reduce generation of structure-borne sound associated with vigorous chalkboard activity. Further, if chalkboards are installed with a slight tilt, sounds reflected from them will be reflected upward rather than directly toward the back wall and side walls in the room.

Heating and air circulation equipment installed within the classroom must be quiet in its operation. Large diameter, slow speed fans rather than small diameter, high speed fans should be used. Centrifugal, so-called "squirrel-cage," type fans usually used in furnaces etc. are quieter than vane-axial or propeller type fans seen in circulating or window fans. The electric motors and fans in such units should be fastened in place with resilient mounts or vibration isolators, and be well maintained in terms of lubrication, replacement of frayed belts, etc. Paths for the air flow should be smooth without sharp edges or corners producing air turbulence (Berendt et al. 1976).

Niemoeller (1981) has stated that the noise levels of classroom heating and air circulation units are easily evaluated with a sound-level meter set to the A scale. Because the noise spectra of most heating, ventilating, and air conditioning units decrease at a rate of 6 to 10 dB/octave in the mid-frequency range, an

A weighted measurement of 30 dBA just meets the NC 25 criterion suggested by Niemoeller.

The disturbing influence of noise from ducts or other air circulation units in the classroom can be reduced further if the room is arranged so that the main instructional areas are away from duct openings or fans (Ross 1972).

REVERBERATION

All rooms, except specially constructed anechoic (echo free) rooms, are reverberant to some extent. In anechoic spaces, wedges of fiberglass or other absorbent materials on all surfaces of the enclosure absorb, rather than reflect the spherical sound waves striking them. (See figure 3.) Hard surfaces in all other rooms reflect sound waves impinging upon them, i.e., reverberating the sound from surface to surface within the space. Thus, in a conventional enclosure, sound waves move spherically away from the sound source at about 1100 feet/second until striking a solid surface from which the sound waves are reflected at the same angle that they struck the surface. Similar reflections continue from surface to surface within the enclosure. Such reflections result in the original spherical sound wave being broken up into many segments traveling in many different directions. (See figure 4.) The reverberation time of a room is defined as the time required for sound to decrease 60 dB after the sound source has abruptly stopped vibrating.

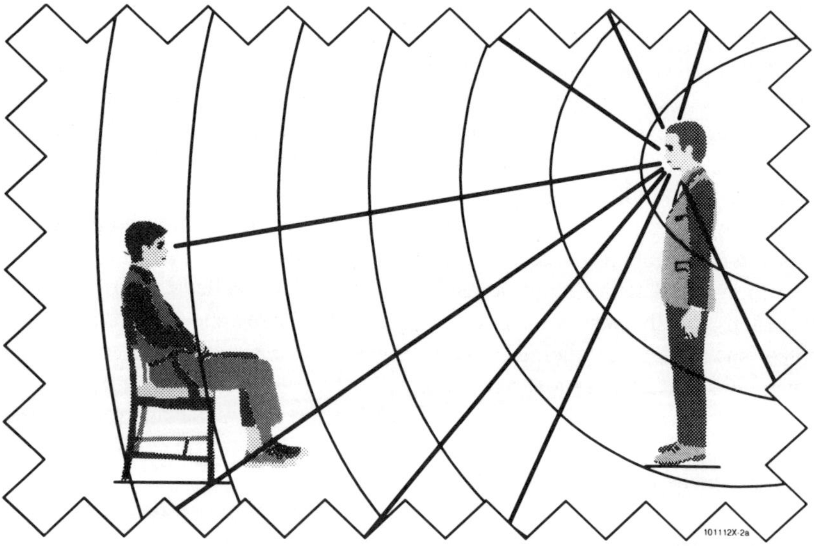

Figure 3. Simplified diagram of sound propagation and sound absorption in anechoic room. Wedges of absorbent material absorb rather than reflect sound waves. Adapted from Dale (1962).

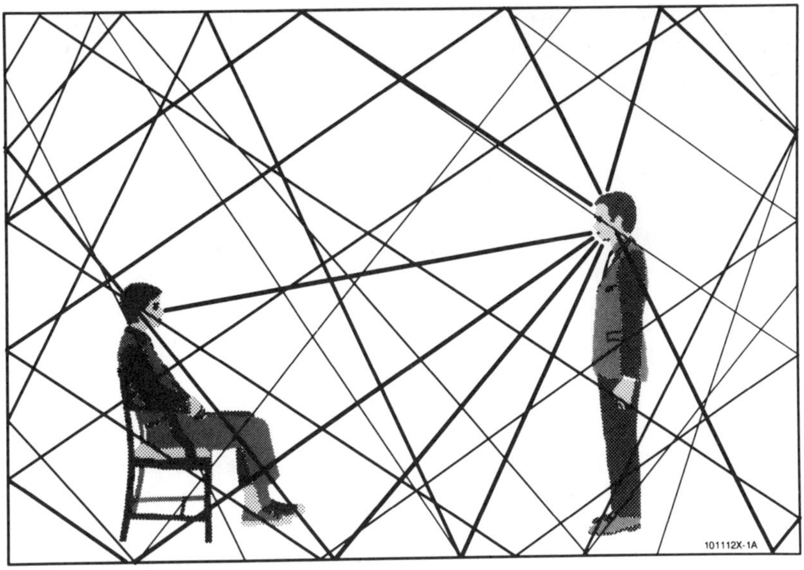

Figure 4. Simplified diagram of sound propagation and reflections in a conventional hard-surfaced room. Sequentially thinner lines for direct sound, 1st, 2nd, 3rd, and 4th reflections indicate some absorption of sound by surfaces and dissipation of sound energy in space. Adapted from Dale (1962).

The disruption of speech intelligibility due to speech sounds reverberating around the room and consequently arriving at the listener's ears at different times is well known. Just as it is well accepted that background noise or other competition is more detrimental to speech understanding for hearing-impaired individuals than for normal-hearing persons, it is well documented that reverberation disturbs speech understanding more severely for persons with hearing losses than for their normal-hearing counterparts (Finitzo-Hieber and Tillman 1978; Moncur and Dirks 1967; Nabelek and Pickett 1974a,b; Nabelek 1980, 1982).

Obviously, one way to counteract the influence of reverberation is to place the talker and listener in closer proximity to one another. As succinctly stated by Nabelek (1980) " . . . the reverberant effect in any enclosure depends not only on the acoustics of the room but also on the distance between the source and listener and directionality of the sound source . . . If we wish to overcome room reverberation we can introduce a highly directional sound source and locate the listener in the field of the direct sound." (p. 36) "Direct sound" is sound received from the sound source within the "critical distance" such that the level of the direct sound is at least equal in level to the level of the reflected sound. Critical distance is defined as the distance at which the intensity of the direct sound is equal in intensity to the reflected sound. Nabelek (1980) cites Peutz (1971) for the formula for critical distance:

$$D=0.2\sqrt{V/T}$$

where D is critical distance, V is volume of the enclosure in meters[3] and T is reverberation time in seconds. She goes on to cite Klein (1971) for adding a directivity factor "Q" to the formula that then becomes:

$$D=0.2\sqrt{VQ/nT}$$

where, as mentioned, Q is the directivity factor, and n is the number of sound sources.

The directivity factor of voice is given as 2.5. Niemoeller (1981) has indicated that the directivity of speech is such that the intensity of speech decreases 4 to 6 dB at 90° to either side of the talker. Thus, talking directly to a listener not only provides him or her with speechreading and facial gesture cues, it also delivers the speech at levels 4 to 6 dB more intense.

Neimoeller (1968) has suggested that reverberation times should not exceed 0.6 seconds for large rooms with a volume on the order of 10,000 cubic feet and 0.4 seconds for small rooms having a volume of about 2000 cubic feet. Critical distance for such rooms, using the first of the two formulas mentioned earlier, would be on the order of 14 feet and 8 feet for the large room and small room respectively. Therefore in rooms having these volumes and reverberation times, talker-to-listener distance should be less than 14 feet for the level of the direct sound to exceed the level of reverberant sound in the large room and less than 8 feet in the smaller room. (As mentioned in Chapter 16 of this book, placing a microphone near the mouth of the talker ensures sound pick up of direct sound at levels well above reverberant sounds, and above the levels of other background noise.)

The reverberation time in a given room can be decreased though modification of the ceiling, wall, and floor surfaces, and probably by rearranging furniture within the classroom. Efforts must be made to soften hard, reflective surfaces. Carpeting on the floor is vitally important in that, as mentioned earlier, it diminishes the noise of footsteps, of sliding chairs and tables, and of sharp impacts, and, to some extent, absorbs a portion of the sounds rather than reflecting them. Acoustic tile on the ceiling and probably part way down the walls also decreases sound reverberation within the room. Hard plaster surfaces absorb only 5 percent of the incident sound, whereas slits and holes and the soft porous materials on the surfaces of acoustic tiling absorb 60 to 70 percent of the sound waves striking it. Because acoustic tile is of soft material it may not be practical to extend acoustic tile to the floor. Even if no acoustic tile is attached to the walls, carpeting on the floor and acoustic tile on the ceiling cover 60 percent of the surface area of the room (Crum and Matkin 1976).

An alternative suggested by Niemoeller (1981) is to leave the front wall and ceiling hard and thereby reflective to direct and reflect sound, but to cover the back wall of the room with absorbent material to avoid reflections from the wall at the back of the classroom. He also suggests that patches of acoustic tile be placed on the side walls in sufficient quantity to reduce the reverberation times to the 0.4 to 0.6 seconds criteria mentioned earlier. He, too, advocated carpeting the floor.

Hard reflective surfaces of windows can be covered with draperies to absorb rather than reflect sound waves. The drapery materials should be hung away from the window surface in order to absorb low frequency energy more efficiently. Reflections of sound waves throughout the classroom can be broken up by placing cork bulletin boards, bookcases, etc., on one or more walls at strategic points, and by positioning mobile pegboards or room dividers at angles not parallel to other walls, so that there are few flat surfaces directly facing one another.

Acoustical engineers should be consulted to assist in the design or modification of a classroom to create an acceptable acoustic environment or "acoustic climate," as Borrild (1978) labeled it. Their knowledge of the sound attenuation that is provided by various construction materials and the sound absorption capacities of various materials, along with their measurements of sound levels and reverberation times within an enclosure, allow them to predict and to determine the sound quality of a given room. Based on such information they can select, design, or modify spaces to be more suitable for the education of hearing-impaired youngsters.

CONCLUSION

Three statements from other writers, with a few words added, are appropriate exhortations for providing the best possible "acoustic climate" in classrooms for hearing-impaired students. "The fundamental purpose in the acoustical design of any classroom is that the speech level must be sufficiently high . . . and the noise level sufficiently low so that the rate at which information can be transmitted to the student is maximized." (Niemoeller 1968, p. 1040) "Undoubtedly the [hearing-impaired] child who is attempting to learn new language concepts as well as academic material, will find typical classroom noises . . . [in most classrooms not specially selected or treated for sound control] more disruptive than would [a normal-hearing child or adult or] a hearing-impaired adult who can synthesize meaning on the basis of past experience even though many sound cues are obscured by background noise." (Olsen and Matkin 1971, p. 8) "One of the main tasks of those who are responsible for the education of most deaf [hearing-impaired] children is to help them get maximum benefit from the use of hearing aids [or auditory training equipment] and this task does not end when the child has been given an aid [or auditory trainer] and has switched it on. Parents, administrators and teachers [as well as clinical audiologists, educational audiologists, architects, acoustical engineers, and electronic engineers] need to recognize the acoustical problems which can arise when [hearing] aids [or auditory trainers] are used and to ensure, as far as possible, conditions which allow them to be used efficiently." (John 1957, p. 160) The acoustic environment must be such that, to the best of their ability, hearing-impaired students can hear and understand speech to learn language structure, new concepts, and information critical to their academic success.

References

Beranek, L. L. 1954. *Acoustics*. New York: McGraw-Hill.

Berendt, R. D., Corliss, E. L. R., and Ojalvo, M. S. 1976. *A Practical Guide to Noise Control. National Bureau of Standards Handbook 119*. Washington, DC: U.S. Department of Commerce/ National Bureau of Standards, U.S. Government Printing Office.

Bess, F. H., Sinclair, J. S., and Riggs, D. E. 1984. Group amplification in schools for the hearing impaired. *Ear and Hearing* 5:138–144.

Borrild, K. 1978. Classroom acoustics. *In* M. Ross and T. G. Giolas (eds.). *Auditory Management of Hearing Impaired Children* (pp. 145–179). Baltimore: University Park Press.

Crum, M. A., and Matkin, N. D. 1976. Room acoustics: the forgotten variable. *Language, Speech, and Hearing Services in Schools* 7:106–110.

Dale, D. M. C. 1962. *Applied Audiology for Children*. Springfield, IL: Charles C Thomas.

Finitzo-Hieber, T. 1981. Classroom acoustics. *In* R. J. Roeser and M. P. Downs (eds.). *Auditory Disorders in School Children* (pp. 250–262). New York: Thieme-Stratton, Inc.

Finitizo-Hieber, T., and Tillman, T. 1978. Room acoustics effects on monosyllabic word discrimination ability for normal and hearing impaired children. *Journal of Speech and Hearing Research* 21:440–458.

Fourcin, A. J., Joy, D., Kennedy, M., Knight, J. J., Knowles, S., Knox, E. C., Martin, M. C., Mort, J., Penton, J., Poole, D., Powell, C. A., and Watson, T. J. 1980. Design of educational facilities for deaf children. *British Journal of Audiology,* Supplement No. 3.

Gelfand, S. A., and Hochberg, I. 1976. Binaural and monaural speech discrimination under reverberation. *Audiology* 15:72–84.

Gengel, R. W. 1971. Acceptable speech-to-noise ratios for aided speech discrimination by the hearing impaired. *Journal of Auditory Research* 11:219–222.

Hawkins, D. B., and Yacullo, W. S. 1984. Signal-to-noise ratio advantage of binaural hearing aids and directional microphones under different levels of reverberation. *Journal of Speech and Hearing Disorders* 49:278–286.

John, J. E. J. 1957. Acoustics and efficiency in the use of hearing aids. *In* A. W. G. Ewing (ed.). *Educational Guidance and the Deaf Child* (pp. 160–175). Washington, DC: The Volta Bureau.

John, J. E. J., and Thomas, H. 1957. Design and construction of schools for the deaf. *In* A. W. G. Ewing (ed.). *Educational Guidance and the Deaf Child* (pp. 176–187). Washington, DC: The Volta Bureau.

Klein, W. 1971. Articulation loss of consonants as a criterion for speech transmission in a room. *Journal of the Audio Engineering Society* 19:920–922.

Moncur, J. P., and Dirks, D. 1967. Binaural and monaural speech intelligibility in reverberation. *Journal of Speech and Hearing Research* 10:186–195.

Nabelek, A. 1980. Effects of room acoustics on speech perception through hearing aids by normal-hearing and hearing-impaired listeners. *In* G. A. Studebaker and I. Hochberg (eds.). *Acoustical Factors Affecting Hearing Aid Performance* (pp. 25–46). Baltimore: University Park Press.

Nabelek, A. 1982. Temporal distortions and noise considerations. *In* G. A. Studebaker and F. H. Bess (eds.). *The Vanderbilt Hearing Aid Report* (pp. 51–59). Upper Darby, PA: Monographs in Contemporary Audiology.

Nabelek, A. K., and Mason, D. 1981. Effects of noise and reverberation on binaural and monaural word identification by subjects with various audiograms. *Journal of Speech and Hearing Research* 24:375–383.

Nabelek, A. K., and Pickett, J. M. 1974a. Monaural and binaural speech perception through hearing aids under noise and reverberation with normal and hearing impaired listeners. *Journal of Speech and Hearing Research* 17:724–739.

Nabelek, A. K., and Pickett, J. M. 1974b. Reception of consonants in a classroom as affected by monaural and binaural listening, noise, reverberation and hearing aids. *Journal of the Acoustical Society of America* 56:628–639.

Niemoeller, A. F. 1968. Acoustical design of classrooms for the deaf. *American Annals of the Deaf* 113:1040–1045.

Niemoeller, A. F. 1981. Physical concepts of speech communication in classrooms for the deaf. *In* F. H. Bess, B. A. Freeman, and J. S. Sinclair (eds.). *Amplification in Education* (pp. 164–179). Washington, DC: Alexander Graham Bell Association for the Deaf.

Olsen, W. O., and Matkin, N. D. 1971. Comments on modern auditory training units and their use. *Bulletin for the Education of the Hearing Impaired* 1:7–15.
Peutz, U. M. A. 1971. Articulation loss of consonants as a criterion for speech transmission in a room. *Journal of the Audio Engineering Society* 19:915–919.
Ross, M. 1972. Classroom acoustics and speech intelligibility. *In* J. Katz (ed.). *Handbook of Clinical Audiology* (pp. 756–771). Baltimore: Williams and Wilkins.

Chapter 18

High-Level Amplification and Potential Hearing Loss in Children

William F. Rintelmann and *Fred H. Bess*

Serious adverse effects on the auditory systems of humans can result from prolonged exposure to high levels of acoustic stimulation. A large body of literature exists documenting the nature and extent of trauma to the auditory system resulting from noise exposure (Ward and Fricke 1969; Kryter 1970; Burns 1973; Miller 1974; Mills 1975). As a consequence of the vast evidence concerning the hazardous effects of noise exposure, federal regulations have been established in an effort to protect workers from excessive occupational noise exposure. According to the U.S. Department of Labor's Occupational and Safety Health Administration (OSHA) regulations (1983), the maximum permissible exposure limit to steady-state noise is 90 dBA Sound Level for an eight-hour work day. Based on a trading relationship between exposure time and intensity, this OSHA regulation permits a 5 dB increase in the noise level by cutting the exposure time in half, (e.g., 90 dBA for 8 hours, 95 dBA for 4 hours, 100 dBA for 2 hours, etc.), with an upper limit of 115 dBA for 15 minutes or less. In other words, according to this regulation, no one should be exposed to steady-state acoustic stimuli above 115 dBA for even brief periods (e.g., 1–2 minutes). Prior to the OSHA regulation becoming a "Final Rule" (U.S. Department of Labor, Occupational Safety and Health Administration 1983), the Environmental Protection Agency (EPA) (1974) submitted considerable scientific evidence in an effort to urge OSHA to reduce the maximum permissible exposure level of an eight-hour time-weighted average of 90 dBA with a doubling rate of 5 dBA to an eight-hour maximum of 85 dBA with a doubling rate of 3 dBA. The EPA took the stand that the OSHA regulation will not adequately protect workers from occupational noise hazards. Further, based on reviewing the literature related to nonoccupational (recreational) noise exposure, Cohen et al. (1970) from the National Institute of Occupational Safety and Health (NIOSH) recommended limiting daily exposure for nonoccupational noise conditions to 75 dBA for eight hours with a maximum exposure of 115 dBA for less than two minutes.

Thus, based on consideration of detailed scientific evidence, departments and agencies of the federal government have recommended that in order to avoid the potential hazard of permanent damage to the auditory system, individuals should not be exposed to steady-state sound levels exceeding 115 dBA for even brief periods of time. In view of these federal regulations, one must question the advisability of using hearing aids with high gain and high-level maximum power outputs (MPO) for hearing-impaired children and adults, since, for example, when a hearing aid user is wearing an instrument that provides 60 dB of gain and a peak-clipping limiting circuit with an MPO of 136 dB, he will receive normal conversational speech at levels ranging from 125 to 135 dB sound pressure level. It should be noted that while the term maximum power output (MPO) was used in the early literature, the more recent term is saturation sound pressure level (SSPL) which ". . . is defined as the sound pressure level developed in a 2-cm^3 earphone coupler when the input sound pressure level is 90 dB, with the gain control of the hearing aid full-on. The abbreviation for this term is SSPL90." (ANSI S3.22–1982, p. 2.) Both terms, MPO and SSPL90, are used in this chapter depending upon which term was employed in the specific study cited or discussed.

The purpose of this chapter is to examine the available evidence regarding whether hearing aids can produce increased loss of hearing among hearing-aid users, particularly children. There have been several reports in the literature of isolated cases and small samples of children showing that pure-tone thresholds have deteriorated in the aided ear but not in the unaided ear. This would suggest that hearing aids may have an adverse effect on hearing sensitivity. Efforts to examine this question with large samples of subjects, however, have produced conflicting, but more frequently negative, results.

Many types of hearing loss are progressive both in children and adults; therefore, it may be difficult to determine whether the further deterioration in hearing is due to spontaneous progression of the hearing loss itself or to the use of a powerful hearing aid. Also, in cases of mixed hearing loss where fluctuating conductive components (as in otitis media) are superimposed on a progressive sensorineural hearing loss, the task of evaluating the reason for increased threshold shifts becomes increasingly difficult. Moreover, this problem of sorting out the cause of progressive deterioration in hearing is further compounded in those cases where binaural amplification, either hearing aids or auditory training units, is employed.

The contradictory results reported in the literature when relatively large samples have been used to investigate the potential harmful effects from powerful hearing aids can undoubtedly be attributed to the contributing variables mentioned above. To overcome these problems, certain strict subject selection criteria should be employed. For example, Jerger and Lewis (1975) suggested that patients suitable for study should (1) have bilaterally symmetrical sensorineural hearing losses; (2) be free from conditions that could cause threshold fluctuation such as middle ear pathology; (3) have worn a powerful hearing aid monaurally for sufficient time to produce noise trauma; and (4) have had valid threshold measurements at least at the beginning and at the end of the clinical investigation.

Recognizing that attempts to evaluate the possible harmful effects from powerful hearing aids have, of necessity, been largely based on the analysis of retrospective clinical data, often contaminated with the problems mentioned above, let us examine the studies reported in the literature. In considering these investigations, it should be mentioned that unlike reports of single cases or small samples, conclusions from large-scale studies can be generalized to a broader population. A distinct advantage of small sample reports over large-scale studies, however, is that the investigators are often better able to avoid the pitfalls of contaminating variables such as those mentioned above.

Review Of Case Reports

A review of the case presentations that have appeared in the literature is shown in table I. The first report of actual cases published in the English language was by Kinney (1953). As part of a large-scale investigation concerning the etiology of hearing loss in children, he observed in 16 children with progressive sensorineural hearing losses that progression was more marked in the aided ear compared to the nonaided ear and that further deterioration in hearing could be dated to the time when the children began wearing hearing aids. Two reports published in Russian at about this same time (1952 and 1953) were cited in a follow-up investigation by Kinney (1961) as supporting Kinney's 1953 observation that hearing aid use resulted in further deterioration of hearing.

Harford and Markle (1955) presented the first report of a single case showing repeated audiograms of both the aided and unaided ear. An eight-year-old girl with a severe congenital, sensorineural hearing loss had worn a hearing aid for three years. At age five, when she first started wearing a hearing aid, her audiogram showed a bilaterally symmetrical loss. Three years later the aided ear (left) displayed an increased loss, ranging from 10 to 25 dB, while thresholds for the unaided ear had remained unchanged. The hearing aid was then switched from the left to the right ear. After two and one-half months the left ear, now unaided, had recovered to its prestimulation level, whereas the right ear, now aided, demonstrated poorer thresholds by as much as 25 dB. At this time, the hearing aid was placed back on the left ear and, after one week, thresholds were obtained again. The right ear, now unaided, showed partial recovery, whereas the aided left ear displayed a greater loss. The hearing aid was then removed for one week, after which another audiogram was obtained. The results showed that after one week, without amplification, thresholds were again bilaterally symmetrical and at essentially the same level as prior to hear-

Table I

Summary of Case Reports Demonstrating Threshold Shifts Following the Use of Amplification

Author(s)	Year	No. of Subjects	Age(s) in Years	Degree of Hearing Impairment†	Hearing Aid Data: *MPO in SPL*	Hearing Aid Data: *Length of Aid Usage*	Results
Kinney	1953	16	2.5–17	Ranging	*	*	Shifts in the aided ear
Harford and Markle	1955	1	8	Severe (70 dB)	*	3 years	Shifts of 10–25 dB in the aided ear
Sataloff	1961	1	7	Left 61 dB	*	4 years	Shifts of 50 dB or more at octaves 250–4000 Hz
Ross and Truex	1965	2	13	Right 68 dB Left 80 dB	139 dB	8 years	Shifts of 20–35 dB in the aided ear
			14	Right 78 dB Left 77 dB		10 years	
Kasten and Braunlin	1970	1	10	Right 46 Left 48	120 dB	14 months	Substantial shifts in aided ear
Roberts	1970	1‡	5	Moderate (20–50 dB)	*	21 months	Marked deterioration in the aided ear with no recovery
Jerger and Lewis	1975	1	9	Left 85 Right 97	135 dB	6 years	Shifts ranging from 10–25 dB in the aided ear
Heffernan and Simons	1979	2	5	Right 52 dB Left 52 dB	135	7 mo. 1 yr.	Shifts of 5–25 dB in the aided ear Shifts of 20–35 dB in the aided ear
			4	Right 38 dB Left 40 dB	125		
Hawkins	1982	1	29	Right 52 dB Left 43 dB	131, 135**	10 yrs.	Shifts of 30-45 dB in the aided ear

*Not reported.
**Max SSPL90 of 1st and 2nd hearing aids
†Three frequency average (500, 1000, and 2000 Hz) shown for those case reports containing audiograms.
‡Although Roberts reported on three cases, specific detail was presented on only one case.
Note: No case reports were located in the literature after 1982.

ing-aid use. Harford and Markle emphasized the importance of additional research in this area and ". . . cautioned against interpreting this report as evidence supporting the concept that hearing aids may cause damage to the ear" (p. 972).

Sataloff (1961) reported similar findings for a seven-year-old boy who had worn a hearing aid in one ear since age three. After two years of hearing-aid use, the child complained that his hearing was getting worse in his aided ear. Audiometric results demonstrated dramatic deterioration in the aided ear (50 dB or more at octave frequencies from 250 to 4000 Hz). The hearing aid was removed, and within two and one-half months, thresholds recovered to pre-hearing-aid use levels. In the next two years, the hearing aid was alternatively put back on and then removed again from the same ear several times. Each time the aid was on the ear, thresholds became substantially worse, and when the aid was removed for a short time, hearing improved considerably. During this entire four-year period, the nonaided ear remained essentially stable. Sataloff believed that the hearing aid was responsible for adversely affecting this child's hearing.

Ross and Truex (1965) reported two cases of progressive deterioration in pure-tone thresholds which they stated possibly resulted from hearing-aid amplification. One case was a 13-year-old boy who had worn a monaural hearing aid in the same ear since age 5. The other case was a 14-year-old boy who had worn a monaural hearing aid in the same ear since age 4. After a few years of hearing-aid use, both children were fitted with powerful body-type aids having maximum power outputs (MPO) of 139 dB according to the manufacturer's specifications. Both children demonstrated substantial threshold shifts (20–35 dB poorer) on the aided ear, whereas the unaided ear for each child remained unchanged. In an effort to minimize the possibility of further trauma from powerful hearing-aid amplification, the authors recommended for both children that hearing aids with automatic volume control (AVC) circuits be fitted for the previously unaided ear.

Kasten and Braunlin (1970) reported on the traumatic effects to hearing resulting from hearing-aid use by a ten-year-old girl with a bilateral, moderate sensorineural hearing loss. After she wore a body-type instrument for 14 months in the same ear, an audiometric evaluation demonstrated marked deterioration in the aided ear with no change in the unaided ear. Her hearing aid was removed, and after seven weeks a reevaluation of her hearing showed substantial threshold improvement (20–30 dB) in the ear that had been receiving amplification. The hearing aid had an average gain of 39 dB and an average MPO or saturation sound pressure level of 120 dB. Kasten and Braunlin recommended that this child be fitted with a less powerful aid (30 dB gain and 100 dB saturation SPL) and that the hearing aid be periodically alternated between ears. By following these recommendations, subsequent audiometric evaluations demonstrated that the temporary threshold deterioration did not recur. The authors concluded that when a child is fitted for a hearing aid, the audiologist should have some means of verifying that the instrument to be worn by the child actually has the electroacoustic characteristics that were recommended, and the status of the child's hearing should be carefully monitored shortly after initiating hearing-aid use.

As part of a large-scale study involving 278 sensorineural hearing-impaired children, all of whom wore hearing aids, Roberts (1970) identified three children for whom serial audiometry provided evidence of deterioration of hearing related to hearing-aid use. He presented the findings of one of these children in detail. A five-year-old boy received pure-tone audiometric threshold tests twice, at six-month intervals. The results of these tests exhibited a bilaterally symmetrical moderate, high-frequency sloping sensorineural hearing loss. The youngster was fitted with an ear-level hearing aid for one ear (no information was given, however, concerning the gain or saturation sound pressure level [SSPL] of the hearing aid). After approximately 21 months, he was retested and demonstrated marked threshold deterioration (e.g., 45 dB at 4000 Hz) in the aided ear, with essentially no change in the unaided ear. The use of the hearing aid was discontinued; but follow-up audiometry 14 months later showed no threshold change. Hence, Roberts concluded: "The acoustic trauma appeared to be permanent" (p. 124).

Jerger and Lewis (1975) presented a case report of a nine-year-old girl with severe bilateral sensorineural hearing loss resulting from rubella. She had been wearing a powerful hearing aid (MPO of 135 dB) in her left ear since age three. In a period of one year, her pure-tone thresholds changed from an essentially bilaterally symmetrical loss to an asymmetrical loss exhibiting substantial deterioration (10–25 dB) in the aided ear, while the unaided ear remained unchanged. As remedial measures for this child, the authors recommended that the aid's MPO be reduced from 135 dB to 125 dB without changing the gain curve. They further advised periodic alternation of the hearing aid from ear to ear to avoid overstimulation of either ear for long periods of time. Finally, as a general comment, they cautioned against the "uncritical advocacy" of high-powered binaural aids.

Heffernan and Simons (1979) described two cases of temporary increases in sensorineural hearing loss following hearing-aid use. In case 1, a boy initially evaluated at age five years, four months, had a moderate bilaterally symmetrical sensorineural hearing loss of probably congenital origin. He was fitted with a body-type hearing aid for the right ear with a reported HAIC gain of 45 dB and a measured peak MPO (SSPL) of 135 dB. Although the family was asked to bring the child back in three months, seven months elapsed before he was returned for evaluation. Pure-tone thresholds in the unaided ear had remained stable, while thresholds in the aided ear became poorer by 5 to 25 dB. Amplification was then removed for 14 days. Upon retesting, thresholds in the aided ear had improved to the levels of the initial evaluation, demonstrating a reversible, or temporary, hearing loss. He was then fitted with a new, less powerful hearing aid for the same ear. After 30 days with no change in his thresholds, he was fitted with the same instrument for his other (left) ear. He continued to wear binaural aids for 1½ years with no change in hearing. Heffernan and Simons also presented a similar case of a boy aged four years, four months, with a mild-to-moderate bilaterally symmetrical sensorineural hearing loss of presumed congenital origin. The authors concluded that both children demonstrated temporary hearing loss resulting from hearing aid use. They recommended: "In cases of mild and/or moderate hearing loss, MPO should be restricted to 120 dB, or less" (p. 90). They also recommended frequent monitoring of thresholds as part of a specific follow-up program for all children fitted with hearing aids.

The last case study discussed in this chapter is a report by Hawkins (1982) of a woman who wore a high-output hearing aid monaurally, in her right ear, for ten years. Her hearing loss, detected in early childhood, was described as a mild-to-moderate bilateral "nerve" loss. She began wearing a hearing aid in 1969 at the age of 29. This hearing aid (with HF-AVE SSPL90 of 122 dB and Max SSPL90 of 131 dB) was worn from 1969–1977 only on the right ear. The left ear was not aided during this time. In 1977 she wanted a more powerful hearing aid, and thus she obtained a new aid for her right ear (with more gain and a HF-AVE SSPL90 of 127 dB and Max SSPL90 of 135 dB). According to Hawkins (1982) ". . . at no time since she began wearing a hearing aid have sounds been uncomfortably loud . . . her most common complaint was that she wanted 'more volume' from the hearing aid" (p. 383).

Hawkins (1982) presented numerous sets of pure-tone threshold data for this woman for a 10-year period (1971–81). During this period, air conduction thresholds in ". . . the right aided ear dropped approximately 30–35 dB at 250 Hz, 40–45 dB at 500 Hz, 40 dB at 1000 Hz, 35 dB at 2000 Hz, and 25 + dB (to the limits of the audiometer) at 4000 Hz" (p. 383). The left unaided ear remained unchanged except for shifts of about 15 dB at 1000 Hz and 10 dB at 2000 Hz. There was no evidence of conductive or retrocochlear involvement. Hawkins (1982) pointed out that even though this patient was receiving audiometric services at two different facilities, ". . . neither took full responsibility for her continued monitoring and care" (p. 384). As a consequence, several years elapsed before the severe increase in her right ear hearing loss was linked to the excessively high output from her hearing aid. Her left ear remained stable with a mild-to-moderate loss, while her aided right ear gradually showed a severe-to-profound loss. Hawkins (1982) concluded that in this case damage to the auditory mechanism occurred from hearing aid output levels below the woman's loudness discomfort level (LDL). This case tends to refute the notion of some writers (e.g., Markides, 1980) that deterioration in hearing from powerful hearing aid use is unlikely because individuals will not tolerate for prolonged periods of time acoustic stimulation that is uncomfortably loud, which according to Markides (1980) for most hearing aid users will be less than 120 dB SPL.

LARGE-SCALE INVESTIGATIONS

A summary of the large-scale investigations on the effects of overamplification appears in table II. Naunton (1957) was the first investigator to report the results of a large-scale study dealing with the question of possible auditory damage from hearing-aid use. He examined the audiometric records of 1480 hearing-impaired adults who had been issued the British government's hearing aid (Medresco). From this patient population, he selected 120 subjects with available audiograms that preceded hearing aid use. Results were evaluated by comparing the relative pure-tone threshold changes in the aided versus the unaided ear. Factors such as duration of hearing-aid use in years and hours per day were considered in the data analysis. Based on a statistical analysis of the results, Naunton could not support the notion that hearing aids may have a detrimental effect on hearing.

Commenting on Naunton's (1957) study, Jerger and Lewis (1975) pointed out that the large number of otosclerotics in the subject sample (38.3 percent) ". . . almost guaranteed negative results. . . . Not only would these patients be expected to show progressive deterioration in one or both ears, but the condition itself probably includes a built-in protection against intense noise" (p. 481). Concerning this later criticism, over 60 percent of Naunton's sample were diagnosed as having some type of middle-ear pathology. Finally, no data were presented regarding the gain or MPOs of the British hearing aids used. In spite of the limitations of Naunton's 1957 study, his findings effectively eliminated the concern over the potentially hazardous effects of hearing aids until 1961, when Kinney reported that use of powerful hearing aids can, indeed, have detrimental effects on children's residual hearing.

Kinney (1961) evaluated the audiometric records of 178 children taken from files of a school hearing conservation program. The sample was divided into two groups: 126 children who had been tested between 1938 and 1958 and 52 youngsters who were examined during 1959 and 1960. Kinney postulated that hearing aids manufactured prior to 1959 were probably less powerful than instruments manufactured after 1959. Hence, although electroacoustic data on the hearing aids were not available, Kinney assumed that the group of children tested in 1959 and 1960 wore more powerful hearing aids than the group tested prior to 1959.

The results of his study showed that in the less powerful hearing aid group (1938–1958), 13 children (10.3%) displayed an average threshold shift (in the speech frequencies) of 10 dB or more in the aided ear and essentially no shift in the unaided ear. Also, 4 subjects (3.2%) in this group showed increased hearing loss in both ears but with greater shifts on the aided ear. Hence, 86.5% of this group showed no threshold change. All children in this group wore monaural hearing aids. In the more powerful hearing aid group (1959–1960), 39 children wore monaural aids, and 19 or nearly half (48.8%) of the cases showed

Table II

Summary of Large-Scale Investigations on Effects of High-Level Amplification

Author(s)	Year	No. of Subjects	Age(s) in Years	Degree of Hearing Impairment	Hearing Aid Data: *MPO in SPL*	Hearing Aid Data: *Length of Aid Usage*	Results
Naunton	1957	120	Young-old	*	*	0-72 months	No significant threshold shifts obtained
Kinney	1961	178	6–16	Varying	*	At least 1 year	Children (15%) who wore less powerful monaural aids exhibited shifts of 10 dB or more; children (nearly 1/2) who wore more powerful aids demonstrated shifts averaging 20 dB
Macrae and Farrant	1965	87	6–16	50–90 dB	119–130 dB	10 months–10 yr, 2 mo	Significantly greater shifts observed in the aided ear for both high-powered and moderately powered hearing aids
Barr and Wedenberg	1965	84	*	Varying	Most<130 dB Nine>138 dB	*	Neither the endogenous or exogenous groups exhibited any significant progression of hearing loss which could be attributed to hearing aids
Ross and Lerman	1967	18	7–19	Moderate	17 S<130 dB 1S—140 dB	1–5 yr	Small but significant shifts observed in the aided ears
Bellefleur and Van Dyke	1968	58	Children	Profound	Powerful	8–10 yr	No substantial shifts observed in the aided ear
Macrae	1968	134	5–18	Mild-severe	115–130 dB	At least 1 year	Substantial shifts in children wearing powerful hearing aids

Madell and Asp	1970	18	2.5–5	Moderate to moderate-severe (3 S's) Severe-profound (15 S's)	*	6 months	No significant shifts were observed
Darbyshire	1976	100	3.5–12	Severe to profound	110 dB or >	apprx. 3 yrs.	No significant deterioration for aided ears
Markides	1976	100	7.9–13.2	Moderate to severe	30S, 130–136 dB 40s, 116–128 dB	3 yrs.	Slight improvement (2–3 dB) for aided ears; slight deterioration (2–3 dB) for unaided ears
Titche, Windrem and Starmer	1977	261	20–90	*	110–142 dB	<1–10 yrs.	No significant shifts were observed
Markides and Aryee	1978**	55	7.9–15.4	Moderate to severe	18S, 130–136 dB 37S, 116–128 dB	4th yr.**	Findings consistent with earlier (1976) study
Kittel and Axmann	1981	55	Grades 6–9, School for Deaf	*	*	4–11 yrs.	Inconclusive (see text)
Reilly, et al.	1981	45	3–21	Moderate to severe	Mean peak SSPL, 130 dB	Variable, approx. 1–8 yrs.	Hearing aid use not implicated in 31 (69%); questionable in 9 (20%); Probably implicated in 5 (11%)

*Not reported
**Follow-up to 1976 study
Note: No studies were located in the literature after 1981.

an average increased loss of 20 dB in the aided ear. Although only one of these 19 children exhibited an increased loss in both ears, the greater shift again was in the aided ear. The remaining 13 children in the more powerful aid group wore binaural aids, and of these, 9 (69.2%) displayed an average increased loss of 25 dB in both ears. Thus, approximately 15 percent of the children who had presumably worn less powerful monaural aids showed increased hearing losses averaging 10 dB or more on the aided ear. In the more powerful hearing-aid group, however, nearly half of the children wearing monaural aids displayed a further deterioration of an average of 20 dB on the aided ear, and over two thirds of the children using powerful binaural aids exhibited increased losses, averaging 25 dB, in both ears.

Based on these findings, Kinney (1961) made three recommendations: (1) for sensorineural hearing-impaired children, hearing-aid gain should not exceed 40 dB; (2) binaural amplification in such children should not be used; and (3) children wearing hearing aids should receive audiometric evaluations at least twice annually.

In a literature review, Ross and Lerman (1967) concurred with Kinney's (1961) recommendation regarding the need for frequent audiological follow-ups; however they disagreed with Kinney's suggestions concerning hearing-aid gain and binaural amplification. Specifically, Ross and Lerman pointed out that to protect the ear from overamplification, the MPO of the hearing aid should be limited—not necessarily the gain. This is a reasonable criticism of Kinney's recommendation, since the method of output limiting can, in general, control the hearing-aid gain. Also, they took exception with Kinney's statement on binaural amplification from the viewpoint, again, that the critical feature lies in the MPO or the SSPL that reaches the ear and not in whether sound is amplified to one or both ears.

The findings of Kinney (1961) were both supported and extended in a well-controlled study published by Macrae and Farrant (1965). It involved 87 Australian children (aged 6 to 16 years) with bilaterally symmetrical sensorineural hearing losses. The children in this investigation had been using either of two types of hearing aids. Thirty-four children wore a hearing aid rated as "high-powered" with a gain (at 1000 Hz) of about 60 dB and an MPO of approximately 126 dB (range = 122–130 dB). The remaining 53 children wore a moderately powered hearing aid having a gain of about 48 dB and an MPO of about 121 dB (range = 119–124 dB). The length of time the hearing aids had been used by these children ranged from 10 months to 10 years, 2 months.

Macrae and Farrant compared the aided to the unaided pure-tone threshold changes. They found that for children fitted with the high-powered aid, statistically significant changes in the direction of poorer thresholds were found for the aided compared to the unaided ear at all frequencies tested (250–4000 Hz). For children using the moderately powered aid, statistically significant changes (poorer thresholds) were found for the aided over the unaided ear only at 500 and 4000 Hz. The results also suggested that children with moderate hearing impairments suffer greater threshold changes from powerful hearing aid use than do children with severe hearing losses. Further, their data showed ". . . the longer the hearing aid is used, and, to a minor degree, the higher its level of acoustic gain, the greater the deleterious effect tends to be. Endogenous deafnesses do not appear to be any more or less susceptible to the deterioration than exogenous deafnesses" (p. 417). Based on their findings, the following recommendations were made: (1) for individuals with sensorineural hearing loss, hearing-aid MPO should be limited to as low a level as practical; (2) periodic audiometric tests should be given to these persons; (3) protective measures, such as switching ears for hearing-aid use, should be initiated if any deterioration in hearing occurs; and (4) use of hearing aids in high levels of ambient noise should be avoided by individuals with sensorineural hearing loss.

Barr and Wedenberg (1965) attempted to sort out the spontaneous deterioration in hearing due to the progressive nature of the hearing loss per se from the risk of auditory damage resulting from overamplification. The audiometric test results of 84 children were monitored for a period ranging from 3 to 15 years. The total sample was classified into two primary groups on the basis of etiology: 40 children diagnosed as endogenous (hereditary) and 44 with exogenous (acquired) hearing impairments. The latter group contained three causal subgroups: (1) maternal rubella, (2) perinatal accident, and (3) meningitis with or without dihydrostreptomycin treatment. In the endogenous group, seven had been using hearing aids; however, only two cases had used the aids with sufficient regularity to permit any conclusions. In spite of this stated limitation, the authors concluded that since more than half (N = 22) of the hereditary cases showed spontaneous progression of the hearing loss, such progression was probably not the result of hearing-aid use but attributable to hereditary factors. In the exogenous groups, all 44 children had been using hearing aids regularly. Hence, in the acquired etiology group, it appears possible to assess the effect of hearing-aid use on progression of hearing loss. Barr and Wedenberg observed that none of the children with hearing impairment caused by maternal rubella or perinatal accidents showed progression of hearing loss even though hearing aids were worn constantly. The meningitis patients, however, either with or without ototoxic drug treatment, exhibited progression of the hearing loss. The authors stated that for these children, it is difficult to determine whether hearing-aid use contributes to hearing loss progression; however, they felt that spontaneous progression is the most reasonable explanation. Thus, Barr and Wedenberg did not observe sufficient evidence in either the hereditary or acquired hearing-impaired groups to support the hypothesis that hearing aids can contribute to progressive hearing loss.

Ross and Lerman (1967) presented the findings of their own investigation of 18 children (ages 7 to 19 years) with moderate, bilaterally symmetrical, congenital, sensorineural hearing impairment. The duration of hearing-aid use was from 1 to 5 years and the aids were worn in only one ear. Following the procedure advocated by Macrae and Farrant, the results were analyzed by comparing the relative pure-tone threshold shift over time between the aided and unaided ears. For all subjects, the initial audiogram had been obtained at the time the hearing aid was introduced. Small (3.6–5.0 dB) but statistically significant relative differences were found at 250, 500, 1000, and 2000 Hz, with the aided ear shifting more than the nonaided ear. Ross and Lerman pointed out that examination of the raw data showed that only half of the subjects exhibited greater shifts on the aided ear and that the other half displayed little or no shift, or negative shifts. Unlike the earlier findings of Macrae and Farrant (1965), this study did not show a significant correlation between MPO and the relative change in threshold. Commenting on this unexpected result, Ross and Lerman stated that this may occur because ". . . it has been our clinic practice to limit the MPO of hearing aids for children. The one child in this study who was fitted with a hearing aid with an output greater than 130 dB (140 dB) showed a substantial shift in the used ear relative to the nonused ear" (p. 643). They commented further that a number of children had been seen recently who were using aids with MPOs greater than 135 dB and that these children displayed 15–25 dB of threshold deterioration in the mid-frequency range since using these powerful aids. Finally, Ross and Lerman recommended that hearing aids fitted for children should be limited in MPO to below 130 dB SPL and that such children should be seen frequently for audiological follow-up.

Bellefleur and Van Dyke (1968) presented a study in which they examined the audiometric records of 58 profoundly hearing-impaired children who had worn powerful hearing aids for eight to ten years. The sample was divided into two groups: 25 "Known" children who had always worn the aid in the same ear, and 33 "Unknown" subjects ". . . for whom the aided ear was not determinable" (p. 345). For the "Known" group, relative threshold changes were computed in a manner similar to the studies reviewed above. For the "Unknown" group the authors attempted to predict the aided ear by examining differences in threshold shifts between ears. No differences between ears were found in either group; hence, the authors concluded that high-gain hearing-aid amplification seems to have little adverse effect on the residual hearing of severely hearing-impaired children. Perhaps this study by Bellefleur and Van Dyke offers indirect support for the notion that there is an inverse relationship between the amount of hearing loss and the deleterious effect of overamplification on residual hearing. We computed the initial threshold average for 500, 1000, and 2000 Hz for the "Known" group from table 2 in the Bellefleur and Van Dyke study. When these children were initially tested (at the beginning of the eight- to ten-year period), the pure-tone average was 93.1 dB HL and 93.9 dB HL for the aided and unaided ears, respectively. Based on the findings of Macrae and Farrant, it appears reasonable that powerful hearing aids may have less deleterious effects on deaf or severely hearing-impaired children than on those with mild or moderate losses. Thus the findings of Bellefleur and Van Dyke need not be regarded as contradictory to the results obtained by Kinney (1961), Macrae and Farrant (1965), and Ross and Lerman (1967).

Primarily because of the conflicting results between the studies of Macrae and Farrant (1965) and of Barr and Wedenberg (1965), Macrae (1968a) reinvestigated the question of the potentially adverse effects from hearing-aid use. Employing a different sample from that used in his earlier study, he compared initial to most recent audiograms for both the aided and unaided ears of 134 children (ages 5 to 18 years) with mild to severe bilateral sensorineural hearing losses. The time span from the first reliable audiogram to the most recent one ranged from 1 to 12 years, with the average length of time being 5.25 years. Throughout the course of the investigation, both the aided ear and the type of hearing aid remained constant for each child.

One important difference between the 1965 study of Macrae and Farrant and the 1968 investigation of Macrae was that in the earlier study the children wore either of two hearing aids: a moderately-powered aid (MPO range, 119–124 dB) or a high-powered aid (MPO range, 122–130 dB). In the 1968 study, in addition to these two aids, two lower-powered aids were added. Some children wore an aid with an MPO range of 117–119 dB, and others used an aid with an MPO range of 115–117 dB. Hence, in the latter study, four different hearing aids were used covering an MPO range of 115–130 dB SPL. The results of Macrae's 1968 study confirmed his earlier (1965) finding that the use of powerful hearing aids (MPO range of 120–130 dB) had an adverse effect upon the residual hearing of children with sensorineural hearing impairment. The less powerful aids (MPO range of 115–119 dB), however, did not show a deleterious threshold effect.

Hence, Macrae's 1968 findings show some evidence suggesting that a hearing-aid MPO limiting factor of approximately 120 dB SPL protects the residual hearing of children with moderate sensorineural hearing losses. Obviously, several other factors besides hearing-aid MPO contribute to the potentially hazardous effects of overamplification on residual hearing. Nevertheless, if a "safe" MPO or saturation sound pressure limiting level can be established, then perhaps "damage risk criterion" guidelines could be developed for hearing-aid use. Clearly, considerable research is needed before a hearing-aid damage risk criterion could be established.

Madell and Asp (1970) investigated the effect of hearing-aid amplification on 18 preschool hearing-impaired children ranging in age from two and one-half to five years. Fifteen of the children were evaluated as having severe or profound hearing losses in their better ear. The other three had moderate to moderately severe losses in their better ear. The children wore one of two types of low-frequency response hearing aids on a regular basis while receiving aural habilitation. Also, most of them wore their aids during their waking hours at home. Pure-tone threshold tests were administered prior to initiating hearing-aid use and then at three-month intervals. Six youngsters were tested before and after three months of hearing-aid use. Twelve children were tested three times, thus covering six months of hearing-aid use. The findings of this study did not show an adverse effect on pure-tone thresholds from hearing-aid use.

Darbyshire (1976) examined test-retest pure-tone thresholds of 100 children over a period of approximately three years during which time they wore hearing aids described as high gain (50 dB or more) and/or high output (MPO over 110 dB). When first tested, the children ranged in age from 3 years 6 months to 12 years. At the time of the first test, 90 children wore monaural body aids and 10 wore binaural body aids. When retested approximately three years later, 45 of the 100 children were wearing binaural aids. Also, some children were now wearing behind-the-ear aids. The average three frequency (500, 1000, and 2000 Hz) hearing loss for all aided ears was 99.1 dB at the first test and was 96.9 dB about three years later at the second test. This 2.2 dB average change in all aided ears was interpreted by Darbyshire to possibly be a very slight improvement in hearing resulting from hearing-aid use. Further support of this notion was the fact that during this same period of about three years, the 54 unaided ears exhibited a slight decrease, 1.8 dB, in the speech frequency pure-tone average. Darbyshire concluded that there was no evidence from his study that amplification was harmful to children with marked hearing losses.

A serious limitation of Darbyshire's study was the lack of control of hearing-aid use (e.g., switching from monaural to binaural aids and body-type to behind-the-ear aids in a large percentage of the children) and no specific information about the power output of the hearing aids. Nevertheless, Darbyshire's study tends to support the findings of earlier studies (e.g., Bellefleur and Van Dyke) that powerful hearing aids may have less hazardous effects on severely hearing-impaired children than on those with less severe losses.

Markides (1976) reported on a three-year longitudinal study involving four groups of hearing-impaired children with 30 children in each of three groups (A, B, and C) and 10 children in group D. The children in group A (age range at the beginning of the study was 8.5–12.6 years) were fitted with hearing aids for one ear (MPO varying from 130–136 dB SPL). Group B children (age range at start was 7.9–13.2 years) were fitted with monaural hearing aids (MPO varying from 116–128 dB SPL). The children in group C (age range at beginning of study was 11.4–15.4 years) were not using hearing aids. Children in group D (age range at start was 8.7–12.9 years) used binaural body-type aids, the same type as those used by the children in group B. All children in this investigation had bilateral sensorineural hearing impairment, some congenital and some acquired, and in most cases the cause of hearing loss was unknown mainly due to unreliable history information. Pure-tone thresholds were measured for all four groups at the start of the study and at six-month intervals for three years. The average pure-tone thresholds in dB HL obtained initially for the aided ears of groups A, B, and D, respectively were as follows: at 500 Hz, 54.5, 50.3, and 58.0; at 1000 Hz, 69.0, 66.3, and 65.0 dB; at 2000 Hz, 81.2, 78.5, and 78.5 dB; and at 4000 Hz, 84.5, 90.5, and 78.0 dB. Average thresholds for the unaided group C were close to those of the aided groups. The findings from the repeated threshold measurement at six-month intervals over three years did not show significant changes in threshold from the initial data; but, a tendency was found for "slight improvement" (2–3 dB) in aided ears at all four frequencies tested while unaided ears (groups A, B, and C) displayed no change or "slight deterioration" (0–2 dB) for all frequencies tested.

In 1978 Markides and Aryee reported as a follow-up study the fourth year of a smaller number of children from the original four groups. The hearing-aid conditions for groups A and B were essentially the same as before; whereas children in group C who were unaided for the first three years of the study were fitted with monaural aids similar to group B (MPO of 116–128 dB SPL), and the children in group D who wore binaural aids for three years were restricted to only one hearing aid for the fourth year of the investigation. The follow-up study supported the findings of Markides' earlier investigation: that is, there was no statistically significant difference between aided versus unaided ears, but aided ears continued to show "slight improvement" (1–3 dB) over the unaided condition. The authors concluded that the children in this four-year longitudinal study did not show any deterioration in thresholds which could be attributed to hearing-aid use. They qualified their conclusion, however, by pointing out that most children only used their hearing aids 3–4 hours per day during school and that very few children used their hearing aids during vacation periods, including summer. It is possible that such limited use served somewhat to protect their auditory systems from the damaging effects of overamplification.

Titche, Windrem, and Starmer (1977) reported their experience of fitting monaural hearing aids over a ten-year period at a Veterans Administration Hospital. A total of 261 patients, ranging in age from 20 to 90+ years with a mean age of 55.2 years, consisted of two subgroups: 175 patients with sensorineural hearing loss and 86 with conductive losses. The amount or degree of hearing loss was not reported. Hearing aids issued varied from a gain of 36 dB and an MPO of 110 dB to a gain of 72 dB and an MPO of 142 dB. The length of time for hearing-aid use ranged from less than one year to ten years. The aided and unaided ears were compared before the aid was fitted and at retest, one to ten years later. The authors compared the relative threshold shifts, aided versus unaided ears, for the entire group and for the two subgroups. No significant differences were found; however, there was a slight trend for poorer thresholds in the aided compared to unaided ear, but only for the small group (N = 9) who had hearing aids for 8–9 years. The conclusion from this study was that prolonged use of hearing aids does not increase hearing loss in the aided ear.

The findings reported by Titche, Windrem, and Starmer (1977) are of questionable value for at least three reasons: (1) patients with conductive hearing loss are, as pointed out earlier, inappropriate subjects for study on this topic; (2) thresholds at 500, 1000, and 2000 Hz were not examined in sensorineural hearing loss subjects; and (3) most importantly, the amount of hearing loss by frequency was not reported. Nevertheless, aside from the above criticisms, it appears that this large sample of sensorineural hearing loss subjects as a whole exhibited little or no threshold shift from using hearing aids for various time periods.

Kittel and Axmann (1981) described the findings of a retrospective study of 55 children in grades 6–9 in a school for the deaf. The degree of hearing loss varied, but absolute values were not reported. Most of the children (number not given) had used binaural hearing aids (gain and SSPL not stated) for a duration of 4–11 years. Seven children exhibited an increase in hearing loss from 15 to 50 dB. By examining the medical histories concerning possible causes of hearing loss for these seven children, along with some information about their hearing-aid use, the authors concluded that for five children, factors other than hearing-aid use (e.g., hereditary progressive loss) probably account for the increase in hearing loss over time. They concluded that in only two cases out of seven, "hearing aid-produced sound pressures can be primarily seen as the cause of threshold deterioration" (p. 113).

The primary problem with the Kittel and Axmann report is that most children wore binaural hearing aids and, therefore, it is not possible to evaluate their report concerning the possible effects of overamplification on hearing. Another serious criticism is that no specific audiometric information was provided.

Several causal factors have been linked to or associated with progressive sensorineural hearing loss. Such a list includes: congenital syphilis, neoplasms, rubella, hypothyroidism, kidney dysfunction, and various hereditary syndromes. Thus, when a child with progressive sensorineural hearing loss wears a high-output hearing aid, it is important to attempt to determine the extent, if any, to which the use of powerful amplification contributes to the progression of the hearing loss. Reilly et al. (1981) reported the results of an investigation to help answer this difficult question. The records of 45 children with progressive sensorineural hearing loss were evaluated. At the time of the first audiogram the age range was 3–17 years, mean age 5.7 years. At the time of the last audiogram the age range was 5–21 years, mean age 12.3 years. Since this was a retrospective study, the number of audiograms evaluated for each child varied from 3 to 11 with a mean of 5.7 audiograms. Concerning progression of hearing loss, the audiometric frequencies analyzed were: 500 Hz, 1000 Hz, 2000 Hz, and 4000 Hz. At the initial test the group mean combined four-frequency threshold was 63.0 dB HL. At the final test the combined-frequency mean threshold was 87.4 dB HL, thus exhibiting a combined-frequency mean threshold progression of 24.4 dB. The mean progression by frequency was greater at 1000 Hz (26.1 dB) and 2000 Hz (28.4 dB) than at 500 Hz (19.4 dB). The authors stated that the mean progression at 4000 Hz (23.7 dB) was an underestimation because most of the thresholds beyond audiometer limits (assigned 100 dB) were at 4000 Hz.

Concerning the relationship between progressive hearing loss and hearing-aid use, the following factors suggested that amplification was not the cause for progression of loss in 31 of 45 subjects (69%): no hearing aid worn in five cases; rapid progression associated with serious illness or neurological degeneration in three subjects; hearing-aid use and progression were "asynchronous" in the remaining 23 cases, that is, the hearing loss had begun to increase well before or after aids were used. In some cases progression was bilateral while aids were used consistently on only one ear. Also, some subjects had histories of progressive loss causal factors, e.g., familial loss, rubella, head injury, or renal disease. Based on consideration of those factors mentioned above, of the remaining 14 subjects the progression of loss due to hearing-aid use was judged "questionable" in nine (20%) and "probably implicated" in five (11%) cases.

Thus, the study by Reilly et al. (1981) suggests that when causal factors other than hearing-aid use are carefully evaluated, overamplification may be responsible, at least partly, for progression of hearing loss in somewhere between one to three out of ten children who exhibit progressive losses. Again, frequent monitoring of thresholds for children wearing hearing aids must be considered an important part of the total aural rehabilitation program.

Temporary Threshold Shift Studies

Noise-induced hearing loss typically occurs gradually, over a period of several months or years, as a consequence of repeated exposure to high levels of noise. The course of progression of noise-induced hearing loss is such that repeated episodes of temporary hearing loss ultimately result in a permanent threshold shift (PTS). Based on this direct relationship between PTS and temporary threshold shift (TTS), investigators have attempted to determine the degree to which TTS can be used as a predictor of PTS. As an outgrowth of studies focusing on the relationship between TTS and PTS, the Committee on Hearing, Bioacoustics and Biomechanics (CHABA) Working Group 46 (Kryter, Ward and Miller 1966) established damage risk criteria (DRC). These criteria indicate that to avoid the risk of permanent auditory damage resulting from daily noise exposure over a period of years, levels of TTS_2 (2 minutes postexposure) should not exceed 10 dB at frequencies of 1000 Hz or below, 15 dB at 2000 Hz, or 20 dB at 3000 Hz or above (higher frequencies). Although DRCs such as the one cited above have merit when applied to groups of noise-exposed individuals (e.g., factory workers), a "neat" one-to-one relationship between TTS and noise-induced permanent threshold shift (NIPTS) does not hold in all cases. For example, Harris (1965) found that when several hundred young men were exposed to noise of 105–110 dB SPL for eight hours per day, TTS measures "vastly overpredicted" the actual NIPTS. Others have also questioned the relationship between TTS and NIPTS (Sataloff, Vasalo and Menduke 1965; Ward and Fricke 1969).

Although the measurement of TTS does not provide a "perfect" predictor of PTS, it remains, for the present, as reliable as any other measure of noise-exposure susceptibility. Even though a large number of experiments has been reported in the literature concerning the relationship between noise exposure and TTS, there is a dearth of information regarding TTS resulting from the use of powerful amplification such as hearing aids.

In a pilot study, Macrae (1968b; 1968c) found substantial amounts of TTS in the aided ears of four children, with not more than 85 dB hearing loss (re: ASA 1951 norm), after use of powerful hearing aids. The children received pure-tone threshold tests on a Friday afternoon, after which their hearing aids were removed until Monday morning at which time thresholds were measured again. Their hearing aids were then returned to them for normal use in the classroom and during play. Their hearing was tested again after one and one-half and three and one-half hours of hearing-aid use. Then the hearing aids were removed for the remainder of the afternoon. Thresholds were obtained two minutes after removal of the aids and subsequent threshold tests were conducted at hourly intervals for up to four hours post-hearing-aid use. The results demonstrated improvement in the children's thresholds between Friday afternoon when the aids were removed and Monday morning before the aids were worn again. Further, after approximately three and one-half hours of hearing aid use substantial amounts of TTS were found over a wide frequency range. Finally, when the TTS_2 data presented by Macrae were compared to the CHABA TTS DRC, all four children exhibited threshold shifts that exceeded the allowable risk level.

Konkle and Rintelmann (1976) conducted a pilot study in order to pursue further the problem of TTS resulting from hearing aid use. The procedures for this investigation have been detailed elsewhere (Rintelmann and Bess 1977). Briefly, seven children, four boys and three girls with essentially bilaterally symmetrical, moderate to severe sensorineural hearing losses had worn hearing aids for at least one year. Two children wore monaural ear-level hearing aids, four used monaural body-type aids, and one child wore binaural body aids. Thus, threshold data were obtained on a total of eight aided experimental ears and six unaided control ears.

Pure-tone air-conduction thresholds were measured both before and beginning two minutes after a one-hour exposure session to tape-recorded, multitalker speech stimuli (75 dB SPL) presented through loudspeakers. During the exposure session, the children wore their hearing aids in the ear(s) that normally received amplification, with the volume control of the aid adjusted to the gain setting for typical everyday use. The children were allowed freedom of movement within the test chamber during the exposure condition, and they were permitted either to read or to play quietly with toys.

Mean thresholds for the unaided ear remained essentially unchanged from pre-exposure to post-exposure. Conversely, mean pure-tone thresholds for the aided ear showed a threshold shift between pre-exposure and post-exposure measurements, with the greatest mean differences occurring at 1000 and 2000 Hz. Although thresholds were essentially unchanged at 250 and 500 Hz, a 6.2 dB mean decrease in hearing sensitivity was noted at both 1000 and 2000 Hz, 5 dB at 6000 Hz, and approximately 3.5 dB at 3000 and 4000 Hz. Based on the CHABA DRC (Kryter et al. 1966) only one subject exhibited a potentially harmful threshold shift in the aided ear, and that occurred at a single frequency, 1000 Hz. Nevertheless, after just one hour of exposure to continuous speech stimuli at normal conversational levels (75 dB SPL), four instances of 15–20 dB of threshold shift were found in aided ears compared to no such shifts in unaided ears. Finally, as hearing aid gain or SSPL increased, threshold sensitivity (at 1000 and 2000 Hz) became poorer. This finding is in agreement with the results of previous investigations.

Humes and Bess (1981) postulated that it is possible to predict NIPTS from TTS data when measured appropriately. They stated that the failure of most studies to show a close relationship between TTS and NIPTS may be due to using a single time course (e.g., TTS_2) for measuring TTS and not that the concept of the relationship between TTS and NIPTS is invalid. Humes and Bess (1981) pointed out that measuring TTS at two-minutes post-exposure (TTS_2) might be appropriate for assessing PTS for continuous exposures to steady-state noise, but exposures to impulse noise or intermittent exposures to continuous noise should be measured at post-exposure times ranging from one hour to 10–12 hours (TTS_{60} to TTS_{600}). Hence, no single time index is appropriate for all noise exposure conditions. They also cited evidence to suggest that measures of threshold shift obtained at frequencies below 1000 Hz tend to underestimate cochlear damage, and hence measuring TTS below 1000 Hz is probably of little value. Based on several studies by Kraak and his associates from 1974–78 (cited by Humes and Bess 1981) a new alternative measure has been proposed " . . . *which considers the whole pattern of TTS growth and recovery.* With this approach, threshold shift is measured periodically throughout the growth and recovery stages of TTS, and the time integral of TTS is then calculated for the period extending from onset of noise exposure to completion of recovery. . . . The resulting measure is known as the integrated temporary threshold shift (ITTS)" (p. 5). Refer to Humes and Bess (1981) for a detailed discussion of ITTS.

Humes (1978) conducted a pilot study in an effort to show that hearing-aid-induced ITTS behaves in a manner similar to other types of noise exposure. A single normal-hearing subject wearing an ear level hearing aid was exposed to tape-recorded four-talker speech babble (Konkle 1976) at 70 dBA for 57 minutes with the hearing aid volume set to the full-on position. Three different exposure conditions were studied by adjusting the aid to three different output settings (HF/AVG SSPL90 = 113, 124, and 132 dB) which resulted in corresponding gain changes (HF/AVG full-on gain = 40.5, 46.2, and 54.3 dB). The findings from this pilot study demonstrated that ITTS produced by hearing-aid use is similar to results obtained " . . . for more typical types of acoustic stimulation. . . . [Further], all other things equal, the greater the hearing aid output, the greater the ITTS (or TTS). A similar relationship has been observed in a more heterogeneous sample of hearing-impaired subjects (Konkle and Rintelmann 1976) " (Humes 1978, p. 7).

Humes and Bess (1981) stated that for controlled or " . . . very restricted exposure conditions TTS_2 may be used in place of ITTS as the index of damage" (p. 10). In order to demonstrate that TTS decreases as pre-exposure hearing level increases they compared the findings of the three studies discussed above, namely: Macrae (1968b, 1968c), Konkle and Rintelmann (1976), and Humes (1978). The exposure conditions of all three studies were sufficiently similar to warrant such a comparison. Recall, two of these studies used hearing-impaired subjects, and one (Humes 1978) employed a normal listener. The data from these three studies (total N = 10) were pooled and are shown in figure 1 (from Humes and Bess 1981). The TTS_2 data from Humes (1978) are for the moderate gain setting which best approximated the mean gain value of Konkle and Rintelmann (1976). Figure 1 illustrates that for both 1000 Hz and 4000 Hz, as pre-exposure hearing level increases, post-exposure TTS_2 decreases. Correlation coefficients showed that the trend seen in figure 1 for group data also holds for the individual thresholds shifts. Thus, the pooled data from the hearing-aid studies confirm further the influence of pre-exposure hearing threshold level on the amount of TTS_2.

The final portion of the Humes and Bess (1981) tutorial article describes and illustrates how one may predict safe limits for output of amplification devices (hearing aids and auditory training units) to avoid further deterioration in threshold for periods ranging from one to fifty years.

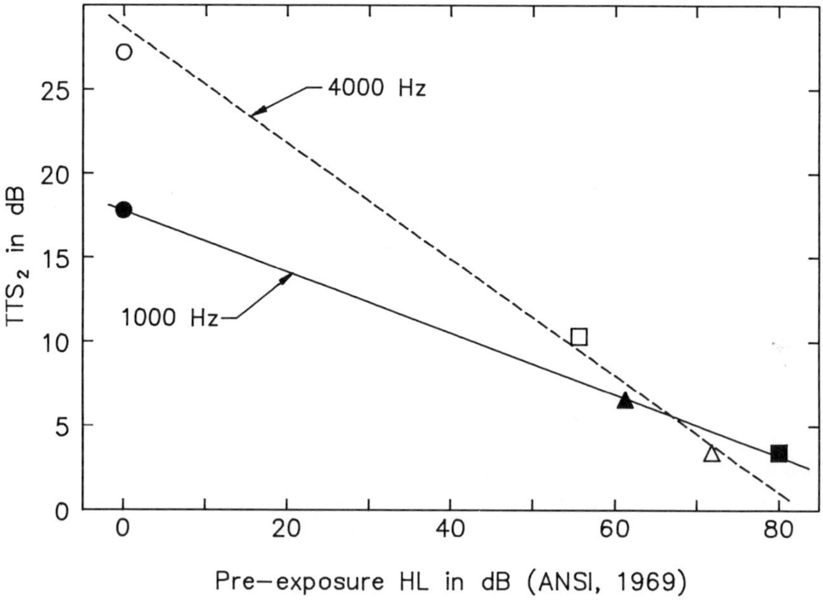

Figure 1. Relation of TTS_2 to pre-exposure hearing level following approximately one hour of hearing-aid use under very similar conditions. Solid symbols illustrate TTS_2 at 1000 Hz while open symbols represent TTS_2 values obtained at 4000 Hz. Circles: Humes (1978); Squares: Konkle and Rintelmann (1976); Triangles: Macrae (1986b). (From Humes and Bess, *Journal of Speech and Hearing Research,* 1981 with permission).

Classroom Auditory Training Systems

Although the focus of this chapter has been on powerful hearing aids, concern over the danger to hearing resulting from high levels of amplification obviously applies equally to high-powered auditory training units. Curiously, however, no reports could be located in the literature regarding the possible deleterious effects on hearing related to the use of auditory training units.

Group amplifying systems of various types are commonly used in classrooms for hearing-impaired or deaf children. In recent years, frequency modulation (FM) auditory training units have become increasingly popular over other types of systems, such as induction loop, because of several reported advantages claimed by manufacturers and supported by the users (educators) (Bess, Sinclair, and Riggs 1984). A discussion of proper classroom acoustics for the employment of auditory training systems is presented by Olsen in this book.

A Clinical Investigation

One of the present authors (Rintelmann 1975) had an opportunity to evaluate the effects of a high-powered FM auditory training system used in two classrooms for hearing-impaired children over a period of a few years. Thirteen hearing-impaired children located in two classrooms began using an FM auditory training system in September 1971. A year later, as part of a routine audiological evaluation, one of these children was found to have substantial deterioration in pure-tone threshold sensitivity in the ear receiving amplification, with no change in the opposite ear. Within the next few months, two additional children from these same two classrooms were found to have marked threshold changes, again in the ear receiving amplification, while their nonamplified ears had remained essentially stable. Partly as a consequence of this finding, 18 months after the FM auditory training system had been installed, we had an opportunity to examine the electroacoustic performance of this FM system as it was routinely being used in the two classrooms. Given this opportunity, a clinical investigation was conducted that involved observing (and measuring) changes in the children's hearing over a three- to four-year period, and measuring the electroacoustic performance of each child's personal hearing aid, as well as the classroom FM auditory training system.

Eight of the 13 children who initially used the FM auditory training system were selected for study. Audiograms had been obtained on each of these children from the same audiology clinic either before or shortly after they started using the auditory training system. All the children had congenital sensorineural hearing losses ranging from moderate to profound. In addition, one child had a conductive component added to the sensorineural loss. When the study began in 1973, except for one child who was 5 years old, the age range of the group was from 8 to 13 years. All the children had worn hearing aids prior to using the school auditory training system, and most of them continued to use their own aids, at least on a part-time basis, when not in school.

Audiological tests were administered at least twice annually. Most of the children received three or four audiological examinations per year. The individual hearing aids of the children were usually analyzed electroacoustically at least twice annually at the same time the child was receiving a hearing evaluation. Details of the testing procedures and the performance of the different amplification systems have been reported earlier in Rintelmann and Bess (1977). Briefly, the children wore either of two types of individual FM training aids (hearing aids). Both types of the FM training aids, according to the manufacturer's specifications, had a saturation output of 132 dB SPL.

Changes in Hearing The primary analysis was focused upon deterioration in pure-tone threshold sensitivity that occurred within approximately the first 18 months after the children began using the auditory training system. Changes in hearing resulting from amplification were computed by comparing threshold shifts in the aided ear to the unaided ear for the period from late 1972 to late 1973; however, subsequent changes until late 1975 were also monitored. As in the case of previous investigators such as Macrae and Farrant (1965), it was reasoned that threshold shifts resulting from such factors as progressive hearing loss and test-retest reliability would influence threshold shifts of the aided and unaided ears essentially equally. Hence, the relative difference between ears, if any, would demonstrate the damaging effects on hearing resulting from over-amplification.

Only three of the eight children satisfied critieria that should be met for the proper evaluation of the effects of amplification on residual hearing. Five children were eliminated from the data analysis for the following reasons: (1) the severity of hearing loss precluded measurement of any threshold shift; (2) the hearing aids were alternated between ears, thus eliminating a control ear; and (3) the use of auditory training units contaminated the nonaided ear data. The remaining three children, who were used as subjects, had moderate bilateral sensorineural hearing impairments. They wore their auditory training aids and their personal hearing aids in the same ear for at least one year between 1972 and 1974. These children used the auditory training unit while in school, approximately six hours per day. The remainder of the time they wore their own hearing aids.

All three children exhibited substantially more pure-tone and speech (SRT) threshold deterioration on the aided ear compared to the unaided ear. In fact, the threshold shifts for two of the three subjects were quite dramatic and are shown graphically in figures 2 and 3. The threshold shifts for a boy, aged ten years in 1972, are shown in figure 2 for a three-year period, from October 1972 to November 1975. During this period, he had three different personal hearing aids that were alternated annually between ears, while in school the auditory training aid was used in the right ear beginning in September 1971. Note that his left ear thresholds remained essentially stable, but his right ear showed

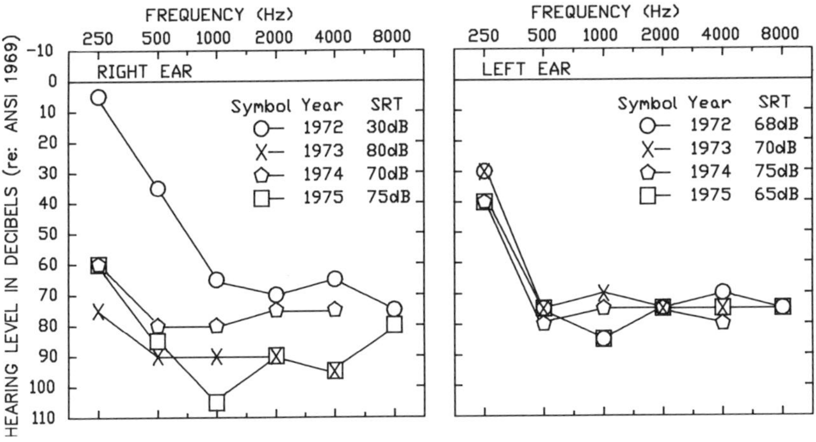

Figure 2. Changes in pure-tone and speech thresholds over a three-year period (October 1972–November 1975) for a boy, aged ten years in 1972, with a bilateral sensorineural hearing loss. During this period, his right ear received amplification at school from a powerful (SSPL = 132 dB) auditory training system. He wore three different personal hearing aids when not in school, which were alternated annually between ears beginning in 1972 with the right ear. (From Bess, F. H. (ed.). 1977. *Childhood Deafness: Assessment and Management*. New York: Grune & Stratton. Used with permission.)

marked deterioration in the six-month period between October 1972 and March 1973, with further reduction in threshold sensitivity during the next two and one-half years. During this three-year period, his SRT also showed marked deterioration from 30 dB to 75 dB.

Figure 3 presents a similar case of a boy aged eight in 1972, who also used the auditory training aid in his right ear for most of the four-year period from September 1971 to November 1975. Note the continued marked right ear threshold deterioration during this four-year period, including a 40 dB loss in his SRT. His left ear, however, demonstrated a 10 to 15 dB improvement in threshold sensitivity from October 1971 to October 1972 and then remained unchanged for the next three years. During this four-year period, his own body-type hearing aid (gain = 64 dB; SSPL = 125 dB) was worn on the left ear from 1971 to 1973 and then switched to his right ear for the next two years. Note that the improvement observed on the left ear occurred while he was using his own body aid in that ear. A possible explanation might be that his own hearing aid was not functioning properly and may not have been worn for several months at a time. This condition was common among the children who wore the auditory training aids at school and did not want to wear their own aids outside the classroom. Nevertheless, his right ear, which received amplification from the auditory training system, exhibited marked deterioration, while his left ear showed improvement.

Personal Hearing Aids and the FM Auditory Training System The children supposedly wore their own hearing aids whenever they were outside the classroom in which the auditory training system was employed. Based on measure-

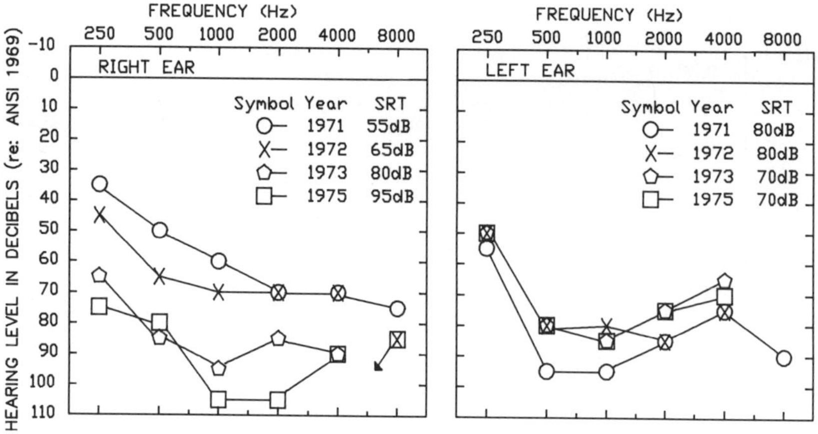

Figure 3. Changes in pure-tone and speech thresholds over a four-year period (October 1971–November 1975) for a boy, aged eight years in 1972, with a bilateral sensorineural hearing loss. During this period, his right ear received amplification at school from a powerful (SSPL = 132 dB) auditory training system. His own body-type hearing aid (SSPL = 125 dB) was worn, when not in school, on the left ear from 1971 to 1973 and then switched to the right ear for the next two years. (From Bess, F. H. (ed.). 1977. *Childhood Deafness: Assessment and Management*. New York: Grune & Stratton. Used with permission.)

ments made in our laboratory, the hearing aids used by the 13 children had an average gain of 61.7 dB with a range from 40 to 79 dB. The average SSPL, or MPO, was 127.7 dB with a range from 118 to 133 dB SPL. These measurements were typical of the gain and saturation output of the instruments worn by these 13 children during the course of this clinical investigation.

Measurements were made of electroacoustic performance of the two auditory training systems, both in our laboratory and in the two classrooms under normal use conditions on three separate occasions. Measurements made at the output of the individual training aids of amplified ambient noise from the boom microphone varied within a range of 71–120 dB SPL, depending upon the volume control setting each child used on his training aid. The average amplified ambient noise was 92.6 dB. The amplified speech also varied considerably from child to child within a range of 94–127 dB SPL and with an average of 111.3 dB. These findings were reasonably consistent on each of the three occasions when measurements were obtained in the classrooms under typical use conditions.

Hence, among the 13 children who received approximately six hours daily of amplified speech and noise in the classroom setting for hearing-impaired children, some were exposed to very high levels of acoustic energy, while others received considerably lower exposure levels. Based on the findings of previous investigations coupled with currently advocated DRC, it is strongly recommended that children who receive such intense acoustic stimulation be frequently monitored audiometrically.

SUMMARY, CONCLUSIONS, AND RECOMMENDATIONS

A review of the literature reveals that, beginning in 1955 with the report of Harford and Markle (1955), several isolated cases have been discovered where hearing-aid use resulted in marked threshold shifts on the child's aided ear with little or no change on the unaided ear (Jerger and Lewis 1975; Sataloff 1961; Ross and Truex 1965; Kasten and Braunlin 1970; Roberts 1970; Heffernan and Simons 1979; Hawkins 1982). Switching the aid to the opposite ear often showed an increased loss in the newly aided ear, with partial or complete threshold recovery in the previously aided ear. Thus, threshold shifts resulting from hearing aid use were sometimes of a temporary nature. In other cases, removal of the hearing aid did not result in threshold improvement, thereby suggesting permanent damage from high-powered amplification.

The findings of investigations involving relatively large samples of hearing-aid users are somewhat contradictory. Although some studies have born out the results obtained in individual case reports, others have not. A number of studies (Naunton 1957; Barr and Wedenberg 1965; Bellefleur and Van Dyke 1968; Madell and Asp 1970; Darbyshire 1976; Markides 1976; Titché et al. 1977; Markides and Aryee 1978; and Kittal and Axmann 1981) reported no evidence to support the hypothesis that amplification from powerful hearing aids produces further deterioration in hearing sensitivity. Investigations conducted by Kinney (1961), Macrae and Farrant (1965), Ross and Lerman (1967), and Macrae (1968a), however, seem to demonstrate that the residual hearing of hearing-impaired children may suffer further damage as a consequence of using high-powered hearing aids. Further, these latter studies suggest that certain factors have an important influence on increasing the risk of further deterioration in hearing resulting from hearing aid use. The amount of hearing loss seems to be a critical variable. Children with moderate to severe hearing losses present a greater risk to increased threshold shifts than do children with profound losses.

A second and probably equally important factor is the maximum power output or SSPL of the hearing aid. The higher the acoustic output, the greater the potential hazard to hearing. Unfortunately, sufficient definitive evidence is lacking to suggest a specific output ceiling for hearing aids. Some experts have recommended limiting the acoustic output of hearing aids to approximately 130 dB SPL. According to the findings of Macrae (1968a), however, children with moderate sensorineural hearing losses may suffer further damage to their aided ears when the saturation output of hearing aids is above 120 dB SPL. On the other hand, some evidence suggests (Bellefleur and Van Dyke, 1968) that children with profound hearing impairments may be able to tolerate high levels of acoustic output without incurring further threshold shifts. Also, some studies suggest that the amount of hearing aid gain may influence threshold deterioration but probably to a less significant extent than saturation output (Ross and Lerman 1967; Macrae 1968a).

Investigators (e.g., Barr and Wedenberg 1965) have attempted to sort out the spontaneous deterioration in hearing due to the progressive nature of the hearing impairment itself from the risk of further auditory damage resulting from hearing-aid overamplification. Most early efforts have produced inconclusive results. Some researchers (e.g., Macrae and Farrant 1965) have found no evidence that endogenous types of hearing impairments are either more or less susceptible to damage from amplification than exogenous hearing losses. More recently, Reilly et al. (1981) concluded that hearing-aid use was not implicated for the majority of children with progressive hearing loss; but for some (ranging from about 10–30 percent), hearing-aid use probably did contribute to progressive threshold deterioration.

The contradictory, and hence inconclusive, findings of the large-scale group studies probably can be attributed to the fact that several of the investigations were poorly controlled retrospective studies. Some studies, however, reported well-controlled longitudinal data (e.g., Markides 1976; Markides and Aryee 1978). Nevertheless, a serious limitation of group studies is that threshold deterioration of individual cases tends to become "lost" when thresholds for large numbers of subjects are averaged.

Although there is a dearth of literature on TTS resulting from hearing-aid use, three pilot studies were reviewed that demonstrated that TTS may occur after as little as one hour of hearing-aid use (Konkle and Rintelmann 1976). Further, after about three and one-half hours of wearing a hearing aid in a classroom setting, all four children in Macrae's pilot study (1968b; 1968c) exhibited threshold shifts that exceeded the allowable risk level of the CHABA TTS DRC. In addition, high positive correlations were found between mean threshold shifts at 1000 and 2000 Hz, average hearing-aid gain, and mean SSPL in the study by Konkle and Rintelmann. A new approach, advocated by Humes and Bess (1981), takes into account the whole pattern of TTS growth and recovery. This measurement procedure, termed integrated temporary threshold shift (ITTS) holds promise for being a better method than the traditional approach of measuring TTS_2 for predicting noise-induced permanent threshold shift. According to Humes and Bess (1981) the use of ITTS studies appears promising for evaluating the potential hazardous effects of high level amplification.

Classroom amplification systems have potential deleterious effects. Although personal hearing aids continue to be the type of amplification used most often in classrooms (34%), the employment of FM-wireless systems (26%) or FM-wireless combined with personal aids (31%) is becoming increasingly popular (Sinclair and Freeman 1981; Bess and Sinclair 1985). Unfortunately, there is limited information available on the selection and evaluation of these types of amplification devices. No satisfactory standard exists for measuring in a practical way the electroacoustic characteristics or the behavioral performance of FM systems (Bess and Logan 1984). Hence, it is not unusual for a group-type hearing aid to be recommended for a child without knowledge of the system's performance characteristics. Such casual practice could result in overamplification of the auditory system. Electroacoustic investigations on FM-wireless devices have reported high levels of output and significant differences in performance between the FM and environmental microphone modes of operations (Freeman, Sinclair and Riggs 1980), marked response differences between the neck-loop FM and environmental microphone of the personal hearing aid (Hawkins and VanTasell 1982), high internal noise levels for teleloop and direct input systems (Hawkins and VanTasell 1982), and inflexible and somewhat unpredictable compression circuitry characteristics (Resnick and Schwartz 1981). Such findings highlight the importance of increasing the research activity associated with educational amplification. This research should include investigation of potential overamplification effects from various types of group systems.

The issue of limiting hearing-aid output is complicated further for young children because the SSPL90 values used for most hearing aid fittings are based on $2cm^3$ coupler measurements. The findings of Jirsa and Norris (1978) and Bratt (1980) support the conclusion that, because sound pressure increases as volume size decreases, the sound pressure output of a hearing aid fitted to a young child's ear may be greater than the output measures in a $2cm^3$ coupler. In other words, because young children have small ear-canal volumes (approximately 0.31–1.36cc), $2cm^3$ coupler measurements typically will underestimate the actual sound pressure delivered by the hearing aid to a young child's ear. This problem recently has been recognized by several writers (Bess and McConnell 1981; Matkin 1986; Mueller and Grimes 1987). As a solution, the latter authors recommended making *in situ* measurements with the presently available probe-tube microphone systems (Harford 1980, 1981).

A final controversial issue is whether a child's loudness discomfort level (LDL) tends to protect his hearing from further damage resulting from overamplification. Some writers (e.g., Markides 1980) argue that hearing-aid users, including young children, will not tolerate " . . . for long periods of time, amplification well above their comfortable listening level which in the great majority of cases will be less than 120 dB SPL" (p. 350). Others, however, including the present authors, do not believe that a person's LDL will necessarily act as a "safety mechanism." In the well-documented case report presented by Hawkins (1982) he stated " . . . damage occurred when output of the hearing aid was limited to levels below the LDL's" (p. 384). He aptly concluded : "Obviously, the variable of importance in setting the SSPL90 in regard to overamplification concerns is the sound pressure level reaching the cochlea, not the LDL's" (p. 384).

In recognition of the seriousness of exposing hearing-aid users to high levels of amplification, the U.S. Food and Drug Administration's document (1977) concerning the sale of hearing aids states that special care should be taken with instruments with SSPLs exceeding 132 dB SPL. Also, in an effort to restrict the maximum output of hearing aids, the American National Standards Institute's (ANSI) document (1982) concerning the electroacoustic performance characteristics of hearing aids states that tolerance for HFA SSPL90 should be within

±4 dB. Such a tolerance restriction can serve at least to keep hearing aids close to their rated saturation output levels.

Based on existing evidence, a reasonable approach to satisfying the amplification needs of hearing-impaired children should include, in our opinion, the following recommendations:

1. Hearing-aid or auditory training unit saturation output should be carefully limited according to the degree (amount) of hearing loss. Wearable amplification for children with mild (25–40 dB) to moderate (40–65 dB) sensorineural hearing losses should probably not exceed an SSPL of 120 dB. Obviously, children with mild losses need less saturation output than youngsters with moderate losses. Children with severe (65–95 dB) or profound (95 dB or more) sensorineural hearing losses can probably safely tolerate SSPLs above 120 dB, but saturation outputs approaching 130 dB SPL should be recommended with extreme caution. Children with conductive or "mixed" losses should be less susceptible to the dangerous consequences of high-level amplification due to the attenuating effect of the conductive pathology. Nevertheless, reasonable caution should also be taken with amplification for these children.
2. Gain should be selected according to the amplification needs of the child, provided that the appropriate SSPL has been chosen.
3. Amplification should be periodically alternated between ears when feasible (for example, if the audiometric configuration is bilaterally symmetrical and speech discrimination is essentially equal in both ears).
4. In the case of young children, a recommendation of binaural amplification should be made with extreme caution. For those professionals who are strong advocates of early binaural amplification, the need to consider careful control of hearing-aid saturation output cannot be overemphasized, particularly if the child is too young to obtain valid and reliable thresholds. In these cases, hearing aid SSPL should not exceed 120 dB. Whenever possible, continued reappraisal of a recommendation for binaural hearing aids should be made via serial audiometry and/or TTS measurements.
5. Periodic audiometric reevaluations should be conducted to monitor possible deterioration in hearing resulting from amplification. Such follow-up testing should be done at least twice annually. For the very young child, audiological surveillance should be even more intense. Presently, monitoring audiometry is the surest way to determine whether or not a child is being subjected to hazardous levels of amplification.

In conclusion, in spite of the potential hazard to hearing posed by the use of amplification, hearing-impaired children must make maximum use of their residual hearing at the earliest possible age. Otherwise, they will suffer in language and speech development, and their educational potential will not be attained. While the use of amplification is indispensable in the aural habilitative process, it must be employed in a cautious and controlled manner.

REFERENCES

American National Standards Institute. 1982. *Specification of hearing aid characteristics* (3.22-1982). New York, NY.

Barr, B., and Wedenberg, E. 1965. Prognosis of perspective hearing loss in children with respect to genesis and use of hearing aid. *Acta Otolaryngologica* 59:462–474.

Bellefleur, P. A., and Van Dyke, R. C. 1968. The effects of high gain amplification on children in a residential school for the deaf. *Journal of Speech and Hearing Research* 11:343–347.

Bess, F. H., and Logan, S. 1984. Amplification in the educational setting. *In* Jerger, J. (ed.). *Pediatric Audiology.* San Diego: College Hill Press.

Bess, F. H., and McConnell, F. E. 1981. *Audiology, Education and the Hearing Impaired Child.* St. Louis: C. V. Mosby Company.

Bess, F. H., and Sinclair, J. S. 1985. Amplification systems used in education. *In* Katz, J. (ed.). *Handbook of Clinical Audiology.* Baltimore: Williams & Wilkins.

Bess, F. H., Sinclair, J. S., and Riggs, D. E. 1985. Group amplification in schools for the hearing-impaired. *Ear and Hearing* 5:138–144.

Bratt, G. 1980. *Hearing aid receiver output in occluded ear canals in children.* Unpublished doctoral dissertation, Vanderbilt University, School of Medicine, Nashville.

Burns, W. 1973. *Noise and Man* (2nd ed.). Philadelphia: Lippincott.

Cohen, A., Anticaglia, J., and Jones, H. H. 1970. "Sociocusis"-hearing loss from non-occupational noise exposure. *Sound and Vibration* 12–20.

Darbyshire, J. O. 1976. A study of the use of high-power hearing aids by children with marked degrees of deafness and the possibility of deteriorations in auditory activity. *British Journal of Audiology* 10:74–82.

Environmental Protection Agency. 1974. *Proposed OSHA occupational noise exposure regulation* (Request for review and report). Washington, D. C.: Federal Register 39:no. 244.

Food and Drug Administration. 1977. *Hearing aid devices* (Professional and patient labeling and conditions for sale). Washington, D. C., Federal Register 42:9286–9296.

Freeman, B. A., Sinclair, J. S., and Riggs, D. 1980. Electroacoustic performance characteristics of FM auditory trainers. *Journal of Speech and Hearing Disorders* 45:16–26.

Harford, E. 1980. The use of a miniature microphone in the ear canal for the verification of hearing aid performance. *Ear and Hearing* 1:329–337.

Harford, E. 1981. A new clinical technique for verification of hearing aid response. *Archives of Otolaryngology* 107:461–468.

Harford, E. R., and Markle, D. M. 1955. The atypical effect of a hearing aid on one patient with congenital deafness. *Laryngoscope* 65:970–972.

Harris, J. D. 1965. Hearing loss trend curves and the damage risk criterion in diesel engine room personnel. *Journal of the Acoustical Society of America* 37:444–452.

Hawkins, D. B. 1982. Overamplification: A well-documented case report. *Journal of Speech and Hearing Disorders* 47:382–384.

Hawkins, D. B., and VanTasell, D. J. 1982. Electroacoustic characteristics of personal FM systems. *Journal of Speech and Hearing Disorders* 47:355–362.

Heffernan, H. P., and Simons, M. R. 1979. Temporary increase in sensorineural hearing loss with hearing aid use. *Annals of Otology, Rhinology and Laryngology* 88:86–91.

Humes, L. E. 1978. Temporary threshold shift resulting from hearing aid usage. *Journal of the Acoustical Society of America* 63:565.

Humes, L. E., and Bess, F. H. 1981. On the potential deterioration in hearing due to hearing aid usage. *Journal of Speech and Hearing Research* 24:3–15.

Jerger, J. F., and Lewis, N. 1975. Binaural hearing aids: Are they dangerous for children? *Archives of Otolaryngology* 101:480–483.

Jirsa, R. E., and Norris, T. W. 1978. Relationship of acoustic gain to aided threshold improvement. *Journal of Speech and Hearing Disorders* 43:348–352.

Kasten, R. N., and Braunlin, R. J. 1970. *Traumatic hearing aid usage: A case study.* Paper presented at the meeting of the American Speech and Hearing Association, New York, NY.

Kinney, C. E. 1953. Hearing impairments in children. *Laryngoscope* 63:220–226.

Kinney, C. E. 1961. The further destruction of partially deafened children's hearing by the use of powerful hearing aids. *Annals of Otology, Rhinology, and Laryngology* 70:828–835.

Kittel, G., and Axmann, D. 1981. Deterioration in hearing caused by hearing aids in children? *Advances in Otorhinolaryngology* 27:130–137.

Konkle, D. F., and Rintelmann, W. F. 1976. *Temporary threshold shift in children after hearing aid use,* unpublished study. The University of Pennsylvania, School of Medicine, Philadelphia.

Konkle, D. F. 1976. *Intelligibility of time-altered CNC monosyllables as a function of contralateral masking.* Unpublished doctoral dissertation. Michigan State, East Lansing.

Kryter, K. D. 1970. *The Effects of Noise on Man.* New York: Academic Press.

Kryter, K. D., Ward, W. D., Miller, J. D., and Eldredge, D. H. 1966. Hazardous exposure to intermittent and steady-state noise. *Journal of the Acoustical Society of America* 39:944–954.

Macrae, J. H. 1968a. Deterioration of the residual hearing of children with sensorineural deafness. *Acta Otolaryngologica* 66:33–39.

Macrae, J. H. 1968b. TTS and recovery from TTS after use of powerful hearing aids. *Journal of the Acoustical Society of America* 43:1445–1446.

Macrae, J. H. 1968c. Recovery from TTS in children with sensorineural deafness. *Journal of the Acoustical Society of America* 44:1451.

Macrae, J. H., and Farrant, F. H. 1965. The effect of hearing aid use on the residual hearing of children with sensorineural deafness. *Annals of Otology, Rhinology, and Laryngology* 74:409–419.

Madell, J. R. and Asp, C. W. 1970. *The effects of hearing aid amplification on pure tone thresholds of preschool deaf children.* Paper presented at the meeting of the American Speech and Hearing Association Convention, New York, NY

Markides, A. 1976. The effect of hearing aid use on the user's residual hearing. *Scandinavian Audiology* 5:205–210.

Markides, A. 1980. The effect of hearing aid amplification on the user's residual hearing. *In* E. R. Libby, (ed.). *Binaural Hearing and Amplification: Vol. 2.* Chicago, IL: Zenetron.

Markides, A and Aryee, D. T.-K. 1978. The effect of hearing aid use on the user's residual hearing: A follow-up study. *Scandinavian Audiology* 7:19–23.

Matkin, N. 1986. Hearing aids for children. *In* W. Hodgson, (ed.). *Hearing Aid Assessment and Use in Audiologic Habilitation.* 3rd ed. Baltimore: Williams and Wilkins.

Miller, J. D. 1974. Effects of the noise on people. *Journal of the Acoustical Society of America* 56:729–764.

Mills, J. H. 1975. Noise and children: A review of literature. *Journal of the Acoustical Society of America* 58:767–779.

Mueller, H. G., and Grimes, A. 1987. Amplification systems for the hearing impaired. *In* J. G. Alpiner and P. A. McCarthy (eds.). *Rehabilitative Audiology: Children and Adults.* Baltimore, MD: Williams & Wilkins.

Naunton, R. F. 1957. The effect of hearing aid use upon the user's residual hearing. *Laryngoscope* 67:569–576.

Reilly, K., Owens, E., Uken, D., McClathchie, A. C., and Clarke, R. 1981. Progressive hearing loss in children: Hearing aids and other factors. *Journal of Speech and Hearing Disorders* 47:328–334.

Resnick, S., and Schwartz, D. M. 1981. Selective amplification: Electroacoustic and clinical considerations. *In* F. H. Bess, B. A. Freeman, and J. A. Sinclair (eds.). *Amplification in Education.* Washington, DC: Alexander Graham Bell Association for the Deaf.

Rintelmann, W. F. 1975. *The potential hazard to hearing from radio frequency auditory training units.* Unpublished study, Michigan State University, East Lansing.

Rintelmann, W. F., and Bess, F. H. 1977. High-level amplification and potential hearing loss in children. *In* F. H. Bess (ed.). *Childhood Deafness: Assessment and Management.* New York, NY: Grune & Stratton.

Roberts, C. 1970. Can hearing aids damage hearing? *Acta Otolaryngologica* 69:123–125.

Ross, M., and Truex, E. H., Jr. 1965. Protecting residual hearing in hearing aid user. *Archives of Otolaryngology* 82:615–617.

Ross, M., and Lerman, J. 1967. Hearing aid usage and its effect upon residual hearing. *Archives of Otolaryngology* 86:639–644.

Sataloff, J. 1961. Pitfalls in routine hearing testing. *Archives of Otolaryngology* 73:717–726.

Sataloff, J., Vasalo, L., and Menduke, H. 1965. Temporary and permanent hearing losses—A ten year follow-up. *Archives of Environmental Health* 10:67–70.

Sinclair, J. S., and Freeman, B. A. 1981. The status of classroom amplification in American education. *In* F. H. Bess, B. A. Freeman, and J. S. Sinclair (eds.). *Amplification in Education.* Washington, DC: Alexander Graham Bell Association for the Deaf.

Titche, L. L., Windrem, E. O., and Starmer, W. T. 1977. Hearing aids & hearing deterioration. *Annals of Otolaryngology* 86:357–361.

United States Department of Labor, Occupational Safety and Health Administration. 1983. *Occupational noise exposure: Hearing conservation amendment; final rule*. Washington, D. C.: Federal Register, *48*, no. 46.

Ward, W. D., and Fricke, J. E. 1969. *Noise as a public health hazard* (Report No. 4). Washington, D. C.: American Speech and Hearing Association.

Chapter 19

Tactual Artificial Hearing for the Deaf

D. Kimbrough Oller and *Rebecca E. Eilers*

Background on Artificial Hearing Through the Skin

Research on tactually based artificial hearing can be traced as far back as Gault (1926), who presented sound as a single channel of vibratory stimulation to the skin. Research with single channel systems indicated that important sound information could be transmitted, but certain limitations of the approach were found to be critical. In particular, the skin is a limited discriminator of frequencies above a few hundred Hz (cf. Békésy 1957), and consequently cannot track much of the key information in the speech code, which heavily utilizes the frequency range from 500 to 3000 Hz. Investigators soon settled on the idea that speech perception through the skin could not be accomplished effectively with a single channel of information but should be modeled after the cochlear frequency-to-locus transform, by which different acoustic frequencies correspond to different locations on the basilar membrane. The devices that accomplish the transform are called "tactual (or tactile) vocoders." They take sound from a microphone, band-pass filter it into channels, and use each channel to drive a stimulator worn on the skin. The stimulators are usually worn in a linear array, presenting a real-time spectral display to the skin.

Wearers of tactual vocoders feel the sounds of speech (and any other sounds that are transmitted through the microphone) as patterns of stimulation on the skin. Different sounds, of course, yield consistently different patterns. A high frequency sound such as /s/, for example, would produce stimulation on one side of the array, while a sound with more low frequency information such as /u/ would produce stimulation on the other side of the array. Dynamic patterns are produced by syllables. The word "sue" (/su/), for example, would produce a pattern moving from the high to the low frequency side of the array. The syl-

The present work has been supported by Rita and Jerome Cohen, Austin and Marta Weeks, Renata Mahan, and by the Mailman Foundation. The authors wish to thank Frank Saunders (Tacticon Corp.), Bill Gavin (Institute of Logopedics), and Ronald Harkness (San Juan Unified School District, Ca.) and the Dade County Public Schools for assistance in the work represented here.

lable /us/ would, in contrast, produce a pattern moving the opposite direction, a highly discriminable event (cf. Gavin 1979). Different durations are often distinguishable. So, for example, the word "to" (/tu/) would produce a pattern moving in the same direction as "sue," but would differ in that stimulation on the high frequency side (resulting from the "t" burst) would be short compared to the fricative "s". Different amplitudes of sounds are also transmitted as different amplitudes of stimulation at the appropriate stimulators. The words "sue" (/su/) and "zoo" (/zu/) differ in amplitude of the high frequency information (in addition to differing in low frequency voicing information), and can be differentiated tactually, based upon the amplitude of the stimulation on the high frequency side of the array.

ROBUSTNESS OF TACTUAL VOCODER FUNCTION

A number of tactual vocoders have been tested for transmission of speech sound contrasts (see reviews in Kirman 1973; Richardson and Frost 1977; Reed, Durlach, and Braida 1982; and Sherrick 1984). The instruments have varied in number of channels (from 8 to 36), in form of stimulation (various vibrotactile or electrocutaneous stimulators have been used), in body locus of the display (fingers, arms, legs, or abdomen), and in various coding parameters. In spite of the considerable differences in hardware, testing results have had much in common. One consistent outcome has been that certain segmental speech sound contrasts are well-transmitted. Tactual vocoders do well on the invisible contrasts of stops vs. homorganic fricatives and affricates, nasals vs. stops, fricatives vs. affricates, voiced vs. voiceless consonants, singleton vs. clustered consonants, etc. (see Pickett and Pickett 1963; Sparks et al. 1978; Oller, Payne, and Gavin 1980; Ozdamar et al. 1985). In general, the contrasts that are especially well-transmitted through tactual vocoders are hard-to-lip-read ones. Consequently, the devices appear to have the potential for filling an important gap in speech reception for the deaf.

The robustness of the tactual vocoder approach is supported by relatively similar speech-transmission performance of two devices that have been tested in our laboratories. In the study in question, the 24-channel Oregon tactual vocoder designed by Rosov (Engelmann and Rosov 1975) was worn by an adult subject on the arm. The 24 solenoid vibrators, housed in four cartridges (each about 3 inches by 1½ inches by 1 inch) with six vibrators each, were linearly arranged on the volar side of the left arm, with the high frequency channels near the wrist and the low frequency channels at the biceps. The stimulators vibrated at 60 Hz with force proportional to the instantaneous channel energy. The vocoder channels were logarithmically spaced across the frequency range from 85 to 9400 Hz. The 32-channel electrocutaneous Telectactor of Saunders (1973), provided electrical stimulation through a belt (about 1½ inches wide) worn about the abdomen. The 32 concentric electrodes (spaced at approximately 1/2 inch intervals) delivered comfortable electrical pulses in bursts, with the number of pulses in each burst proportional to the instantaneous channel amplitude. As with the Oregon device, the channels were logarithmically spaced and the frequency range covered was similar (60–8000 Hz).

The adult hearing subject in the study comparing the two devices had experienced 30 to 40 hours of training with the Oregon vocoder in a vocabulary acquisition study to be described in a later section. In addition, he had trained in speech perception exercises for 10 to 15 hours with the Teletactor. After the training on both devices, the subject opined that the two devices were substantially similar in that both delivered a linear pattern of stimulation, and that different phonetic elements were displayed in similar relative locations, even though different body sites were used. Differences in the type of stimulation were noticed but seemed to the subject to have little effect on the delivery of speech information. Knowledge of transmission on one device appeared to generalize quickly to the other.

To examine the relative performance more systematically, the subject was seated in a sound-proof chamber, wearing one of the two devices, and a speaker was seated outside with a microphone connected to the subject's vocoder. The speaker presented two-choice identification trials for a variety of speech sound contrasts: a fricative-stop pair ([sa]/[ta]), a sibilant pair ([sa]/[ʃa]), a glide-stop contrast ([wa]/[ba], a nasal-oral distinction ([na]/[da]), a fricative-affricate pair ([tʃa]/[ʃa]), a high vowel contrast ([us]/[is]), and three contrasts using real words where the two members of each pair represented opposite orders of the same phonetic elements, "soon"/"noose" ([sun]/[nus]), "sought"/ "toss" ([sɔt]/[tɔs]), and "bomb"/"mob" ([bɔm]/mɔb]). The pairs were presented in the same order for both types of devices. Twenty randomly determined trials were presented with correction for each pair (i.e., subjects were informed of errors), first in a training session, and then in a testing session.

The results of the tests are indicated in figure 1. Tests of both devices produced at least 80% correct performance by the subjects on all the contrasts. Some contrasts resulted in perfect performance on both devices. The vibrotactile device was superior on three contrasts, the electrocutaneous device on two. These results represented the optimal performance with both devices in the experiment. Performance was deleteriously affected by deviations from the stimulation amplitude that was chosen. For example, the overall optimal performance of approximately 90% on the Teletactor was reduced by 10 to 15 percent if amplitude of pulses was increased (pulse width) to a level that the subject judged "strong." "Medium" and "weak" levels produced relatively similar performance. In separate testing not indicated in the figure, both devices failed to transmit (voiced) stop and nasal consonant place of articulation contrasts above a chance level.

The same two devices were also compared for performance with a single subject on recognition of Swedish numbers (Spens 1980). Results also indicated

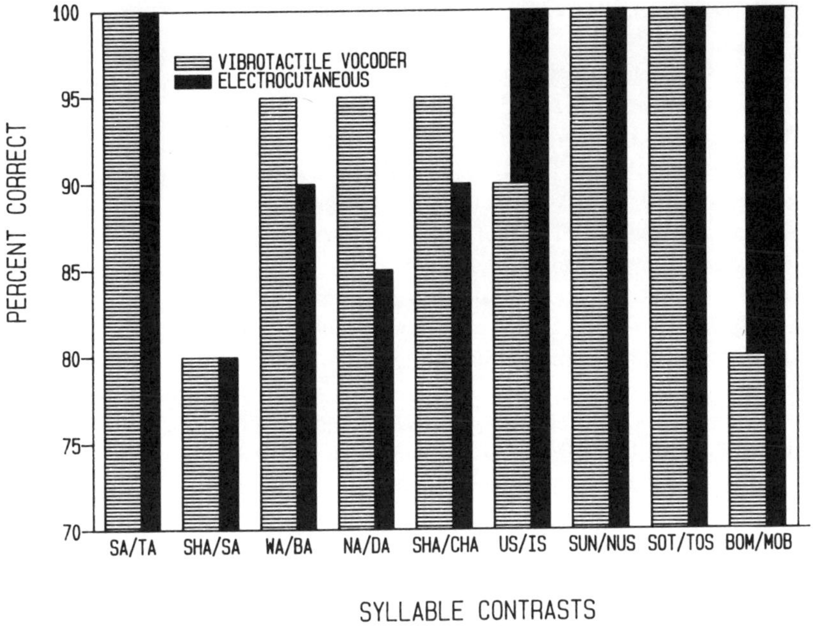

Figure 1. Vibrotactile & electrocutaneous device comparison.

relatively similar performance. Both studies are supportive of the idea that the tactual vocoder approach is relatively robust with regard to transmission of certain speech-sound contrasts to a subject with less than 60 hours experience in tactually presented speech. The general similarity of patterns of speech-sound transmission across such different devices suggests that useful applications of such tactual vocoders will not depend on delicate fine tuning of systems. Yet while the studies support the notion that the vocoder approach is robust, they do *not* address the question of whether or not different tactual vocoders may differ in ultimate performance. First of all, only a few contrasts were tested, and running speech reception was not compared. Further, the subject involved in the reported study had experienced speech tactually for an amount of time that might be thought of as trivially short when compared with the thousands of hours of auditory experience a human infant has before general speech reception is possible. While the results for the two devices were rather similar, performance with the vibrotactile device seemed somewhat less sensitive to slight changes in the stimulation level—perhaps an indication of superior dynamic range of the vibrotactile method. It is uncertain at present how much difference it will make for long-term subjects if they use an electrocutaneous or vibrotactile method. A variety of additional questions regarding optimal processing strategies and body locations remain unresolved.

Similarities in Tactual and Auditory Processing of Speech

A key issue in the processing of speech sounds through the skin is whether or not the pattern and style of perception can be similar to that of the auditory system. Certain speech perception theorists (e.g., Liberman et al. 1968) have suggested that effective speech perception is necessarily linked to the human auditory system. The view of such theorists depends in part on the well-established finding that identification and discrimination of a variety of consonant contrasts are "categorical" (Liberman et al. 1967). For example, identification and discrimination of a continuum of synthesized speech-like syllables ranging from /sta/ to /sa/ (depending on the duration of the silence duration between /s/ and /a/) shows that maximum discriminability is near the boundary of identification. Within-category discrimination is relatively poor and near chance if the duration differences are small (Bastian, Eimas, and Liberman 1961). On the other hand, vowel discrimination has been shown to be relatively good even for within-category synthesized pairs (Pisoni 1971).

The categorical pattern of consonant perception paired with the less-categorical pattern of vowel perception has been taken to be a uniquely human auditory response to speech stimuli in spite of counterevidence based on work with nonhumans (e.g., Kuhl and Miller 1975). Similar reasoning about the uniqueness of audition leads to the expectation that tactual perception would not mimic the auditory pattern.

In fact, recent work by Eilers, Ozdamar, Oller, Miskiel, and Moroff (1986) indicates that a synthetic consonant (/sta/-/sa/) and vowel contrast (/a/-/ ə /) show a tactual perception pattern that distinctly resembles the auditory one. Adult hearing subjects were presented with both an identification and a discrimination task; they showed a categorical pattern both auditorily and tactually (through a 32-channel electrocutaneous vocoder) on the consonant contrast, while showing a "non-categorical" pattern on the vowel contrast for both sensory modalities. The results of this work represent the first attempted comparison of categoricalness of speech perception in audition and taction. Other results (Ozdamar et al. 1985) indicate that for several additional contrasts, the patterns of identification in auditory and tactual modalities are notably similar. The results of these studies contradict the assumption that categorical perception is unique to the auditory modality and further suggest that, at least for some contrasts, it may be unnecessary for subjects to have long-term experience in the tactual modality in order to show a pattern of perception that may be necessary for optimal speech perception performance.

Limitations of Current Tactual Vocoders in Transmitting Speech Sound Contrasts

In spite of excellent results on certain speech-sound contrasts, the tactual vocoders currently available have important apparent limitations, some of which may be due to inherent limitations of the skin as a reception system (see Kirman 1973). In other realms the devices manifest limitations that may be remediable. An area of potential improvement concerns restricted dynamic range of amplitudes when compared with audition (cf. Sachs, Miller, and Grant 1980; Bull et al. 1985). Consequently, the devices are quite sensitive to noise and even in conditions of low noise, speech contrasts that depend upon subtle amplitude discriminations or the tracking of rapid low amplitude events may not be possible. Another problem is that the stimulus delivery rate (often 60 Hz or lower) of tactual vocoder stimulators imposes restrictions on the rate of information reception.

Consequently, rapid acoustic events such as those represented by format transitions in rapid speech, may be difficult to track through tactual vocoders due to insufficient stimulation (numbers of electrocutaneous pulses or cycles of mechanical vibration) presented during the brief acoustic events (cf. Eilers, Bull, and Oller 1984).

Another important problem in development of tactual devices is that there is insufficient empirical information upon which to optimize vocoder configuration designs. Most tactual vocoder scientists have used logarithmic channel spacings, or near-log spacings based on critical bands data, but extensive tests of the assumptions underlying these designs are lacking, and many additional signal processing questions related to vocoder design have never been addressed experimentally (Ozdamar et al. 1985).

One empirical indication of limitations is that available tactual devices have thus far been relatively unsuccessful in transmitting effectively the common place of articulation contrasts for voiced stops and nasals (cf. Sparks et al. 1978). Considerable effort has been directed to determining the reasons for the difficulty of place of articulation reception. Research in our own laboratories shows that synthetic place contrasts are not discriminable if the formant transitions are fast, as in rapid speech, but become discriminable when slowed down by a factor of two. These and other results have inspired interest in improving dynamic range and increasing effective rate of information delivery to the skin. Our laboratory research continues in the attempt to improve transmission capabilities (cf. Mandalia et al. 1983; Eilers et al. 1984). Fortunately, place of articulation contrasts are often visible on the lips, a fact that reduces the practical urgency of improving tactual vocoders' transmission of the place feature.

Other tactual vocoder problems have been seen in the transmission of suprasegmentals. Ozdamar et al. (1985) found that fundamental frequency was transmitted relatively poorly through a 32-channel electrocutaneous system, and Carney and Beachler (1986) found that suprasegmental features were not well-transmitted by the Oregon vibrotactile machine. Improvements in transmission of suprasegmentals may require improvements in rate of stimulation, dynamic range, and vocoder configuration designs. One attempt to deal with the problem of fundamental frequency tracking has resulted in development of a multichannel tactual device that transmits fundamental frequency only (Boothroyd 1985).

Prior to the 1970s, researchers generally expressed disappointment at the failure of tactual vocoders to provide information that could immediately be used to interpret real speech (see e.g., Kringelbotn 1968). One approach to study of word and sentence reception had been to give subjects a few hours of training with tactually presented speech and then present them with a speech tracking task in two conditions—lip reading alone and lip reading plus vocoder. A failure to improve the tracking rate substantially in the lip reading plus vocoder condition was taken to mean that tactual vocoders were not effective speech transmission aids (cf. Sparks et al. 1979). In general, studies that have tested real speech recognition after short-term training have not produced impressive performance (Yeni-Komshian and Goldstein 1977).

THE NECESSITY OF LONG-TERM, INTENSIVE TRAINING WITH ARTIFICIAL HEARING

The fallacy of the reasoning that concluded tactual vocoders could not be effective in running-speech transmission lies in the assumption that minimal training is sufficient to realize the potential of perceivers to use the tactual signal. Normal-hearing babies do not even begin to speak meaningfully until they have already had many hundreds, perhaps thousands of hours of experience with auditorily presented speech. Fluent comprehension of meaningful speech develops over years, not hours, of experience. Consequently it seems unreasonable to assume that a tactual vocoder user, who has never previously felt sound as systematic patterns on the skin, could learn to understand running speech through the skin in a few hours. It is worthwhile to consider the analogy of long-term sensory deprivation. Adult victims of congenital cataracts have excellent visual acuity shortly after surgical correction. However, excellent visual acuity is insufficient to produce good visual interpretation of the world. Post-surgical patients show an inability to understand what they see even though they see it clearly. They continue to function as blind and only gradually improve as they experience the visual world over months and years. The need for experience to learn the perception of complex information in a new sensory modality is also seen in data on tactile learning of reading by the blind. It takes hundreds of hours of training and practice for blind people to learn to read effectively using a tactile device (the Optacon) that transmits alphabetical symbols to the fingers (Linvill 1973).

The necessity of long-term experience for tactual reception of speech was recognized by Englemann and Rosov (1975) who developed a systematic vocabulary acquisition task that has produced excellent results in several laboratories. In the Engelmann and Rosov paradigm, subjects, either deaf or hearing, are provided with tactual input only. On each trial the trainer, speaking into a microphone connected to the vocoder, says "ready" followed by a word from the subject's training list. The subject, who cannot hear (due to sound isolation or deafness) or see the speaker, tries to recognize the word based upon the tactual pattern, and responds by pronouncing a word from the list. If it is correct, the trainer says "yes," the subject repeats "yes" and they go on to the next trial. If the guess is incorrect, the trainer says "no, not X," inserting the word the subject mistakenly guessed. The subject repeats "no, not X," the trainer repeats the correct word, and the subject again attempts to recognize it.

In this training paradigm the word list begins small (usually five or six words) and is added to as subjects reach a criterion, commonly near 70% correct identification. Thus, if 70% of the words are identified correctly on the first attempt in a particular session, the criterion is satisfied, and the word list is increased by 1 to 6 additional words for the next session. Sessions are usually from one-half to one hour in duration. Ideally, sessions are at least daily, but in practice the paradigm has been used with more widely-spaced training.

Learning patterns of subjects who have been trained in this paradigm are quite stable across different subjects, laboratories, and device types. Subjects acquire from slightly less than one to more than three words per hour, and more importantly, the learning curves do not level off across time, even up to 80 hours of training. Englemann and Rosov (1975) tested four adult hearing subjects and four deaf children in the paradigm using the 24-channel Oregon vibrotactile vocoder described above. The device was placed on the arms of adults, and on the legs of children (two of the four cartridges of vibrators on each leg). All the subjects made excellent gains, and there was a tendency for learning curves to accelerate across time, especially for subjects trained beyond a 30–40 word initial set. The most trained deaf subject acquired a vocabulary of 150 words (that could be correctly recognized at a 70% level) after 48 sessions of one-hour or less.

Brooks (1982) and Brooks and Frost (1983), using a very similar training approach, showed similar results for two hearing adults and three deaf adolescents using the 16-channel Queen's University vibrotactile vocoder strapped to the arm. The hearing subject who had trained the most (to 80 hours) had acquired a 250 word vocabulary. Again no subjects showed levelling off of learning patterns.

The same paradigm has been applied in our own laboratories in work with the Oregon 24-channel vocoder worn by four adult hearing subjects. Subjects were trained as described above in three to four sessions weekly. Training sessions lasted from one-half to one hour and consisted of two parts—the vocabulary acquisition part as described above, and a sentence recognition task that was administered concurrently with the individual word vocabulary training in each session after the sixth. The same persons who served as subjects were also trainers, with the schedule set up in a rotating fashion, so that each subject was trained roughly equally by three different speakers. As can be seen in figure 2, across 26–33 sessions of training, subjects acquired vocabularies ranging from 25 to 36 words. More recent work by Lynch (1986) with two adult deaf subjects over a 40–50 hour period using a 16-channel miniaturized electrocutaneous vocoder (by Tacticon) worn on the abdomen has also shown consistent, though slower, learning rates.

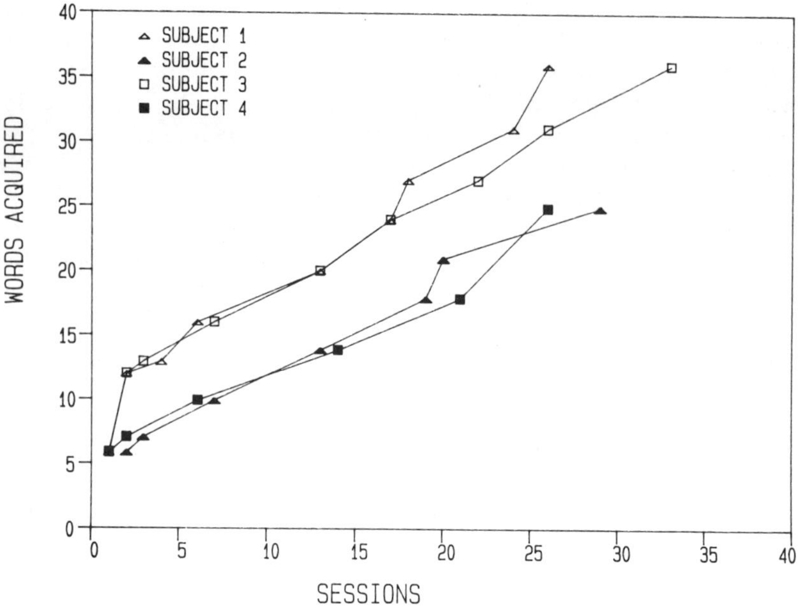

Figure 2. Vocabulary acquisition with a tactual vocoder.

It is important to recognize that vocabulary acquisition that continues with no deceleration in rate suggests a powerful learning strategy, rather than rote learning of a particular pattern for each word. If subjects were learning each word independently by rote, one might expect to see asymptotic learning as subjects reached a maximum number of potentially recognizable individual word patterns. Instead learning curves are stable or accelerating, suggesting that subjects are learning patterns not for words but for phonetic features and segments. Since the number of possible segments and features is relatively small, it is possible to apply the recognition knowledge of the segments and features more and more effectively as time passes. What the subjects appear to be learning is not word patterns per se, but rather generalizable phonetically oriented strategies for recognizing words presented to the skin.

In addition to the stability of learning across long time periods, several other kinds of data support the view that subjects trained in the vocabulary acquisition task learn by developing tactually based phonetic knowledge. One kind of data is introspective. Subjects report that they can recognize fricatives, voicing information, nasality, and different vowel qualities by particular patterns. Empirically, subjects in the vocabulary studies show an excellent capability to recognize certain features (cf. Brooks and Frost 1983); but even more telling are the data on recognition of new words. Engelmann and Rosov (1975) employed a "rhyming" format to present new words. The trainer would say, for example, "rhymes with at" ("at" being on the subject's acquired list), and the subject would repeat "rhymes with at." The trainer would then produce an isolated consonant, for example "mmmmm," and the subject would repeat "mmmmm." Then the trainer would put the "m" and "at" together, saying "mat," and the subject would repeat "mat." This approach worked very well for words that rhyme with other words already in the subjects' vocabularies.

Brooks et al. (1986a) went even further, presenting an open-set word recognition task to the subject who had trained in the vocabulary recognition task to 80 hours. The subject had had over 200 hours of total experience working with the 16-channel vibrotactile vocoder, much of it obtained in tasks conducted during tests of various device modifications. After the 200 hours of total experience, she was able to recognize words from an unfamiliar 3000 word list at a rate of 9% on the first trial with vocoder input alone, a pattern of performance that was stable across numerous trial blocks. Chance performance would have been one correct response in 3000 trials—consequently, the subject performed 270 times better than chance. It is consequently quite certain that she had learned to recognize vocabulary by means of a phonetic strategy that could be applied to recognition of any speech signal presented.

SENTENCE RECOGNITION THROUGH TACTUAL VOCODERS

An important concern about the use of any sensory aid for the deaf is that it must be capable of transmitting full sentences in addition to isolated phonetic elements or words. All the studies referred to in the discussion of vocabulary acquisition included training and test results using sentences composed over the tactual vocabulary known to subjects. In our own laboratories sentence recognition training began in the sixth training session, and occurred thereafter in most sessions for periods ranging from five to twenty minutes. Sentences were composed of from three to five words from the known vocabulary (e.g., "I can see the book." or "Today you can understand.") pronounced slowly at first, but more rapidly as time passed. At the end of twenty-five sessions, subjects had reached a point of responding to sentences pronounced at a normal rate of articulation, with no decrement in recognition performance. Figure 3 indicates that correct identification of words in sentences averaged about 60% with vocoder input alone. This rate represents only a small decrement from the 70% criterion that was used for determining acquisition of words produced in isolation. Subjects with longer training periods continue to show excellent abilities to recognize sentences composed of known vocabularies (see Engelmann and Rosov 1975; Brooks and Frost 1983).

GENERALIZATION AND INTEGRATION OF LEARNING WITH TACTUAL VOCODERS

Another key question about the use of tactual vocoders concerns the potential ability of users to integrate information across the visual and tactual modalities.

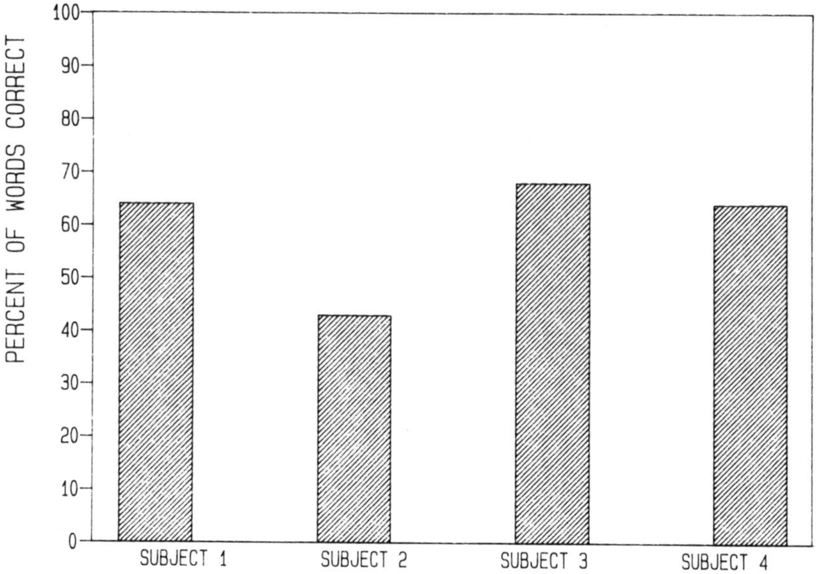

Figure 3. Sentence recognition with a tactual vocoder.

After short-term experience with speech discrimination tasks (but not the vocabulary acquisition paradigm), Sparks et al. (1979) for example, found that speech tracking rates were improved only a small amount with a 36-channel tactual vocoder plus lip reading over lip reading alone. This failure appears, however, to have been due to lack of systematic training in vocabulary and sentence recognition. Brooks et al. (1986a) have shown excellent integration of visual and tactual information by the previously mentioned 200-hour subject. In open-set recognition of words presented randomly from a list of 3000, the subject identified 40% correctly with lip reading alone and 69% correctly with lip reading plus tactual vocoder. The nearly 75% gain in recognition with the vocoder indicates a high level of phonetic integration of visual and tactual information presented simultaneously.

In a separate study Brooks et al. (1986b) presented their most trained subject with open-set sentences from a list of 2000 unfamiliar to the subject. The sentences, averaging 5.9 words in length, were presented in two conditions—lips alone and lips plus vocoder at a normal speaking rate. In the lips alone condition, 58% of the words in the sentences were identified correctly on the first try, while in the lips plus vocoder condition, 80% were correct. Perhaps even more significantly, the tracking rate for sentences presented in the lips plus vocoder condition (49 words per minute) was more than three time faster than in the lips alone condition. Again the results indicated that for a subject with substantial experience in speech recognition through a tactual vocoder, visual and tactual information can be effectively integrated in a real-speech recognition task.

In additional work in our laboratories, Lynch (1986) showed integration across the auditory and tactual modalities by two deaf adults trained in a vocabulary acquisition task for 40–50 hours. The subjects were presented with an inventory of words twice the size of their acquired inventories and were asked to recognize the words in an auditory (hearing aids turned on) condition alone, and in an auditory plus vocoder condition (both hearing aids and vocoder on). Results showed a 25 times better than chance performance for both subjects in the auditory alone condition. Performance in the combined condition was 60% better than that with hearing aids alone.

The Brooks et al. (1986a and 1986b) and Lynch (1986) work indicates that integration of information can occur after intense unisensory training with tactual recognition of speech. Another sort of integration of information appears to occur in learning of speech recognition through simultaneous bisensory training. Such training (with all trials providing input through lip reading and tactual vocoder) was given to a six-year-old profoundly deaf boy in a two-choice speech recognition task in our laboratories. Twenty-two sessions (45 minutes to an hour in length) were scattered over a period of four months. The child was prelingually profoundly deaf, and he made little use of his hearing aids, which in any case were turned off during training and testing.

The stimulus materials consisted of a set of noun pairs and corresponding pictures. The noun pairs were specially chosen to meet the following requirements: group 1 consisted of word-pairs that were expected to be easy to distinguish tactually (gas/can, bell/belt, pan/man, key/knee), group 2, of pairs expected to be easy to lip read (dog/ball, arm/barn, mail/whale, car/fan), and group 3, of pairs expected to be easy both visually and tactually (bus/sun, ship/bed, feet/meat, pail/nail). The words were all familiar to the child (he knew appropriate signs and had basic reading knowledge of the words) although his pronunciations of them were largely unintelligible. The child's visual discrimination of the spoken word-pairs was evaluated in a pretest with lip reading alone, followed in later sessions by training with both modalities of information presented simultaneously, and finally by post-testing with lips alone and vocoder alone. On each trial of all sessions the child was presented with two pictures representing the word-pair to be tested, e.g., dog and ball. The trainer would say, for example, "show me the ball" and the child was expected to respond by pointing to the ball. On each trial, presentation of words and physical location of pictures were randomized. Word-pairs used in each pretesting, training and post-testing session were counterbalanced. During all sessions the subject was rewarded for correct responses with a token that he put in a cup to redeem later for prizes. The subject was very cooperative and eager to learn.

During training, each word pair was tested with a sequence of not less than 8 trials. If the child correctly identified 8 in a row, criterion was reached. If not, additional trials (up to 20) could be given. The goal was for the child to reach an 80% correct criterion. After three consecutive sessions of reaching the criterion on a particular word-pair, post-testing began on that pair. In post-testing, 10 trials were presented in a lips alone condition (vocoder turned off) and ten trials in a vocoder alone condition (vocoder on, face of speaker obscured). The presentation of the two conditions was counterbalanced across word-pairs.

Results of the study are shown in figure 4. The subject showed excellent improvements in performance after training based on comparisons of the pre- and post-test data displayed. Perfect performance was achieved with lip reading in the post-tests on the "easy visual" and "easy both" pairs. At the same time excellent gains were also made on all the types of word-pairs in the tactual condition. Data not displayed in the figure indicate that in the "easy tactual" condition, the average number of sessions to criterion was 8 while for the "easy visual" and "easy both" conditions the average was 5. The data suggest that for these words the subject found learning the relevant lip reading information easier than learning the relevant tactual information, perhaps due to greater familiarity of the visual signal. The surprising indication of the study is that bisensory training seemed to have substantial effect on both lip reading *and* tactual performance. The results suggest that the subject used the tactual information effectively as a supplement to lip reading during training, ultimately enhancing lip reading performance. The subject apparently was integrating information across the two modalities during training.

A Model Program Training Speech and Speech Reception in Deaf Children with Tactual Vocoders

The abilities of various subjects, deaf and hearing, to make excellent gains in speech recognition with systematic training has inspired the development of a regular deaf education approach incorporating tactual vocoders. At the University of Miami's Mailman Center for Child Development a model program has been established in collaboration with the Dade County Public Schools and with support from private donors. The program has been running for over four years, housed at the Mailman Center's Debbie Institute and includes full-time classrooms for elementary school deaf children and preschoolers. Additional work is ongoing with toddlers and infants.

Various devices have been used in the classroom training program. For the first three years the training employed the 24-channel Oregon vocoder (worn on the legs) with most of the children, and the 32-channel electrocutaneous Teletactor for the others. More recently, since the development of the 16-channel miniaturized electrocutaneous system by Tacticon (Saunders 1985), the program has moved to utilization of that system with all the children. The amount of training with the vocoders has varied across the years. Prior to the miniaturization developments, preschool and elementary school-aged subjects were given vocoder training only during speech and language therapy (about 30 minutes daily at school). Since the availability of the miniaturized system, the devices are worn whenever possible and tactual experience time has been in-

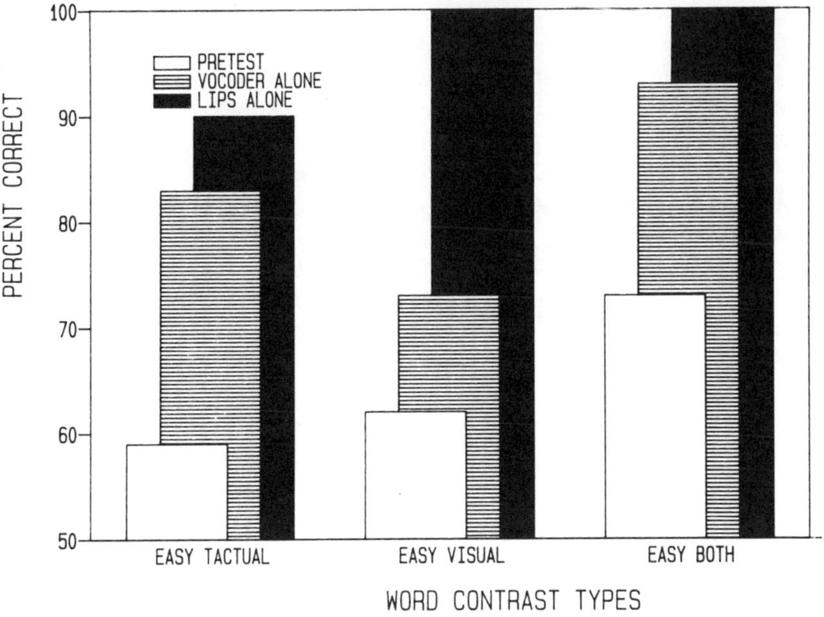

Figure 4. Speech recognition in a 6-year-old deaf subject.

creased by a factor of three or more, and is now limited mainly by availability in the program of sufficient numbers of devices. Work with the younger children in the program also uses tactual vocoders although training time is less extensive.

The goal of the classroom project is to demonstrate the use of tactual vocoders with deaf children and to develop appropriate training methods for use of miniaturized systems as full-time prostheses and training aids. One important difference between the goals of the classroom work and goals of other tactual vocoder training studies, is that in the classroom, speech production as well as speech perception improvement is emphasized. Because children who wear tactual vocoders feel their own voices as well those of their teachers, they are in a position to learn to pronounce speech appropriately by matching the tactual patterns produced by other speakers against patterns produced by their own voices. Previous research with short-term experience through a tactual vocoder display on the fingers of deaf preschoolers had indicated gains in syllable production (Goldstein and Stark 1976).

Results of the first full year of operation of the Miami classroom project can be found in Oller et al. (1986). The study indicated excellent gains in speech production and speech perception during a one-year training period in which 13 deaf children (ages 3–6) received approximately 60 hours of speech and speech reception instruction (mostly one-to-one) using a tactual vocoder. Two kinds of vocoders were available. Some children used the Oregon vocoder and others, the electrocutaneous Teletactor. At the beginning of the school year the children had only the most limited speech skills.

The children increased their consonant inventories by a factor of eight during the year and nearly tripled their vowel inventories. Speech reception improved markedly and language usage also improved.

While the progress of the children was considerable, it was not possible to assign all the gain to the tactual vocoder training, since similar children might have progressed similarly in an intense training program without tactual vocoders. Subsequent work compared the gains made by the children in the tactual training group during the year with gains of similar children (matched for ethnicity, hearing loss, secondary handicaps, etc.) in a regular public school setting (Oller et al. 1986). The comparison children were tested across a year's time on speech production skills in a manner that paralleled the testing of the children in the tactual training program. Results indicated that the tactually trained children made consistent progress in speech production while the children in the traditional program made very little progress at all. Intelligibility of the tactually trained children improved by 17% (of phonetic information in words) during the year while children in the traditional program gained only 1%. Projecting into the future, it could be said that if the tactually trained children could continue a comparable level of progress for several years they would reach a point of substantially intelligible speech by adolescence. The same optimistic projection was not possible for the children in the traditional program.

The excellent gains of the children in the training program suggest that the use of tactual vocoders may be of substantial benefit in deaf education. At the same time, the results do not indicate unequivocally that the better performance of the children in the tactual training program was due to vocoders to the exclusion of other teaching variables. A variety of potentially confounding teaching and teaching environment variables could not be controlled in the study. In order to achieve greater certainty about the contribution of tactual vocoders in the program, additional comparisons with progress of comparable children in intense oral training settings are being developed.

Progress of the children in subsequent years of work in the program with tactual vocoders has offered further encouragement for the approach (Oller et al. 1986). Of five children (now aged 7–10) who have been engaged in the training for over four years, three have made such excellent progress that they are now partially mainstreamed (without interpreters) in a Dade County Public Schools classrooms. Their English language development (as opposed to speech development) as well as reading and mathematics skills are so extensive that they have been judged by independent school testers to be at, or near, age level. Their performance on standardized tests such as the Grammatical Analysis of Elicited Language (GAEL) show speech scores above the 90th percentile. The other two children who have been in the program for four years have also made excellent progress, but have progressed more slowly in some areas owing to substantial secondary learning disabilities.

While the overall gains of children studying in a program using systematic artificial hearing training are very encouraging, additional results of the work have suggested the need for some important adjustments in procedure. Through most of the four years of work, the bulk of training with tactual vocoders has been multisensory, i.e., using lip reading, auditory amplification, and tactual signals simultaneously. The assumption was that with many hours of training, the deaf children would absorb so much knowledge of skin sensations corresponding to sounds that they would come to depend upon the tactual signal for speech perception (even in running-speech situations) without a large amount of specific unisensory tactual training. However, empirical results do not support that expectation. Eilers et al. (1985) showed that while the deaf children had learned to use tactual vocoder input effectively as a speech reception aid in limited circumstances (such as 2–5 choice recognition tasks, or speech articulation training exercises), they showed little increase in rate of speech tracking (of specially prepared stories written at the children's reading levels) with vocoder plus lip reading as opposed to lip reading alone. One reason for this lack of difference may have to do with the synergistic effect of the multisensory training on the lip reading performance of the children, who are, as the data indicate, extremely good lip readers. But whatever the enthusiasm about lip reading improvements, the results call into question the assumption that deaf children can learn to adapt sufficiently to the tactual vocoder signal itself in a classroom situation where vocoders are used most often with simultaneous visual (lip reading) and tactual presentation of speech information. Eventually, if the devices are to be used to their full potential, the children must show improvements in running-speech perception performance that are specifically attributable to the tactual devices.

Two kinds of adjustments seem appropriate, one involving classroom procedure and one involving instrumentation. In the classroom a new emphasis on unisensory tactual vocabulary training has been instituted. The basic format for the vocabulary training is an adaptation of the Engelmann and Rosov (1975) method (described above). The approach is only recently underway and the children are progressing rapidly, as expected. The goal is to teach the children tactual recognition of a substantial vocabulary (50 or more words) and then to progress towards generalization (sentences, rhyming tasks, and larger word sets) and integration tasks involving recognition of speech with hearing and lip reading plus vocoder input.

The instrumentation adjustments that seem appropriate would make the tactual signal useful in a wider variety of circumstances. Because the dynamic range of perceived amplitudes of stimulation is rather limited in currently available devices, noise severely limits their effectiveness. Thus far, the available devices have lacked adequate noise limitation circuitry and have not incorporated FM transmission. Such adjustments in addition to any improvements in the devices' dynamic range may substantially enhance device performance and accelerate the learning process. Engineering and psychophysical work in our own laboratories (see for example Bull et al. 1983; Mandalia et al. 1983; Ozdamar et al. 1985) and elsewhere is directed towards improving dynamic range, while noise suppression and FM adaptations are being developed by corporations in the tactile devices area (e.g., Tacticon, Audiological Engineering, and Artificial Hearing Systems).

SUMMMARY

Empirical research has provided support for the use of sensory substitution as a strategy for helping the deaf to perceive and acquire speech. Studies have indicated that a number of speech-sound contrasts that are difficult to transmit to the deaf through lip reading or hearing aids can be transmitted effectively through tactual vocoders. With systematic unisensory training in the tactual modality, subjects learn to recognize substantial vocabularies of words with no levelling off of learning as training proceeds up to at least 80 hours. The success is dependent, not upon the rote learning of individual tactual patterns for words, but rather upon the development of tactually based phonetic identification strategies. After substantial training, it is possible to recognize many words and sentences that have not been specifically taught. Generalization of learning to bisensory recognition tasks after unisensory training is also possible, as shown by substantial improvements in open set word and sentence recognition as well as tracking rates in a lip reading plus vocoder over lip reading alone condition.

Children in a model training program using tactual artificial hearing devices have made excellent progress in speech and language development. The results for children in the model program show much better speech and language gains than in matched children in traditional programs. Future work will be directed both to device improvements and to development of classroom training procedures based on the outcomes of psychophysical and classroom research.

REFERENCES

Bastian, J., Eimas, P. D., and Liberman, A. M. 1961. Identification and discrimination of a phonemic contrast induced by a silent interval. *Journal of the Acoustical Society of America* 33:842.

Békésy, G. von 1957. Neural volleys and the similarity between some sensations produced by tones and by skin vibrations. *Journal of the Acoustical Society of America* 29:1059–1069.

Boothroyd, A. 1985. Tactile presentation of fundamental frequency as an aid to lip reading. Presented at the Tactual Communications Conference, The Institute of Logopedics, Wichita, KS.

Brooks, P. L. 1982. Evaluation of running speech on a vibrotactile vocoder. Presented at the Tactual Communications Conference, The Institute of Logopedics, Wichita, KS.

Brooks, P. L., and Frost, B. J. 1983. Evaluation of a tactile vocoder for word recognition. *Journal of the Acoustical Society of America* 74:34–39.

Brooks, P. L., Frost, B. J., Mason, J. L., and Gibson, D. M. 1986a. Continuing evaluation of the Queen's University tactile vocoder. I: Identification of open set words. *Journal of Rehabilitation Research and Development* 23:1, 119–128.

Brooks, P. L., Frost, B. J., Mason, J. L., and Gibson, D. M. 1986b. Continuing evaluation of the Queen's University tactile vocoder. II: Identification of open set sentences and tracking narrative. *Journal of Rehabilitation Research and Development* 23:1, 129–138.

Bull, D. H., Eilers, R. E., Oller, D. K., and Mandalia, B. D. 1985. The effect of frequency change on discrimination of pulse bursts in an electrocutaneous tactual vocoder. *Journal of the Acoustical Society of America* 77:1192–1198.

Carney, A. E., and Beachler, C. R. 1986. Vibrotactile perception of suprasegmental features of speech: A comparison of single-channel and multichannel instruments. *Journal of the Acoustical Society of America* 79:131–140.

Eilers, R. E., Bull, D. H., and Oller, D. K. 1984. Tactual perception of speech-like stimuli with an electrocutaneous vocoder. *Artificial Organs* 8:494–497.

Eilers, R. E., Ozdamar, O., Oller, D. K., Miskiel, E., and Moroff, D. 1986. Comparison of tactual and auditory discrimination of speech. *Journal of the Acoustical Society of America* 79:s74.

Eilers, R. E., Turner, R., Oller, D. K., Ozdamar, O., and Saunders, F. 1985, November. An analysis of deaf children's speech tracking with tactual vocoders. Presented at the American Speech Language and Hearing Association Convention, Washington, D.C.

Engelmann, S., and Rosov, R. J. 1975. Tactual hearing experiment with deaf and hearing subjects. *Exceptional Children* 41:243–253.

Gault, R. H. 1926. Touch as a substitution for hearing in the interpretation and control of speech. *Archives of Otolaryngology* 3:121–135.

Gavin, W. J. 1979. Discrimination of vibrotactile patterns: Length of pattern as a major variable for success. Doctoral dissertation, University of Miami.

Goldstein, M. H., and Stark, R. E. 1976. Modification of vocalizations of preschool deaf children by vibrotactile and visual displays. *Journal of the Acoustical Society of America* 59:1477–1481.

Kirman, J. H. 1973. Tactile communication of speech: A review and an analysis. *Psychological Bulletin* 80: 54–74.

Kringelbotn, M. 1968. Experiments with some visual and vibrotactile aids for the deaf. *American Annals of the Deaf* 113:311–317.

Kuhl, P. K., and Miller, J. D. 1975. Speech perception by the chinchilla: Voiced-voiceless distinction in alveolar plosive consonants. *Science* 190:69–72.

Liberman, A. M., Cooper, F. S., Shankweiler, D. P., and Studdert-Kennedy, M. 1967. Perception of the speech code. *Psychological Review* 74:431–461.

Liberman, A. M., Cooper, F. S., Shankweiler, D. P., and Studdert-Kennedy, M. 1968. Why are speech spectrograms hard to read? *American Annals of the Deaf* 113:127–133.

Linvill, J. G. 1973. *Research and Development of Tactile Facsimile Reading Aid for the Blind (the Optacon).* (Final report, project #142112, grant #OEG-08-071112-2995). Washington, DC: Office of Education.

Lynch, M. 1986. Speech perception by congenitally deaf subjects using an electrocutaneous vocoder. Master's thesis, University of Miami.

Mandalia, B. K., Tapia, M. A., Oller, D. K., Bull, D. H., and Eilers, R. E. 1983. A non-real time software vocoder for tactual communication. *Proceedings of the Southeastern Symposium on System Theory,* Huntsville, AL.

Oller, D. K., Eilers, R. E., Vergara, K., and LaVoie, E. F. 1986. Tactual vocoders in a multisensory program training speech production and reception. *Volta Review* 88:21–36.

Oller, D., K., Eilers, R. E., Vergara, K. C., and Saunders, F. 1986, June. Training speech in deaf infants and children with tactual vocoders. Presented as a miniseminar at A. G. Bell Association for the Deaf, Chicago.

Oller, D. K., Payne, S. L., and Gavin, W. J. 1980. Tactual speech perception by minimally trained deaf subjects. *Journal of Speech and Hearing Research* 23:769–778.

Ozdamar, O., Eilers, R. Oller, D. K., Miskiel, E., and Moroff, D. 1985, October. Empirical considerations for vocoder design in tactual artificial hearing. Presented at the Tactual Communications Conference, Wichita, KS.

Pickett, J. M., and Pickett, B. H. 1963. Communication of speech sounds by a tactual vocoder. *Journal of Speech and Hearing Research* 5:207–222.

Pisoni, D. B. 1971. On the nature of categorical perception of speech sounds. Doctoral Dissertation, University of Michigan.

Reed, C. M., Durlach, N. I., and Braida, L. D. 1982. Research on tactile communication of speech: A review. *American Speech and Hearing Association Monograph* No. 20:1–23.

Richardson, B. L., and Frost, B. J. 1977. Sensory substitution and the design of an artificial ear. *Journal of Psychology* 96:259–285.

Sachs, M., Miller, J. D., and Grant, K. W. 1980. Perceived magnitude of multiple electrocutaneous pulses. *Perception and Psychophysics* 28:255–262.

Saunders, F. A. 1973. Electrocutaneous displays. *In* F. A. Geldard (ed.). *Conference on Cutaneous Communication Systems and Devices,* Austin, Texas: The Psychonomic Society.

Saunders, F. 1985, October. Wearable multichannel electrotactile sensory aids. Presented at the Tactual Communications Conference, Wichita, KS.

Sherrick, C. E. 1984. Basic and applied research on tactile aids for deaf people: Progress and prospects. *Journal of the Acoustical Society of America* 75: 1325–1342.

Sparks, D. W., Kuhl, P. K., Edmonds, A. E., and Gray, G. P. 1978. Investigating the MESA (Multipoint Electrotactile Speech Aid): The transmission of segmental features of speech. *Journal of the Acoustical Society of America* 63:246–257.

Sparks, D. W., Ardell, L. A., Bourgeois, M., Wiedmer, B., and Kuhl, P. K. 1979. Investigating the MESA (Multipoint Electrotactile Speech Aid): The transmission of connected discourse. *Journal of the Acoustical Society of America* 65:810–815.

Spens, K. E. 1980. Tactile speech communication aids for the deaf: A comparison. *Speech Transmission Laboratories Quarterly Progress Status Report* 4:23–39.

Yeni-Komshian, G., and Goldstein, M. H. 1977. Identification of speech sounds displayed on a vibrotactile vocoder. *Journal of the Acoustical Society of America* 62:194–198.

Chapter 20

The Children's Cochlear Implant Study: Review and Update

Jeannette Seloover Johnson

The past five years have been exciting and productive ones in the study and use of implantable auditory prostheses for humans. We are moving from an era of speculation regarding the benefits and limitations of cochlear implants to one of increased knowledge and technical sophistication—yet all the time maintaining a healthy degree of skepticism and an attitude of scientific inquiry. The issues have become more focused, particularly with the use of cochlear implants in children. Many questions have been answered, some are provisionally answered but require further investigation, and, as expected, new ones have arisen. Nonetheless, we hope we have reached the point where we can examine, on a rational basis, the various aspects of this non-traditional treatment of profound deafness.

The early detection of auditory impairment in children and intervention with appropriate amplification and habilitation have long been considered critical to the reduction of the multiple and far-reaching effects of hearing loss (Pollack 1981; Ross 1977). Unfortunately, some hearing-impaired persons are unable to benefit significantly from the use of even the most powerful standard amplification systems. They cannot use sound through hearing aids in any practical manner. The cochlear implant is intended for use in those persons with the degree and type of hearing impairment that cannot be ameliorated to any useful extent by other more conventional procedures or devices.

The author is grateful to the following: The House Ear Institute for their leadership in the Children's Cochlear Implant Program; the seven co-investigator teams for their critical contributions to the study; the Houston School for Deaf Children for their innovative approach to education of profoundly hearing-impaired children; Martha Ellison, Charlene Kanniainen, and Jan Nelson for their industry in data monitoring, management, and statistical analysis; my colleagues in the 3M Otologic Products Program for their labors on behalf of the hearing impaired and to the children and their families who have been our inspiration and our teachers.

The study of children with the 3M Cochlear Implant System/House Design (Fretz and Fravel 1985) was undertaken following extensive experience with adult patients and demonstration of device safety and efficacy in that population. At this time, it is the only system approved by the United States Food and Drug Administration for clinical use in both prelingually and postlingually deafened adults (marketing approval granted to 3M by FDA, November 1986) or for investigation in both prelingually and postlingually deafened children, and children between the ages of 2 and 18 years.

The influence of the study has gone far beyond its original purpose. It has revived interest in work on a variety of "aids to hearing" for the profoundly deaf. Further, it has reawakened interest in the development of materials, educational procedures, and the management of profoundly hearing-impaired children. And, perhaps most importantly, it has revitalized an attitude of professional responsibility for this very special group.

Certainly, extraordinary human and financial resources have been brought to bear upon development of wearable cochlear prostheses. A significant outcome is that a segment of the population once considered outside the realm of learning through audition now has access to sound and can participate in habilitative procedures designed to maximize the development of auditory skills.

The Children's Cochlear Implant Study is a multidisciplinary, multicenter one, designed to investigate the benefits and limitations of the implant in this young population. The study was initiated by the House Ear Institute in 1980 and later extended to other centers in a variety of settings. (See Appendix for list of co-investigators.) The co-investigators have met several essential criteria. They all have had experience with adult cochlear implant patients. The team members have met the qualifications and standards of their own professions and are skilled in evaluation and diagnosis of profoundly deaf children. The co-investigators have accepted a long-term commitment of facilities, staff, and financial resources in order to assure regular monitoring and assistance for the implanted children.

The Candidate Selection Process

The candidate selection process begins well before the child visits the clinic. Inquiring families receive basic descriptive information about the cochlear implant study and a profile of the type of children for whom the implant may be appropriate. Should the family decide to continue the process, they are requested to provide detailed historical information regarding their child's general health, auditory, speech and language skills, academic status, previous treatment of hearing impairment, and so on.

When children are referred to an implanting center, they are viewed as children with possible communication and other disorders, and not only as potential implant candidates. The focus is on determining individual abilities, skills, and needs. For most children, this does not constitute the first evaluation. Ordinarily the children already have been assessed by a variety of professionals and are enrolled in intervention programs. Most children in the study have had a history of hearing aid use and share a failure to show progress in the development of auditory skills. Some children have no useful expressive or receptive means of communication; others have acquired some communication skills, but clearly need assistance in maintaining or improving those skills.

Determination of candidacy for the cochlear implant includes a full medical/otolaryngology evaluation; a comprehensive patient history; polytomography to establish the patency and other conditions of the cochlea; audiology, speech-language, and psychology assessments; and a review of information provided by the child's educational program. The family is given the opportunity to talk with other parents whose children have had cochlear implants.

Following the extensive selection procedures, the family, other caregivers, and the implant team consider a variety of options for future management of the child. Recommendations might include new hearing aids, hearing aid trial with auditory training, speech therapy, speech-reading instruction, special class placement, family counseling or other assistance, and education appropriate to the child's requirements. For a few children, the cochlear implant may be one of the options.

Whenever there are any doubts about the diagnosis or questions about auditory or other behavior, the child either is not recommended for implantation or the decision is delayed pending confirmatory information. In some instances, an extended trial with hearing aids and auditory training may be warranted. Further, diagnostic teaching may more clearly establish the child's status and needs (Brookhauser and Moeller 1986).

CANDIDATE SELECTION CRITERIA

Children selected for participation in the study must be between 2 and 18 years of age. There must be no medical contraindications to the surgery such as congential absence of a cochlea, poor general health, or any active infectious process. Profound bilateral sensory hearing loss must be established. Children should be unable to benefit from hearing aids as demonstrated in auditory tests and in their history of failure to achieve progress in auditory perceptual skills. Their performance must be poorer than that which would be expected with the cochlear implant. There should be no psycho-neurologic aspects such as personality aberrations, organic brain damage, or psychosis, which would interfere with the child's ability to benefit from the cochlear device.

The family, and the child if old enough to understand, receive extensive counseling so that they may make an informed decision about the cochlear implant. They learn about its benefits and its limitations, and the known and possible adverse effects (Berliner and Eisenberg 1985; House, Luxford and

Courtney 1985; Luxford and House 1985). The risks of the implant procedure are essentially the same as those of chronic ear surgery: infection, facial paralysis, cerebrospinal fluid drainage, meningitis, and anesthetic risks. These risks are remote in chronic ear surgery and have proven to be so in implant surgery as well. The family is given information about the average performance and the range of performance of children with cochlear implants. Because deaf children are a heterogeneous group, it is necessary for professionals and parents to be aware of what is reasonable to expect across this broad and varied population. Beyond a logical statement of prognosis, guarantees of performance for individual children with the cochlear implant are inappropriate.

As a further prerequisite, parents should show commitment to follow-up activities, both at the implant center and in the educational setting. Appropriate intervention resources and support systems should be available; liaison with the child's school and/or rehabilitation specialist is critical.

Characteristics of the Study Population

As of August 1986, over 230 profoundly deaf children had received 3M House cochlear implants in the FDA approved clinical trials.

AGE AT ONSET OF DEAFNESS

For the 200 children reported at time of data lock, the mean age at time of onset of profound deafness was 1.7 years, the median was 0.9 years and the range, birth to 11.2 years. In 63% of the children, the hearing loss was adventitious as compared to 37% wherein the hearing loss was congenital. The early loss group, that is, those less than 3 years of age, is the largest—81%. Approximately 13% experienced hearing impairment between the ages of 3 and 6 years while only 6% had been deafened between 6 and 12 years of age.

DURATION OF AUDITORY DEPRIVATION

The number of years of profound deafness before cochlear implant surgery covered a broad range, from 6 months to nearly 18 years with a mean of 6.4 years and a median of 5.5 years. Approximately 23% had been deaf for fewer than 3 years, 33% for 3 to 6 years, 19% for 6 to 9 years, 9% for 12 to 15 years, and 4% for 15 to 18 years.

AGE AT TIME OF SURGERY

The mean age at time of surgery was 8.1 years with a median of 7.0 years and a range from 2.2 to almost 18 years. The preschool group, those younger than 6 years, accounted for 40% of the children in the study. About 41% were elementary school age, 6 to 13 years, and only 19% were secondary school age, that is, older than 13 years.

ETIOLOGY

A review of the etiologies of hearing impairment among the study population shows that meningitis accounts for 57% of the total. Another 33% had sensory deafness of unknown origin, that is, the specific etiology could not be determined from the medical history or examination. Other causes such as cytomegalic inclusion disease, Mondini deformity, trauma, maternal toxemia, and heredity account for 10%.

CONDITION OF THE COCHLEA AT TIME OF SURGERY

An important factor among this young population which includes a large proportion of post-meningitic children is the patency of the cochlea. One of the sequelae of meningitis is new bone growth in the cochlea. Some degree of ossification was present in approximately 47% of the children implanted. Many of these were undetected by preimplant radiographic studies. Fortunately, this condition does not preclude placement of the 6 mm electrode. An opening may be drilled into the scala tympani through the new bone. Interestingly, all but 3% of the more than 200 children were able to respond to the electrical stimulation provided by the implant. Furthermore, the children with cochlear ossification were able to obtain auditory thresholds and discrimination scores essentially equivalent to those who had unobstructed cochleas.

MODE OF COMMUNICATION

Most of the children, 70%, used total communication (TC); approximately 22% were classified as oral/aural communicators (O/A); 4% used cued speech (CS); and 4% had no formal mode of communication. Significantly, the mean age at onset of deafness was considerably younger for children using TC, 1.4 years, as compared to those who used O/A, 3.2 years. For CS children, the mean age at onset was 0.8 years and for those unclassified, 0.5 years.

DURATION OF USE OF THE COCHLEAR IMPLANT

The length of time that children have used the 3M House cochlear implant ranges from less than four months to nearly four years. The mean duration of use is 23 months; the median, 22 months. Approximately 9% have had the system for fewer than 6 months, 26% for 6 to 18 months, 36% for 18 to 30 months, 22% for 30 to 42 months, and 7% for 42 to 48 months.

The majority of the children use the cochlear implant system on a regular basis. In most cases the use is all day, every day. A few children limit use of the device to school hours or speech-language therapy sessions. A few teenagers choose not to wear the system because of concern with cosmetic issues and/or peer group pressures; one of these children has returned to use of the implant now that he has entered a college program. Another child receives sound awareness only at the lower frequencies and does not use the device routinely. One other child experiences a facial twitch with the electrical stimulation and has decided not to use the implant.

Audiologic Measures

WARBLE-TONE THRESHOLDS, IMPLANT EAR BEFORE SURGERY

Tables I and II display mean, standard deviation, median, range, and percentage of *no response* for preimplant auditory thresholds unaided and with the use of powerful hearing aids. For the purpose of statistical analysis, 130 dB SPL was assigned to represent *no response* in the unaided condition; 100 dB was used in the aided condition. As unaided threshold data indicate, the children participating in the cochlear implant investigation were profoundly deaf; median thresholds were *no response* across the test frequency range. Most of the children did not respond to test stimuli in the unaided condition.

Median thresholds with hearing aids were 82 dB SPL at 250 Hz, 96 dB at 500 Hz and *no response* at all higher test frequencies. Most hearing aids are driven into saturation at this level. Although improved somewhat over the unaided condition, aided thresholds consistently were outside the range of normal conversational speech and many environmental sounds. Many of the children were responding to vibrotactile rather than to auditory sensations at the high intensity levels.

WARBLE-TONE THRESHOLDS, NON-IMPLANT EAR

In most cases, the poorer ear is selected for implantation. However, the children in the study were bilaterally profoundly deaf. Thresholds for the con-

Table I

Mean, Standard Deviation, Median, Range, and Percentage of No Response for Preimplant Unaided Warble-Tone Thresholds in Preoperative Implant Ears, dB SPL

	Frequency (Hz)					
	250 (n = 193)	500 (n = 188)	1000 (n = 183)	2000 (n = 182)	3000 (n = 182)	4000 (n = 179)
Mean	122.5	126.1	128.9	130+	130+	130+
SD	12.2	7.9	4.2	1.7	1.9	1.1
Median	NR	NR	NR	NR	NR	NR
Range	70-NR	80-NR	105-NR	109-NR	105-NR	115-NR
% NR	49	65	90	97	99	98

Table II

Mean, Standard Deviation, Median, Range, and Percentage of No Response for Preimplant Aided Warble-Tone Thresholds in Preoperative Implant Ears, dB SPL

	Frequency (Hz)					
	250 (n=196)	500 (n=194)	1000 (n=185)	2000 (n=185)	3000 (n=182)	4000 (n=175)
Mean	82.0	89.4	92.5	97.2	99.0	99.5
SD	11.7	13.5	13.3	8.5	5.6	3.4
Median	82.0	96.5	NR	NR	NR	NR
Range	48-NR	55-NR	54-NR	58-NR	60-NR	66-NR
% NR	10	39	69	94	98	98

tralateral ears were only slightly better, either unaided or with hearing aids, than the presurgical implanted ears in the same conditions. The median unaided threshold was 125 dB SPL at 250 Hz with *no response* across the remainder of the frequency range. Median thresholds with hearing aids were 77 dB SPL at 250 Hz, 82 dB at 500 Hz and *no response* at all higher test frequencies. These children received very little help from hearing aids in either ear.

WARBLE-TONE THRESHOLDS, IMPLANTED EAR, 1ST POSTOPERATIVE SESSION

Median thresholds for the cochlear implant at the time of first stimulation with the system appear in Table III. Thresholds average 60 dB SPL across the frequency range. With the implant, nearly 100% of the children respond to all of the test frequencies, 500 to 4000 Hz. The average improvement of median thresholds with the implant as compared to unaided median thresholds in the same ear is greater than 70 dB; average improvement over thresholds with hearing aids is 36 dB. When compared to the contralateral ear, average improvements for the implant are only slightly less, that is, 69 dB and 32 dB improvement over the unaided and aided conditions, respectively. Additionally, thresholds with the implant show some improvement over time as the children adjust to the unusual stimulation so that differences between the implant and preoperative measures become greater.

For most of the children, thresholds with a hearing aid in either ear did not permit detection of speech at average conversational levels. The cochlear im-

Table III

Mean, Standard Deviation, Median, Range, and Percentage of No Response for Warble-Tone Thresholds in Implanted Ears at the First Postoperative Test Session, dB SPL

	Frequency (Hz)					
	250 (n=182)	500 (n=185)	1000 (n=186)	2000 (n=186)	3000 (n=173)	4000 (n=161)
Mean	62.2	58.7	58.4	61.4	63.0	66.2
SD	7.8	7.8	8.3	10.1	10.8	12.1
Median	62	58	57	59	61	63
Range	41–85	42–93	41–98	42-NR	40-NR	49-NR
% NR	0	0	0	3	4	6

plant, however, provides detection of sound, though not necessarily pitch discrimination, at useful levels. Functionally this means that with the implant, children can detect most medium and high intensity sounds, including speech, that would occur in the environment.

Auditory Perception

Once provided with awareness of sound at levels encountered in daily life, children are able to make increasingly more difficult auditory discriminations over time. One of the demonstrations of this growing skill is the improved ability to perform on the *Discrimination After Training Test* (DAT), developed by Thielemeir (1982). It is specifically for use with prelingually impaired, profoundly deaf adults and children who, because of their early onset of hearing loss, usually cannot respond to conventional auditory discrimination tasks. The DAT determines the auditory capability to learn progressively more subtle discriminations following a brief intense interval of training. The DAT stimuli are drawn from the *Monosyllable-Trochee-Spondee* (MTS) test, developed by Erber and Alencewicz (1976), which has been used with adult cochlear implant patients.

The test progresses in a hierarchy of difficulty, from a simple visual discrimination task to determine that the child understands and is able to make the appropriate response (Level 1), and proceeds to auditory-only detection of the presence of speech (Level 2), and auditory-only perception of non-linguistic (Levels 3–5) or linguistic (Levels 6–12) stimuli. Of the speech items, Level 2 is a detection task; Levels 3 through 5 require perceptions of gross durational and timing differences; and Levels 6 through 8 are discriminations of different word stress patterns. Levels 9 and 10 each contain two spondees; Level 11 contrasts three spondees and Level 12, four spondees.

Table IV presents means, medians, and ranges of DAT scores (levels) for non-implant ears with the help of conventional hearing aids, and for implant ears preoperatively with hearing aids and postoperatively at six month intervals. The number of children in each category varies because the children had been implanted at different times and therefore are on different retest schedules. With hearing aids, the majority of children could demonstrate the cognitive skill required to perform the task, that is, they passed Level 1, the visual discrimination item. But many of them could not even detect the test stimuli presented at approximately 70 dB SPL. These children were not included in the statistical analyses. If their scores had been entered as zero, mean scores for the hearing-aid condition would appear even poorer. For the children who could detect the stimuli with their hearing aids, the mean score was Level 2.1 for the preoperative implant ear in the hearing aid condition and Level 3.2 for the non-implant ear in the same condition.

With the cochlear implant, the mean score at the first postoperative visit, the session at which children received the external system and had been using the

Table IV

Mean, Median, and Range of DAT Levels for Preoperative Implant Ears with Hearing Aids, Non-Implant Ears with Hearing Aids and Implant Ears at 6 Month Intervals, dB SPL

	DAT Levels				
	n	Mean	SD	Median	Range
Preoperative implant ear with hearing aid	165	2.1	2.4	1.0	0–12
Non-implant ear with hearing aid	154	3.3	3.6	1.0	0–12
Implant					
Initial Session	65	5.5	3.0	6.0	0–11
6 Months	110	6.1	3.1	7.0	0–12
12 Months	61	7.1	2.8	8.0	0–12
18 Months	38	7.5	2.2	8.0	0–12
24 Months	31	8.3	2.1	8.0	4–12
30 Months	17	8.7	1.9	8.0	5–12
36 Months	10	9.9	1.7	11.0	8–12

implant for only a few hours, is Level 5.5, discrimination of one versus two syllables. The implant mean scores increase over time reaching a level of 9.9, discrimination between two spondees, for the children tested at 36 months. The lower end of the range of scores also improves over time so that at 36 months, the lowest scoring child is at Level 8, discrimination of monosyllables versus trochees.

Paired comparisons of children at each test session indicate that mean scores with the cochlear implant are significantly better than preimplant scores with the hearing aid in either ear.

The DAT scores demonstrate that the cochlear implant enables these previously profoundly deaf children to detect human voice at a conversational level, to perform auditory discriminations of different stress patterns, to discriminate between two spondees and later among four spondees without the use of visual cues. These achievements should be considered in the light of the degree of preimplant auditory impairment, the early onset of deafness, and the relatively long periods of auditory deprivation.

With this heterogeneous population, one would expect different factors to have an impact on performance. Several variables were evaluated for correlation with test scores at any given test session and also with the rate of change in scores across sessions: (a) preimplant baseline scores, (b) duration of use of the cochlear implant, (c) age at onset of deafness, (d) age at time of surgery, (e) duration of hearing loss, and (f) mode of communication.

In the multivariate analysis, the preimplant baseline scores and months of use of the cochlear implant were the two factors accounting for the greatest variability among children at any postimplant test session. Months of use of the implant accounted for much of the change by individual children. Two additional factors account for some, but a smaller amount of the variability: age at onset of profound deafness and mode of communication.

The children who begin with higher scores improve over time and tend to maintain higher scores at successive test sessions than other children in the group. The longer they use the implant, the higher the levels they achieve. Children who were deafened later and who use an oral mode of communication tend to score higher.

In terms of amount of improvement, the children who have worn the cochlear implant system longer show more improvement at successive test periods. Of great interest is the fact that children who were deafened earlier in life and who use Total Communication show the greatest amount of improvement over time. It is particularly encouraging that, although they begin at lower levels, these children improve at a faster rate.

In summary, the differences in baseline scores, that is, where the child starts, account for much of the difference seen among children at any given time. How far and how fast they will advance depends in great part on how long the implant is used and to a lesser extent on the age at which they were deafened and the mode of communication that they employ.

Of course, a certain amount of variability in scores is unaccounted for in our models; certainly one would expect that the child's cognitive skills, intervention programs, parent support, and other factors would have additional influence on developing auditory abilities.

In a recent presentation, Berliner and Eisenberg (1986) viewed the DAT levels as five perceptual categories: (a) no auditory detection, (b) auditory detection only (Level 1), (c) pattern perception (Levels 3–8), (d) partial word recognition, closed set (Levels 9–11), and (e) consistent word recognition, closed set, (Level 12). This scheme categorizes children according to their ability to process time-intensity and spectral information. According to Geers (1986), prelingually deafened children who receive only pattern perception have substantially poorer speech intelligibility than those who have spectral or intonation perception. Residual hearing is considered the major variable in predicting competence in verbal language.

With the implant, Berliner and Eisenberg (1986) report, only 2 of the 73 children in their study fall into category 1. Both had occluded cochleas secondary to meningitis and had not responded to the implant. Fifty-three percent of the children currently are performing in category 2, while 40% are in categories 3 or 4. Because the trend is toward improvement over time, it is expected that some of the children in the lower categories would move into the higher categories in the future.

For the majority of the children—83%—the implant is superior to the hearing aid by at least one perceptual category; 60% of the children improved by two or more categories. Further, 37% moved up from lower levels into word recognition categories.

According to Berliner and Eisenberg (1986), "a small but growing number of cochlear implant children are now demonstrating some open-set recognition of phonemes, words, and simple phrases." They used the Glendonald Auditory Screening Procedure (Erber 1982) to assess children who had speech intelligible enough to be understood by the clinician. They tested 10 children on open-set word recognition and 18 on sentence comprehension. Nine of the 10 showed auditory-only open-set word identification, with a mean score of 43%. Ten of the 18 children showed open-set sentence comprehension, with a mean score of 31%. Though the sample thus far is limited, it indicates the potential of the cochlear implant system in providing speech recognition without the aid of visual cues for both prelingually and postlingually deafened children. Berliner and Eisenberg point out that increasing numbers of children are exceeding previous expectations for performance with the 3M House implant system and that we do our clients a disservice in limiting our expectations for their success.

Speech Production and Language Development

There are expectations and hopes, as for other kinds of aids to the hearing impaired, that the cochlear implant will benefit deaf children in speech production, in language development, and in educational progress. None of the new or conventional treatments, whether hearing aids, teaching methods, cued speech, computerized interactive rehabilitation programs, or the cochlear implant can solve the problems of deafness consistently or in isolation (Markides 1983; Quigley and Paul 1984). What they do achieve is to open additional opportunities for developing communication skills. In the case of the cochlear implant, it provides possibilities for learning through the auditory channel (Brown, Eisenberg, and Tonokawa 1986; Eisenberg et al. 1986; Sperling, Kirk, and Brown 1985).

Speech Production

In the Children's Cochlear Implant Study, the Phonetic Level Speech Evaluation (imitative speech) and the Phonologic Level Speech Evaluation (spontaneous speech), described by Ling (1976), are used to monitor changes in speech production. The children show progress in all areas over time, in both the non-segmental and the segmental aspects of speech. In a multivariate analysis of the variables correlated with performance, as with speech perception, the preimplant baseline scores and months of use of the cochlear implant are the two most important factors. When these two factors are held constant, then mode of communication and age at onset of profound deafness become important. Children who were deafened later in life and who use an oral mode of communication score higher; however, those deafened earlier in life and who employ Total Communication make more progress over time.

Language

Language skills are included in the patient evaluation process, but do not serve as part of the selection criteria per se. Receptive and expressive language are assessed preimplant and at regular intervals postimplant in order to chart the children's progress. Specific tests are selected for individual children on the basis of age and skill levels. When appropriate, they are tested using their usual modes of communication.

Preimplant results show that the children were severely delayed in language skills relative to their hearing peers, as would be expected for children with this profound degree of hearing impairment (Geers et al. 1981; Kretschmer and Kretschmer 1978; Moeller et al. 1986). Nonetheless, they consistently show improvement above baseline data on receptive and expressive language tests at each successive postimplant session. Surprisingly, the gap between language age and chronologic age tends to narrow over time, just the reverse of what typically is observed in profoundly deaf children (Moeller et al. 1986; Clarke and Rogers 1981). It will be of great interest to discover whether cochlear implant children will maintain this growth or will eventually reach a plateau in language learning or begin to demonstrate a widening gap between chronologic and language ages.

THE BASIC GUIDANCE PROGRAM FOR CHILDREN

The initial days of use of the cochlear implant are carefully guided by the implant team. The House Ear Institute calls this period "Basic Guidance," a multisensory program that provides an orientation for the child and family on beginning use of the cochlear implant system (Eisenberg 1986). The program attempts to make listening activities enjoyable and motivating as it progresses in a hierarchy of difficulty. Early on, the concept is taught that specific actions and objects create sound; later lessons stress more abstract concepts about sound as experiences with the cochlear implant increase.

The goal of the Basic Guidance Program is to establish meaningful everyday use of sound through the cochlear implant. The critical elements of the program are: (a) insure proper adjustment of the external system, (b) orient the child and family to the care and use of the implant, (c) introduce the child to processed sound, (d) develop the use of minimal auditory cues, (e) establish patterns of practice, (f) encourage participation in communicative situations, (g) promote speech-reading strategies, (h) teach voice monitoring, and (i) provide counsel and support.

LONG-TERM INTERVENTION

Following basic guidance, most children continue in their current educational settings. It is essential that educational staff and the child's special teachers be involved in the evaluation and selection process. Close cooperation must be maintained between the implant center and the school. The center offers information about the cochlear implant system itself, about the child's performance with the new device, and assistance in programming for auditory skills development and speech-language intervention. The school has valuable historical information about the child's performance and provides the day-to-day educational and special needs programming.

We recognize, as Brookhauser and Moeller (1986) expressed in a recent article, "that the efforts of professionals attempting to habilitate these children [referring to prelingually deaf infants] more effectively has [sic] been hampered by the paucity of substantive research dealing with the effects of early intervention and the consequent lack of accepted benchmarks for judging acceptable habilitative progress" (p. 51). In this regard, we are pleased to note that clinical trials of cochlear implants have played a role in reactivating interest in developing "valid, objective, and measurable criteria for use in selecting the most appropriate habilitative track for children with early profound hearing impairment, in measuring progress and in designing materials for use with these children" (Brookhauser and Moeller, p. 51).

AURAL REHABILITATION PROGRAM FOR THE PROFOUNDLY DEAF CHILD; INTEGRATING SOUND INTO THE HOME: STRATEGIES FOR PARENTS

Eisenberg (1985) has developed materials for home use by families to enable children to achieve competency in listening abilities and to increase reliance on the auditory modality. Awareness of sound is introduced and reinforced in association with contextual and situational cues. The program then moves on to higher level auditory processing activities using environmental sounds and prosodic elements of speech. It integrates overall communication skill development into the auditory training process.

THE DEVELOPMENTAL APPROACH TO SUCCESSFUL LISTENING

The *Developmental Approach to Successful Listening* (DASL), was developed by Windle and Stout (1984) at the Houston School for Deaf Children. It is based on the *Auditory Skills Curriculum* developed by the Los Angeles County Schools (1976). The program provides a hierarchy of auditory skills along with suggestions for developing those skills at home and at school. It is a means of guiding auditory training and of measuring progress over time. The DASL may be employed with children of any age, at any level of auditory proficiency, and is appropriate for children with various degrees of hearing impairment who are using hearing aids or cochlear implants (Maddox, Stout, and Jorgensen 1986; Maddox, Jorgensen, and Stout 1986).

The DASL program contains an auditory checklist of broad guidelines for observation of children's responses to sound. Sections on sound awareness, phonetic listening, and auditory comprehension proceed from simple sound detection activities to highly complex listening skills (Stout, Smith, and Clark 1986).

THE COCHLEAR IMPLANT—A TOOL FOR LEARNING

Sensory experience exerts a powerful influence on learning and overall development of children. The importance of auditory experience is well recognized (Conrad 1979; Emerton et al. 1979; Gentile and DiFrancesca 1969; Meadow and Trybus 1979). Sound is the primary source of information regarding events that occur in the environment, even those outside the visual field. Deaf children with a cochlear implant can gain an appreciation of the environment via auditory contact. Common sounds lost or not heard previously or ignored because of the very low loudness level now can be given meaning, made exciting and become an important part of everyday experience. Life's activities are enriched by the addition of sound.

The Children's Study has demonstrated that, for properly selected children, the cochlear implant is a tool for aiding learning through the auditory sense. For children who do not benefit from conventional amplification, attempts to develop auditory skills through conventional techniques are futile; there is a serious gap in the habilitation process. The cochlear implant opens the door to intervention using the auditory sense, thereby facilitating improvement of functional communication.

The gains children make with the cochlear implant are influenced by various factors including the age at onset of deafness, the duration of auditory deprivation, the age at identification of the hearing loss, innate abilities and motivations, current language base and method of communication, auditory memory, auditory nerve survival, the intervention program, personal motivation, and family support. In this sense the cochlear implant is much like hearing aids, media materials, or language teaching methods. It should be viewed as part of the special educational process.

The greatly improved auditory detection levels provided by the cochlear implant create opportunities for children to develop critical links between sound and communication. With audition, speech and environmental sounds can take on meaning, significance, and purpose. The children's own production of sound causes responses in others. Sound thus becomes important as they learn that it can be used for the communication of needs and feelings. It becomes possible to secure their attention through audition. They learn to contact people by using their voices. The children's vocalizations are acknowledged with reciprocol activity, thereby reinforcing the use of their own voices (Brown, Eisenberg, and Tonokawa 1986).

The level of audition provided through the implant ensures that the speech of others is heard and that the children's own vocal attempts are audible to them. Rate, rhythm, pitch, and intensity levels of speech become more appropriate as the children use audition to monitor their own speech output (Eisenberg et al. 1986; Sperling, Kirk, and Brown 1985). Establishment of the auditory-vocal loop occurs and enables children to form a strong association between the auditory impression and the movements of the speech muscles (Brown, Eisenberg, and Tonokawa 1986). Furthermore, sounds now may be associated with the visual language of speechreading. Children can use a combination of auditory, visual, tactile, and kinesthetic information to aid in communication. The implant allows a program of intensive auditory education based on sequential and interrelated development of audition, speech, and language, and utilization of the new cues available through the implant (Bilkovec et al. 1986; Clark and Marshall 1986).

Teachers and caregivers report that children make more rapid and more consistent progress in communication skills with the cochlear implant when compared with earlier hearing aid use (Bilkovec et al. 1986; Jorgensen 1986). There is increased interest and pleasure in auditory training for both children and their parents which results in better follow-up in practicing auditory goals at home. Enhanced listening skills and attending behaviors, especially in the classroom, lead to increased socialization. More frequent initiation of peer interaction occurs as the children respond to their friends' communicative attempts and as others respond to their attempts (Jorgensen 1986; White and Clark 1986).

With the cochlear implant, the use of more age-appropriate social skills and a decrease in behavior problems has led to diminishing frustration on the part of children, teachers, and families. Older children report that they feel new confidence in communication situations and, further, that they feel less isolated from the world around them. Both children and families express increased feelings of safety and security because the children can perceive attention-getting and warning sounds via the implant system (Jorgensen 1986).

The Future

Unquestionably the ultimate cochlear implant has yet to be developed. Future cochlear implant systems may offer more or different benefits. Depending upon their design intent and population served, they may not necessarily eliminate present systems. There will be a broader variety of devices and they will be more patient-specific. Improved diagnostics and predictors of neural reserve will aid in selection of candidates and prescription of devices with particular characteristics. The cochlear prostheses themselves will become more durable with greater longevity. Size and power requirements will be reduced.

With children, the emphasis in cochlear implants already shows signs of shifting from engineering and medically dominated aspects to educational and habilitative ones. New diagnostic materials, therapy programs and teaching techniques for profoundly deaf children will be tailored to the unique signals provided by the implants. Perhaps younger children may be implanted as well as persons with more residual hearing.

For patients of all ages, the ultimate system would provide for cochlear stimulation without surgical intervention. The signals from this device would differentially target the auditory nerve, perhaps from a remote transmitter. Furthermore, the system would more closely mimic the function of the missing or damaged cochlear elements, thereby providing a more complete and more natural signal for the brain to interpret.

REFERENCES

Berliner, K. I., and Eisenberg, L. S. 1985. Methods and issues in the cochlear implantation of children: An overview. *Ear & Hearing* 6(3) (Suppl.):6S–13S.

Berliner, K. I., and Eisenberg, L. S. 1986. Our experience with cochlear implants: Have we erred in our expectations? Paper presented at the 2nd International Symposium and Workshops. Snowmass-Aspen, Colorado.

Bilkovic, T., Hillman, C. G., Smith, A. H., and Marshall, E. 1986. Management of the cochlear implant child in the classroom. Paper presented at the International Convention of the A. G. Bell Association for the Deaf. Chicago, IL

Brookhauser, P. E., and Moeller, M. P. 1986. Choosing the appropriate habilitative track for the newly identified hearing-impaired child. *Annals of Otology, Rhinology and Laryngology* 95:51–59.

Brown, C. H., Eisenberg, L. S., and Tonokawa, L. 1986. Perceptual capabilities with the cochlear implant: Influences on speech production and auditory discrimination. Paper presented at the International Convention of the A. G. Bell Association for the Deaf. Chicago, IL.

Clark, J. G., and Marshall, E. 1986. Benefits of interfacing speech and auditory training. Paper presented at the International Convention of the A. G. Bell Association for the Deaf. Chicago, IL.

Clark, B. R., and Rogers, W. T. 1981. Correlates of syntatic abilities in hearing-impaired students. *Journal of Speech and Hearing Research* 24:48–54.

Conrad, R. 1979. *The Deaf Schoolchild: Language and Cognitive Function.* London: Harper & Row.

Eisenberg, L. S. 1985. *Aural Rehabilitation Program for the Profoundly Deaf Child; Integrating Sound in the Home: Strategies for Parents.* Los Angeles: House Ear Institute.

Eisenberg, L. S. 1986. *Basic Guidance for Children with the Cochlear Implant* (Rev. ed.). Los Angeles: House Ear Institute.

Eisenberg, L. S., Kirk, K. I., Thielemeir, M., Luxford, W. M., and Cunningham, J. A. 1986. Cochlear implants in children: Speech production and auditory discrimination. *In* T. J. Balkany (ed.). *Otolaryngologic Clinics of North America* 19(2) (pp. 409–421).

Emerton, R. G., Hurwitz, T. A., and Bishop, M. E. 1979. Development of social maturity in deaf adolescents and adults. *In* L. J. Bradford and W. G. Hardy (eds.). *Hearing and Hearing Impairment* (pp. 451–460). New York: Grune & Stratton.

Erber, N. P. 1982. *Auditory Training.* Washington, D.C.: A. G. Bell Association for the Deaf.

Erber, N. P., and Alencewicz, C. M. 1976. Audiologic evaluation of deaf children. *Journal of Speech and Hearing Disorders* 41:256–267.

Fretz, R. J., and Fravel, R. P. 1985. Design and function: A physical and electrical description of the 3M House cochlear implant system. *Ear and Hearing* 6(3) (Suppl.):14S–19S.

Geers, A. E. 1986. A presentation to the Food and Drug Administration; Ear, Nose and Throat Devices Panel. Washington, D.C.: Food and Drug Administration.

Geers, A. E., Kuehn, G., and Moog, J. S. 1981. Experimental project in instructional concentration: Evaluation and results. *American Annals of the Deaf* 126:929–964.

Gentile, A., and DiFrancesca, S. 1969. *Academic Achievement Test Performance of Hearing Impaired Students—United States: Spring, 1969.* Washington, D.C.: Gallaudet College.

House, W. F., Luxford, W. M., and Courtney, B. 1985. Otitis media in children following the cochlear implant. *Ear & Hearing* 6(3) (Suppl.):24S–26S.

Jorgensen, S. 1986. Clinical endpoints in cochlear implants for children. A presentation to the Food and Drug Administration; Ear Nose and Throat Devices Panel. Washington, D.C.: Food and Drug Administration.

Kretschmer, R., and Kretschmer, L. 1978. *Language Development and Intervention with the Hearing Impaired.* Baltimore: University Park Press.

Ling, D. 1976. *Speech and the Hearing Impaired Child: Theory and Practice*. Washington, D.C.: A. G. Bell Association for the Deaf.
Los Angeles. Office of the Los Angeles County Superintendent of Schools; Audiologic Services and the Southwest School for the Hearing Impaired. 1976. *Auditory Skills Curriculum*. North Hollywood, CA: Foreworks.
Luxford, W. M., and House, W. F. 1985. Cochlear implants in children: Medical and surgical considerations. *Ear & Hearing* 6(3) (Suppl.):20S–23S.
Maddox, H. E., Jorgensen, S., and Stout, G. 1986. Cochlear implants in children: A model for successful educational habilitation. Paper presented at the International Convention of the A. G. Bell Association for the Deaf. Chicago, IL.
Maddox, H. E., Stout, G. G., and Jorgensen, S. 1986. Educational aspects of cochlear implants in children. *In* T. J. Balkany (ed.). *Otolaryngologic Clinics of North America* 19(2) (pp. 267–274).
Markides, A. 1983. *The Speech of Hearing-Impaired Children*. Oxford: Manchester University Press.
Meadow, K. P., and Trybus, R. J. 1979. Behavioral and emotional problems of deaf children: An overview. *In* L. J. Bradford and W. G. Hardy. (eds.). *Hearing and Hearing Impairment* (p. 395–403). New York: Grune & Stratton.
Moeller, M. P., Osberger, M. J., and Eccarius, M. 1986. Receptive language skills. *In* M. J. Osberger (ed.). *Language and Hearing Skills of Hearing-Impaired Students*. Rockville, MD: American Speech-Language-Hearing Association.
Pollack, D. 1981. Acoupedics: An approach to early management. *In* G. T. Mencher and S. E. Gerber (eds.). *Early Management of Hearing Loss* (pp. 301–318). New York: Grune & Stratton.
Quigley, S. D., and Paul, P. V. 1984. *Language and Deafness*. San Diego: College-Hill Press.
Ross, M. 1977. Hearing aids. *In* B. Jaffe (ed.). *Hearing Loss in Children* (pp. 676–698). Baltimore: University Park Press.
Sperling, T. B., Kirk, K. I., and Brown, C. H. 1985. Amount of vocalizing in cochlear implant children using total communication. Paper presented at the Annual Convention of the American Speech-Language-Hearing Association. Washington, D.C.
Stout, G., Smith, A., and Clark, J. G. 1986. The developmental approach to successful listening. Paper presented at the International Convention of the A. G. Bell Association for the Deaf. Chicago, IL.
Thielemeir, M. A. 1982. *Discrimination After Training Test*. Los Angeles: House Ear Institute.
White, E., and Clark, J. 1986. Successful mainstreaming for the hearing-impaired child. Paper presented at the International Convention of the A. G. Bell Association for the Deaf. Chicago, IL.
Windle, J. V. E., and Stout, G. G. 1984. *The Developmental Approach to Successful Listening*. Houston, TX: Houston School for Deaf Children.

APPENDIX

List of Co-Investigator Teams in the Children's Cochlear Implant Study

W. F. House, M. D. and W. Luxford, M.D.
The House Ear Institute, Los Angeles, CA

J. V. D. Hough, M.D.
Otologic Medical Clinic, Oklahoma City, OK

H. E. Maddox, III, M.D.
The Houston Ear Research Foundation, Houston, TX

R. T. Miyamoto, M.D.
Indiana University, Indianapolis, IN

S. C. Parisier, M.D.
The Children's Hearing Institute, New York, NY
C. M. Luetje, M.D.
Midwest Ear Institute, Inc., Kansas City, MO
S. E. Kinney, M.D.
Cleveland Clinic Foundation, Cleveland, OH
D. Goin, M.D. and R. Mischke, M.D.
Denver Ear Institute, Denver, CO

Chapter 21

Otitis Media: Models of Effects and Implications for Intervention

Lynne Feagans, Ingrid Blood, and *Jonathan G. Tubman*

Introduction

Our current knowledge about the consequences of otitis media in children is surprisingly meager, given the scope of the disease and the massive literature that is now developing on the possible long-term cognitive and language effects of the disease. Some have argued that we have become alarmed about the developmental effects of this disease too quickly (Paradise and Rogers 1986) since knowledge is so weak. This chapter will review the important literature that purports to show an association between otitis media and later developmental delays. This research is fraught with problems and individually none of the studies is definitive. Therefore, we will attempt to synthesize the current status of the literature in a piecemeal way in order to formulate various models of the possible effects of otitis media that could have implications for the development of specific intervention programs.

There are no data to indicate a clear causal relationship between otitis media, subsequent hearing loss, and immediate or long-term developmental effects. The studies presented indicate an association between these processes from a series of flawed studies. This does not mean these studies cannot be used to argue for a causal relationship. Truth in this area will continue to be elusive because we are studying human beings who cannot always be randomly assigned and/or manipulated medically to satisfy our thirst for truth. Thus knowledge must come slowly and with much caution about specifying cause and effect relationships. Yet, it is the number of studies on various populations of children and the number of different measures that show an effect which now make possible the development of some causal models that can be tested systematically.

The effects of this disease, which are real and serious, may seem clear; yet, when we begin to describe what these effects are—at what ages and at what hearing levels they occur—we find how little we really know about the effects of the mild to moderate hearing loss that fluctuates in early childhood as a result of this disease. Even less clear is what intervention should be recommended.

Definition

Physicians often distinguish between acute otitis media (often called suppurative otitis media) and otitis media with effusion (OME) (called nonsuppurative otitis media). Differentiation of these two types of otitis is often difficult (Paradise 1980). Acute otitis media is associated with an acute infection and is considered the precursor to otitis media with effusion. Otitis media with effusion is characterized by fluid that accumulates in the middle ear. This fluid is associated with a mild to moderate hearing loss in some children.

The symptoms of the disease are variable. In the acute phase, children may have a fever, complain of pain, or merely exhibit irritability. In otitis media with effusion children may exhibit some symptoms or no overt symptoms at all. It has been reported that up to 75% of episodes of OME are silent, with no presenting symptoms (Marchant et al. 1984; Schwartz et al. 1981). These silent episodes have made estimates of the prevalence difficult to establish.

The diagnosis of the disease has taken many forms. The authors of most of the studies have used otoscopy or pneumatic otoscopy as their primary diagnostic tool. The otoscope used to examine the eardrum contains lenses and an internal light source. The pneumatic otoscope contains, in addition, a bulb and tubing attached to the otoscope. When the physician examines the eardrum with this instrument he can assess the degree of mobility of the eardrum by creating an air-tight chamber. By pressing the bulb, the mobility of the eardrum can be assessed in response to both positive and negative pressure.

Although this technique is widely used, the exact criteria used in the formal diagnosis vary considerably. Hayden (1981) reviewed 43 studies of otitis media between 1955 and 1979. He found that the authors used 18 different criteria to diagnose otitis media and that the use of identical criteria was usually the result of multiple publications by the same authors rather than replication by different researchers. The most consistent single criteria for otitis media was a red tympanic membrane. Other criteria that are commonly cited in the literature are distortion of the light reflex and the disappearance of the concave shape of the tympanic membrane (Schwartz et al. 1981). Paradise (1980) has written extensively on this issue and admits he trusts few to follow the careful guidelines he sets out for diagnosis (personal communication). He characterizes the eardrum findings with regard to discharge, contour, color, luster, translucence, and mobility.

Recently another technique—immittance testing—has been used in addition to pneumatic otoscopy in the diagnosis of the disease. This technique is an easy, quick, and objective measure that provides assessment of the function of the eardrum and is highly correlated with middle ear effusion. Problems reside in the rather large number of false positive results. Thus, alone it is not a completely reliable diagnostic tool. In conjunction with pneumatic otoscopy, it appears to be an excellent tool.

The medical treatment of otitis media has not altogether been successful. Antibiotics have decreased markedly the number of secondary infections that often result from otitis media, including mastoiditis and infections in the brain itself. Attempts to reduce fluid in the middle ear have been much less effective. A number of antibiotic treatments have been tried but none has shown great effectiveness (Paradise 1980), although Schwartz (this volume) has indicated some success with low dosage long–term antibiotic treatments.

For the purposes of this paper we will be most concerned with otitis media with effusion because it is the fluid in the middle ear that is correlated with the hearing loss that in turn may cause developmental problems in children. In addition, since the fluid is somewhat impervious to traditional medical interventions, it is a problem not easily dealt with by physicians. This hearing loss is usually intermittent and only occurs during an episode of otitis media. The episodes may last only a few weeks or as long as nine months. The hearing loss, usually between 10 dB and 50 dB, is the proposed cause of developmental delays in otitis-prone children, even though the hearing loss is not permanent.

PREVALENCE

One of the reasons that this rather mild disease has received so much attention is that it is such a common disease in infancy and early childhood. The most commonly diagnosed disease by pediatricians, it accounts for up to 15% of office visits (Hayden 1981). Although this seems quite large, it is probably a considerable underestimation of the prevalence because many episodes are silent ones that would be likely to go undiagnosed unless the parents bring their child into the clinic for another reason. In a study that we just completed on day-care-attending children, only one child out of 44 did not suffer an episode of otitis media in the first three years of life (Feagans et al. 1987). Unlike children seen in a clinical practice, those in our study were observed daily by medical staff for signs of illness and monitored for upper respiratory infections, including otitis media. Other studies in private practice clinics have reported two-thirds of their children having an episode within the first two years of life (Howie 1975; Schwartz et al. 1981).

RISK GROUPS

Since so many children get this disease, interventions for otitis-prone children must be aimed at those at greatest risk and at those with the sequelae of the disease. Studies have clearly delineated some of the factors that appear to be important. They are summarized here in order to develop an argument about which children should be targeted for intervention.

Age. Otitis media is most prevalent in the first two years of life and then decreases over the later preschool years (Paradise 1980). Children who suffer episodes in the first year of life are those who are most likely to continue to have recurring episodes (Lundgren, Ingvarrson, and Olofsson 1984). Thus, the later the child suffers his first episode the less likely he is to become a chronic otitis media child. Some of these children suffer a hearing loss with the episodes at an age when they are acquiring language and other important cognitive skills.

Social Class. Children from lower socio-economic status homes tend to have more episodes of otitis media than children from middle-income homes. This has been pointed out in a number of studies in both the United States and other countries (Cambon, Galbraith, and Kong 1965; Pukander, Sipila, and Karma 1984). Children who live in single family dwellings or in rural areas are less likely to contract otitis media than children in urban settings or children in apartments. Children from larger families are more at risk for otitis media than those from smaller families. It is estimated that children from the lower socio-economic groups have five to six times the incidence of otitis media, indicating that this is an important risk factor.

Day-care. Day-care has consistently been shown to increase the risk of contracting otitis media. Large scale studies in Denmark (Fiellau-Nikolajsen 1979) and Sweden (Lundgren et al. 1984) reported that children in day-care were three times more likely to have an abnormal tympanogram than children at home. This same trend was evident in studies using otoscopic examinations. Children in family day-care were at intermediate risk, since they resembled day-care-attending children in the winter and home-care children in the summer. Similar studies found that these effects remain even after social class, living conditions, and other factors were controlled (Vinther, Brahe-Pedersen, and Elbrond 1984).

Sex. Most epidemiological studies indicate boys at higher risk than girls (Feingold, Klein, and Haslam 1966; Pukander, Sipila, and Karma 1984; Teele, Klein, and Rosner 1984), but some recent studies have not found this sex difference (Diamant and Diamant 1974; Lundgren et al. 1984). Although it is difficult to reconcile these findings, it may be that boys are only at increased risk for more serious otitis media complications. Vinther et al. (1984) report no sex differences in the incidence of otitis media but they do report significantly more adenoidectomies in boys.

Handicapped children. Several groups of handicapped children have been identified as having higher rates of otitis media than normal children. In two of these groups, the medical problems related to their handicap clearly seem to predispose the children to more otitis media. Cleft palate children almost universally have otitis media and it is even more severe in those with unrepaired palates (Paradise 1980). Down syndrome children also have high rates of otitis media, although it is not clear what physiological and health differences might predispose them to the disease.

The last group of children who have high rates of otitis media are children with learning problems (Zinkus and Gottlieb 1980). In this group the cause-

and-effect relationship is difficult to establish. As will be seen in the next sections, most would argue that the otitis media caused the learning problems; but since most of the studies are retrospective in nature, whether this is the case or whether other predisposing factors are implicated, as with other handicaps, cannot be firmly established.

Other factors. A variety of other factors are also associated with increased incidence of otitis media. For instance, otitis media appears to be much more frequent in the winter months than the summer months. This is true whether the child is at home, in family day care, or in center-based day care (Fiellau-Nikolajsen 1979). There is some speculation, but no real evidence, that there may be a certain genetic predisposition toward otitis media since it appears in some families more than others (Paradise 1980). Premature infants appear to be at increased risk (Berman, Balkany, and Simmons 1978) as well as infants who are bottle fed. Feeding an infant a bottle while he is in a supine position is postulated to allow milk to collect in the back of the throat which may promote infection (Beauregard 1971).

HEARING LOSS AND OTITIS MEDIA

The most frequent clinical course of otitis media for children, no matter what their risk, is fluctuating, mild to moderate, conductive hearing loss. Although the assessment of this hearing loss is critical to the causal models, only a handful of studies have documented the hearing loss associated with otitis media and related this loss to concurrent or later functioning. In addition, several factors differ considerably from child to child and probably have an effect on whether the hearing loss will have a short or long term effect. The onset of otitis media may be acute or insidious, age of onset may vary, the number of episodes and their duration may vary, variations in degree of hearing loss may occur with different stages of the disease, and there may be unilateral or bilateral involvement. All of these variations influence the hearing loss and its effect on development.

The environment in which the child spends the majority of the preschool years (day care, home, etc.) will differ in terms of ambient noise level, individual interactions with adults and peers, and instruction. Each of these variables may determine how receptive the child is to auditory stimulation and how conducive the child is to speech and language learning. Thus we can describe the hearing loss, but its effect may be different for different types of children in different environments.

THE AMOUNT AND DEGREE OF HEARING LOSS

Estimates of the prevalence of hearing loss due to otitis media range from 25% to 95% of children (Jerger and Jerger 1981). Similar ranges in estimates are found for the degree of hearing loss associated with otitis media (Fria, Cantekin, and Eichler 1985). Reasons for the wide range are numerous. Presence or absence of hearing loss, as well as degree of impairment and audiometric configuration, will vary with type of otitis media and progression of the disease. Hearing impairment associated with otitis media is typically mild and unsustained. Existing screening programs establish differing criteria for what decibel level constitutes a critical level for hearing loss. The suggested criteria of 15 dB for the frequencies 500, 1000, and 2000 Hz are the beginning of a significant hearing loss (Kessner, Snow, and Singer 1973) and would make pure tone screening ineffective because the majority of screening programs test at 20 dB or higher.

An additional contributing factor to the discrepancies regarding the presence of a hearing loss is related to whether the condition is symptomatic or not. Acute suppurative or purulent otitis media, which refers to the sudden onset and short duration characterized by a middle ear infection behind a reddened eardrum, is often symptomatic. Yet, otitis media with effusion or serous or secretory otitis media, which refer to clinically noninfectious forms of otitis media, can be asymptomatic. McCandless and Thomas (1974) suggest that 50% to 80% of hearing losses resulting from otitis media are undetected.

Audiologically, abnormalities of the middle ear due to otitis media produce conductive hearing loss. Audiometric measurements obtained by air conduction show the loss of sensitivity. Measurements obtained by bone conduction generally show normal hearing because the condition does not effect the inner ear. The differences between the air- and bone-conduction thresholds indicate the amount of conductive impairment. The amount of air conducted hearing loss is directly related to the type and amount of accumulation of material in the middle ear.

Instances of otitis media with effusion are related to inadequate ventilation of the middle ear cavity because of eustachian tube blockage or dysfunction. When tympanic cavity ventilation is impeded, the air trapped within the middle ear becomes absorbed by tissue. Negative air pressure is created in comparison to atmospheric pressure and a vacuum is created causing the eardrum to contract. At this stage, if any hearing loss exists, it is slight. Eventually, the fluids normally secreted by the mucosal lining of the middle ear will accumulate because of lack of aeration, resulting in serous effusion. As fluid continues to build in the middle ear cavity, the tympanic membrane will move from a retracted position to an outward position. The amount of hearing loss is usually dependent on the amount of the serous fluid. Because serous fluid affects the mass of the system, the air conduction audiometric contour will show a greater hearing loss for higher frequencies and spread to lower frequencies as the duration of the disorder lengthens. Eventually the audiogram assumes a flat configuration (Martin 1986). Bone conduction responses may be depressed slightly in the higher frequencies but this air-bone gap may be an artifact due to middle ear fluid.

Thick mucosal secretions are sometimes blown into the middle ear through the eustachian tube. This condition has been referred to as secretory otitis media or glue ear. Both mucosal and suppurative otitis media produce similar audiometric results because of the thick density of fluids. The audiometric contour is usually flat demonstrating similar hearing across all frequencies with the amount of loss again in direct proportion to the amount of fluid accumulation, typically between 20 to 40 dB hearing level (Jerger and Jerger 1981). More advanced stages and thicker fluids produce pure tone sensitivity greater than 40 dB. Losses may be unilateral or bilateral. Some have found that hearing impairment is dependent on whether one or both ears were affected. An average of 10 dB increment to hearing impairment was found by infection of a second ear (Fria, Cantekin, and Eichler 1985).

Regardless of type of otitis media or degree of hearing loss, speech discrimination in quiet is usually excellent. Additional audiological procedures such as Bekesy audiometry, tone decay, SISI and uncomfortable loudness levels indicate non-sensorineural involvement.

Immittance audiometry is characterized by absent acoustic reflexes, abnormal tympanograms, and lower than normal static compliance measures. Tympanometric shapes often differentiate suppurative from serous otitis media and change as the disease progresses. Tympanograms may reveal the presence of middle ear effusion when observation via otoscopy may not.

Recent evidence suggests that children with unilateral sensorineural hearing loss may experience difficulty in communication (Bess, Tharpe, and Gibler 1986) and academic achievement (Bess and Tharpe 1986; Culbertson and Gilbert 1986; Klee and Davis-Dansky 1986). Poorer performance may be attributed, in part, to the loss of binaural summation, squelch effects, localization, and binaural release from masking. Although this is a relatively unstudied area, children with constant, unilateral conductive hearing loss may also have similar problems. The issue of unilateral versus bilateral involvement is still unresolved.

DOCUMENTATION OF HEARING LOSS

The most persistent problem with research on the possible developmental sequelae associated with otitis media has been inadequate documentation of the hearing loss associated with this disease (Ruben 1984). Otitis media with effusion is fluctuant and recurrent in probably 40% of cases (Lim, Bluestone, and Klein 1984); therefore, frequent evaluations appear warranted prior to, during, and following bouts of middle ear effusion. Furthermore, most studies have not monitored hearing sensitivity to determine the effect of changes in hearing on subjects' performance.

Current trends in methods used for identification of hearing loss in otitis media include immittance audiometry, evoked response audiometry, pure tone screening, and/or plotting of thresholds, visual reinforcement audiometry, to name a few. There has been a lack of a uniform approach in assessment, and routine screening for hearing loss and middle ear effusion is not typically carried out during preschool years. Additional problems have included lack of qualified and experienced examiners and audiological facilities, high cost of equipment, limited specificity and sensitivity for certain measures, and few tools appropriate for evaluating very young children. Thus, the literature is somewhat disappointing in this area, but we will review some of the current techniques available to assess hearing.

Evoked response audiometry. Recent advances in computer technology have facilitated the use of Auditory Brainstem Response (ABR) as a routine approach for assessing hearing. ABR is a safe, reliable, objective, and appropriate clinical tool in evaluating children, yet limited data are available on the role of evoked potential audiometry in children with recurrent middle ear disease.

Fria and Sabo (1980) and Mendelson et al. (1979) studied the effectiveness of ABR in predicting the presence or absence of middle ear disease, and found certain components of the response, such as the latency of Wave I, to be sensitive in identifying otitis media. This provided support for utilizing ABR as a tool in assessing hearing loss due to middle ear disease. ABR predictions of otitis media were validated by myringotomy in the Fria and Sabo study, while Mendelson et al. confirmed the presence of middle ear disease by otoscopy.

Friel-Patti et al. (1982) obtained ABR measurements to estimate hearing loss in 28 otitis media prone children longitudinally from birth to 24 months of age. During this period, language development was assessed using the Receptive-Expressive Emergent Language Scale (Bzoch and League 1971) and the Sequenced Inventory of Communication Development (Hedrick, Prather, and Tobin 1975). ABR and language measurements were taken at six-month intervals. A high correlation was found for both expressive and receptive language delay and degree of estimated hearing loss from ABR measures.

Auditory evoked brainstem response audiometry has also been used to determine if transient reduced auditory input may have an effect on neural development. Folsom, Weber, and Thompson (1983) measured auditory brainstem responses from 15 elementary-aged children with early histories of recurrent middle ear disease. Significant differences between the experimental group and a control group of children with no history of middle ear disease were found. Results support a connection between recurrent otitis media and neurological development.

Based on the preceding documentation, ABR measures may be promising in documenting hearing loss in a pediatric population and could prove useful in monitoring the progression of transient hearing loss due to otitis media. Finally, longitudinal investigation of brainstem maturity using ABR as a clinical tool in otitis-free and otitis-prone children may provide information regarding the effects of reduced auditory input on neurological function.

Immittance audiometry. Middle ear effusions can be identified by immittance procedures in children not known to have otitis media. Immittance techniques are well suited for use with children since they require little cooperation, provide objective results, are cost-effective, are quick and easy to administer, and are extremely sensitive to the presence of middle ear disease in children. Immittance audiometry is a critical component of screening programs because it is well established that standard audiometric screening alone may miss as many as 70% of ears with pathology (Melnick, Eagles, and Levine 1964).

Routine immittance testing for otitis media includes tympanometry and acoustic reflex measures. Tympanometry is the measurement of the acoustic impedance of the ear as a function of ear canal air pressure. A graph, or tympanogram, is plotted showing how the impedance of the ear is altered when the ear canal is pressurized above and below atmospheric pressure. A variety of tympanometric patterns are now associated with various pathologic conditions. Tympanometry will not only identify those with otitis media with effusion but the technique is also sensitive to complications or sequelae of the disease. However, the extent to which continual, periodic, tympanometric monitoring can be used to improve diagnosis and prognosis needs more systematic study.

Acoustic reflex measures are made by introducing an acoustic stimulus loud enough to elicit contraction of the middle ear muscles. The contraction of the stapedius muscle in the ear with the immittance measuring device will suddenly increase the compliance of the eardrum synchronously with signal presentation. This acoustic reflex response is absent in ears with middle ear effusion. Optimal clinical assessment of otitis media is achieved when both tympanometry and acoustic reflex measures are made. Although this tool is extremely useful, it has often been found to produce a number of false positive readings. In the identification of disease the pneumatic otoscope has been used in conjunction with this technique to reduce false positives.

Behavioral threshold testing. Selection of behavioral identification techniques will be dependent on the age, maturation, and cooperation of the child. Generally, operant conditioning procedures have been used in assessing infants and young children. Tests of localization are most commonly employed in sound field for children between the ages of four months and three years. Visual (Visual Reinforcement Audiometry) and tangible (Tangible Reinforcement Operant Conditioning) reinforcement have been used (Northern and Downs 1984). Conventional audiometric approaches using earphones are employed with children three years and older. Threshold procedures utilize pure tone, noise, warble tone, and speech stimuli. Supra-threshold auditory assessment for young children includes speech discrimination testing and assessment of central auditory processing skills.

Studies of the Effects of Otitis Media

The vast majority of studies concerning the effects of otitis media on child development are currently retrospective in nature. These studies attempt, in general, to document several factors in constructing associations between otitis media and deficits in several domains of children's cognitive and language development. First, the studies attempt to establish a history of otitis media in a particular sample. Second, they attempt to demonstrate that samples exhibit or have exhibited significant hearing losses using actual hearing data or by assumption. Third, these studies attempt to demonstrate that the samples are characterized by a range of deficits in academic, cognitive, behavioral, intellectual, or language skill domains.

The authors of many of these articles suggest causal linkages between otitis media, hearing loss, and deficits in child development outcomes. Yet, the associations reported are confounded by threats to internal and external validity (Paradise 1981; Ayukawa and Rudmin 1983; Ventry 1980). These may include any of the following: inaccurate diagnoses of otitis media, lack of data on early hearing ability, small sample sizes, inadequate matching of subjects, and selective bias in data already collected. There are, however, some consistent findings in these retrospective studies. While the literature on the effects of otitis media on child development may be seriously flawed, the associations suggested by this body of research are invaluable in proposing causal models to be tested.

RETROSPECTIVE STUDIES

General learning problems. A number of authors have suggested that the hearing losses associated with otitis media will expose afflicted children to a higher risk for developmental disorders or learning disabilities. For example, Battin (1978) and Howie (1980) briefly reviewed relevant otitis media literature and concluded that a large portion of school-age language- or learning-disabled children had auditory processing deficits that were associated with early experience with otitis media. They also concluded that children suffering from otitis media experience temporary and long-term intellectual impairments such as inattentiveness, reduced retention, and hyperactivity. Leviton (1980) reviewed literature on the effects of otitis media and proposed seven hypotheses that relate otitis media with effusion to increased risk of hearing impairment and, in turn, relate hearing losses to increased risk of learning disorders like those discussed by Battin and Howie. Kirkwood and Kirkwood (1983) in a more recent review article attempted to make a similar association between otitis media with effusion and learning disabilities like deficits in auditory language skills. These authors related otitis media to hearing deficits. They then proposed a critical period for the acquisition of auditory learning skills, during which otitis media could cause irreversible damage in the ability to receive and process auditory input. The authors cited as indirect evidence studies of children with hereditary deafness and studies suggesting associations between histories of otitis media and academic underachievement. A review of empirical retrospective studies revealed a wide range of potential learning disabilities or problems to which otitis media was at least tentatively associated.

While some studies of the effects of otitis media on the developing child are concerned with specific abilities or skills purported to have been retarded due to early childhood experience, some authors have concentrated on a more global picture of the effects of this disease. For example, Gottlieb, Zinkus, and Thompson (1979) examined associations between an early history of otitis media and such outcome measures as language development, intelligence, educational progress, and behavioral problems and found lower performance levels associated with auditory processing deficits. Similarly, Brandes and Ehinger (1981) administered no less than 12 auditory perceptual tests along with measures of academic achievement, nonverbal intelligence, and visual perception and found lower overall performance and lower performance in specific auditory perceptual measures of selective attention, sequence memory, spelling, etc. In short, some investigators approached otitis media as having a fairly general effect on child development. Rational choice, however, of outcome measures to test specific hypotheses concerning the effects of otitis media will result in a more precise and therefore more meaningful picture of these effects.

Academic problems. A number of contemporary investigators claim to find associations between subjects' histories of early childhood experience of otitis media and academic achievement. Zinkus, Gottlieb, and Shapiro (1978) and Zinkus and Gottlieb (1980) examining school-age children explored the relationship between early otitis media, auditory processing deficits, and academic deficits. Otitis media histories were constructed from medical records and parent interviews. These authors found that a high incidence otitis media sample had lower scores on the Wide Range Achievement Tests (WRAT) subtests for reading, spelling, and math skills. They concluded that experience of otitis media in early childhood was associated with later academic underachievement and slowed academic progress. Sak and Ruben (1981) found that when tested against a control group of well siblings, a sample of school children with a history of three or more episodes of otitis media before age five scored significantly less well at spelling as measured by the WRAT. Yet, Brandes and Ehinger (1981) in a sample of school children with disease histories before age three of three or more episodes found no significant differences beween clinical and control samples on measures of math ability, reading comprehension, and word recognition. In this case, school records indicate that the clinical subsample received more supportive services from school personnel.

Intelligence. A wide range of studies has indicated that children experiencing otitis media with effusion early in life suffer deficits in general intellectual functioning, especially verbal intelligence. Gray (1983) raised three issues with respect to the impact of otitis media on the child's developing cognitive capabilities. The first involved the notion of a critical period in the development of cognitive skills. Was there a critical period in which otitis media produced deficits in a child's cognitive capabilities? Second, it was not known whether experience of otitis media in early childhood would produce a delay in development or permanent damage to the child. Third, it was not known whether these deficits were real or perceived. The majority of the evidence reported in retrospective studies seemed to indicate that the deficits in cognitive or intellectual skills were long-lasting and real.

Gottlieb, Zinkus, and Thompson (1979) found significant differences between otitis media afflicted and control groups on the Wechsler Intelligence Scales for Children—Revised Edition (WISC-R), including Full Scale, Verbal, and Performance subtests. They did not, however, find any significant group differences on the Nonverbal subtest. Brandes and Ehinger (1981) also found no significant group differences on measures of nonverbal intelligence. Yet, Lewis (1976) found differences between clinical and control groups on culturally biased measures of nonverbal intelligence. Significant group differences were found between clinical and control school-age groups on the verbal subtest of the WISC-R by Sak and Ruben (1981). In addition, Battin (1978) documents lower than normal scores on the WISC-R and Stanford-Binet intelligence tests for school samples with early childhood experience of otitis media.

Behavioral and attention problems. The existence of behavior problems in children with current diagnoses of otitis media has only recently been documented by several authors. Silva et al. (1982), in a cross-sectional study comparing five-year-old children with current bilateral otitis media to an otologically normal sample, found that the children with otitis media were significantly deficient in speech articulation ability. In addition, these children scored lower on measures of verbal comprehension, motor development, and intelligence at levels that approach significance. More interesting, however, was the manner in which the mothers of these children rated them. These children received maternal ratings that distinguished them as being significantly more dependent, restless, destructive, fidgety, and disobedient than the control sample. These children were also maternally rated as being significantly less attentive, less oriented toward goals, and less well liked by other children. The authors did not offer a clear explanation of this association between otitis media and behavior problems in children. It was not clear whether these differences were related to otitis media or to a background of general illness. While the association was unambiguous in the data, it might have been moderated by low grade pain and discomfort or simply by the child's inability to hear.

Battin (1978) supported the findings of this study by noting that children with histories of early otitis media were often characterized as hyperactive, easily distracted, or inattentive by teachers. In addition, these children often scored poorly on measures of selective attention. Hersher (1978) compared 22 hyperactive children and 772 normal children age 7–13 matched for background characteristics. He found that the hyperactive group had a signficantly higher percentage of children (54%) who had more than six episodes of otitis media in comparison to the normal group (15%). In addition, McGee, Silva, and Stewart (1982) found that 90 children identified as having behavioral problems by parents and teachers had significantly more otitis media in early childhood than a control group.

Language development. The most frequently cited effect of otitis media has been on language development. Berko-Gleason (1983) characterized the language development of children with early histories of chronic otitis media in three ways. First, these children produced normal sounding speech. Second, when these children acquired language skills, they were delayed rather than deviant. Third, compared to control groups, children with early histories of otitis media had limited vocabularies and problems in reading. Most of the retrospective studies support the notion that the groups with a history of early chronic otitis media exhibit delayed development of language skills compared to controls but there is no consistent evidence about what areas of language are affected.

Gottlieb, Zinkus, and Thompson (1979) found significant associations between auditory processing deficits related to experience of chronic otitis media and delays in a number of outcome measures including speech and language development in children with an average age of 8.3 years. The authors used a four-group design and administered standardized instruments including the Illinois Test of Psycholinguistic Abilities (ITPA) and the WRAT. Holm and Kunze (1969) administered a battery of standardized language measures and a language development scale to an experimental and control group of children ages 5 to 9 years. The experimental group, with a history of otitis media, did significantly worse on all the combined tests, as well as a majority of the individual instruments. Zinkus, Gottlieb, and Shapiro (1978) and Zinkus and Gottlieb (1980) found that a sample of children (average age of 8.5 years) with a history of early experience of otitis media did significantly worse on specific verbal tasks that heavily involve auditory processing than did a control group. Yet there was little difference between performance in the groups if the tasks tested did not involve a great degree of auditory processing.

Speech. A number of investigators have studied the effect of conductive hearing loss due to otitis media on the development of speech processing skills (Bergstrom 1980; Brandes and Ehinger 1981; Dalzell and Owrid 1976; Jerger et al. 1983; Lewis 1976; Needleman 1977; Sak and Ruben 1981). These studies present a variety of auditory skills tests including speech discrimination in quiet, speech hearing in noise with various signal-to-noise ratios, and speech tests with degraded messages as in dichotic listening and filtered speech. For an extensive bibliography of references dealing with speech perception and communciation disorder studies associated with otitis media see Gabbard (1982). The results of all these studies point to minor hearing losses as being responsible for depressed linguistic and auditory processing abilities. However, most previous studies were limited to older children with a history of otitis media or to a single session of testing. Few pediatric speech discrimination test materials are available because of the difficulty in selecting appropriate vocabulary items and response protocol.

More recently Jerger et al. (1983) found a significant difference in speech discrimination between 25 normal preschool children and 25 children with recurrent otitis media on the Pediatric Speech Intelligibility (PSI) test which consists of word and sentence messages applicable for preschool speech discrimination testing. Results were obtained during a single session of testing, measurements were made while the children were otitis media free, and the investigators did not indicate whether they had obtained serial hearing and middle ear effusion data on the otitis media children prior to the experimentation date.

LIMITATIONS

While these retrospective studies, in general, offer clues to the direction in which longitudinally based research should move, the conclusions reached by a number of these retrospective studies are suspect due to confounds with various threats to internal and external validity (Ayukawa and Rudmin 1983; Paradise 1981). It may be difficult to draw uniform conclusions from this body of studies because the age and number of members in the subject population varies widely across the studies. For example, Brandes and Ehinger (1981) employed an experimental group/control group design in which each group contained 15 members. Similarly, Holm and Kunze (1969) used clinical and control comparison samples that contained only 16 members each. These studies, with so few members per sample of subjects, cannot be expected to have good randomization of subject attributes. Yet, retrospective studies with large numbers of subjects do exist, e.g., Silva et al. (1982) which included 402 subjects from a larger examination of 879 children.

As did the number of subjects, the ages of subjects may vary widely among studies of the effects of otitis media on the development of children. For this reason it is also difficult to make interstudy comparisons. This is especially true if one sees the effect of otitis media on the development of children's language and cognitive skills as dependent on certain critical periods. If children are tested at wide age ranges after impact of otitis media, then the effects recorded could look qualitatively or quantitatively different at different points after the critical period. In contemporary retrospective studies, the ages of the children serving as subjects may be anywhere from five to eleven years of age (Holm and Kunze 1969; Hutton 1984; Lewis 1976; Sak and Ruben 1981; Zinkus, Gottlieb and Shapiro 1978; Zinkus and Gottlieb 1980).

The demographic characteristics of samples involved in retrospective studies of otitis media may also vary widely. For example, Zinkus, Gottlieb, and Shapiro (1978) and Zinkus and Gottlieb (1980) include only white, middle-class children in their sample. Battin (1978) studied children initially defined as learning disabled. Some "primitive population" studies include Lewis' (1976) study of Australian Aborigines and Kaplan et al.'s (1973) study of Eskimo children. It is not hard to imagine that other factors might have some influence on the developmental outcomes in these widely ranging samples. Again, interstudy comparisons may be more difficult if samples are so different on background characteristics. It is certainly difficult to generalize beyond such select populations.

In the majority of retrospective studies on the effects of otitis media on children's development of language and cognitive skills, the diagnosis of otitis media is made from doctors' records, as well as from parental reports of middle ear infections. These methods are known to be highly unreliable. Yet a number of studies rely on either physicians' records or parental reports (or both) to establish a child's history of otitis media (Brandes and Ehinger 1981; Gottlieb et al. 1979; Holm and Kunze 1969; Lewis 1976; Sak and Ruben 1981; Zinkus and Gottlieb 1980; Zinkus et al. 1978).

Retrospective reliance on physicians' records to construct a history of otitis media is unreliable because the length of time spent with otitis at a critical age may not be adequately noted. Holm and Kunze (1969) note only that their subjects had chronic otitis media from before the age of two to the time of testing. Sak and Ruben (1982) evaluated subjects between the ages of eight and eleven years who had experienced otitis media before the age of five years. Brandes and Ehinger (1981) use the criteria for study participation of at least three episodes of otitis media per year, starting before the second year. Zinkus and Gottlieb (1980) required their severe otitis media group members to have experienced their first episode before the age of six months and to have had an average of four episodes a year until age three years. None of these studies, however, controlled the length of episodes of otitis media, that is, days per year with otitis media.

Some of the retrospective studies that examine the relationship between early childhood otitis media, auditory deficits, and delayed language development, report the administration of hearing tests to subjects at the time other testing takes place. Yet, the investigators quite often do not have complete audiometric histories for the study participants. While Brandes and Ehinger (1981) assessed current conductive hearing losses as part of a larger battery of auditory perceptual tests, Gottlieb et al. (1979), Zinkus et al. (1978), and Zinkus and Gottlieb (1980) have no data on hearing. None of these authors have data on their subjects' audiological competence during the period of early chronic otitis media. While at least a partially accurate history of otitis media might be constructed from physician records, audiological histories are much harder to construct without hearing assessments across the early part of the lifespan.

The outcome measures employed in retrospective studies of the effects of otitis media on children's intellectual and language development are widespread. They range from classroom and home behavior problems to measures of academic achievement. A host of indices of language development have been used as dependent measures, as have a great number of measures of intelligence. Indeed, it has frequently seemed that contemporary investigators have adopted a "shotgun approach" in specifying developmental outcomes of early experience of otitis media. That is, if a large number of outcome measures are administered to two groups of subjects, a certain proportion of those measures is bound by chance to uncover at least marginally significant differences between the groups. Yet, the majority of these authors gave little rationale for the outcome measures that they were using. Significant group differences might easily be attributed to factors left uncontrolled by inadequate matching procedures rather than by the effects of otitis media.

In contemporary literature on the effects of otitis media on child development, the procedures used to match control and clinical groups are largely undiscussed. What is revealing is that investigators routinely fail to match subjects on important variables that could very well pose threats to internal validity (Ayukawa and Rudmin 1983; Paradise 1981). For example, Holm and Kunze (1969) match subjects for sex, race, and age but fail to match them for IQ, environmental stimulation, motivation, or language experience in the home. In fact, scarcely any attention is given to family or home-centered variables and how they may serve as possible confounding influences in the mediation of the effects of otitis media. Sak and Ruben (1981) assume that environmental factors are controlled by matching children who have histories of otitis media with their siblings who have no histories of otitis media. Although this is certainly an advance over most matching procedures, this stance supposes that the home environment has remained stable in the interval between the birth of the two children.

PROSPECTIVE STUDIES

While the results of retrospective studies may be confounded for a number of reasons (Ayukawa and Rudmin 1983; Paradise 1981; Ventry 1980) the results nevertheless offer suggestions for prospective and longitudinal research. Recent (ongoing) prospective studies of the effects of otitis media on speech and language development have attempted to find the same type of detrimental effects so commonly found in retrospective studies. Yet these studies (Feagans et al. in press; Fischler, Todd, and Feldman 1985; Roberts 1986; Teele, Klein, and Rosner 1984) provide only mixed support for associations between experience of otitis media and language development found in the retrospective studies.

Fischler et al. (1985) studied a group of 167 Apache Indian children from birth to eight years of age. Otitis media was documented carefully over the infancy and early childhood period. Four subtests of the Test of Language Development were administered to the children, two receptive and two expressive subtests. Results indicate a consistent but rather modest association between otitis media and language development on some subtests. The authors suggest that these findings show weak if not counter evidence to the prevailing view of an effect. The Roberts et al. (1986) study attempted to find associations between standardized measures of both verbal and nonverbal intelligence, as well as academic performance and the number of days which the child spent with otitis media in the first three years of life. They carefully documented otitis media in a day-care-attending group of 61 low-income children. This was an exploratory study with no a priori specific hypotheses like the Fischler et al. study. No significant correlations were found between number of days with otitis media and any of the outcome measures, which included the Stanford-

Binet Intelligence Scale, the McCarthy Scale of Children's Abilities, the WPPSI, and the Peabody Individualized Achievement Test (PIAT).

The Teele, Klein, and Rosner (1984) study attempted to find associations between the time with otitis media and standardized measures of speech and language development in a sample of over 200 children. These authors, in contrast to Roberts et al. found significant associations between length of time with otitis media and progress in speech and language development. Specifically, children from a high SES group scored significantly less well on standardized instruments like the Peabody Picture Vocabulary Test, the Auditory Comprehension Quotient, and the Verbal Ability Quotient when they had a great deal of otitis media in comparison to children from the same SES group who had experienced little illness. This effect was not seen in low SES children, as they seemed to do less well on the measures of speech and language development in general.

Feagans et al. (1987) tested the hypothesis that otitis media and its subsequent hearing loss would affect only higher order language processes in the long term. This was hypothesized to be due to problems in sustained attention caused by reduced levels of hearing in early childhood. This study used the same sample as the Roberts et al. study (1986) but used regression to predict narrative storytelling skills at five and seven years of age from potent developmental predictors in early childhood. These included such factors as mothers' IQ, the home environment in infancy, the child's IQ at five years of age, and the number and length of otitis media episodes. The only variable in early childhood that remained in the final model was experience with otitis media. The other variable in the final model was the child's IQ at age five. Thus, otitis media accounted for variance beyond IQ in the prediction of a higher order language skill, i.e., narrative ability. In addition, this study found that the long term effect of otitis media was evident only in children with nine or more episodes in the first three years of life and that those children with nine or more episodes were found to be off-task twice as often as other children in their kindergarten classrooms when we observed them during academic learning activities. Poor attention, it could be argued, is the mediating variable that accounts for long-term developmental problems from otitis media.

Otitis media was diagnosed by using relatively strict criteria in all of these studies and each used pneumatic otoscopy to establish the presence of otitis media. In addition, the Roberts et al. (1986) and the Feagans et al. (1987) studies employed tympanometry to validate otoscopic findings. Hearing tests were not administered in the studies, so that otitis media could only be used as a marker for hearing loss. Only the Feagans et al. study tried to test a specific hypothesis.

There is only one study to date that has examined otitis media, its immediate effect on hearing loss, and later language functioning (Friel-Patti et al. 1982). This study followed a small group of 28 infants from birth to 24 months. Correlations were found between hearing loss (using ABR measures) and general language development at 24 months. More extensive studies of this nature are needed if the relationship is to be deemed causal.

Models of Effects

There are a variety of ways in which otitis media might have an effect on concurrent and/or later development which could be deduced from the literature just reviewed. We will present three major models as possible ones to test, although there certainly may be others that are plausible. These models can be seen in figures 1, 2, and 3.

First, the developmental effects found in both retrospective and prospective studies possibly are due not to early otitis media but to illness in general. Since it has been demonstrated that upper respiratory infections are associated with

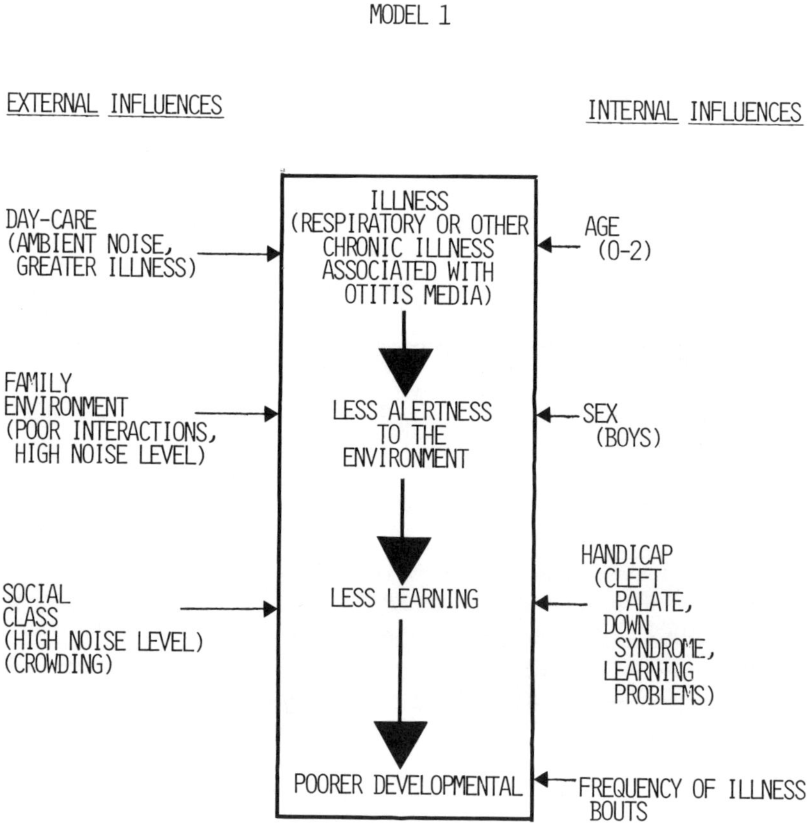

Figure 1. Effects of otitis media: Model 1.

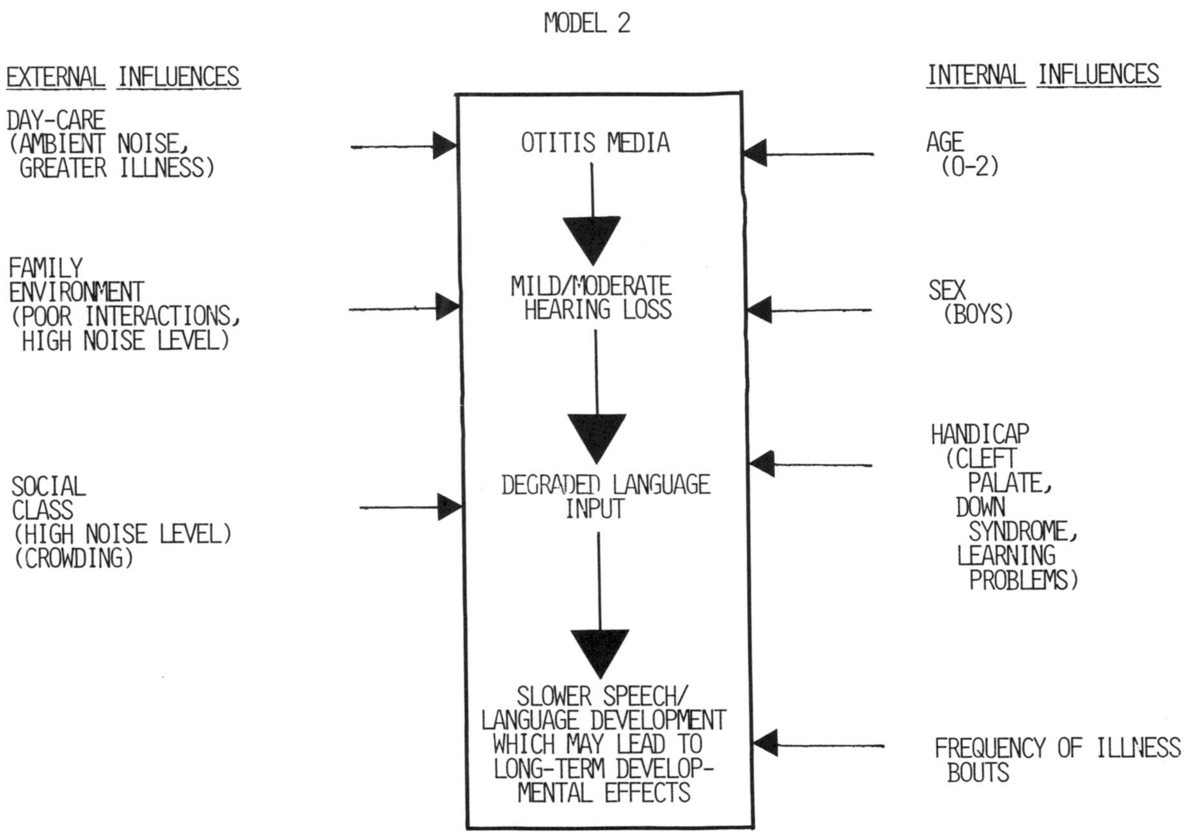

Figure 2. Effects of otitis media: Model 2.

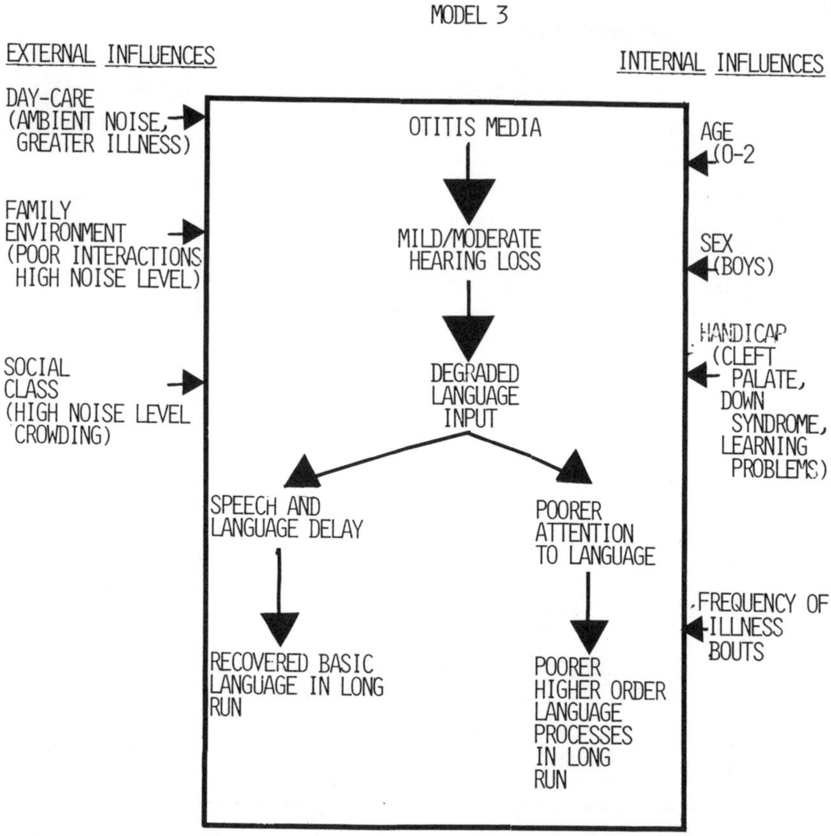

Figure 3. Effects of otitis media: Model 3.

otitis media (Henderson et al. 1982), children with more otitis media incidents may simply be showing the effects of illness. There are currently no studies that examine children's general illness apart from otitis media specifically. General illness, and chronic illness in particular, has been associated with a host of family and developmental problems for children (Hobbs, Perrin, and Ireys 1985). Even the common cold has been shown to reduce performance on achievement tests for children during the time when they have symptoms of the cold (Heazlett and Whaley 1976). Figure 1 illustrates how the child with much illness may not be able to attend to his environment as carefully, and thus may not learn at the same rate, as well children.

Second, as Menyuk (1980) has discussed, otitis media may cause effects through the child's experience with fluctuating hearing loss. Although there is really no good evidence about the effects of fluctuating hearing loss except through the otitis media literature, it has been hypothesized that the changing base on which otitis-prone children depend, forces them to base deductions about the rules of the language or degraded stimuli which may lead to deficits in language in many areas. In this way rather direct effects of the fluctuating hearing loss should be seen in the short-term and also in the long-term. These effects would be rather broad-based and affect a number of areas of language and speech (see figure 2).

Third, the fluctuating hearing loss may have only a temporary effect on the acquisition of language and other processes, but because of the inconsistency of the input, children may learn not to attend to language input as consistently as normal-hearing children. This attention problem may be the mediating variable that leads to poorer developmental outcomes in a variety of areas. This may be the most plausible model for long-term effects after hearing has returned to normal. This model would postulate only short-term problems in basic language and speech and long-term problems in higher order language processes that require sustained attention (Feagans 1986). These higher-order language skills include the ability to engage in sustained dialogues with others or to produce narrative sequences. Both of these language processes require sustained attention and are related to school performance and other important developmental markers (Feagans 1982). Let us take one example of such skill. In order to tell a coherent story, a child must be able to listen carefully to examples of such stories. If attention wanders because of difficulty in hearing or because of the habit of not listening, it will be more difficult for that child to tell a story in comparison to children who are able to sustain attention to language sequences like these narratives. Thus attention problems may indirectly affect such higher level language processes.

In all of these models, there are factors within and outside the child that influence the severity of the effect seen. In all the models those factors on the right of the figure represent influences within the child and those on the left influences that are outside the child in the environment. Each of the factors may be critical in determining the amount and frequency of the effects and will help determine which children are at most risk for detrimental developmental effects.

Although difficult to depict in the models, there is probably a threshold effect operating in the experience of this disease. One episode of otitis media in early childhood will most probably have no effect on the child's development but at some number more than one an effect may be seen, depending on the context in which it occurs. As has been suggested by others, three episodes a year for the first three years has been found to be associated with an effect (Feagans et al. 1987; Teele et al. 1984).

Intervention

Each of the models presented has implications for the kind of intervention needed. The models are similar with respect to the types of influences within and outside the child that may intensify an effect or put the child at greater risk for a developmental effect. The interventions will be discussed within a framework of intervention seen in figure 4. This intervention model can be used to discuss all the models. Only the last part of the intervention model differs for each causal model. Different strategies are used, depending on the causal influences.

The basic rationale for the first part of the intervention model is that parents and professionals outside speech and hearing who deal with young children on a daily basis lack information about what otitis media is and what the possible effects are on the child. Thus, the first step in any intervention model would be the development of information about the disease for people who deal with young children. Brochures, workshops, and other information-dissemination efforts are necessary to alert people about the identification of the disease, its treatment, and ways to prevent long-term effects.

Once information is conveyed, a mechanism needs to be in place so that adults can act on the information they have obtained. Screening children for otitis media needs to be a routine procedure performed by physicians, audiologists, speech pathologists, and nurses as well as paraprofessionals. With the advent of immittance testing, measures can be obtained on children quickly and cheaply if the equipment is available for use. Even though acoustic immittance may give some false positive results, it is an excellent screening device for further otoscopic examination and hearing testing (Paradise 1980).

Otoscopic examination may require the assistance of a skilled physician. This is somewhat costly but could be carried out effectively if children who were screened by tympanometry were seen by physicians only if they indicated abnormal tympanograms on several occasions. For instance, day-care centers with tympanometry available could screen children once a month and refer children to physicians only when they showed two abnormal tympanograms in a row. A speech and hearing specialist in the public schools could supervise such an activity.

Threshold hearing testing is valuable but, as already discussed, there are problems with obtaining these measures. Children below the age of three are very difficult to test and, even with advanced techniques, getting true thresholds on young children is a difficult and time-consuming task. Evoked potential audiometry is one possible approach to document hearing loss in infants, but this is expensive and has shortcomings in terms of the frequency range of hearing measured. It may even require some sedation of the infant in order to obtain accurate data. Hearing testing must be done to determine the degree of hearing loss and to rule out any sensorineural hearing loss but this can take time. Most physicians who are concerned about an otitis-prone child will refer them to an ENT clinic. In turn the ENT physician will refer the child for an audiological evaluation. In many cases this can take months. Assessment of auditory thresholds then may be necessary but initial intervention may begin before this has

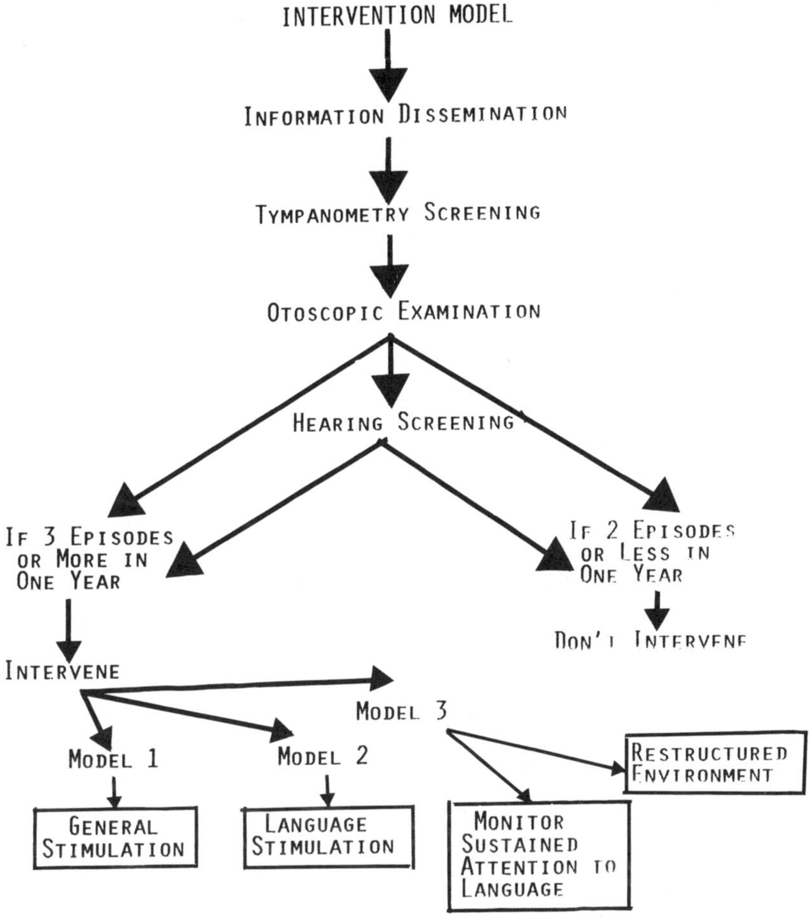

Figure 4. Diagram of proposed intervention.

been completed. This is in contrast to the testing of models in research where it is critical to understand the conditions, i.e., the degree of hearing loss, at what frequencies it occurs, at what age, etc., that make a difference for the child. In the model presented, intervention may begin before hearing testing can be completed.

After this monitoring of the disease, the question of when to intervene must be answered. Evidence is scant in this area but, as was mentioned earlier, an effect may be evident when a physician has seen a child three times in one year for otitis media. Thus, it could be a continuation of one bout of otitis media or three separate bouts. This criteria is a conservative one for intervention.

TYPES OF INTERVENTION

If the above procedure or variant on the procedure are in place in pediatric clinics and in day-care settings, interventions can be implemented in a number of areas. There may be a number of very specific interventions based on thorough language and speech testing of the children, but when this is not feasible there are a number of aspects of the child's life that can be changed relatively easily and inexpensively (Feagans 1986).

Based on the first model, children who are generally ill need general stimulation and more carefully monitored input in all areas of development. This model suggests an undifferentiated program of language, cognitive, and social development programs that might be patterned after programs devised for children from deprived home environments.

The second model concentrates efforts on specific areas of speech and language. These include specific speech discrimination or phonological training, as well as specific strengthening of morphological, syntactic, and semantic skills. This intervention might resemble programs designed for language-impared or mild hearing-impaired children.

The third model, and the one emphasized in this paper, focuses on two aspects of the child's environment. The first is to restructure the child's environment to foster adequate hearing and listening during times of otitis media. The other focuses on adult strategies to foster sustained attention to language. A few examples in each domain may help to demonstrate the thrust of such a program.

The restructuring of the child's environment is not an unreasonable task for parents or day-care staff. For instance, if a child is known to have constant otitis media and meet the threshold criteria, ambient noise, which often permeates many places children play, can be reduced by the use of rugs, by making sure the child plays in small groups of children, by placing the child close to the teacher during instruction, and by the selective use, especially during the otitis-high winter months, of techniques to make the environment more quiet for all children.

The other strategy is for adults who interact with the otitis-prone child to engage in as much one-to-one interaction as possible, especially interaction that requires sustained attention to language. In this way the child can get practice in listening carefully and enjoying it. This strategy can be employed in large groups by making sure the otitis-prone child is not looking out the window during story time or ignoring language when it is directed to him. These strategies could be taught to teachers and parents as an effective strategy with all children but especially those who are identified as otitis-prone. Some of these activities are described by Tough (1982) as meaning-extending activities. The adult engages the child in extended dialogue on a topic, encouraging the child to use language to explain, predict, or elaborate. Joint book reading (Ninio 1980; Snow, Dubber, and DeBlauw 1982) has also been shown to foster vocabulary development as well as to help the child learn the conventions of dialogue out of context. These activities seem particularly appropriate for children who need to concentrate on higher-order language processes, like the otitis-prone child.

These interventions are not new, nor are they appropriate only for the otitis-prone child. They are strategies that may help prevent later problems for these children no matter what the cause of their inattention and language problem. At the present time we do not have definitive evidence for a causal relationship between otitis media and developmental problems, but the evidence is mounting that something should be done now, even if the evidence is not complete. The cost of losing a child to poor school achievement and poor language is great in comparison to the cost of these modest programs. Although some have argued persuasively for a moratorium on tympanostomy tubes as treatment for otitis media (Stickler 1984; Paradise and Rogers 1986), they have done so because of the risks involved for the child in such an invasive operative procedure. In the interventions proposed here, there are no such risks, but the benefits may be great.

It will be up to informed professionals to devise intervention programs for these otitis-prone children. They will need to convince local communities to institute monitoring programs and to help develop new programs. Until more definitive evidence has been obtained so that we have more confidence about the nature of the effects or non-effects of early otitis media, our efforts at solutions must be rather tentative and less specified than we would like. Although causal evidence is far from definitive, it seems clear that better monitoring of the disease, professional and parent education, and general intervention programs can do nothing but improve the lives of these otitis-prone children.

REFERENCES

Ayukawa, H., and Rudmin, F. 1983. Does early middle ear pathology affect auditory perception skills and learning? Comments on Brandes and Ehinger (1981) [Letter to the editor]. *Journal of Speech and Hearing Disorders* 48:222–224.

Battin, R. R. 1978. Developmental effects of early middle ear pathology. *Texas Speech and Hearing Journal* 111:11–12.

Beauregard, W. G. 1971. Positional otitis media. *Journal of Pediatrics* 79:294.

Bergstrom, L. 1980. Continuing management of conductive hearing loss during language development. *International Journal of Pediatric Otorhinolaryngology* 2:3–9.

Berko-Gleason, J. 1983. Otitis media and language development. *In* C. D. Bluestone, J. O. Klein, and J. L. Paradise (eds.). Workshop on the effects of otitis media on the child. *Pediatrics* 71:639–652.

Berman, S. A., Balkany, T. J., and Simmons, M. A. 1978. Otitis media in the neonatal intensive care unit. *Pediatrics* 62(2):198–201.

Bess, F. H. 1983. Hearing loss associated with middle ear effusion. *In* C. D. Bluestone, J. O. Klein, and J. L. Paradise (eds.). Workshop on the effects of otitis media on the child. *Pediatrics* 71:639–652.

Bess, F. H., and Tharpe, A. 1986. Case history data on unilaterally hearing-impaired children. *Ear and Hearing* 7(1):14–17.

Bess, F. H., Tharpe, A., and Gibler, A. 1986. Auditory performance of children with unilateral sensorineural hearing loss. *Ear and Hearing* 7(1):20–26.

Brandes, P., and Ehinger, D. 1981. The effects of early middle ear pathology on auditory perception and academic achievement. *Journal of Speech and Hearing Disorders* 46:250–257.

Bzoch, K., and League, R. 1971. *Receptive-expressive Emergent Language Scale*. Baltimore: University Park Press.

Cambon, K., Galbraith, J., and Kong, C. 1965. Middle ear disease in Indians of the Mount Currie reservation, British Columbia. *Canadian Medical Association Journal* 93:1301.

Culbertson, J. L., and Gilbert, L. E. 1986. Children with unilateral sensorineural hearing loss: Cognitive, academic, and social development. *Ear and Hearing* 7(1):38–51.

Dalzell, J., and Owrid, H. 1976. Children with conductive deafness: A follow-up study. *British Journal of Audiology* 10:87–90.

Diamant, M., and Diamant, B. 1974. Abuse and timing of use of antibiotics in acute otitis media. *Archives of Otolaryngology* 100:226–230.

Feagans, L. 1982. The importance of the development of narratives for school-age children. *In* L. Feagans and D. C. Farran (eds.). *The Language of Children Reared in Poverty: Implications for Research and Intervention* (pp. 95–116). New York: Academic Press.

Feagans, L. 1986. Otitis media in children: A model of effects and implications for intervention. *In* J. Kavanaugh (ed.). *Otitis Media and Child Development* (pp. 192–208). Parkton, MD: York Press.

Feagans, L., Sanyal, M., Henderson, F., Collier, A., and Appelbaum, M. 1987. Middle ear disease in early childhood and later language skills. *Journal of Pediatric Psychology* 12(4):581–594.

Feingold, M., Klein, J. O., and Haslam, G. E. 1966. Acute otitis media in children. *American Journal of Diseases of Children* 111:361–366.

Fiellau-Nikolajsen, M. 1979. Tympanometry in 3-year-old children: Type of care as an epidemiological factor in secretory otitis media and tubal dysfunction in unselected populations of 3-year-old children. *Otolaryngology* 41:193–205.

Fischler, R. S., Todd, W., and Feldman, C. M. 1985. Otitis media and language performance in a cohort of Apache Indian children. *American Journal of Diseases of Children* 139:355–360.

Folsom, R. C., Weber, B. A., and Thompson, G. 1983. Auditory brainstem responses in children with early recurrent middle ear disease. *Annals of Otology, Rhinology, and Laryngology* 92:249–253.

Fria, J. J., Cantekin, E. I., and Eichler, J. A. 1985. Hearing acuity of children with otitis media with effusion. *Archives of Otolaryngology* 111:10–16.

Fria, J. J., and Sabo, D. L. 1980. Auditory brainstem responses in children with otitis media with effusion. *Annal of Otology, Rhinology, and Laryngology* 68:200–206.

Friel-Patti, S., Finitzo-Heber, T., Conti, G., and Brown, C. K. 1982. Language delay in infants associated with middle ear disease and mild, fluctuating hearing impairment. *Pediatric Infectious Disease* 1:104–109.

Gabbard, S. A. 1982. References for communication disorders related to otitis media. *Seminars in Speech Language and Hearing* 3:351.

Ginsberg, I. A., and White, T. P. 1985. Otologic considerations in audiology. *In* J. Katz (ed.). *Handbook of Clinical Audiology* (3rd ed.). Baltimore: Williams & Wilkins.

Gottlieb, M. I., Zinkus, P. W., and Thompson, A. 1979. Chronic middle ear disease and auditory perceptual deficits: Is there a link? *Clinical Pediatrics* 18(12):725–732.

Gray, S. W. 1983. Cognitive development in relation to otitis media. *In* C. D. Bluestone, J. O. Klein, and J. L. Paradise (eds.). Workshop on the effects of otitis media on the child. *Pediatrics* 71:639–652.

Hayden, G. F. 1981. Acute suppurative otitis media in children. *Clinical Pediatrics* 20:99–104.

Heazlett, R. N., and Whaley, R. F. 1976. The common cold: Its effects on perceptual ability and reading comprehension among pupils of a seventh-grade class. *The Journal of School Health* 46:145–147.

Hedrick, D. L., Prather, E. M., and Tobin, A. R. 1975. *Sequenced Inventory of Communication Development*. Seattle, WA: University of Washington Press.

Henderson, F. W., Collier, A. M., Sanyal, M. A., Watkins, J. M., Fairclough, D. L., Clyde, W. A., and Denny, F. W. 1982. A longitudinal study of respiratory viruses and bacteria in the etiology of acute otitis media with effusion. *The New England Journal of Medicine* 306:1377–1383.

Hersher, L. 1978. Minimal brain dysfunction and otitis media. *Perceptual and Motor Skills* 47:723–726.

Hobbs, N., Perrin, J. M., and Ireys, H. T. 1985. *Chronically Ill Children and Their Families*. San Francisco: Jossey-Bass.

Holm, V. A., and Kunze, L. K. 1969. Effect of chronic otitis media on language and speech development. *Pediatrics* 43:833–839.
Howie, V. M. 1975. Natural history of otitis media. *Annals of Otology, Rhinology, and Laryngology Suppl.* 19:67–72.
Howie, V. M. 1980. Developmental sequelae of chronic otitis media: A review. *Developmental and Behavioral Pediatrics* 1(1):34–38.
Hutton, J. B. 1984. Incidence of learning problems among children with middle ear pathology. *Journal of Learning Disabilities* 17(1):41–42.
Jerger, S., and Jerger, J. 1981. *Auditory Disorders: A Manual for Clinical Evaluation.* Boston: Little, Brown and Company.
Jerger, S., Jerger, J., Alford, B. R., and Abrams, S. 1983. Development of speech intelligibility in children with recurrent otitis media. *Ear and Hearing* 4(3):138–145.
Kaplan, G. H., Fleshman, J. K., Bender, T. R., Baum, C., and Clark, P. S. 1973. Long-term effects of otitis media: A ten-year cohort study of Alaskan Eskimo children. *Pediatrics* 52:577–585.
Kessner, S. M., Snow, C. K., and Singer, J. 1973. Assessment of medical care in children. *In* Contrasts in health status (Vol. 3). Washington, DC: Institute of Medicine, National Academy of Science.
Kirkwood, C. R., and Kirkwood, M. E. 1983. Otitis media and learning disabilities: The case for a causal relationship. *The Journal of Family Practice* 17(2):219–227.
Klee, T. M., and Davis-Dansky, E. 1986. A comparison of unilaterally hearing-impaired children and normal-hearing children on a battery of standard language tests. *Ear and Hearing* 7(1):27–37.
Leviton, A. 1980. Otitis media and learning disorders. *Developmental and Behavioral Pediatrics* 1(2):58–63.
Lewis, N. 1976. Otitis media and linguistic incompetence. *Archives of Otolaryngology* 102:387–390.
Lim, D. J., Bluestone, C. D., and Klein, J. O. (eds.). 1984. *Recent Advances in Otitis Media with Effusion* (pp. 5–44). Burlington, Ontario, Canada.
Lundgren, K., Ingvarrson, L., and Olofsson, B. 1984. Epidemiologic aspects in children with recurrent acute otitis media. *In* D. J. Lim (ed.). *Recent Advances in Otitis Media with Effusion.* Philadelphia: B. C. Decker.
Marchant, C. D., Shurin, P. A., Turczyk, V. A., Wasikowski, D. E., Tutihasi, M. A., and Kinney, S. E. 1984. Course and outcome of otitis media in early infancy: A prospective study. *The Journal of Pediatrics* 104:826–831.
Martin, F. N. 1986. *Introduction to Audiology* (3rd ed.). Englewood, NJ: Prentice-Hall.
McCandless, G. A., and Thomas, G. K. 1974. Impedance audiometry as a screening procedure for middle ear disease. *Transactions of the American Academy of Ophihalmology and Otolaryngology* 78:98–102.
McGee, R., Silva, P. A., and Stewart, I. A. 1982. Behaviour problems and otitis media with effusion: A report from the Dunedin Multidisciplinary Child Development Study. *New England Medical Journal* 95:655–657.
Melnick, W., Eagles, E. L., and Levine, H. S. 1964. Evaluation of a recommended program of identification audiometry with school aged children. *Journal of Hearing Disorders* 29:75–78.
Mendelson, T., Salamy, A., Lenoir, M., and McKean, C. 1979. Brainstem evoked potential findings in children with otitis media. *Archives of Otolaryngology* 105:17–20.
Menyuk, P. 1980. Effects of persistent otitis media on language development. *Recent Advances in Otitis Media with Effusion* 89 (3, Pt. 2).
Needleman, H. 1977. Effects of hearing loss from early recurrent otitis media on speech and language development. *In* B. Jaffe (ed.). *Hearing Loss in Children* (pp. 640–649). Baltimore, MD: University Park Press.
Ninio, A. 1980. Picture-book reading in mother-infant dyads belonging to two subgroups in Israel. *Child Development* 51:587–590.
Northern, J. L., and Downs, M. P. 1984. *Hearing in Children* (3rd Ed.). Baltimore, MD: Williams and Wilkins.
Paparella, M. M., Morizono, T., Le, C. T., Mancini, F., Sipila, P., Choo, Y. B., Liden, G., and Kim, C. S. 1984. Sensorineural hearing loss in otitis media. *Annals of Otology, Rhinology, and Laryngology* 93:623–629.
Paradise, J. L. 1980. Otitis media in infants and children. *Pediatrics* 65:917–943.
Paradise, J. L. 1981. Otitis media during early development: How hazardous to development? A

critical review of the evidence. *Pediatrics* 68:869–873.

Paradise, J. L., and Rogers, K. D. 1986. On otitis media, child development, and tympanostomy tubes: New answers or old questions? *Pediatrics* 77(1):88–92.

Pukander, J., Sipila, M., and Karma, P. 1984. Occurrence of risk factors in acute otitis media. *In* D. J. Lim (ed.). *Recent Advances in Otitis Media with Effusion*. Philadelphia: B. C. Decker.

Roberts, J. E., Sanyal, M. A., Burchinal, M. R., Collier, A. M., Ramey, C. T., and Henderson, F. W. 1986. Otitis media in early childhood and its relationship to later verbal and academic performance. *Pediatrics* 78:432–440.

Ruben, R. 1984. An inquiry into the minimal amount of auditory deprivation which results in a cognitive effect in man. *Acta Otolaryngologica* 414:157–164.

Sak, R., and Ruben, R. 1981. Recurrent middle ear effusion in childhood: Implications of temporary auditory deprivation for language and learning. *Annals of Otology, Rhinology, and Laryngology* 90:546–551.

Schwartz, R. H., Stool, S. E., Rodriguez, W. J., and Grundfast, K. M. 1981. Acute otitis media: Toward a more precise definition. *Clinical Pediatrics* 20(9):549–554.

Silva, P. A., Kirkland, C., Simpson, A., Stewart, I. A., and Williams, S. M. 1982. Some developmental and behavioral problems associated with bilateral otitis media with effusion. *Journal of Learning Disabilities* 15:417–421.

Snow, C. E., Dubber, C., and DeBlauw, A. 1982. Routines in mother-child interactions. *In* L. Feagans and D. C. Farran (eds.). *The Language of Children Reared in Poverty* (pp. 53–72). New York: Academic Press.

Stickler, G. B. 1984. The attack on the tympanic membrane. *Pediatrics* 74:291–292.

Teele, D. W., Klein, J. O., and Rosner, B. A. 1984. Otitis media with effusion during the first three years of life and development of speech and language. *Pediatrics* 74:282–287.

Tough, J. 1982. Language, poverty, and disadvantage in school. *In* L. Feagans and D. C. Farran (eds.). *The Language of Children Reared in Poverty* (pp. 3–18). New York: Academic Press.

Ventry, I. M. 1980. Effects of conductive hearing loss: Fact or fiction. *Journal of Speech and Hearing Disorders* XLV:143–156.

Vinther, B., Brahe-Pedersen, Chr., and Elbrond, O. 1984. Otitis media in childhood: Sociomedical aspects with special reference to day care conditions. *Clinical Otolaryngology* 9:3–8.

Zinkus, P. W., and Gottlieb, M. I. 1980. Patterns of perceptual and academic deficits related to early chronic otitis media. *Pediatrics* 66:246–253.

Zinkus, P. W., Gottlieb, M. I., and Shapiro, M. 1978. Developmental and psychoeducational sequelae of chronic otitis media. *American Journal of Diseases of Children* 132:1100–1104.

Chapter 22

Speech and Language Development in Hearing-Impaired Children

Harry Levitt and Nancy McGarr

Background

It is well known that the language and communication skills of hearing-impaired children are, on the average, much poorer than those of their normal-hearing peers. What is not well known is the nature of the inter-relationships between communication skills, language skills, and hearing impairment and, more importantly, to what extent these relationships are affected by educational and environmental factors. In an attempt to answer these questions, a longitudinal study was undertaken examining the development of speech and language skills in a relatively comprehensive sample of hearing-impaired children at schools for the deaf. A smaller sample of mainstreamed children was also studied.

The data reported here are extracted from a monograph soon to appear on the development of language and communication skills in hearing-impaired children (Levitt, McGarr, and Geffner 1987, in press). The study summarized here, as well as several related studies, are described in detail in that monograph.

The children participating in the study were hearing-impaired children, 10 to 11 years of age at the start of the study, attending schools for the deaf in New York State. The sample was comprehensive in that it included all children satisfying the age requirement and attending state-supported or state-operated schools for the deaf. It is estimated that over 95% of the children satisfying the age requirement and attending schools for the deaf in the state of New York participated in the study.

An important population of hearing-impaired children not included in the longitudinal study were hearing-impaired children who had been mainstreamed into the regular school system. In order to obtain some comparative data on these children, a one-year study was undertaken on a representative

This study was supported by the State of New York Education Department, Bureau for Special School Supervision, Office for the Education of Children with Handicapping Conditions.

sample of hearing-impaired children attending regular schools in the New York City school system.

The longitudinal study spanned a period of four years, and covered an age range from 10 to 14 years. Roughly 120 children were tested in each year of the longitudinal study. The study of the mainstreamed children was for one year only and involved 38 children. The ages of the mainstreamed children were comparable to those of the children at schools for the deaf during the first year of the longitudinal study.

The children attending schools for the deaf had hearing levels of 80 dB (pure tone average, 0.5, 1, and 2 kHz) or higher. The mainstreamed children were equally divided between those with hearing levels above 80 dB and those with hearing levels below 80 dB.

A wide range of tests was administered to each of the children in each year of the study. These included tests of speech reception and speech production at both the segmental and suprasegmental (prosodic) levels, a rating of each child's overall speech intelligibility, a lip reading test, a measure of written language ability, and an experimental version of the Test of Syntactic Abilities[1] (Quigley et al. 1976). The syntactic forms covered by the last-mentioned test included negation, question formation, verb forms, pronominalization, determiners, conjunctions, and embedding of clauses in complex sentences. In addition to the above tests, data were obtained on hearing level, age at onset of hearing impairment, years of special education, and other relevant educational and clinical information.

EXPERIMENTAL RESULTS

The inter-relationships between the various speech communication measures, language measures, and hearing level were analyzed using two separate techniques. The first was a factor analysis which showed that two factors accounted for most of the variance in the data. The first factor, referred to as the Language Factor, showed very high weights for all of the language measures (the various subtests of the Test of Syntactic Abilities, and the written language measure). These weights[2] ranged from just under 0.5 for the subtest on possessive pronouns to over 0.9 for the subtest on question formation. The weight for the written language measure was also close to 0.9. The second factor, referred to as the Communication/Hearing Level Factor, showed moderate to heavy weights for the various speech communication measures. These weights ranged from 0.2 for the speech reading measure to just under 0.9 for the overall rating of the child's speech intelligibility. Hearing level also showed a large

---

[1]We are extremely grateful to Stephen P. Quigley for allowing us to use the experimental version of his test and for the very helpful cooperation provided by Dr. Quigley and his staff.

[2]The weights reported here are for the factor analysis performed in the final year of the study.

negative weight for this factor. A negative weight is to be expected since the greater the hearing level the poorer the child's performance on the speech communication measures.

An important difference between the language and speech communication measures was that the language measures showed high weights on only one factor (the Language Factor) and low weights on the Communication/Hearing Level Factor, whereas the speech communication measures showed moderate to high weights on the Communication/Hearing Level Factor as well as moderate weights (roughly 0.2 to 0.6) on the Language Factor. Of the various speech communication measures, speech reading showed the greatest weight on the Language Factor.

The factor analysis was repeated for each of the four years of the longitudinal study. Only minor longitudinal changes were observed in the relationships among the various measures. Perhaps the most important change was that the degree of separation into two factors increased over time. During the first year of the study, the first two factors accounted for 76% of the variance in the data. In the last year of the study, 90% of the variance was accounted for by these two factors. A related longitudinal change showed a systematic increase over the years in the weights of the language measures on the Language Factor. This was particularly noticeable for those language tests that were very difficult and involved much random guessing during the early years of the study. A similar increase was observed over the years in the weighting of overall speech intelligibility on the Communication/Hearing Level Factor.

An alternative approach to analyzing the interrelationships among the various measures is that of the analysis of proximities (Shepard 1962). The left side of figure 1 shows the results of this analysis for children attending schools for the deaf. Each point in the diagram represents a different measure. The distance between any two points is inversely related to the correlation between the measures represented by the two points. For example, the point SC (an acronym for syntactic comprehension) represents the average score on the Test of Syntactic Abilities and the point W represents the written language measure. The points SC and W are closely spaced in the diagram indicating a high degree of correlation ($r = 0.83$) between these two measures. In contrast, the point HL, representing hearing level, is relatively far from the point SC indicating a very low correlation ($r \approx o$) between hearing level and syntactic comprehension.

As noted above, the left side of figure 1 shows the proximity plot for children at schools for the deaf (10 to 11 years of age). The right side of figure 1 shows the proximity plot for mainstreamed hearing-impaired children of comparable age. The measures represented in the two diagrams include hearing level (HL), reception of prosodic features of speech (Rpros), production of prosodic features (Ppros), reception of segmental features (Rseg), production of segmental features (Pseg), ratings of the child's overall speech intelligibility (Isp), and speech reading ability (SR). Since several of the tests were modified after the first year of the study, the suffices indicate which version of the test was used.

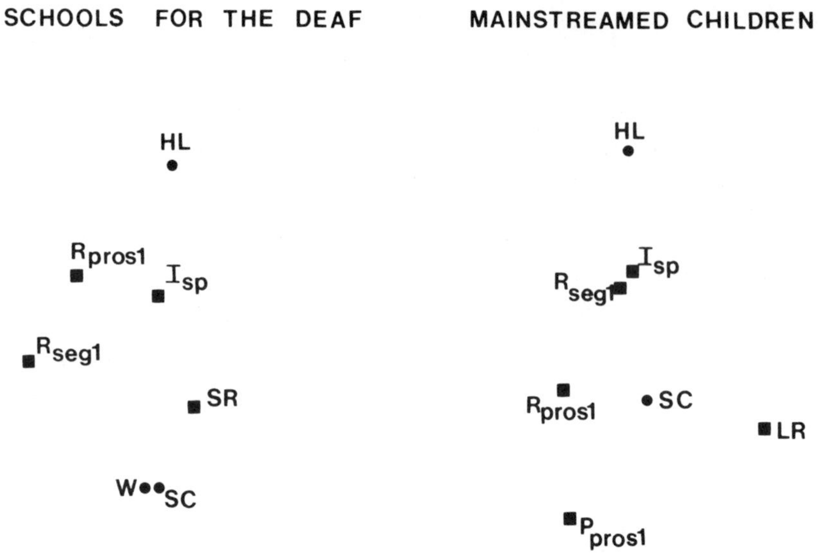

Figure 1. Proximity plots for language and speech communication measures. Each point represents one of the measures used. The distance between any two points is inversely related to the correlation between the measures represented by the two points (i.e., closely spaced points represent highly correlated measures).

HL = hearing level
Isp = speech intelligibility rating
Ppros = production of prosodic features
Rpros = reception of prosodic features
Rseg = reception of segmental characteristics
SC = syntactic comprehension (average score, Test of Syntactic Abilities)
SR = speech reading
W = written language rating

From Levitt. 1987. Used with permission of the American Speech-Language-Hearing Association.

The two proximity plots show similar inter-relationships among the various measures. In both cases, hearing level (HL) shows a higher correlation with measures of speech communication (e.g., Rpros, Rseg, Isp, SR) than with measures of language ability (W, SC). Of the communication measures, speech reading (SR) shows the highest correlation with the language measures and the lowest correlation with hearing level. The ratings of speech intelligibility (Isp) show a moderately high correlation with hearing level, but an even higher correlation with the measures of speech reception ability (Rpros, Rseg). A similar result was obtained by Smith (1975).

The most important difference between the two proximity plots is that the mainstreamed children showed a small but significant correlation ($r = 0.25$) between hearing level and the measure of syntactic ability (SC), whereas the children at schools for the deaf showed no significant correlation between hearing level and the language measures ($r \approx o$).

A proximity plot summarizing the inter-relationships among relevant educational and clinical variables is shown in figure 2. The variables shown in this

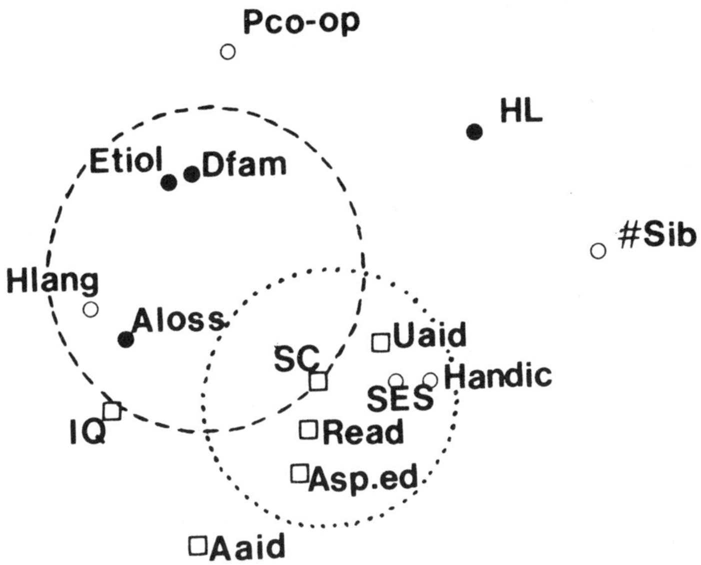

Figure 2. Proximity plot for background variables. Each point represents a separate variable. The distance between any two points is inversely related to the degree of interdependence between the two variables (i.e., closely spaced points show a high degree of interdependence). The variables enclosed within each circle show a statistically significant interdependence with each other (as obtained from chi-square contingency tables).

Aaid = age hearing aid first fitted
Asp.ed = age special education began
Aloss = age at onset of loss
Dfam = deafness in family
Etiol = etiology
Handic = other handicaps
HL = hearing level
Hlang = home language (includes sign)
IQ = intelligence quotient
Pco-op = parental cooperation
Read = reading score
SC = syntactic comprehension
SES = socioeconomic status
Uaid = use of hearing aid
#Sib = number of siblings
● = etiological variable
□ = educational variable
○ = other variables

Figure reproduced from Levitt. 1987. Used with permission of the American Speech-Language-Hearing Association.

diagram have been subdivided into three groups, *etiological, educational,* and *other.* The etiological variables, represented by solid discs, are: age at onset of hearing loss (Aloss), deafness in the family (Dfam), etiology of impairment (Etiol), and hearing level (HL). The educational variables, represented by open squares, are: age when hearing aid first fitted (Aaid), age at onset of special education (Asp.ed), intelligence quotient (IQ), reading score (Read), syntactic comprehension (SC), and use of hearing aid (Uaid). The other variables, represented by open circles, are: home language (Hlang), other handicapping conditions (Handic), parental cooperation (Pco-op), socioeconomic status (SES), and number of siblings (#Sib). Some arbitrariness was necessary in order to subdivide the variables into these three groups; the resulting breakdown was nevertheless very useful in interpreting the results.

The data summarized in figure 2 were obtained from school records and from assessments provided by the teachers. Unfortunately, it was very difficult (and in many cases, impossible) to obtain reliable information on the early audiological and educational history of the mainstreamed children. As a consequence, figure 2 relates only to children at schools for the deaf.

Two clusters of points are evident in figure 2. The first cluster, encircled by a dashed line includes most of the etiological variables (Etiol, Dfam, Aloss), as well as home language (Hlang) and syntactic comprehension (SC). With few exceptions, each of the inter-point distances within this cluster indicate a statistically significant inter-dependency ($p < .05$ in a chi-square contingency table). In contrast, the inter-dependencies between variables lying inside and outside of the dashed circle were negligibly small.

The second cluster, encircled by a dotted line, involves most of the educational variables including the two measures indicative of language development, SC and Read. As before, almost all of the variables within the cluster showed statistically significant inter-dependencies, while there were no significant inter-dependencies between those variables lying within the dotted circle and those lying without.

Most of the significant inter-dependencies shown in figure 2 were consistent with expectation. Children with good reading scores also scored well on the Test of Syntactic Abilities, as shown by the close spacing between Read and SC in the diagram. Similarly, children who had the benefit of special education at an early age showed higher reading scores and, to a lesser extent, higher scores on the Test of Syntactic Abilities.

The diagram also shows several significant inter-dependencies which are not immediately obvious. For example, Hlang and Aloss are closely spaced, indicating a significant relationship between home language and age at the onset of deafness. The reason for this interaction is that all the children with sign as their home language were born of deaf parents and were typically deaf at birth.

Of particular interest are the relationships between hearing level and language skills and between hearing level and speech communication skills. The solid curve in figure 3 shows the average score for children 10 to 11 years of age on the Test of Syntactic Abilities. The curve shows the mean test score (averaged over successive 10 dB increments in hearing level) for prelingually hearing-impaired children without additional handicapping conditions and whose first language was either English or sign. The dashed curves show average scores for particular sub-populations of the hearing-impaired children. These include postlingually deafened children, children who had the benefit of special education early in life (prior to three-years of age), children with other handicapping conditions, children from a non-English speaking home, and

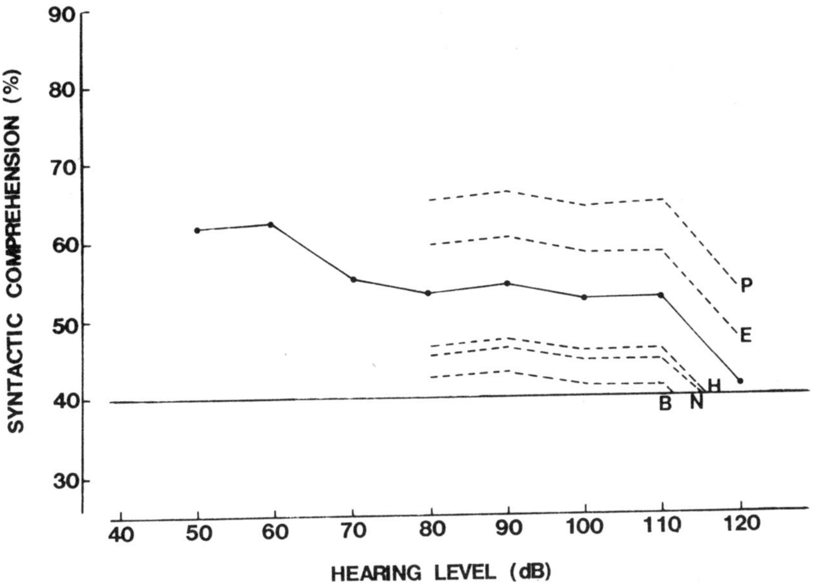

Figure 3. Syntactic comprehension as a function of hearing level. The solid curve shows average score on the Test of Syntactic Abilities (Quigley et al. 1976) for prelingually hearing impaired children 10 to 11 years of age without additional handicapping conditions and whose first language was either English or sign. The dashed curves are for specific sub-populations of hearing-impaired children showing significant differences in average performance. These curves have been estimated from an additive, multiple linear regression model Levitt 1987.

P = postingually hearing impaired
E = early special education
H = other handicapping conditions
N = non-English-speaking home (excluding sign language)
B = severe behavioral or emotional problems

children with severe behavioral or emotional problems. With the exception of the early special education group, the above sub-populations of hearing-impaired children are typically not considered in studies of this type. The mainstreamed children, for example, were all prelingually hearing impaired with no additional handicapping conditions and without severe behavioral or emotional problems. As a consequence, the average curves for these special sub-populations are only for children at schools for the deaf. These children all had hearing levels of 80 dB or higher.

It is important to note that the sample of children within each sub-population was small and hence the dashed curves should be regarded as rough estimates only. An additive, linear regression model was used in estimating these curves. For further information, see Levitt (1987).

The postlingually hearing-impaired children showed substantially higher scores on the Test of Syntactic Abilities. Their scores were over 10 percentage points higher, on the average, than those of the typical prelingually hearing-impaired child. Those children who had the benefit of early special education also showed significantly higher test scores, on the average. The curves for children with other handicapping conditions, or from non-English-speaking homes, or with severe behavioral or emotional problems, showed significantly poorer test scores, on the average. The poorest scores of all were obtained by children with severe behavioral or emotional problems. These children were particularly difficult to test and their low scores reflect the combined effects of poor syntactic skills and a lack of co-operation during testing.

Two other important sub-populations were hearing-impaired children of deaf parents, and mainstreamed children. Both of these groups of children showed significantly higher test scores, on the average. Separate curves are not shown for these two sub-populations for statistical reasons. For children of deaf parents, there were too few data points to derive a reliable curve. A problem in representing the mainstreamed children with a separate curve is that all of the children with hearing levels less than 80 dB were mainstreamed and most of those with hearing levels above 80 dB were concentrated in the region of 80 to 90 dB.

The relationship between speech intelligibility and hearing level is shown in figure 4. As before, the solid curve is for prelingually hearing-impaired children without additional handicaps and whose first language was either English or sign. The dashed curves show average performance for postlingually hearing-impaired children, children with significant high-frequency hearing[3], children who had the benefit of early special education, children from non-English-speaking homes, and children with severe behavioral or emotional problems. The first three of these special sub-populations showed signficantly higher intelligibility ratings, on the average. The remaining two sub-populations showed significantly poorer speech intelligibility ratings, on the average. Although not shown as a separate group in the diagram, the mainstreamed hearing-impaired children showed significantly higher intelligibility ratings (by roughly 1 rating point, on the average).

The association between hearing level and speech communication skills other than speech intelligibility is similar to that shown in figure 4. As noted earlier, there is a fairly high correlation between speech reception skills (e.g., Rseg, Rpros) and speech intelligibility (Isp). These skills also show a moderately high correlation with hearing level. Similar correlations also exist between hearing level and the production of specific speech features (Pseg, Ppros). The correlation between speech reading and hearing level is not as great and the average curve relating these two variables is not as steep as that shown in figure 4 (Isp vs HL) but steeper than that shown in figure 3 (SC vs HL).

---

[3]Children with hearing levels at 8 kHz greater than that at 4 kHz were defined as having significant high-frequency hearing. Note that the conventional pure-tone average does not distinguish between children with or without high-frequency hearing.

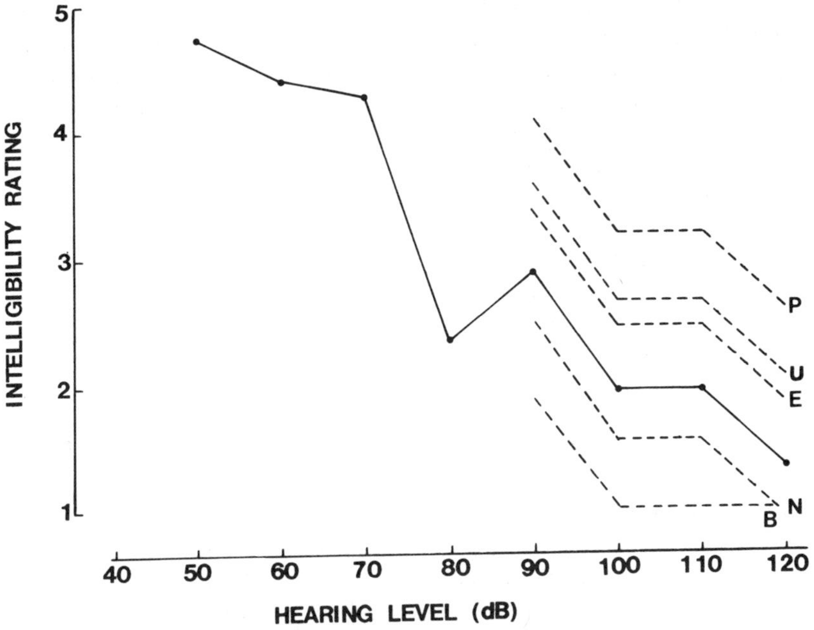

Figure 4. Intelligibility rating as a function of hearing level. The solid curve shows the average intelligibility rating (1 = unintelligible, 5 = completely intelligible) for hearing-impaired children 10 to 11 years of age without additional handicapping conditions and whose home language was either English or sign. The dashed curves are for specific subpopulations of hearing-impaired children showing significant differences in average performance. These curves have been estimated from an additive, multiple linear regression model Levitt 1987.

P = postlingually hearing impaired
U = significant high-frequency hearing (U-shaped audiogram)
E = early special education
N = non-English-speaking home (excluding sign language)
B = severe behavioral or emotional problems

DISCUSSION

One of the most surprising results obtained in this study was the low correlation between hearing level and the two language measures (SC and W). This correlation was virtually zero for children at schools for the deaf. It would be erroneous to conclude, however, that hearing level and language skills are unrelated. Examination of figure 3 shows that the curve relating syntactic comprehension (SC) to hearing level (HL) is essentially flat over the range from 80 to 110 dB. (W also shows very little variation with HL over this range of hearing levels.) Since the vast majority of children at schools for the deaf have hearing levels within this range it is not surprising that a negligibly small correlation was obtained between hearing level and the language measures for children at schools for the deaf.

Very few hearing-impaired children have hearing levels poorer than 100 dB. These children are often referred to as "feelers" since they are presumably feeling rather than hearing the test stimuli. Only five children were found to fit this category and although their language skills were measurably below those of other profoundly hearing-impaired children their numbers were too few to have a noticeable affect on the statistical correlation between hearing level and language skills.

For the mainstreamed hearing-impaired children the correlation between hearing level and language skills was small but statistically significant (r = 0.25 for HL and SC). By design, half of the mainstreamed hearing-impaired children had hearing levels of less than 80 dB, and as is evident from figure 3, there is a gradual decrease in the average score on the Test of Syntactic Abilities with increasing hearing level for hearing levels below 80 dB.

The shallow slope of the average (solid) curve in figure 3 indicates that even children with only moderate hearing losses scored relatively poorly on the Test of Syntactic Abilities. If language skills are already well below normal for children with hearing losses of 40 to 50 dB, as shown in the figure, then children with less severe losses should also show a significant correlation between language skills and hearing level over the range 0 to 40 dB. More attention should be paid to this group of children who are typically not thought of as being seriously impeded by their hearing impairment.

The many factors found to have a significant effect on the development of language and communication skills in hearing-impaired children can be subdivided into two broad groups; those factors over which clinicians and educators have no control (e.g., age at onset of hearing impairment) and those factors that are a direct result of clinical and/or educational intervention (e.g., age when special education began). Of the latter group of factors, the age at which special education began showed the largest effect. Those children who had received special education from the age of three years or younger showed significantly higher speech and language scores, on the average. Further, the improved performance shown by these children was evident more than a decade after their early start in special education.

Educators and clinicians have long championed the need for early intervention. The data presented here provide strong quantitative evidence of the association between superior speech and language skills and early intervention. It is important to bear in mind, however, that the observed relationships are correlational in form and are not necessarily causal. Although the children who had received early special education showed superior speech and language skills, it does not necessarily mean that early intervention was the cause of the measured improvement. Other factors which, in turn, are correlated with early intervention may also have contributed. For example, a child who has received special education from a very early age is also likely to come from a home environment with a high degree of parental involvement, motivation, and concern for the child's development. These factors do not operate independently and it is difficult to assess the role of each in facilitating the development of language and communication skills. It is our view that these factors act symbiotically and that early intervention is only one facet of the whole. In encouraging early intervention, it is important not to lose sight of other relevant factors.

A second important caveat is that early intervention is, of itself, insufficient to guarantee improved performance. Although the majority of children who received early special education showed better than average test scores, there was nevertheless a significant number whose scores were below average. In contrast, the children who did not have the benefit of early special education, with few exceptions, showed poorer than average scores. (The most notable exceptions here were those children with hearing impairments acquired postlingually.) These results indicate that early intervention may be necessary but, of itself, insufficient for long-term gains in speech and language development. Obviously the quality of the special education provided and other relevant factors, such as the child's home environment, play an important role.

As expected, children with hearing-impairments acquired postlingually showed superior speech and language skills. Although this result is well known, there is a paucity of data on expected levels of performance for postlingually hearing-impaired children. The data obtained here provided useful quantitative information on the magnitude of the differences in speech and language skills between pre- and postlingually hearing-impaired children. The relatively high scores shown by the postlingually hearing-impaired children, impressive as they are, should be regarded as relatively conservative since data were only obtained for postlingually hearing-impaired children at schools for the deaf. Postlingually hearing-impaired children who have been mainstreamed successfully would be expected to show even higher levels of performance than those reported here.

An observation of particular interest was that, on the average, hearing-impaired children of deaf parents did relatively well on the language measures but not on the speech-communication measures. Several reasons have been proposed to explain these differences. Firstly, there are fewer problems of adjustment for deaf parents of a hearing-impaired child. Secondly, inherited hearing impairment is usually entirely peripheral whereas other forms of hearing impairment may often involve additional central impairments. Thirdly, and perhaps most importantly, the deaf infant is immersed in an environment where some form of signing is the home language, and hence the earliest stages of language are acquired without impediment.

As noted by Levitt, McGarr, and Geffner (1987) it is important to bear in mind that the acquisition of sign as a first language is very different from learning sign language later in life. Also, although the children of deaf parents in this study showed superior language skills, on the average, the language skills of the best of these children were no better than the language skills of the best of those hearing-impaired children who had the benefit of effective special education very early in life. Exposure to language at an early age thus appears to be the critical factor, rather than the type of language.

A relatively neglected group of hearing-impaired children are those with measurable high-frequency hearing. It is not common practice to measure residual hearing at frequencies above about 4 kHz in "deaf" children; also, very few hearing aids provide amplification at these high frequencies. Yet, as shown in this study, at least 10% of the children at schools for the deaf and an even higher proportion of mainstreamed hearing-impaired children had significant high-frequency hearing. None of these children had hearing aids designed for high-frequency amplification. Nevertheless, despite the inadequacies of their hearing aids, these children showed superior communication skills. Much more needs to be done to identify children with significant high-frequency hearing, to provide appropriate amplification for these children, and to provide more effective auditory and speech training to take full advantage of their high-frequency residual hearing.

Another neglected group of children are those with no measurable hearing. Although, as noted earlier, the number of such hearing-impaired children is relatively small, they present a challenge that must be met. As shown by the final portion of the average (solid) curves in figures 3 and 4, both the speech and language skills of these children are well below those of profoundly hearing-impaired children with some measurable hearing.

A question that is often asked is whether language development in hearing-impaired children is delayed or deviant. The data obtained in this study indicate that the question itself is inappropriate. All of the children in the study showed both delays and differences (not necessarily deviations) in their language development. Developmental delays were far more noticeable, however, than differences in patterns of development, although the two appear to be closely related.

The children who scored least well on the language measures showed extremely long delays in their language development as well as marked differences in patterns of development with even simple syntactic forms. In many cases, these children developed non-standard syntactic forms that could be attributed to their slow development of other emergent forms. The children who scored relatively well on the language tests showed measurable delays in their language development but only subtle differences in their pattern of development for the simpler syntactic forms. It was only for the more advanced syntactic forms, such as those involving complex sentences, that systematic differences in patterns of development were clearly evident.

A question of great practical importance is the effect of mainstreaming on the development of language and communication skills in hearing-impaired children. Although this study was not designed to address this issue, the data nevertheless provide several revealing insights. It is to be expected that mainstreamed children should have language and communication skills that, on the average, are superior to those of their peers at schools for the deaf. The differences in relative performance are due, in large measure, to the selection process whereby children are mainstreamed. Hearing-impaired children with good language and communication skills are much more likely to be placed in a regular school environment than children with relatively poor skills.

The data obtained in this study showed that the speech-communication skills of the mainstreamed children were well above the average level of performance for children at schools for the deaf. The language skills of the mainstreamed children, however, were not uniformly better than those for children at schools for the deaf. Those mainstreamed children who did well on the language tests did very well, but those who did poorly did very poorly. In particular, there there were several mainstreamed children who were not profoundly hearing-impaired, but whose level of performance was below that of profoundly hearing-impaired children at schools for the deaf.

It should be remembered that the sample of children from schools for the deaf was comprehensive and included children with additional handicapping conditions, as well as children with severe behavioral or emotional problems. In contrast, the sample of mainstreamed children excluded such "problem" children. Considering the differences between the two samples of children and the inherent bias in the selection process for mainstreaming, serious questions should be raised regarding the effect of mainstreaming on those hearing-impaired children at regular schools who are not performing as well as their peers at schools for the deaf.

The data obtained in this study support the view that mainstreaming can be of great benefit to those children who manage to succeed in a regular school environment but that it can also be detrimental to the development of language and communication skills for those hearing-impaired children who are unable to function effectively in a mainstreamed environment. Greater care needs to be given to the selection process for mainstreaming and, if a child has been mainstreamed, much greater attention needs to be paid to that child's relative progress. The many successes that have been obtained with mainstreaming should not be allowed to obscure the many failures that have also resulted from mainstreaming.

An educational issue that was not addressed was the relative effect of the various educational philosophies (oral, total, manual) in facilitating the development of language and communication skills. This was done deliberately since it was apparent at the outset that the size of the study, large as it was, was insufficient to provide a reliable answer. In order to perform such an investigation properly, all factors (other than education philosophy) known to affect the development of language and communication skills should be balanced out. Considering the large number of such factors, such an investigation would need to be extremely large. The data obtained in this study supported this view in that the children who did best came from a variety of educational programs and the children who did poorly were distributed among all of the schools.

Acknowledgements

Many researchers, teachers and clinicians contributed to the research reported here and we would like to thank them most sincerely for their assistance. In particular, we would like to thank Toni Gold for her help on this project as well as our research assistants, Cheryl Barry, Jane Carp, Sister Rosemary Gaffney, Lisa Rothman-Freeman, Everett Leiter, Adriana Oleksuik-Velez, and Susan Wurtzel. We would also like to thank Harvey Stromberg and Marian MacEachron for their expert assistance in computing and analyzing the data and Linda Ashour for her valuable help in preparing the manuscript.

We are indebted to Stephen Quigley for allowing us to use his Test of Syntactic Abilities before its final publication and also for his advice and that of his staff in using and interpreting the many subcomponents of that test. The supervisors and staff of the schools for the deaf were also most helpful and encouraging. Their assistance is gratefully acknowledged. The participating schools were:

Bureau for Hearing Impaired Children, Manhattan
The Cleary Deaf-Child Center, Ronkonkoma
Lexington School for the Deaf, Jackson Heights
Mill Neck Manor School for the Deaf, Mill Neck
New York School for the Deaf, White Plains
New York State School for the Deaf, Rome
School for the Deaf-J.H.S. #47, Manhattan
Rochester School for the Deaf, Rochester
St. Francis de Sales School for the Deaf, Brooklyn
St. Joseph's School for the Deaf, Bronx
St. Mary's School for the Deaf, Buffalo

Most important of all, we would like to thank the children who participated in the study.

References

Levitt, H. 1987. Interrelationships among the speech and language measures. *In Development of Language and Communication Skills in Hearing-impaired Children,* H. Levitt, N. McGarr, and D. Geffner (eds.). Chapter 9, ASHA Monograph #26, Washington, D.C.: American Speech-Language-Hearing Association.

Levitt, H., McGarr, N., and Geffner, D. 1987. *Development of Language and Communication Skills in Hearing-impaired Children,* ASHA Monograph #26, Washington, D.C.: American Speech-Language-Hearing Association.

Quigley, S. P., Wilbur, R. B., Power, D. J., Montanelli, D. S., and Steinkamp, M. W. 1976. *Syntactic Structures in the Language of Deaf Children* (Final Report, Project #233175). Urbana: Institute for Child Behavior and Development, University of Illinois at Urbana-Champaign.

Shepard, R. N. 1962. The analysis of proximities: Multidimensional scaling with an unknown distance function. *Psychometrika* 27:125–140, 219–245.

Smith, C. R. 1975. Residual hearing and speech production in deaf children. *Journal of Speech and Hearing Research* 18:795–811.

Chapter 23

Management of Preschool Hearing-Impaired Children: A Cognitive-Linguistic Approach

Mary Pat Moeller

The primary objective of early intervention programs for hearing-impaired children is reduction of the effects of their sensory deficits on language acquisition. Programs strive to provide the child access to communicative competence through comprehensive habilitation, including amplification, parent guidance, perceptual and cognitive skill development, and aggressive language intervention. In recent years, the proliferation of research in early childhood language has prompted reconceptualization of the language intervention process. This changing body of literature has numerous implications for the management of the preschool-aged hearing-impaired child. Key principles in cognitive/linguistic management, based on the contemporary psycho- and sociolinguistic issues, will be the focus of this paper.

Two major shifts in conceptualization of children's language acquisition have occurred since the 1960s, when syntactic models, such as transformational grammar, dominated (deVilliers 1983). The mid-1970s brought understanding of the importance of semantic and cognitive aspects of the language acquisition process (Bloom and Lahey 1978). In the late 1970s language use (pragmatics) was determined to have a predominant role in language learning (Bates 1976). Most recently, the child's learning of social rules governing language use in various contexts has been investigated (Bates 1976; Bruner 1975; Corsaro 1984; Halliday 1975). Contemporary theories view the child's developmental task as learning to use language to encode cognitive knowledge in social situations (Friel-Patti and Lougeay-Mottinger 1985). An integrated perspective of language has evolved—one that recognizes the interdependent contributions of linguistic, social, and cognitive learning to communicative development.

How have theoretical changes influenced the language intervention process? In the 1960s, the language therapy process was characterized by a behavioristic orientation. Snow et al. (1984) noted that such approaches elicited imitation and emphasized drill and extrinsic reinforcement. The drills were product-oriented and focused primarily on the structure of expressive language. Psycholinguistic models of the 1970s generated semantically-based approaches that sought to elicit meaningful comments from the child. These were then expanded by the clinician to provide complete language models. More recently the literature has recommended that clinicians approach the young child with the recognition that discourse is the proper forum for developing language (Boothroyd 1982). Ethnographic research has revealed that children learn language through meaningful dialogues. Certain facilitative characteristics of normal caregiver/child interactions have been identified (Cross 1977, 1978; Waterson and Snow 1978). Attempts have been made to extend these productive features to clinician/child exchanges (Snow et al. 1984). (One might argue that this objective remains elusive to some clinicians.) This latest shift in intervention approach is both meaning-based and function-based. Emphasis is placed on turn-taking and learning language within social/conversational contexts. Rather than requesting imitation or merely expanding utterances, the clinician seeks to engage the child in dialogue by following the child's lead and reinforcing his verbal or nonverbal initiations with semantically contingent responses. The emphasis on semantically tied responses emerged from research implicating the negative effects of adult utterances that change a child's topic or fail to relate to the child's focus (Cross 1977; Snow et al. 1984).

The current emphasis on replicating, as closely as possible, normal facilitative interactions has also brought into question the role of imitation and constant correction of children's errors. These strategies are generally seen as counterproductive to the establishment of meaningful dialogue (Anderson 1979; Cross 1984; White and White 1984). The over-use of these strategies with hearing-impaired children has been challenged, especially when the child's intention and social interaction is thwarted. Earlier language "bombardment" approaches have given way to interpersonal, conversational approaches. No longer is it "talk, talk, talk," but rather "converse, converse, converse."

The charge to the clinician, then, is to provide the child with natural interactions, while placing emphasis on turn-taking and extended conversations, semantically contingent responses, and integrated focus on semantic, syntactic, social and cognitive goals within pragmatically appropriate contexts. Given the integrative nature of this "ideal" approach, it is no wonder that practice often lags behind theory. The interdependence of form, content, and use behaviors in language acquisition is not fully understood. Integration of these areas throughout preschool language curricula is indeed challenging. In practice, actualization of an integrated approach may be thwarted by: (a) restricted therapy contexts; (b) limitations of evaluation materials used to develop goals; (c) need to provide a hearing-impaired child with repetitive exposure, often resulting in overly directive approaches; (d) individualized educational plans that are product-oriented or that view form, content, and use as discrete areas, and/or (e) tradition.

Are there ways that programs for young hearing-impaired children may better achieve an integrative, pragmatically-based approach? The following premises are proposed in response to this question. These perspectives are based on clinical attempts to implement an integrative approach, critical review of traditional approaches, and implications from the normal language literature.

Premise One: Language intervention approaches should incorporate the view that the child is an active participant in the language learning process.

In the past, preschool hearing-impaired children were treated as passive recipients of knowledge imparted didactically by adults. Adults assumed a directive role to "teach" language. The "teachability" of language has been seriously questioned, and directiveness has been associated with impedance to language-learning and creativity (Cross 1984). Studies have underscored the importance of adult assumption of a facilitator's role. Such a role is felt to encourage the child's active attempts to construct meaning through dialogue.

Consider the following parent/child exchange:

Adam: Mom, 25 is the Olimik, right?
Mom: I think so. What's "Olimik," Adam?
Adam: It's when the police come . . . see like that sign—25 Olimik.
Mom: Oh, I see. 25 is the speed limit.
Adam: Yeah, Mom. If you go more than 25 the police give you a ticket!

In this example, the child applies his language skills to investigate and shape his world knowledge. He checks his notion with the adults, and assimilates the feedback to reshape his concept of reality. Hearing-impaired children need to be provided with language-learning environments that motivate active exploration and adult encouragement to encode their thoughts verbally.

A framework that is well-suited to active learning is a cognitively oriented approach. It is important that the child's language needs not be addressed in isolation, but rather, within a broad, developmental framework. Boothroyd (1982) asserts that a central ability that hearing-impaired children must acquire is that of representing thoughts, internally, by language patterns. The child also needs to develop a detailed and accurate understanding of his world. These important language skills have their roots in cognition. In many respects, cognition and language are inseparable.

Several preschool programs for hearing-impaired children have promoted a cognitive/linguistic approach to learning (Grammatico and Miller 1974; Stone 1980; Moeller and McConkey 1984; Moeller, Osberger, and Morford 1986). In such an approach, language and thinking skills are emphasized in synchrony. Primary emphasis is placed on helping children construct relationships and develop representational skills on increasingly abstract levels. Justification for cognitively oriented approaches comes from:

—recognition of the importance of the child's active, explorative role in learning—his need for opportunities to manipulate, create and notice relationships—and to apply his knowledge to solving daily problems.

—Recognition of the importance of verbal reasoning and problem solving skills to future academic and social functioning.

—Recognition of the necessity of laying a foundation for verbal/conceptual reasoning and logical thought in the preschool years.

Cognitively oriented approaches share certain features, and may be characterized by:

1. Methods of presentation that lend organization to the child's learning.
2. Active learning that involves mental, as well as physical, manipulation. (e.g., the children's observation of the cooking time for potatoes baked in a microwave and a regular oven prompts mental comparison of *fast* vs. *slow*). Active learning also implies child-directed activities and provision of toys and materials that promote multiple possibilities for representation, experimentation, attention to and comparison of attributes and properties (Boothroyd 1982; Weikart, et al. 1971).
3. Provision of opportunities to solve nonverbal and verbal problems in flexible ways; the teacher can capitalize on those opportunities (e.g., child runs out of masking tape he was using to build (represent) a road. Teacher prompts, "I see you want a longer road. The tape is gone. What will you use?").
4. Use of thought-provoking and divergent questions to prompt children's discovery of relationships. This goal is facilitated by pairing linguistic and nonlinguistic cues to assist the child in developing comprehension skills. Nonlinguistic/contextual cues are initially numerous, but are gradually lessened to encourage the child's reliance on lingustic input (Boothroyd 1982; Moeller and McConkey 1984).
5. Use of a daily routine that encourages decision-making, prediciting, and reasoning (e.g., provision of opportunities for child to plan his playtime by selecting play areas and tools he will use first, second . . .).
6. Provision of a curriculum content in key experience areas to support the emergence of logical thinking (e.g., the child is exposed to activities that promote classification, seriation, temporal relations, spatial relations, and numeric concepts; see Hohmann, Banet, and Weikart [1979], Weikart et al. [1971], and Moeller et al. [1986] for further discussions).

Curriculum materials from early childhood education have been successfully adapted for use with preschool hearing-impaired children in a self-contained, experimental program (Moeller and McConkey 1984; Moeller et al. 1986). Results to date have been encouraging, particularly in the children's concept applications, flexible and creative thinking, and spontaneous initiation of language. Considering points made earlier, cognitive/linguistic strategies also have the advantage of providing conversations that emerge from the child's perspectives and from his mental and physical manipulations.

Premise Two: In order to facilitate cognitive/linguistic development, clinicians must give up some control. That is, attention should be given to a balance between adult-directed and child-directed activities.

Premise Three: Play provides a rich context for social and cognitive learning.

Another recent development in child language research is the study of how children learn to use language for social interaction (sociolinguistics). Prutting (1982) has suggested that pragmatics be defined as social competence. Her position is that the most competent communicators know more than grammar, meaning, and function rules. They are sophisticated in their knowledge of the subtle and changing social rules that govern human interactions. Thus, being an effective communicator requires more than formulating thoughts into well constructed, grammatically correct utterances. Competence requires that the communicator respect elusive and changing social conventions.

Ethnographic studies of children's worlds (e.g., their interactions with parents or peers in nursery schools) have begun to describe how hearing children gain social knowledge that is critical to communicative competence (Corsaro 1984). McCune-Nicolich and Carrol (1981), Westby (1980), and Corsaro (1984) suggest that clinicians consider peer interaction play settings as rich therapeutic contexts for developing social cognition and language. Although hearing-impaired children have been observed to lag behind their hearing peers in verbally mediated symbolic play, routine applications of goal-directed play experiences suggest that this characteristic is amenable to change (Moeller et al. 1986). Corsaro (1984) suggests that social cognition may be facilitated in children when adults extend their traditional roles in play settings and become partners, observers, and mediators of peer interaction. Observation of problems children encounter repeatedly in social and communicative interactions with their peers will suggest intervention priorities.

Darbyshire (1977) expressed concern at the underutilization of play in preschools for hearing-impaired children. When play periods are provided, they often lack structure or goals, and are considered "free" time. An attractive approach to goal-oriented play has been described by Weikart and his colleagues at the High/Scope Educational Research Foundation (Weikart et al. 1971). The staff of the experimental preschool at the Boys Town National Institute turned to the use of goal-directed play experiences in response to a self-study that revealed: (1) less than adequate frequency of spontaneous initiations (teachers usually controlled the topic); (2) language "stalled" in the here and now; (3) limited imaginative uses of language by the children. Play experiences that would reinforce representational behavior, fantasy, and cooperation, we felt, would be a preferred route to program goals.

This play therapy approach, derived from early childhood education, incorporates a process-oriented daily routine known as "Plan - Do - Recall." In the *planning* phase, children receive structured guidance, enabling them to use language to make and express choices regarding their upcoming playtime. Planning time provides the child with consistent opportunities to express himself and see himself as one who can act upon decisions (Hohmann et al. 1979; Weikart et al. 1971). The teacher helps the child extend and elaborate his plan through directive questioning. The cumulative effect of the child's repeated encounters with this systematic routine is his ability to initiate dialogue, express choices, describe his plan in detail, and gradually incorporate peers in his planning behavior.

To illustrate, early in the school year one child's plan was limited to gesturing toward the building area and saying "fireman with tinker toy." As the year progressed, the child learned about his environment through exploration and gained the skills to verbalize his actions. His plans became elaborate, and he began to include social negotiation and extension of his plans into the future. The following scenario illustrates this process.

Child: First I will play in building area.
Teacher: Oh, and what will you do there?
Child: Build a fire station!
Teacher: Really? A fire station! What will you use to build it?
Child: Tinker toys and three towels for beds.
Teacher: Oh, you will have several firemen?
Child: Yeah (directs comment to peer) Matt, get Josh and we'll build. You can be chief, okay?
Matt: Ok, I'll get the ladder (The day before the boys had hidden their tinker toy ladder when they negotiated a plan to play with it again tomorrow).

Planning is followed by a period of *doing*. Here, children implement their plans during an active play period. Adults become play partners, but the context and play are child-directed. The adult reacts to ideas, encourages verbal and nonverbal representations, and uses comments and questions to prompt children to notice relationships or expand their play. For example, one child represented a tinker toy rod as a fishing pole. The clinician responded, "Oh, I see you are fishing. This string is your line. What will you use for bait?" The child thought and then announced "maybe macaroni will work."

Clinician: Good idea. Macaroni looks like a worm. How will you keep it on your string?
Child: I think tape will work.

Corsaro (1984) has described several interesting dimensions in children's construction of social play contexts. He reported that hearing children use several verbal and nonverbal "ploys" to gain entry to play groups. Because their social awareness is developing, they are often subtle in their entry behaviors. They have learned that direct requests (e.g., "Can I play?") too often result in denial of permission. Corsaro (1984) also notes that a common "script" in children's play is the creation of some crisis (e.g., a fire, a monster, or an injury) that calls the play partners into cooperative action to resolve the conflict. Kretschmer and Kretschmer (1984) suggest that children's knowledge of story grammar may have its roots in these rich, early discourse experiences.

Observation of hearing-impaired children in two cognitively oriented programs revealed emergence of similar phenomena as noted by Corsaro, especially when adults promoted such fantasy and helped children extend it. Children in one group were observed to gain entry in subtle ways (by knocking on imaginary doors; by timing their entry and offering a novel toy or role-appropriate comment). The strong emphasis on language use prepared them to engage in sociodramatic play, much of which, of necessity, is mediated linguistically. One child, for example, spent the play period meticulously arranging chairs. When questioned, he told his teacher he was building an airplane. Once his task was completed the child summoned the other children, asking, "Will you come on my airplane and fly to California?" As the children entered the imaginary aircraft, several donned fire hats. This made little sense to the adult play partner, whose apparent liability was viewing the world from an adult frame of mind. The child who was first to bring along a fire hat for the ride imagined and suggested a fire on the runway shortly after take off. Their play then took a spontaneous, creative shift toward resolution of the problem. Prompting by the teacher assisted the children in verbally mediating their cooperative play encounter.

The final step of the process is *recall*. This is a conversationally based review of the play period. Children are helped to recall verbally their play experience. The teacher supports and extends their descriptions of what they enjoyed, problems they encountered, etc. This is another example of a conversational context that is tied closely to the child's interest and frame of reference. It becomes a natural situation in which to reinforce the use of past tense in conjunction with the informational function of language. The open-ended nature of the Plan - Do - Recall process builds on children's representational abilities, and encourages them to create and socialize. The context of play should be given serious consideration as a medium for establishing natural and facilitative conversational exchanges.

Premise Four: The diversity among children who are learning language needs to be considered in program planning and implementation.

Along with increased understanding of the interdependence of form, content, and use behaviors has come an appreciation for the wide variability and diversity in individual children's language/learning styles. Measurements used commonly to equate children's language levels, e.g., mean length of utterance (MLU) are now seen as potentially misleading, as important differences in the pragmatic domain are underrepresented by such measures (Wollner 1983). As noted earlier, pragmatic development results from linguistic, social, and cognitive experience. Intervention programs must respect the number of variables that contribute to diversity in language learning and use. Programs must be tailored to the uniqueness of individual children.

This suggests that clinicians need to apply problem-solving strategies in routine case management. Kamhi (1984) recommends consistent use of clinical science techniques, such as hypothesis testing, critical analysis of treatment outcomes, and application of single subject design.

Hearing-impaired children have long been recognized as a heterogeneous group, requiring individualized management (Brackett 1982; Moeller, McConkey, and Osberger 1983). Yet, there is inconsistent application of diagnostically oriented treatment approaches. Too often, the hearing-impaired child is expected to "fit" into the existing curriculum. Considering the increasing numbers of hearing-impaired children with multiple-handicapping conditions, the challenge to consider diversity within language learning is of paramount importance.

The systematic application of techniques to validate intervention approaches empirically is overdue with the hearing-impaired population. Especially when difficult decisions need to be made about communication modalities, options must be selected objectively, based on evidence from the child's response to systematic learning trials. A brief example illustrates this point. A six year old female presented with a steeply sloping moderate-to-profound sensorineural hearing loss of unknown etiology (figure 1). She was followed by a neurologist

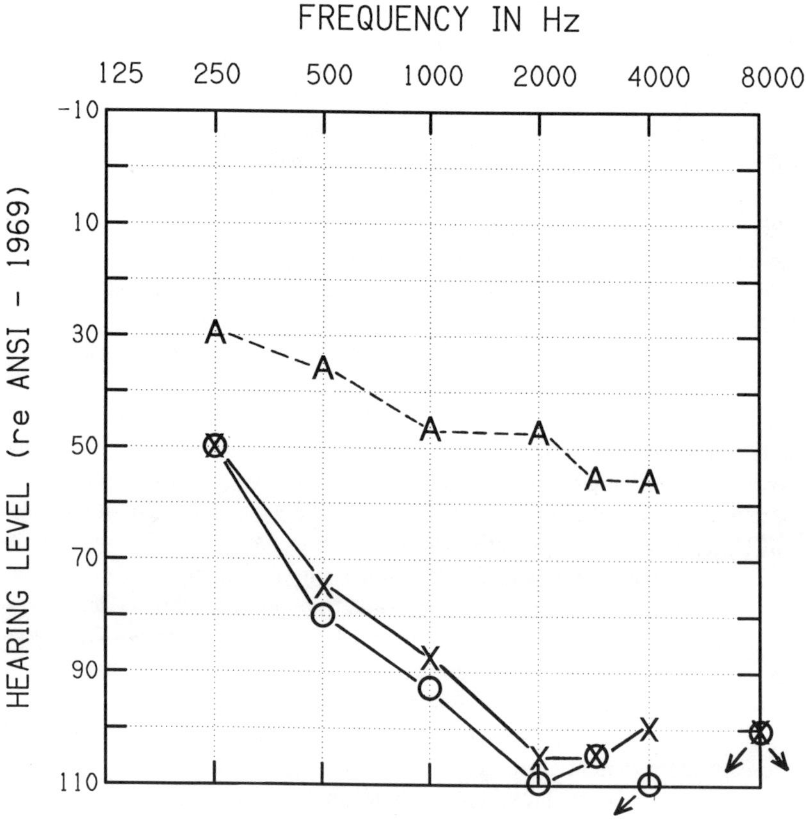

Figure 1. Pure-tone audiological results for six-year-old female.

for treatment of a seizure disorder. In spite of 5 years of intensive, quality oral education, she failed to progress beyond rudimentary communication skills. She was referred for multidisciplinary evaluation by her teachers, who felt that augmentation with a visual communication system was needed. The parents were attracted to the cued speech system, given their commitment to the development of the child's spoken language skills.

Multidisciplinary evaluation revealed borderline nonverbal intellectual skills, significant verbal memory deficits, attention deficits, severely delayed language, unintelligible speech, and poorly controlled seizures. Following medical intervention, the child was enrolled in a diagnostic teaching program, designed to assess her learning rates in cued speech in comparison to signs. Figure 2 shows the results of the child's vocabulary learning. Her initial receptive learning rates in cued speech vs. sign were similar. Two weeks into the program, the child recognized 50% of the target vocabulary presented in cued speech and 60% presented in sign. The relative efficacy of the systems became clear, however, only when retention of trained information was probed. The child demonstrated enhanced retention in the sign mode, with continued progress toward mastery. Retention of words presented receptively through cued speech was discouragingly low. Parental observation of the child's performance provided them with objective input for decision making. Given the multiplicity of issues and diversity among learning styles, efforts should be made to base educational management decisions objectively on data from the child's performance. This goal will be facilitated by research describing processing strategies and constraints within various modalities.

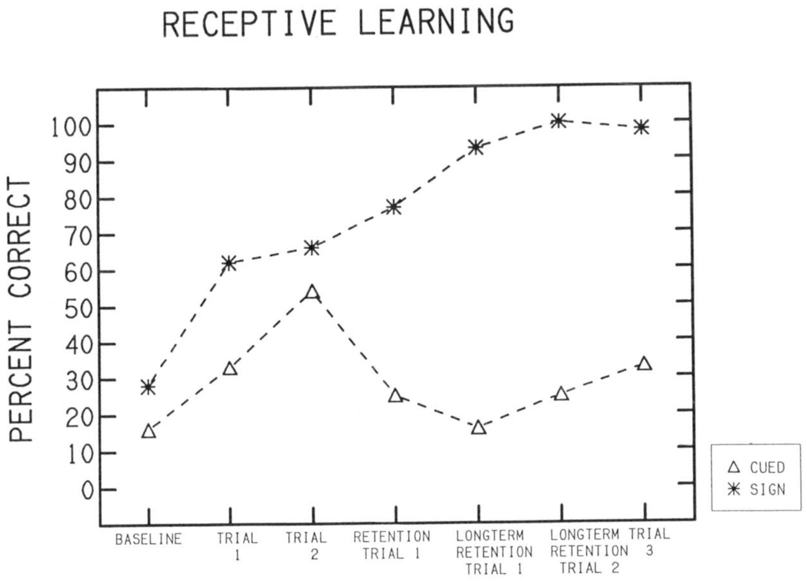

Figure 2. Comparison of a child's vocabulary learning rates with cued speech versus signed input.

Premise Five: "Parents' Power" is often an untapped resource. Parents should participate in substantive ways in the language-intervention process.

Intensive parental involvement has been recognized as an integral component of quality programs for hearing-impaired children. With the advent of successful parent/infant programs, parents often enter the preschool experience with excellent skills—an outgrowth of multifaceted support systems. Yet, critical evaluation of patterns of service delivery to parents suggests the need for continued expansion of services to parents of preschoolers. In particular, the following are seen as priorities:

1. Given significant societal changes (e.g., dual career families; single, working parents) creative models of service delivery are needed. Are parent programs serving only a select few?
2. Parents should be given opportunties to extend therapy principles in natural ways to numerous social and experiential contexts. Periodic workshops that orient the parents to process-oriented curriculum goals would be useful. Videotapes that contrast directive vs. supportive/open-ended teaching strategies are recommended.
3. Parents may be better able to extend dialogue if they receive information about the child's daily school experience. A daily communication diary that travels to and from school can provide the parents with enough shared background to understand and elaborate upon the child's attempts to relay events that happened at school.
4. Parents of signing children need special and aggressive assistance if they are to provide a nurturing linguistic environment for the child. Research studies (Bornstein, Saulnier, and Hamilton 1980; Swisher and Thompson 1985) show that most hearing parents gain only minimal sign competencies and tend to delete critical linguistic features in their signed messages. In part, sign language teaching strategies may be implicated. The complexities of the parent's sign language learning needs have been underestimated (Swisher and Thompson 1985). Creative approaches to intervention are needed if nurturing dialogue is to be established between hearing parents and their signing children (Moeller and Luetke-Stahlman in press).

SUMMARY

This paper has reviewed several recent developments in language theory and their implications for intervention with the hearing impaired. The need for an integrative approach has been highlighted. A truly integrative approach focuses on: (a) goal-oriented experiences within natural social contexts; (b) provision of dialogue as the context for learning semantic and syntactic rules; (c) opportunities for social, linguistic, and cognitive learning; and (d) an active role on the part of the child.

If current psycholinguistic and sociolinguistic theories are to be effectively incorporated into intervention programs, several needs remain: (1) increased appreciation of how form, content and use behaviors interact in language learning; (2) strengthening of evaluation theories and practice; (3) wider dissemination of theoretical information to generate revision of traditional approaches; and (4) programs that will accommodate the diverse needs of hearing-impaired children by providing methodological options selected in an objective manner.

The influx of knowledge in the area of child language has generated exciting changes in intervention strategies. Consequently, preschool programs for the hearing impaired are undergoing a face lift. Remodeling includes donning a child-oriented perspective, a concern with process instead of product, and an integrated, individualized sociolinguistic approach.

REFERENCES

Anderson, B. J. 1979. Parents' strategies for achieving conversational interactions with their young hearing-impaired children. *In* A. Simmons-Martin and D. R. Calvert (eds.). *Parent-Infant Interaction*. New York: Grune and Stratton.

Bates, E. 1976. Pragmatics and sociolinguistics in childhood language. *Language Deficiency in Children: Selected Readings*. Baltimore: University Park Press.

Bloom, L., and Lahey, M. 1978. *Language Development and Language Disorders*. New York: Wiley & Sons.

Boothroyd, A. 1982. *Hearing Impairments in Young Children*. Englewood Cliffs, N.J.: Prentice-Hall.

Bornstein, H., Saulnier, K., and Hamilton, L. 1980. Signed English: A first evaluation. *American Annals of the Deaf* 125:467–481.

Brackett, D. 1982. Language assessment protocols for hearing-impaired students. *Topics in Language Disorders* 2(3):46–55.

Bruner, J. 1975. The ontogenesis of speech acts. *Journal of Child Language* 2:1–20.

Corsaro, W. A. 1984. The development of social cognition in preschool children: Implications for language learning. *Topics in Language Disorders* 4(4):77–95.

Cross, T. 1977. Mother's speech adjustments: The control of selected child listener variables. *In* C. Snow and C. Ferguson (eds.). *Talking to Children: Language Input and Acquisition*. Cambridge: Cambridge University Press.

Cross, T. 1978. Mother's speech and its association with rate of linguistic development in young children. *In* N. Waterson and C. Snow (eds.). *The Development of Communication*. New York: Wiley & Sons.

Cross, T. 1984. Habilitating the language impaired child: Ideas from the studies of parent-child interactions. *Topics in Language Disorders* 4(4):1–13.

Darbyshire, J. 1977. Play partners in young children with impaired hearing. *Volta Review* 79:19–26.

deVilliers, P. 1983. Semantic and pragmatic factors in the acquisition of syntax. *Volta Review* 85:10–28.

Friel-Patti, S. and Lougeay-Mottinger, J. 1985. Preschool language intervention: Some key concerns. *Topics in Language Disorders* 5(2):46–53.

Grammatico, L., and Miller, S. 1974. Curriculum for the preschool deaf child. *Volta Review* 79: 19–26.

Halliday, M. A. K. 1975. *Learning How to Mean: Exploration in the Development of Language*. London: Edward Arnold.

Hohmann, M., Banet, B., and Weikart, D. 1979. *Young Children in Action*. Ypsilanti, Michigan: High-Scope Press.

Kamhi, A. 1984. Problem solving in child language disorders: The clinician as clinical scientist. *Language, Speech, and Hearing Services in the Schools* 15:226–234.

Kretschmer, R., and Kretschmer, L. 1984. Habilitation of language of deaf children. *Current Therapy of Communication Disorders*. New York: Thieme-Stratton, Inc.
McCune-Nicolich, L., and Carroll, S. 1981. Development of symbolic play: Implications for the language specialist. *Topics in Language Disorders,* 1(1):1–14.
Moeller, M. P., McConkey, A., and Osberger, M. 1983. Evaluation of the communicative skills of hearing-impaired children. *Audiology* 8:113–127.
Moeller, M. P., Osberger, M. J., and Morford, J. 1986. Enhancing the communicative skills of hearing-impaired children. *In* J. Alpiner and P. McCarthy (eds.). *Aural Rehabilitation: Adults and Children.* Baltimore: Williams and Wilkins.
Moeller, M. P., and Luetke-Stahlman, B. in press. Are parents trained to sign to their deaf children? *American Annals of the Deaf.*
Moeller, M. P., and McConkey, A. J. 1984. Language intervention with preschool deaf children: A cognitive/linguistic approach. *In* W. H. Perkins (ed.). *Current Therapy of Communication Disorders: Hearing Disorders.* New York: Thieme-Stratton.
Prutting, C. 1982. Pragmatics as social competence. *Journal of Speech and Hearing Disorders* 47:123–134.
Snow, C., Midkiff-Borunda, S., Small, A., and Proctor, A. 1984. Therapy as social interaction: Analyzing the contexts for language remediation. *Topics in Language Disorders* 4(4):72–83.
Stone, P. 1980. Developing thinking skills in young hearing-impaired children. *In* S. A. Kirby (ed.). *Curriculum, Content and Change, Volta Review:* 82(6):345–353.
Swisher, V., and Thompson, M. 1985. Mother's learning simultaneous communication: The dimensions of the task. *American Annals of the Deaf* 130:212–218.
Waterson, N., and Snow, C. 1978. *The Development of Communication.* New York: Wiley & Sons.
Weikart, D., Rogers, L., Adcock, C., and McClelland, D. 1971. *The Cognitively Oriented Curriculum,* Urbana, IL: University of Illinois Press.
Westby, C. 1980. Assessment of cognitive and language abilities through play. *Language, Speech and Hearing Services in Schools* 11:154–163.
White, S., and White, R. 1984. The deaf imperative: Characteristics of maternal input to hearing-impaired children. *Topics in Language Disorders* 4(4):38–49.
Wollner, S. 1983. Communicating intentions: How well do language-impaired children do? *Topics in Language Disorders* 4(1):1–14.

Chapter 24

Management of the School Age Child: A Psychosocial Perspective

Julia M. Davis

The population of hearing-impaired children designated as "school-aged" is a heterogeneous one, ranging in age from 5 to 18 years and in degree of hearing impairment from 20 dB to 110 dB. These children also differ regarding their speech and language skills, academic abilities, and the extent to which their families are involved in their educational lives. Furthermore, the age of onset and type of hearing loss vary across children, as does the prevalence of other handicapping conditions. Therefore, any discussion of the management of this diverse group of children must be based on the assumption that there are some central issues affecting hearing-impaired children in school settings that can be discussed for the group as a whole in spite of the diversity it represents. Because my own research and experience involves hard-of-hearing rather than deaf children, and because so much less has been written about them, I will limit my remarks to the management of children with mild to moderately severe hearing losses.

I would like to propose the following assumptions about school-aged hard-of-hearing children.

First, hearing-impaired children who require special services have some general characteristics in common. Their hearing losses have resulted in speech and language deficits of varying degrees, which in turn have affected either their academic achievement or their social adjustment or both.

Second, the communicative demands associated with school life are particularly difficult for hearing-impaired children to meet.

Third, failure to meet the demands and expectations of teachers and fellow students often results in damaged self-esteem and social isolation.

Finally, educational placement and other management decisions affect hearing-impaired school children significantly; unfortunately, they are not always based on the individual characteristics of the children in question or on the interaction between those characteristics and the educational environment in which they must go to school.

The purpose of this chapter is to describe the communication and educational problems faced by children with hearing impairment, the communicative demands associated with school activities, and strategies for the management of the difficulties that result.

Characteristics of Hearing-Impaired School Children

There are no good estimates of the number of hearing-impaired children between the ages of 5 and 18. Published estimates tend to vary widely, probably because different criteria for hearing loss are used by different investigators. If mild unilateral or conductive losses are included, the numbers tend to be high. If only permanent, bilateral hearing losses are included, estimates will be significantly lower. Unfortunately, criteria are not given for most of the estimates that appear in the popular press, and careful demographic studies of the population have not been published. The number of children served in educational programs usually includes only those children who require special classroom placement at least part of the time. It is possible that fewer than half the hearing-impaired children in the country fall into that category, because there are many more children with mild hearing losses than there are children with severe hearing impairments. The less severely hearing-impaired children are not likely to be found in special classes or schools. Some estimates suggest that there are 20–30 times as many mildly hearing-impaired children as severely hearing-impaired (Bess and McConnell 1981); Silverman and Lane (1970) have estimated that at least 2.5 million school children exhibit hearing impairment, whereas the number of children being served in special programs in the United States in 1983 was reported to be 45,496 (American Annals of the Deaf 1984).

Describing the characteristics of a population that is difficult to even count because of its diversity is a challenging task. Three published studies of school children in Iowa attempted to provide both demographic and psychoeducational data for hard-of-hearing children (Davis et al. 1981; Shepard et al. 1981; Davis et al. 1986). In the first two studies, hearing-impaired children were chosen randomly from the population of children who failed hearing screening in their schools. Their records were examined and the characteristics of children who fell into certain hearing-loss categories were described. The third study described the characteristics of a much smaller sample of hearing-impaired children who had undergone a special standardized assessment protocol. Members of the same investigative team have recently collected additional data on 376 Iowa school children who are enrolled in the itinerant teaching programs of the 15 Area Education Agencies in the state of Iowa (Davis, Elfenbein, and Pratt 1986). Results of these studies will be summarized briefly in the following sections.

COMMUNICATION CHARACTERISTICS

One of the difficulties in describing the communication characteristics of hearing-impaired children as a group occurs because there appears to be so little correlation between their speech and language skills and other relevant factors, such as the degree of hearing loss (within a wide range), use of amplification, or extent of professional intervention. Therefore, it is not possible to estimate accurately the specific speech and language deficits a given child may have by examining an audiogram or by referring to average data obtained on similar children. Nevertheless, within a broad range of actual performance, there are certain characteristics that are more or less typical of children with hearing losses that range from mild to moderately severe (20–80 HL).

Production and perception of speech. The speech characteristics of profoundly hearing-impaired children have been described extensively in the literature. They include phonatory, articulatory, and prosodic problems that are unique to this population. Difficulty with the coordination of respiration and phonation is common, resulting in poor ability to sustain phonation and produce a consistent vocal tone during speech. Pitch breaks and nasal or pharyngeal resonance are common. The articulation of vowels as well as consonants is often inaccurate, and the intelligibility of speech by deaf children is often extremely poor. The severity and uniqueness of these speech problems sets deaf speakers apart from their peers.

The speech of hard-of-hearing children is much less affected and not well described in the literature. Elfenbein, Hardin, and Davis (1985) reported that hard-of-hearing children exhibit speech that is much more like that of normal-hearing children than deaf children. Voice quality and resonance are rarely affected by moderate hearing loss and speech prosody is usually normal. The primary area of difficulty for hard-of-hearing children lies in the development of articulation skills. They exhibit misarticulations consisting primarily of phoneme substitutions and distortions. The phonemes on which errors are made vary with the degree of hearing loss; a mild loss of hearing causes difficulty with the production of fricatives, whereas hearing losses between 45 and 60 dB affect affricates and, to a lesser extent, glides as well. Children with hearing losses greater than 60 dB usually exhibit a significant number of misarticulations on all phoneme types except plosives and nasals. Table I shows the performance of 40 hard-of-hearing children on the *Fisher-Logemann Test of Articulation*. Many of the children demonstrated normal or near normal articulation. In contrast to deaf children, hard-of-hearing youngsters do not misarticulate vowels. This fact, combined with their ability to use normal prosody and phonation, results in speech that is highly intelligible (Conrad 1979).

Table I

Mean Performance by Children With Mild to Moderate Hearing Impairment On the Fisher-Logemann Test of Articulation Competence						
	Percent Correct					
Degree of Loss	Total Score	Nasals	Plosives	Glides	Affricates	Fricatives
<45dB	88.65	98.07	93.58	96.15	91.02	77.92
45–60dB	85.19	96.87	96.52	89.84	73.95	73.09
>60dB	84.14	98.86	96.96	82.62	68.18	73.27

Although their speech production is characterized by relatively mild articulation problems, hard-of-hearing children view this as a major deficit. They dislike being singled out for speech therapy, but they consider their speech problems to be the most serious effect of the hearing loss (Peterson 1972). Certainly, it is the most obvious one, and it sets them apart from their peers in an embarrassing way. It may be that this aspect of their performance interferes more than any other with normal social interactions with hearing classmates, although failure to perceive speech accurately would seem to be a more serious communication deficit.

During interviews, hard-of-hearing children seemed unaware or unconcerned about problems perceiving the speech of others (Davis et al. 1986). Indeed, the speech recognition skills of the children who were interviewed were excellent. Their average NU CHIPS scores are shown in table II. Their auditory skills in quiet were well-developed, allowing them to listen to a story and re-tell it, often with minimal use of visual cues. When asked if they ever had difficulty understanding others, the children almost always said yes, but then described failure to *comprehend* what was said because they didn't "know enough." It is interesting to note that the children interviewed by these investigators did not often report failure to understand adults; they seemed to see peer communication as more important and to respond to questions about communication solely from that perspective. In this context they believed their attempts at communication were hampered by personal flaws that were not always related to hearing impairment. They described the people with whom they did not communicate well as "smarter" or "higher education kids," and themselves as "dumb" or not "knowing as many words" (Davis et al. 1982).

Vocabulary skills. For many hard-of-hearing children, none of the perceptions reported above are accurate. Not only were the children in that study as

Table II

Means and standard deviations for NU CHIPS scores for three groups of hard-of-hearing children (adapted from Davis et al. 1986)				
	Quiet, Aided		Noise, Aided	
Hearing Loss	Mean	SD	Mean	SD
<45 db	97.67	3.60	87.27	11.27
45–60 dB	96.86	3.57	86.00	12.12
>60 dB	90.50	6.74	72.50	16.76

intelligent as their classmates, some of them had equally strong vocabularies and were achieving as well in school. As a group, however, these hard-of-hearing children exhibited more deficits in vocabulary knowledge than any other language skill measured. Children with sharply sloping hearing losses seemed especially vulnerable to have reduced vocabularies. On the average, hard-of-hearing children's word knowledge appears to be delayed by 2–3 years relative to their peers (Young and McConnell 1957; Davis 1974; Brannon 1968; Davis et al. 1986). Table III shows a summary of several studies of vocabulary usage by hearing-impaired children.

Not only are overall vocabulary skills influenced by hearing impairment, certain other aspects of vocabulary knowledge that contribute directly to the problems these children face in communicating with their peers are also affected. Hearing-impaired children do not learn as much incidental vocabulary as do normal-hearing children. In addition, the most common meaning of a word is usually learned first and well, with other meanings of that word being learned poorly or not at all. Consequently, slang use of common words may be confusing to hearing-impaired children, making it more difficult for them to follow casual conversations among classmates and friends. Even when slang or unusual meanings of words are understood, the ease with which they are incorporated into daily usage varies and may lag significantly behind that of other children. Although relatively minor problems with the learning of vocabulary may not seem of major importance as we view the overall development of a given child, they could be a major deterrent to easy communication between

Table III

Summary of Studies of Vocabulary Knowledge of Hard-of-Hearing Children

Investigator	Subjects	Measures	Results
Young and McConnell (1957)	Matched pairs of normal and hearing impaired children (8–14 years)	Ammons Full Range Picture Vocabulary Test	No hearing-impaired child scored as high as the matched pair
Davis (1974)	Hard-of-hearing and normal 6–8 year olds	Boehm Test of Basic Concepts	91% of hard-of-hearing children scored below the 10th %ile
Brannon (1968)	30 normal-hearing, 15 deaf, and 15 hard-of-hearing	Analysis of spoken language samples	Hard-of-hearing (27–66 dB) showed reduced number and type of words. Total number of words was less than half that of normal-hearing children. Hard-of-hearing did not use adverbs, pronouns, or auxiliary verbs correctly.
Davis, et al. (1986)	40 hard-of-hearing children, 5–18 years	Peabody Picture Vocabulary Test, Revised	Only 6 children scored within normal range; mean age deviation was −2.18 years

children, further setting the hearing-impaired child apart in the important area of socialization.

Other Language Skills. The syntactic skills of hard-of-hearing children also vary widely. The errors that appear in language samples produced by these children involve primarily the bound morphemes of the language (Brown 1984; Elfenbein et al. 1985). Word endings such as plural, tense, or adjectival markers are omitted frequently. Serious errors of grammar are not common, although the use of modal or auxiliary verbs is sometimes affected along with omission of prepositions, infinitives, and determiners. Complex sentence structures (passive voice, relative clause, complementation) may not be comprehended accurately or produced (Brannon and Murry 1966; Pressnell 1973; Wilcox and Tobin 1974; Davis and Blasdell 1975). Nevertheless, the overall impression is that most of the common grammatical forms are used accurately by hard-of-hearing children. The casual observer would probably be unaware that there was poor comprehension of complex sentences or that the sentences produced by these children were simpler in construction than those of their peers. It is unlikely, therefore, that grammatical problems influence the success of oral communication efforts although they almost surely interfere with academic success, especially with the development of reading skills.

In summary, the communication skills of hard-of-hearing children are characterized by relatively good auditory speech recognition in quiet, mild to moderate articulation problems, somewhat reduced vocabularies, and delayed development of the ability to use complex grammatical structures. Of these, only the articulation disorder is obvious to classmates and educational personnel.

EDUCATIONAL CHARACTERISTICS

The data available suggest that hard-of-hearing children are academic underachievers (Kodman 1963; Quigley and Thomure 1968; Peterson 1972; Conrad 1979; Davis et al. 1981; Davis et al. 1986). They exhibit poorer reading skills than their normal-hearing peers, and reduced performance in those academic subjects that are based on the ability to learn new information through reading. Even mathematics performance is affected, but to a lesser extent than other subjects (Davis et al. 1981; Wood, Wood, and Howarth 1983, Davis et al. 1986). Verbal skills and academic achievement are highly correlated, regardless of whether the former are measured by vocabulary tests, language arts tasks, or verbal I.Q. measures (Davis et al. 1986).

Some individual hearing-impaired children may achieve very well academically. However, as a group they fall into three major categories: those performing at grade level, those performing slightly below grade level, and those whose performance is significantly below grade level. As a rule, then, any degree of hearing impairment can put a child at risk for reduced academic achievement.

One measure of the educational problems of hard-of-hearing children is the proportion who have repeated grades in school. Our recent survey of 376 children enrolled in the itinerant teaching program of the 15 Area Educational Agencies in Iowa revealed that 27.5 percent of them had repeated a grade (Davis et al. 1986). The range was from first grade to 11th, but failure of the fourth, fifth, and sixth grades was most common. Bess (1982) reported an even higher proportion of grade failures by children with unilateral hearing losses. It seems clear that hearing loss interferes with educational achievement, often to a significant degree.

SOCIAL AND BEHAVIORAL CHARACTERISTICS

Only a few studies have reported data concerning the social behavior and emotional adjustment of hard-of-hearing children (Goetzinger, Harrison, and Baer 1964; Fisher 1966; Peterson 1972; Kennedy and Bruininks 1974; Reich, Hambleton, and Houldin 1977; Davis et al. 1986; Loeb and Sarigiani 1986). In general, hard-of-hearing children exhibit social problems characterized by less acceptance by their peers, a tendency to be more aggressive in their behavior, and serious difficulty making friends. The result is a high degree of social isolation.

SUMMARY OF CHILDREN'S CHARACTERISTICS

The most common problems experienced by hard-of-hearing children in the schools are the inability to hear in the school setting, articulation problems, vocabulary deficits, delayed development of reading skills, and social isolation. These are not independent problems that can be attacked and solved separately; each influences another and interferes with its resolution. Furthermore, all children do not exhibit these problems to the same degree. Careful assessment of the performance of individual children is necessary before an appropriate management program can be developed.

CHARACTERISTICS OF SCHOOLS

When children enter school they encounter a world full of new experiences, complex heirarchies, and varied rules and regulations. Adjustment to the behavior, academic, and social expectations involved requires a certain level of maturity, comprehension of social mores, language skill, and self confidence. Such is the resiliency of youth that the vast majority of young children are able to make a smooth transition from the protected environment of the home to the relatively unfamiliar jungle of the school. This is especially true when parental expectations are reasonable and the family is accepting and supportive. The normal level of anxiety associated with testing one's self against the system and one's peers soon decreases as success occurs and new friends are made.

If a normal level of academic success does not take place at once, but friends are made and social acceptance occurs, anxiety is not likely to increase and the child's sense of accomplishment may be undiminished. If academic success occurs but friendships develop more slowly, self-esteem may suffer slightly but solace can be found in the rewards that come from high achievement. For children who achieve little academic success, perhaps even requiring special placement, tutoring, or other forms of assistance, and who find it difficult to make friends as well, the school experience may be a very unhappy one.

COMMUNICATION DEMANDS

From the moment a child enters school, certain expectations are made clear. Group activities abound and although certain types of originality are rewarded, others are not. Children are expected to conform to both spoken and unspoken rules. Indirect requests are common. Such pragmatic aspects of communication are not taught overtly; those that have not been learned before school age must be absorbed through observation of the behavior of older children or teachers. Children learn from the mistakes of their peers, and everyone settles into the routine of school pretty quickly. The children who do not adapt to the rhythm and rules of school are almost immediately noticed, not only by alert teachers but by their rapidly maturing classmates.

Furthermore, a certain level of linguistic knowledge is assumed. The language of instruction requires comprehension of terms such as "more than," "on top of," "next to," and other items depicting quantity, location, or some other common language concept. Curriculum materials are controlled for vocabulary but not for syntactic structure, and the usual vocabulary may be a higher level than hearing-impaired children can comprehend easily. Therefore, whereas the task for normal-hearing children is to use previously learned language as a basis for learning new material, the hard-of-hearing child must learn the prerequisite, but unfamiliar, language and the curriculum material at the same time.

EFFECTS OF ENVIRONMENT ON COMMUNICATION

Further examination of the communicative demands faced at school make clear the disadvantages to being hearing impaired. Instead of depending on one major individual as a source of important information, the child must attend to several speakers and to a large number of peers. It takes time to adjust to the speech of all of the teachers, playground attendants, lunchroom workers, and classmates with whom the child comes in contact. During the period of adjustment hearing-impaired children need small special considerations (such as seating, noise control, position of the teacher) of which most school personnel are unaware. By the time the hard-of-hearing child shows clear evidence of having communication problems and solutions are developed, a pattern of "being different" and possibly of failure has been established. In some cases, children withdraw from interactions or become aggressive in an attempt to gain control over the uncertainties of the school situation.

Not only are children expected to adjust to a variety of speakers quickly, they must do so in an impossibly noisy setting. Most adults are appalled at the sound levels that exist in the average school classroom. The average signal to noise ratio (S/N) is +10 dB, not a very favorable ratio for any child, much less one who is hearing impaired. This ratio results from the fact that teachers raise their voices to a level of about 85 dB SPL that allows their speech to be louder than the noise in the classroom.

The actual S/N ratio at a child's ear depends on many factors, including distance from the speaker, type of amplification used, and positioning of the child relative to the speaker. Most young children have no idea about how to maximize their hearing in a noisy setting, and most educators are unaware that the problem exists. As a result, hearing-impaired children are placed in an almost impossible listening situation from the moment they enter school. Even if the hearing loss is characterized by good speech recognition skills in a quiet environment, the interaction of the noise in the classroom and the use of amplification may result in a drastic decrease in the ability to perceive speech, perhaps as much as a 60% reduction in speech recognition scores (Finitzo-Hieber and Tillman 1978). However, Hawkins (1984) has shown that the detrimental effects of an unfavorable S/N ratio can be reduced significantly by use of an FM amplification system.

Interaction between the Characteristics of Children and Schools

Try to imagine the confusion and anxiety that being plunged into a sea of unfamiliar speakers, whose voices are buried in a babble of noise, would cause a young child with hearing loss. Well-established strategies for communicating become inadequate. For most children, direct assistance for modifying communication patterns is not available, and the child must sink or swim alone. Thus, the stage is set early for anxiety and failure.

The overall picture of hard-of-hearing children that emerges from the data available is one of varied levels of performance, most of which fall below the norm for their peers. Unlike deaf children, the average hard-of-hearing child is not severely delayed or deficient in any area of development, although most skills are affected to some degree. The reason for the problems encountered by the child—hearing impairment—is not obvious, however. Although the children may recognize their hearing losses as the cause of whatever deficits they exhibit, they tend not to want other children to know they are hearing impaired (Peterson 1972; Davis et al. 1982). Therefore they may not routinely do the things that would make communication easier, such as asking for clarification, requesting changes in the environment, or discussing openly the limitations imposed by the hearing loss. Consequently, failure to respond to a greeting or misunderstanding comments made by others are behaviors that have no obvious cause. Opportunities to interact may occur less often because other children find these communication encounters either difficult or slightly embarrassing. The end result is one of social isolation. Hard-of-hearing children report unsuccessful attempts to communicate that are frustrating and disappointing. When asked about their experiences in school, they rarely mention academic problems but talk instead about difficulty making friends or being unpopular with other children (Davis et al. 1982; Davis et al. 1986).

Why should such relatively mild communication problems cause such widespread social isolation? When compared to deaf children, hard-of-hearing children show far fewer educational problems, but significantly more social problems (Peterson 1972; Northcott 1973; Reich et al. 1977). Data are scarce and do not address the reasons directly, but it is tempting to hypothesize that much of the social isolation experienced by hard-of-hearing children comes about because they are so much like normal children without being *enough* like them. Attempts to behave exactly like their peers only serve to make hard-of-hearing children seem strange, because they cannot quite carry them off. They misunderstand, they are inconsistent in their responses, they sound different when they speak, and they make "dumb mistakes" in class. They are just unusual enough to call attention to themselves, but not different enough to elicit concern, pity, or empathy. Because most school children value being just like their peers, they are unlikely to be completely comfortable with children who are different in small but significant ways. Therefore, although they may not be disliked by anyone, hard-of-hearing children may make their classmates faintly uncomfortable. The result is social isolation and the reduced self-esteem that occurs when a child feels rejected by those children with whom daily interaction is necessary (Loeb and Sarigiani 1986).

According to Erikson (1968), a six year old has already moved through three important developmental stages related to emotional growth and development since birth. A sense of trust in the world has developed; the child has developed awareness of being an individual, independent person; and a sense of purposefulness has occurred. Many rules of social behavior have been learned through the same kind of observation that is so important to perceiving the particular regulations that govern school behavior. Children whose observational skills are hampered by sensory deficits may be at a disadvantage from the beginning of the school years.

Erikson states that the child's developmental tasks for the years between 6 and 11 involve developing feelings of competency and industriousness. School tasks offer a way to test one's problem-solving skills as well as one's ability to complete tasks, engage in cooperative effort, learn new material, excell at some activity, sharpen social skills, and make parents proud. Children who do not have the requisite language skills to compete with other children or to benefit easily from instruction may develop a view of themselves as less than capable, slower to learn, marginally competent, or dumb. Attempts on the part of educators or clinicians to help by orienting classmates to the hearing problem, providing a "buddy" to be sure the hearing-impaired child understands directions, or obtaining tutorial help for the child may exacerbate feelings of incompetence by calling further attention to the child's struggle to perform. On the other hand, failure to inform classmates about the effects of hearing loss may also be detrimental to a child's adjustment. There are no clear guidelines by which decisions of this sort can be made.

Between the ages of 11 and 18, children develop a true sense of their identities as separate individuals (Erickson 1968). As they participate in activities within and outside the school community, they develop increased autonomy and competency. Gradually they take more control of their lives and develop private aspirations and plans for achieving them. The degree to which they develop a positive self-image is influenced by earlier experiences, their perceptions of the competence with which they have accomplished tasks, and the level of success achieved. Unfortunately, much of a given child's perception of self-worth comes from the evaluations of others or, more important, the child's *perception* of the opinions of others. Years of struggling to keep up with classmates, to make friends, and to satisfy the expectations of teachers and parents often result in a self-image that is less than positive.

Developing Appropriate Treatment Programs

Keeping the characteristics of hearing-impaired children and those of the public schools in mind, what kind of programs might offer the greatest probability of successful management of the problems these children face? To be most effective, a treatment program should have two major characteristics. It should be based on the needs of the individual child as they relate to the school environment, and it should be designed to prevent some of the major difficulties that develop in the school setting. The first goal requires that we assess the needs of each child thoroughly. This is easier said than done. Most evidence suggests that thorough psychoeducational assessment is rarely carried out within school systems (Davis et al. 1981). There are probably many understandable reasons for this, ranging from a lack of personnel to philosophical objections to standardized testing. The most common reason for inadequate assessment is probably a combination of time constraints and the fact that hard-of-hearing children as a group have no designated advocates. Their problems and needs require the services and expertise of several different professionals, such as audiologists, speech-language pathologists, special educators, psychologists, and so on. None of these groups has primary responsibility for meeting the educational needs of hearing-impaired children. This fact contributes to the dearth of information about the actual services received by hearing-impaired children and effectiveness of such services. Studies of Iowa children show that the professional most likely to spend time with hard-of-hearing children is the speech-language pathologist, but these children represent only a small proportion of the speech clinician's case load (Davis et al. 1981).

The second goal would require a change in the way we conceptualize support services for children with hearing impairment. Instead of viewing their language problems in terms of the structures misused or the vocabulary that is not yet known, clinicians would have to analyze individual problems as they relate to the overall developmental and educational needs of the children to be served. It is one thing to describe children's achievement in terms of norms that have been established; it is quite another to describe it in relation to the particular tasks that face a child on a daily basis. The first approach might lead to a program designed to teach a child specific vocabulary, sentence structures, or facts involved in subject matter; the second might include efforts to teach children problem-solving strategies and pragmatic communication skills that can be used to discover the meaning of words, the different ways of expressing messages, or ways of establishing dialogue with their peers.

MATCHING DEFICIT WITH TREATMENT: COMMUNICATION STRATEGIES

Using what we know about the interactions among children's deficits and school circumstances, we can identify some major approaches toward management. The first difficulty faced by the hard-of-hearing child is hearing and understanding what is said in the school setting. Although audiologists have been writing and speaking for years about the need for sound treatment of classrooms and/or use of special amplification devices, recent surveys indicate that fewer than a third of the children enrolled in itinerant teaching programs, and therefore assumed to spend most of their time in regular classrooms, use any form of auditory training unit (Davis et al. 1986). Surveys of the noise levels in classrooms indicate how unusual it is to encounter a classroom that does not have high levels of noise and reverberation present. It makes no sense to continue to sound the alarm concerning the detrimental effects of these noisy environments, unless we also teach children how to take responsibility for manipulating the environment to the best advantage possible.

During our interviews with the children involved in our studies, we were struck repeatedly by the observation that few of the hard-of-hearing children knew how to troubleshoot their hearing aids or what to do if the hearing aid malfunctioned. The most common response was to remove the aid and wait until they got home so mother could determine the problem. Many of the children did not carry spare batteries to school routinely. At the time of their interview, 22% of the children's hearing aids were malfunctioning even though their parents were asked to be sure the hearing aids were working properly before their appointments. Twenty-three of the 40 children wore binaural aids and 12 of them were wearing one aid that did not meet the manufacturer's specifications.

These children gave little evidence of the pragmatic ability to determine strategies to foster communication beyond asking the speaker to repeat, speak louder, or slow down. A common reaction to communication failure was to "just let it go," or to try to "listen harder" or "read lips better," but few children suggested changing position, moving away from noise sources, or other simple requests that might have enhanced their ability to function auditorily in the school setting. One child expressed bitterness that he always had to sit in the front row in the first grade, with no apparent understanding as to why this might have been beneficial.

One important aspect of a treatment program for school aged children certainly should be training in the effects of noise, distance, angle and speaker characteristics on their perception of the speech signal, and development of practical strategies for maximizing their ability to hear. This will undoubtedly require a form of assertiveness training, because hard-of-hearing children resist calling attention to themselves and their disabilities either because of embarrassment or shame or because they assume that any failure to communicate effectively is due to a personal fault. The principles of good communication can be discussed and the responsibilities of the communicators (speakers and listeners) should be stressed. If hard-of-hearing children can become knowledgeable about communication in general and their own communication problems in particular, they should be able to take greater responsibility for their own abilities to participate in school and playground activities. At the very least, hearing-impaired children must be taught to troubleshoot their hearing aids, encouraged to carry extra batteries to school, and trained to request listening checks of their hearing aids at least daily.

If hearing-impaired children can become better communicators in the school setting, their confidence in their abilities to participate in school activities should increase. It may be that some of the social isolation that occurs comes about because of a tentativeness on the part of the hearing-impaired child that is rooted in uncertainty. Furthermore, any improvement in self concept is likely to have an effect on participation in academic activities, possibly leading to improved performance in a variety of activities. The most successful hearing-impaired children I have known have been those whose social skills are good and who have a strong self-concept that allows them to try anything, often with surprising success.

MATCHING DEFICIT WITH TREATMENT: PREVENTING SPEECH AND LANGUAGE DELAYS

Obviously, simply teaching children to use their hearing aids effectively and to seek more control over communication situations will not solve all the problems they face in school. If we know, and we do, that hearing loss places children at risk for speech, language, and academic deficits, why not concentrate on programs designed to prevent, rather than remediate, such problems? It is not unusual for audiologists to evaluate young hard-of-hearing children whose development of language and speech skills is still within the normal range. Many of us hestiate to recommend remedial services for these children, preferring to select amplification for them and monitor them for an extended period of time. In many cases, we lose contact with these children, either because their families relocate or because parents see no advantage to continued monitoring if other services do not appear to be necessary. Would it not be far more beneficial to parents and to children if we enrolled them in programs designed to prevent speech and language problems? We should include in such programs language stimulation, articulation therapy, and auditory training, in addition to activities designed to foster awareness of the limitations imposed by hearing loss and the development of strategies to overcome them. The procedures suggested by Moeller (Chapter 23) have great potential for preventing many of the most common language problems faced by hard-of-hearing children.

A major advantage of prevention rather than remediation is the likelihood that many of the social and academic problems experienced in school might not occur at all if children were more confident in their abilities to talk and behave like other children. Instituting communication strategy training, articulation therapy, and hearing-aid management activities as soon as a child begins school has the potential of either preventing or alleviating some of the major social and academic problems experienced later on.

I do not mean to suggest that hearing-impaired children should not receive direct language therapy or academic tutoring if these activities will contribute to their overall development and achievement levels. I am suggesting, however, that there are equally important aspects of communication and learning that are largely ignored at present. Many hearing-impaired children are passive consumers of educational and remedial procedures; their teachers concentrate on the teaching of facts because there are so many facts the children do not know. Baron (1975) discussed the prerequisites for becoming a literate, educated person; these included five "domains of linguistic consciousness" that are developed more or less sequentially by children as they grow up. Only the first two of these are concerned with the knowledge of words and sentence structures. The others require a clear understanding of what communication is about and the ability to unravel ambiguity, determine the style of communication that is appropriate for various people and situations, and interpret the communication patterns of others. It is important that we learn how to help hearing-impaired children develop this level of linguistic consciousness, especially as it relates to the educational demands they will face throughout their school years.

REFERENCES

Annual demographic data report 1984. *American Annals of the Deaf* Volume 129.

Baron, N. 1975. Linguistic consciousness: Prerequisites for learning to read and write. Address delivered to the Summer Institute on Applied Linguistics, Rhode Island School for the Deaf.

Bess, F. 1982. Children with unilateral hearing loss. *Journal of the Academy of Rehabilitative Audiology* XV:131–143.

Bess, F., and McConnell, F. 1981. *Audiology, Education, and the Hearing Impaired Child.* St. Louis: C. V. Mosby Co.
Brannon, J., and Murry, T. 1966. The spoken syntax of normal, hard of hearing, and deaf children. *Journal of Speech and Hearing Research* 9:604–610.
Brannon, J. 1968. Linguistic word classes in the spoken language of normal, hard of hearing, and deaf children. *Journal of Speech and Hearing Research* 11:279–287.
Brown, J. 1984. Examination of grammatical morphemes in the language of hard-of-hearing children. *Volta Review* 86:229–238.
Conrad, R. 1979. *The Deaf School Child.* London: Harper and Row.
Davis, J. 1974. Performance of young hearing impaired children on a test of basic concepts. *Journal of Speech and Hearing Research* 17:342–351.
Davis, J., and Blasdell, R. 1975. Perceptual strategies employed by normal hearing and hearing-impaired children in the comprehension of sentences containing relative clauses. *Journal of Speech and Hearing Research* 18:281–295.
Davis, J., Shepard, N., Stelmachowicz, P., and Gorga, M. 1981. Characteristics of hearing impaired children in the public schools: Part II—Psychoeducational Data. *Journal of Speech and Hearing Disorders* 46:130–137.
Davis, J., Elfenbein, J., Lansing, C., and Dixon, E. 1982. Experiences with mainstreaming: The view from the other side, Paper presented at the American Speech-Language Hearing Association annual convention, Toronto.
Davis, J., Elfenbein, J., and Pratt, S. 1986. *Survey of Children Enrolled in Itinerant Programs for the Hearing Impaired in 15 Area Education Agencies in Iowa.* Report submitted to the Department of Public Instruction, State of Iowa.
Davis, J., Elfenbein, J., Schum, R., and Bentler, R. 1986. Effects of mild and moderate hearing impairments on language, educational, and psychosocial behavior of children. *Journal of Speech and Hearing Disorders* 51:53–62.
Elfenbein, J., Hardin, M., and Davis, J. 1985. Oral communication skills of hard of hearing children. Paper presented at the American Speech-Language Hearing Association annual convention, Washington, D. C.
Erikson, E. 1968. *Identity, Youth and Crisis.* New York: Norton.
Finitzo-Hieber, T., and Tillman, T. 1978. Room acoustics effects on monosyllabic word discrimination ability for normal and hearing-impaired children. *Journal of Speech and Hearing Research* 21:440–458.
Fisher, B. 1966. The social and emotional adjustment of children with impaired hearing attending ordinary classes. *British Journal of Educational Psychology* 36:319–321.
Fisher, H., and Logemann, F. 1971. *The Fisher-Logemann Test of Articulation Competence.* Boston: Houghton-Mifflin.
Goetzinger, C., Harrison, C., and Baer, C. 1964. Small perceptive hearing loss: Its effect on school-age children. *Volta Review* 66:124–131.
Hawkins, D. 1984. Comparisons of speech recognition in noise by mildly to moderately hearing impaired children using hearing aids and FM systems. *Journal of Speech and Hearing Disorders* 49:409–418.
Kennedy, P., and Bruininks, R. 1974. Social status of hearing impaired children in regular classrooms. *Exceptional Children* 40:336–342.
Kodman, F. 1963. Educational status of hard of hearing children in the classroom. *Journal of Speech and Hearing Disorders* 28:297–299.
Loeb, R., and Sarigiani, P. 1986. The impact of hearing impairment on self-perceptions of children. *Volta Review* 88:89–100.
Northcott, W. 1973. *The Hearing Impaired Child in a Regular Classroom.* Washington, D.C.: A. G. Bell Association.
Peterson, M. 1972. Achievement of hard of hearing students in regular public schools, Ph.D. Dissertation, Wayne State University, Detroit, MI.
Pressnell, L. 1973. Hearing impaired children's comprehension and production of syntax in oral language. *Journal of Speech and Hearing Research* 16:12–21.
Quigley, S., and Thomure, R. 1968. Some Effects of a Hearing-Impairment on School Performance. Champaign-Urbana: Institute of Research on Exceptional Children, University of Illinois.
Reich, C., Hambleton, D., and Houldin, B. 1977. The integration of hearing impaired children in regular classrooms. *American Annals of the Deaf* 122:534–543.
Shepard, N., Davis, J., Gorga, M., and Stelmachowicz, P. 1981. Characteristics of hearing-

impaired children in the public schools: Part I—Demographic data. *Journal of Speech and Hearing Disorders* 46:123–129.
Silverman, R., and Lane, H. 1970. Deaf Children. *In* H. Davis and S. R. Silverman (eds.). *Hearing and Deafness* (3rd ed.). New York: Holt, Rinehart, and Winston.
Wilcox, J., and Tobin, H. 1974. Linguistic performance of hard-of-hearing and normal-hearing children. *Journal of Speech and Hearing Research* 17:286–293.
Wood, D., Wood, H., and Howarth, P. 1983. Mathematical abilities of deaf school-leavers. *British Journal of Developmental Psychology* 1:67–73.
Young, C., and McConnell, F. 1957. Retardation of vocabulary development in hard of hearing children. *Exceptional Children* 23:368–370.

Chapter 25

The Impact of a Child's Hearing Impairment on the Family: A Parent's Perspective

Stanley J. Maliszewski

Introduction

This paper is an attempt to focus attention on parents of hearing-impaired children. Placing emphasis on the parent perspective provides an opportunity for the reader to become more aware of the impact of having a deaf child on everyday family life, and, moreover, makes the insights of selected parents available to others who are in a similar situation.

A child's hearing loss and the constraints imposed by deafness not only affect the life of a deaf child but also can cause parents of deaf children to structure their lives in fundamentally different ways from parents of hearing children. Those who have never been exposed to deafness within their families cannot completely understand what it is to be the parent of a deaf child. Indeed, parents of deaf children may even have a difficult time comprehending how the unique complexities of life experienced by other parents of the deaf are vastly different from their own.

Each child is a unique individual and generates unique concerns. Personalities differ as do the degree and type of hearing loss. Also, all parents are not the same. Perhaps the only shared significance understood by all parents of deaf children is an "underlying sorrow" often manifested throughout their lives.

If understanding appears to be elusive, what can educators of the deaf, speech therapists, audiologists, and physicians strive towards in order to more appropriately meet the needs of parents of a deaf child? As the father of two profoundly deaf children, it has been my experience that awareness, empathy, and competence appear to be the characteristics most desired when seeking out professionals who are willing to assist parents in the development of their deaf child.

Hearing parents who have recently been informed that their child is deaf, often feel fright and guilt. These parents search for a "savior" to guide them toward finding solutions to many questions and concerns experienced throughout the development of their deaf child. This much sought after "savior" is usually found in the role of audiologist, speech therapist, or educator of the deaf. The short-lived feeling of salvation is often followed by discouragement and perhaps anger because the "saviors" are only experts and not gods. Experts are available to lend assistance and offer guidance; they must not be expected to perform the impossible. In seeking the best professionals and educational programs for both profoundly deaf children, I was fortunate to find a number of professionally dedicated, sensitive, and astute men and women working with deaf children and their parents.

These contemporary heroes to parents of deaf children can accentuate feelings of hopelessness or provide a sense of warmth and nourishment that enhances the confidence necessary to build a trusting relationship between parents and professionals who work with hearing-impaired children. Consider how the differences in attitudes between two audiologists affected the lives of our family when it was announced that our children had profound hearing losses.

When our daughter was one year old a hearing loss was suspected. Our family physician felt that the child was simply being stubborn and refused to immediately respond to environmental sounds. However, to pacify us, he gave us the name of an audiologist. At the time my wife and I were in our early twenties and had recently moved to Southern California. The audiologist was on the staff of a hospital for the multiple-handicapped located in the San Gabriel Valley area. After what appeared to be a comprehensive audiological examination, the audiologist briefly visited with us inside an acoustically treated room and proceeded to say that "a profound hearing loss was evident, nothing could be done to repair the nerve loss, and restoring hearing or expecting any means of oral communication would be having false expectations." He suggested that Karen be enrolled in the educational program at the hospital which provided an "excellent program" for children displaying a variety of handicapping conditions.

While I was sitting bewildered in the hall waiting for forms to be processed another parent asked what was wrong with Karen. When the parent learned that Karen had just been diagnosed as being deaf, the parent suggested that Karen be taken to the John Tracy Clinic in Los Angeles. A whole new world was opened to Karen largely because of a concerned parent. Until this conversation, the John Tracy Clinic was never mentioned and no one encouraged us to express our thoughts or feelings or to ask questions.

Ten years later, our second child was born in Omaha, Nebraska. As a result of the older child's profound hearing loss, a thorough audiological examination was scheduled at the Boys Town National Institute for Communication Disorders in Omaha. Arrangements were made to have Ryan formally tested two days after he was brought home from the hospital. A hearing loss was already suspected twelve hours after his birth.

As we sat patiently during the audiological tests, the look on the audiologist's face indicated that the test results were not going to be favorable. When the diagnostic tests were completed, the audiologist touched us and with tears in his eyes said, "After knowing how hard you worked with Karen, I feel a sense of despair thinking that you may have to go through it all again." He went on to say: "My entire family prayed for the two of you and little Ryan during the weekend." Finally, he specifically stated, "Ryan has nerve damage which has resulted in a profound hearing loss, almost identical to Karen's." Then he just sat with us and provided a sense of comfort.

Another time and another place made a difference to the parents. Perhaps most of all the genuine humanism and caring of a dedicated professional provided us with the encouragement we needed to work through our loss of the fantasy of having a hearing child.

Tension and Family Disruption

Children who are deaf represent potentially significant burdens to their families. Between the stress experienced by parents having a child who is deaf and the limitations imposed by the hearing loss of the child, deaf children and their families are at risk throughout their lives. Due to the variety of societal forces acting on marriages in the United States today, the degree of risk for families with deaf children may well be heightened. When initial reactions to having a deaf child are not adequately resolved by parents, they continue to exert a negative influence not only on the marriage, but also on the child's adaptation to life (Mindel and Vernon 1971). As harsh as it may sound, I believe that parents must place the importance of their marriage above the needs of their deaf child; ultimately the child will benefit.

Parents of deaf children are faced with a multitude of problems. In addition to the instrumental concerns of providing appropriate hearing aids, initial auditory training, educational rehabilitation, speech therapy, and corrective treatment required for the child, there are strong feelings related to guilt, denial, or anger, feelings of incompetence or self-doubt, and chronic sorrow (Davis 1960; Cummings 1966). The dynamics of the entire family may be threatened and relationships destroyed (Farber 1960; Jordan 1962).

Emerging parent-centered services and programs for the hearing-impaired infant have helped to prepare parents for their role as parents of a deaf child. The family's adaptation to having a child who is deaf can often be accomplished most effectively by non-professional persons who have made the same "passage through crises" (Davis 1963).

PAST STUDIES

A review of literature finds several studies that focus on the parents of handicapped children. This study deals specifically with parents of the hearing impaired. Perhaps one of the problems with publishing in this area is the lack of a theoretical base, although Meadow (1968), and Bronfenbrenner (1979) have provided two useful models appropriate for parents of the hearing impaired. Also, Buboly and Whiren (1984) described a framework for understanding the roles and functions of families who have handicapped children. A basic tenet of their theory is that a change in any part of the system affects other parts of the system and the system as a whole. For the family unit, the immediate and enduring stress of giving birth to a handicapped child tests the family's capacity to adapt.

Parents experience various stages of grief in response to the diagnosis of hearing-impairment in their child. The birth of a child who is deaf is sometimes viewed as the death of the fantasy of having a normal-hearing child. To help explain parental responses to the diagnosis of a handicapped child, several authors have sought to describe the reactions of parents (Epperson 1971; Goodman 1964; Ross 1972; Seligman 1979; Solnit and Stark 1961). A theory describing parental mourning was developed by Fortier and Wanlass (1984).

With a few exceptions (Chinn, Winn, and Walters 1978; Ross 1972; Seligman 1983), the majority of the professional literature on parents of handicapped children has been contributed by special educators and by parents who write about their personal experiences with their handicapped sons and daughters.

Recently the medical profession has come to recognize the potential stresses and conflicts that can exist in families when a deaf child is present. Regrettably, mental health professionals, including clinical and rehabilitation counselors, have not kept pace with professionals in other fields; articles focusing on parents are just now beginning to appear in counseling and psychology journals (Opirhory and Peters 1982; Wasserman 1983).

SIGNIFICANT CONCERNS OF PARENTS

A study reported by Erting (1982) reveals that the majority of deaf children have hearing parents—92% according to Schein (1982) and 91% according to Rawlings (1977); only 3% have two hearing-impaired parents (Rawlings 1977). Families with deaf children tended to have a larger mean number of children (3.2) when compared with the general population (2.09). Hearing-impaired children tended to have fathers who are less well-educated than fathers in the general population with 21% having an elementary education or less, compared with 15% of the general population; and 27% having one or more years of college, compared with 32% of the general population. Mothers of deaf children were not as likely to be employed outside of the home as mothers in the general population (Rawlings 1977).

COMMUNICATION: THE REAL PROBLEM

Relatively little attention has been paid to determining how parents and their hearing-impaired children communicate with each other. A study was conducted based on questionnaire responses (self-report) from the parents of 557 hearing-impaired students eight years of age and older (Jensema and Trybus 1978). The investigators found that speech alone or in combination with other modes of communication is most often used by both parents and their hearing-impaired children. The parents' reports indicate that signs are used by more of the children (41%) than the parents (32%), and that speech is used by fewer of the children (70%) than the parents (80%). Speech alone is the single channel of communication reported most often by the parents and consists of nearly 40% of the communication between parents and children (Erting 1982).

The questions and concerns of parents are as varied and confusing as the meaning behind the numbers and data about deaf children. Consider the debate between oralism and total communication as simply one point of confusion for parents of deaf children. There appear to be as many "research" studies reported that favor oralism as there are favoring total communication. Even such an important "basic for living" as establishing a means of communication cannot be reported to parents with credibility.

With such a point of contention as oralism vs. total communication in mind, I reviewed one report on academic achievement of deaf children. The 1986 study conducted by the Center for Assessment and Demographic Studies indicated that only 10% of hearing-impaired students at age 18 read at or above the eighth-grade level. The average hearing child reaches this level at age 13. In math only the top 10% of hearing-impaired students can compute as well as the average hearing child of the same age. Nowhere in this study was it indicated whether the participants used oralism or total communication as a means to communicate. Obviously something more than just being able to speak must be considered when parents decide the most appropriate means of communication for their child. When a hearing person describes another hearing person, the statement "he talks" is not addressed but rather, the total person is described. Parents of deaf children want to know what is best for the total child and not just one aspect of their development. The individual child's needs must be considered when advocating a specific mode of communication.

Deaf children look "normal," and yet the handicap of deafness is very real. For individuals who have never met a hearing-impaired child, it is difficult to understand how much difference it can make. One might think of what a person who cannot hear normal conversations misses—chimes blowing in the wind, or the sounds of animals.

Even though environmental sounds are important, it is not missing the sounds of everyday life that constitutes the real problem. It is learning to send and receive information that is the real area of difficulty. Parents of hearing-impaired children mentioned the following "worries" they have for their children:

If they get lost how will they communicate?
How will they communicate at summer camp, in little league, or in a restaurant?
What will their reaction be when neighborhood children exclude them from games because they don't understand the rules?
Will they pass a driving test?
How will they interview for a job?
Will they be safe when they leave home?

One mother of a 16 year old deaf daughter expressed the thoughts she had when her daughter did not make the swimming team at the public high school she attends:

> I didn't think she would make the team, she isn't that good of a swimmer . . . I am proud of the fact that she at least tried. What does bother me is that she didn't understand when she was told that she was 'cut' from the team . . . She showed up the next day for practice and was quite embarrassed when she discovered she wasn't supposed to be there. It's hard not to blame the teacher . . . but I don't. Maybe my daughter needs to say 'I don't understand' when she is confused.

EXPRESSION OF FEELINGS

There are various "stages of loss" that parents pass through when they first learn their child is deaf. The first stage occurs when the parent suspects that "something is wrong." Feelings of confusion and anxiety remain until a diagnosis has been confirmed (Meadow 1968). During this time, the parent looks to the physician as the "expert." Feeling that the parents are not qualified to exercise objective judgment in reporting symptoms, the pediatrician may be reluctant to make a referral to a specialist, even though each day is so important to a deaf child's development.

The second stage of the process occurs when the diagnosis is confirmed by a specialist. At that moment, the parent becomes the true patient. Perhaps the fortunate parents are those who go into shock immediately. One parent remembered when his wife called him at the office to tell him that his son had just been diagnosed as being deaf. "I left my office, in a daze, started to drive my car without any destination and ended up in a bank parking lot . . . I just sat there . . . tried to cry, but couldn't."

> The first reaction to any devastating news is shock. Parents reported: The audiologist told us our child was deaf but it didn't really sink in. In most cases a confirmed diagnosis is a relief. Consider the parents who have suspected a hearing loss for over a year before a positive diagnosis. Throughout the year they struggled to think positively, doing their best to suppress their fears. Every now and then, the feelings that their child was deaf would surface at very peculiar times, such as at a family

> gathering, and they would have to begin again the struggle against believing it. This kind of an emotional tug-of-war is exhausting. (Ogden and Lipsett 1982).

A parent of a sixteen year old deaf son replied, "You never seem to completely get over the shock, or fully accept your child's deafness . . . feelings come out in subtle ways."

In addition to shock, hearing parents experience feelings of grief. The grief is very similar to the grief one feels with the loss of a loved one. In a sense, the child the parents thought they had has died.

Grief is often manifested in feelings of denial, anger, bargaining, and depression—ideally culminating in some form of acceptance. Denial takes on many forms. Most recognizable is the outright refusal to accept certain facts that can prolong corrective treatment to the child. Parents may put off obtaining hearing aids for their child, delay making arrangements for further testing, refuse to take part in the important individualized educational plan, or in some cases, refuse to learn sign language; all may be a means of denying the child's hearing loss.

Anger often is directed toward the child for being deaf and/or toward God for causing the child to be deaf. One father became aware of his anger while at a visit to the fair. "I kicked a rock and it hit a barn door, a horse stabled in the barn immediately turned around . . . I thought, why does God allow animals to hear and not people."

There are no answers, even for parents who choose to put those questions to God. Rabbi Harold Kushner reasons that God has nothing to do with what happens everyday in the real world. Perhaps, bad things happen just because they do and no one is to blame (Dickman and Gordon 1985).

A father felt that he was experiencing "bargaining" when he purchased only one hearing aid for his deaf son. "Thinking back, maybe I was trying to compromise my feelings by only having one hearing aid fitted for my son. I always knew I didn't completely accept his deafness . . . sort of like all right, if he is deaf he only needs one aid . . . Two hearing aids will produce sounds too loudly."

Depression is perhaps the hardest feeling to work through. To overcome depression, it is first necessary to "own the feeling" and express it, either verbally or non-verbally. In an effort to overcome depression it is necessary to put meaning back into life by establishing goals unrelated to the child's deafness. Parents do have a right to life and to be happy again.

Amazingly, one morning a parent wakes up to discover his child's deafness is not the first thing on his mind. When this occurs, acceptance is within reach. In the same moment a parent may realize that a child is separate from the life of a parent. This realization is extremely beneficial to the parent as well as to the child. When there is an honest understanding of the hearing loss and an acceptance of the child, parents can more readily address their child's needs and progress.

As feelings are identified and confronted, thoughts and questions emerge such as: Will the deafness necessitate a change in family life style?, or, Should having another child be considered? Financial worries also are of concern to parents. Doctors, audiologists, speech therapists, hearing aids, and special schools must be paid for from limited budgets. At times money concerns can cause parents to feel guilty, yet they are real considerations. Thinking about them is natural and understandable.

SUPPORT GROUPS

Parents of deaf children can provide invaluable assistance to other parents, particularly those who recently were informed of their child's deafness. Simply knowing that other parents have similar concerns and feelings tends to validate the unexpressed emotions of parents who have recently learned their child is deaf. It is important for these parents to know that they will laugh again, and given the appropriate assistance, their child will be capable of being independent. How a child is perceived can enhance everyone's personal growth. Children who are deaf can be marvelous teachers to their parents.

EDUCATION

Most hearing-impaired children need special programs for learning. Those deaf children who successfully enter the mainstream in the public schools need supportive services and continuous monitoring of their progress. Parents must decide which educational placement is best for their deaf child. At times the options are overwhelming and at other times local educational agencies are willing to provide only minimal support services.

In a number of school districts, the type of support services reflects the philosophy of the director of special education. This is particularly true regarding the means of communication. One parent reflected on the debate between oralism and total communication:

> I feel like I'm caught in the middle. Some say I should send my daughter to the state school for the deaf where they teach students to sign . . . others say she needs to learn to speak and sign. The deaf school is supposed to teach total communication. When I visited I saw students signing; not using their voice. When I visited the public school in our area I observed the resource teacher using oral communication with very few signs . . . she admitted that she didn't know how to sign very well . . . This is total communication?

The dilemma faced by parents can often result in far-reaching changes effecting where the family lives and what type of work to pursue.

For many years educators of the deaf have demonstrated considerable interest in families who have deaf children. Their interest and involvement with parents increased significantly with the passage in 1975 of Public Law 94-142, the Right to Education Act (Strickland 1983). Under this legislation educators are required to develop, with parents, individualized educational plans (IEPs) for the handicapped children they teach. The IEP process necessitated more parent involvement than in the past and the document often reflects the services required of other professionals such as speech therapists and audiologists.

Despite the positive changes that PL 94-142 was supposed to effect on the operating policies of local agencies, some seemed to disregard the intent of the law. When a father of a 10 year old deaf girl requested an interpreter to accompany his daughter to a math class, local district officials informed him that funds were not available. Although the district subscribed to a philosophy of total communication they were not willing to provide interpreters when needed. When the parent mentioned PL 94-142, the director of special education replied, "The district doesn't have to provide the 'cadillac' of services for the hearing impaired." Finally protests voiced by several parents ultimately resulted in interpreters being hired for mainstreamed classes.

Ultimately, parents must decide which educational setting is best for their child. The decision-making process can result in a great deal of stress for the entire family. The choices are many: state schools for the deaf; private schools advocating oralism; private schools with a total communication approach; public schools which subscribe to oralism and those believing in total communication; some public schools with an interpreter available and some without this resource. All educational settings can be appropriate for the unique needs of the child. Parents must be "wise consumers" and know what they are looking for prior to observing the educational programs and deciding on the most appropriate placement.

THE SIGNIFICANCE CONTINUES . . .

The emotional, educational, social, medical, and financial frustrations are different for each family. However, the theme of underlying sorrow for parents remains the same. It would appear that mentally healthy parents can disassociate their feelings from what is happening to the child. Perhaps this "ideal" is a goal to work towards. However, striving toward this goal is most difficult for parents as they encounter, almost daily, such events as are so very well described in a poem by a 17 year old deaf girl who is attending a regular public high school:

> How do you feel today?
> I'm upset mostly!
> Everyday I go learning in school and it's fun
> but I can't stand being alone most of the time
> inside my feeling crying hardly
> outside I have a bad mood
> my face hurts me alot
> At first I thought I'm happy at the beginning
> but the second beginnings I feel unhappy
> I walked in the crowded hall filled with students
> to see if I could make friends; no one notices me

Students who I know in the past years said,
"Hi" to me as I thought they want me to make happy
Why a single word sound making me happy?
One word? Everyday they continue to say the same word
I'm tired of it
Again, I walk alone when I'm free
Looking for new friends as I try to
but they seem to ignore me and walk away from me
Is something wrong with me . . . (Naiman and Schein 1978)

PARENTS HAVE RIGHTS AND NEED ENCOURAGEMENT

Perhaps the most common self-defeating emotional response of a parent who has a deaf child is a perception that the parent is guilty of somehow causing the child's deafness and that the parent is inadequate at providing the educational experiences necessary for the child to develop academically, emotionally, and socially. This parental negative self-image can be quite detrimental to the hearing-impaired child. Professionals who work with the deaf can assist parents by becoming more aware of the impact of a child's hearing-impairment on the family and by sensitively confronting parents who have illogical ideas about their child's deafness. Being honest with parents and providing them with the necessary information to "take charge of their own lives" can be of great value not only to the parent but ultimately to the child.

Professionals who interact with parents of deaf children must not only be experts in their own particular field, they also need to be aware of referral agencies such as local, state, and national associations of the deaf, parent support groups, sources of financial aid, educational opportunities in the area, genetic counseling and personal counseling services. Medical and educational professionals must believe and recognize that parents of handicapped children have certain "rights." If the challenge of having a deaf child in the family is going to be met successfully, parents must accept the following rights, as stated by Dickman and Gordon (1985):

—The right to cry
—The right to be angry and not be ashamed of it
—The right to not feel guilty
—The right to feel you're doing the best you can
—The right to make your own decisions
—The right to respect
—The right to get help
—The right to have and be a family
—The right to go on living
—The right to be only human
—The right to laugh
—The right to believe in miracles

THE STRUGGLE FOR A SIGNIFICANT MEANING

The old expression "when life gives you lemons, make lemonade," is very reflective of the manner in which some parents arrive at the acceptance of their child's deafness. Having a handicapped child doesn't have to result in the family living a handicapped life. Often it is a person's perception of a problem, rather than the problem itself, that results in personal suffering. Obstacles in life can be growth-producing. Parents have a choice: they can look on their child's hearing loss as a learning experience, or they can view it as an obstacle that hinders further personal growth.

Professionals should not be hesitant about challenging parents with the idea of a potential meaning behind having a deaf child. This is not to say that professionals should linger on the "whys" of a child's deafness. The child is deaf. *Why* may very well be unanswerable beyond a given medical explanation. However, for parents, many personal growth-enriching experiences can be found when the words *how* and *what* are kept in focus. *How* parents can help their hearing-impaired child and *what* can be learned to enhance personal growth through living with a deaf family member can certainly provide enough personal growth opportunities to last a life-time.

Having a deaf child can cause parents to question their own personal significance. In order to "adjust" to the life-changing demands of deafness in the family, parents must own their feelings—knowing that feelings aren't wrong or right, they just *are*—and to forgive themselves for perceived guilt. Forgiveness is the vehicle for changing perceptions and letting go of fears, condemning judgments, and grievances (Jampolsky 1979).

Viktor Frankl (1963) and others in humanistic psychology believe that every human being carries within his or her own life the only real and possible standard by which to measure adjustment—the actualization of selfhood. Parents who strive towards this end attempt to "actualize" their selfhood as fully as possible while keeping a realistic understanding of the unique demands made upon them by having a child who is deaf. This often calls for compromise in behavior, though not always for compromise in thought and attitude.

During a recent presentation, Dr. Sol Gordon expounded on the requirements that individuals must meet in order to retain their significance as people and continue to strive towards personal growth. They include:

—Risk taking
—Quiet time
—Counseling outlet
—Openness to change
—Intellectual stimulations
—Disregarding toxic people
—Re-creation program
—Nuturing support group
—Loving one other person and being loved

—Having meaning in one's life
—An abundance of laughter
—Involvement in a cause
—Sense of integrity

RECOMMENDATION

This paper does not suggest that physicians, audiologists, educators of the deaf, speech therapists, or mental health professionals are not assisting parents with deaf children. It does recommend that such professionals be well aware of the impact that a child's hearing loss has on the family. Of course, parents have choices to make and that is one responsibility they can't refuse.

Preparing the parent for having a major role in the deaf child's development cannot be accomplished by generalizations. Two important tasks are necessary: First, professionals who work with the deaf and their parents must become aware of the devastating and life changing consequences of having a hearing-impaired child; and then at the time of diagnosis, there must be trained staff, and ideally a parent-support system available to give the parent, who is the real patient, proper care and attention.

Both parents have emotions that must be acknowledged; and both need instruction in what deafness is and how it varies. The Boys Town National Institute for Communication Disorders provides this service superbly but carries the attention one step further—beyond information giving. Through other parents who have benefited from the Institute, parents of newly diagnosed hearing-impaired children are led to some insight of their own feelings. This type of parental support, along with the institute's dynamic professional team of physicians, audiologists, speech therapists, educators, and psychologists has been of tremendous assistance to parents as they journey through the growth experiences of having a child who is deaf.

For those parents and professionals who are in need of referral assistance or have questions about raising and educating a deaf child, help is only a phone call away! Located in Los Angeles, the GRAPEVINE is a national toll-free hotline for information on deafness (1-800-352-8888 V/TDD or in California 1-800-346-8888 V/TDD). Through their national network of parents and professionals, they will put the caller in touch with resources in the local community. Trained volunteers answer the GRAPEVINE phones and research each response individually.

The GRAPEVINE is one of the services provided by TRIPOD, a laboratory school founded by parents and professionals committed to helping families interact with their hearing-impaired children in an informed and positive way. TRIPOD's seventeen-member National Advisory Board—made up of professionals, parents, and deaf adults from across the U.S.—contribute their expertise and are available to callers for individual counseling.

References

Bronfenbrenner, V. 1979. *The Ecology of Human Development: Experiments by Nature and Design.* Cambridge, MA: Harvard University Press.

Buboly, M. M., and Whiren, A. P. 1984. The family of the handicapped: An ecological model for policy and practice. *Family Relations* 33:5–12.

Center for Assessment and Demographic Studies. 1986. *Educational Achievement and Personal Characteristics of Hearing Impaired Children.* Washington, DC: Gallaudet Research Institute.

Chinn, P. C., Winn, J., and Walters, R. H. 1978. *Two-Way Talking with Parents of Special Children.* St. Louis: Mosby.

Cummings, T. S. 1966. Effects of the child's deficiency on the mother. *American Journal of Orthopsychiatry* 36:395–608.

Davis, F. 1960. Uncertainty in medical prognosis, clinical and functional. *American Journal of Sociology* 66:41–47.

Davis, F. 1963. *Passage Through Crisis.* Indianapolis: Bobbs-Merrill.

Dickman, I., and Gordon, S. 1985. *One Miracle at a Time.* New York: Simon and Schuster.

Epperson, M. 1971. Families in sudden crisis. *Social Work in Health Care* 2:265–273.

Erting, C. J. 1982. Deafness, communication, and social identity: An anthropological analysis of interaction among parents, teachers, and deaf children. Unpublished manuscript. American University.

Farber, B. 1960. Family organization and crisis. *Society for Research In Child Development* 25:1–3.

Fortier, L. M., and Wanlass, R. L. 1984. Family crisis following the diagnosis of a handicapped child. *Family Relations* 33:13–24.

Frankl, V. 1963. *Man's Search for Meaning.* New York: Washington Square Press.

Goodman, L. 1964. Continuing treatment of parents with congentially defective infants. *Social Work* 9:92–97.

Jampolsky, G. G. 1979. *Love is Letting Go of Fear.* New York: Celestial Arts.

Jensema, C., and Trybus, R. 1978. *Communication Patterns and Educational Achievement of Hearing Impaired Students.* Washington, D.C.: Office of Demographic Studies, Gallaudet College.

Jordan, T. E. 1962. Research on the handicapped child and the family. *Merrill-Palmer Quarterly* 8:243–260.

Meadow, K. P. 1968. *Parental Response to the Medical Ambiguities of Congenital Deafness.* Unpublished manuscript. University of California, Berkeley.

Mindel, E. D., and Vernon, M. 1971. *They Grow In Silence: The Deaf Child and His Family.* Silver Spring, Md.: National Association for the Deaf.

Naiman, D. W., and Schein, J. D. 1978. *For Parents of Deaf Children.* Washington, D. C.: National Association for the Deaf.

Ogden, P. W., and Lipsett 1982. *The Silent Garden.* New York: St. Martins Press.

Opirhory, G., and Peters, G. A. 1982. Counseling intervention strategies for families with the less than perfect newborn. *Personnel and Guidance Journal* 60:451–455.

Rawlings, B. 1977. The family unit: A basic to be considered. *In Two Studies of the Families of Hearing-Impaired Children.* Washington, D. C.: Office of Demographic Studies, Gallaudet College.

Ross, A. 1972. *The Exceptional Child in the Family.* New York: Grune & Stratton.

Schein, J. 1982. The demography of deafness. *In* P. Higgins, and J. Nash (eds.). *The Deaf Community and the Deaf Population.* Washington, D. C.: Sociology Department, Gallaudet College.

Seligman, M. 1979. *Strategics for Helping Parents of Exceptional Children: A Guide for Teachers.* New York: Free Press.

Seligman, J. 1983. *The Family with a Handicapped Child: Understanding and Treatment.* Orlando, FL: Grune & Stratton.

Solnit, A. J., and Stark, M. H. 1961. Mourning and the birth of a defective child. *Psychoanalytical Study of the Child* 16:523–537.

Strickland, B. 1983. Legal issues that affect parents. *In* M. Seligman (ed.). *The Family with A Handicapped Child: Understanding and Treatment.* Orlando, Fl.: Grune & Stratton.

Wasserman, R. 1983. Identifying the counseling needs of the siblings of mentally retarded children. *Personnel and Guidance Journal* 61:622–627.

Chapter 26

Enriching the Partnership

Laura Knox

When I started teaching, I had little use for parents. They got in my way. I used to think, "If only my children didn't have to go home with those people. If only they could go home with me, instead." Then I had the humbling experience of having three children of my own, and I realized my students were not a whole lot better off with me than they were with their parents.

In my years in the classroom I went to bat for those children, out on many limbs for them. I was their advocate, their strong right arm. Now, 30 years later, I barely recall a few faces, and fewer names. But, during all this time, their parents have been their most enduring support. That realization impressed me with the critical need to strengthen my relationship with parents when working with their children. This was my first awakening about parents.

Now, how many of you are parents? What kind of training have you had to be one?

Isn't this outrageous? In our society, we talk so much about the importance of parents. Yet, we have few opportunities to learn about skills, attitudes, and ways of relating to children that would make our lives together more pleasant.

When we become parents, we have two concepts to fall back on: one is the way that we ourselves were brought up, which may or may not be useful to us; the other is trial and error, which, I suggest, is too costly a way to raise children. There is something else: common sense. However, the longer I live the more convinced I am that common sense is not "common"; it is very rare. I think few of us stop and listen to ourselves long enough to know what it is *we* think is appropriate for ourselves and for our children, in a given situation. I think, even fewer of us trust ourselves enough to act on what we hear.

At the same time, we are somewhat leery of other people who tell us what to do—even suspicious, and perhaps hostile. I do not believe any parent walks into a clinic and thinks: "Which of these professionals shall I become angry at today? Which shall I blame for my child's lack of progress? Which shall I accuse of not caring about my child?" Yet, occasionally, we perceive that that is the way some parents act.

Now I do not think that professionals fare a great deal better than parents in their training. Not one moment of any course I ever took taught me about how to listen to a young child, how to talk with—not at—a young child, or how to understand his feelings. And, of course, working with parents was not a main focus either.

Two months ago I held a workshop with 90 directors of day-care centers from all over the country. Most of those people are a good 20 years younger than I am. I mention this fact only to stress that their training is much more recent than mine. Yet several of those people said that they had been taught that a way to maintain control over parents—MAINTAIN CONTROL OVER PARENTS—was to be sure, when having a conference, to seat the parents in a small chair while they sat in a regular-sized chair. If they did not have two sizes of chairs, they were to seat the parent in a chair and *they* were to stand.

I do not think any professional looks at the appointment schedule for the day and thinks, "Which of these parents can I intimidate, and reduce, literally, to tears? Which shall I blame for their child's lack of progress and which shall I accuse of not caring about their children?" Yet, some parents think that some professionals act in this way.

I want to put aside the notion of blame. Given the inadequacies of our training both as parents and as professionals, I think we all do the best we can. At any given time along the path of my life if I could have done better, Lord knows I would have.

There have been so many turning points for me in working with parents. Shortly after I started teaching in the Bill Wilkerson Home Program, I was with a young woman who drove up each Thursday morning from Alabama. She had a two-year-old severely hearing-impaired child and a four-year-old youngster. One day she said to me, "I was so angry at Jason this morning I almost threw him down the basement steps." Feeling, intensely, her pain and wanting so desperately to help, I said, "That's really rough, Martha. I understand how you feel." She looked me straight in the face and said to me more kindly than I deserved, "Laura, you don't understand. You never will, and don't you ever say that to me again." I have often thought what an incredible gift that young woman gave me—the opportuntity to look inside myself and to learn something valuable. It was impossible for me to understand, because I had not had the same experience.

Shortly afterwards I was working with a different family and I said to the mother, "Now, Susie, what you need to do is go home and read to Bubba every day." She would return the next week and I would say, "How did the reading go?" "Fine." Some time passed before I had earned her trust so she felt she could be honest with me. One day she said, "Laura, you know all those times you told me to read to Bubba? I never read to him once." "You didn't! Why?"

"Because I don't like to read to him. But you know what I do? I go out in the yard and play with him every day and you can get in just as much language development over a ball as you can over a book."

In my ignorance it had never occurred to me to say, "Susie, what do you enjoy doing with Bubba that we could use to build language?" I said to the graduate students I was working with then, "The next time you sense you are about to say to a parent, 'Now what you need to do is . . . ' Please know that I am somewhere haunting you, because we do *not* know what any other human needs to do. I have enough difficulty, sometimes, knowing what *I* need to do."

Recently I held a workshop in Nashville with the parents and staff of a center for exceptional children. I recognized one of the teachers as having had a child in our Infant Program years ago, but I could remember neither her name, nor her child's. She showed me his picture, said he was 18 and when she mentioned his name I recalled very well who he was. Though I had not worked with him, he was a child we had all discussed a good bit because he had so many problems and we knew so little to do to help. As that recent workshop ended, the mother said, "Laura, I'm glad to be with you today because I sense you are so warm and caring and that is not the way I remember you from the past. One day, many years ago, Todd's teacher was sick and you met with us. I thought you were cold, unfeeling. Your questions seemed so clinical. You know of course, that may have been only my perception. You were talking to me about some things I did not want to hear, but I'm so glad to see you in a different light today."

I have racked my brain and still cannot recall the event that mother talked about. But she had remembered it, *for sixteen years*. I think that often we have a session with a parent, go on to the next one, and eventually some of those sessions begin to blur and fade from our memory. Not so for the parents. They ponder our every word, and agonize over many of them. They recall our gestures, our looks, our tone of voice.

Do we communicate, not just with words, but with our eyes, our touch, our demeanor, that we care for the parents we are talking to? And for their children? A wise person once said to me, "I don't love every child I meet. I don't even like a lot of them. But I feel such compassion for them because I know the rough spots they will face down the road." Do we extend this same compassion to parents?

There are a thousand familiar reasons why we charge ahead, planning *for* parents instead of *with* them. Some parents are said not to care about their children, and to be too close to them to be objective. Parents are assumed not to know enough techniques, or are thought to be undependable. Nicholas Hobbs, founder of Project Re-Ed, in speaking of the need for professionals to change their attitudes toward parents, wrote:

> Teachers tend to have the same view of parents as psychologists, pediatricians, social workers, and many other professional people—condescension and poorly disguised assumptions of incompetence. The professional is the expert. It is the rare professional person who recognizes that the parents are the true experts on their children.

He often told of the time when, preparing a paper, he wrote, "We at Project Re-Ed make parents full partners with us in our efforts to help their children." He said he was rather pleased with this statement until a secretary who was typing his notes, said, "Nick, don't you think that's a little bit arrogant?"

When we change our attitude, and ask parents to let *us* be *their* partners, we realize they are a walking storehouse of information that we need if our efforts with their children are to be fruitful. Parents may not have the skill, at first, to observe their children, but they can quickly learn to tell us what they see without being judgmental. When parents say their child is "lazy" or "afraid" or "mean" we do not gain any useful information. When we ask parents, "What do you see your child do, what do you hear him say that leads you to believe he is "lazy," or "afraid," or whatever? then we have something concrete to work with. Conversely, I say to parents, don't let any professional tell you your child is "immature," "not motivated," "has a short attention span." Ask the professional, "What is it you see my child do, what do you hear him say—that leads you to believe he is immature . . . or whatever?"

I think one of the reasons some parents say, "I don't know why I go to that clinic. I leave feeling this big!" or "I don't know why I go there, they don't tell me anything," relates to all of this. If much of what we tell parents, particularly about a child's behavior, are our judgments, our opinions, our assumptions, each statement invites the parent to respond, "Well, my child's not like that at home!" Then, both parent and professional may feel blamed, attacked, put down, and a conference may degenerate into a needless confrontation.

Sometimes, parents *do* come in angry. And they unload all that anger on us. We have several choices about how we respond. We can choose to react in anger, we can choose to become defensive, but we have a vast array of other choices, also.

Neil Welliver is an artist whose work I have lately come to know and enjoy. I read an interview with him last summer that mentioned that within the course of a short time his wife died, his infant daughter died and the barn burned in which many of his paintings were stored. When asked how he handled that terrible period in his life, he replied, "I didn't take it personally."

No matter what parents say to us, we can choose not to take it personally. Often their anger builds from all the fears, all the frustrations, all the unknowns they are facing, compounded by the feeling that "no one's listening." Their anger often has nothing to do with us.

Sometimes, though, it is directed at us, rightfully. Instead of becoming defensive we can choose to ask, "What is there here for me to learn about myself? How can I change *my* behavior?" This is a new learning for me. I would not have said it a few years ago. A long time ago, I heard a speaker say, "Everytime I point my finger at you, accusing you of something, blaming you for something, being disappointed with you, my thumb is pointing back at me, pointing out that same thing within me." When I first heard that statement, I thought it was pretty ridiculous and definitely corny. But I have learned that often when I become upset with a parent, blame a parent, accuse a parent, put a parent down, it is because what I see in him or her is a red flag, pointing out something in me that needs healing, something I am not even aware of. If I can stop, and search my heart, that moment can become a time of insight and growth for me.

I find it extremely valuable to offer parents opportunities to come together in groups, not as a requirement but as an option. When I am involved in a parent group, I have two purposes in mind: to help create an atmosphere of acceptance so parents feel comfortable to say whatever is in their hearts, and to work myself out of a job as soon as possible. By this I mean to encourage parents to see that, within themselves, they have the potential to become their own best resource. They may not believe this at first. And as long as I continue to do *for* them what they are capable of learning to do for themselves they will never know it.

Many people, I think, have been so influenced by fear of what others think that they are often on guard, unwilling to trust. We have not always learned how to support and enable each other. But when we create a safe climate, when parents know they will not be judged nor blamed, we find they are hungry to talk. They will tell us about themselves, if they sense that we want to know.

Always in parent groups that continue over several sessions, I ask for a written evaluation at the end of each session:

The most valuable part today for me was . . .
A part that was not valuable for me was . . .
What I wanted to say, but didn't, was . . .
What I will work on this week is . . .

Usually the most valuable part was not anything I did or said but the realization from the parents that they are not alone, that other people have the same feelings, and that, finally, someone understands. When those moments occur, they are nurturing for the whole group.

I do not begin a group, hoping to change anyone. This is another new learning for me. In my eagerness I used to think I could change almost anyone. But I have learned, slowly and painfully, that there is only one person I can change . . . and that, with the greatest of difficulty. But I find that when I change, changes happen around me.

Much of what we offer people is, I think, conditional love. I will love you when . . . you do what I want you to do. I will love you if . . . you become the person I want you to be. Of course, we are much too sophisticated to say that in words, but we express that attitude in subtle and not so subtle ways. But love, with strings, is not love. It is a bribe. When we accept parents, or anyone, as they are, without insisting or even suggesting that they change, the exciting paradox is that they are free to change themselves.

I see this happening, and I see parents leave group meetings feeling lighter, less burdened, feeling more valued, more worthwhile and confident—thus, more competent people.

And all of this takes time. Several years ago I was meeting with a state association of speech and hearing professionals and we were discussing how important it is to allow parents time to go through whatever emotional stages they may be experiencing. One participant said, "I always give parents plenty of time to accept what's happened to their child." "Great," I said. "How long do you allow?" "At least three months," was the reply.

Some parents tell us it takes four to five years to accept the fact their child will never hear normally. One young woman said, "I've looked 'acceptance' up in the dictionary. It means 'to receive gladly and willingly, to endure without protest, to regard as proper and right' and I will *never* do any of these things. I think that's too much to ask of a human being!"

In a group this past spring at Bill Wilkerson a parent said, "I realize now that every retest, at least in the early stages, brought hope that my child's hearing would have improved. Each time, the disappointment seemed to start the grieving process all over again." Encouraging parents to express these feelings, not keep them inside, is healing.

In that same group, a parent said, "Sometimes I feel so inadequate. It's not that I'm passing my responsibility on to someone else, though it may appear that way. It's just that I want some qualified person to help me, and it's reassuring to know that help is there!" At that moment, the opportunity is ripe for parent and professional to work together effectively.

Occasionally, though, a parent may say to us, "You're the expert. You've had all the training, all the experience. I'm just a parent. Tell me what to do and I'll do anything you say." Depending on our own ego needs, at the time, we may think, "Yes, I *am* the expert. Glad you recognize that," and then assume the responsibility of telling the parents what they need to do. How much *more* useful it is, I think, to say to that parent, "Look, you know your child in ways I will never know him. And I need *your* help. Yes, I have had training and experience. I have ideas and suggestions, but don't leave *your* brain outside the door when you come in here. I need your observations and your ideas, too."

Years ago I was working with a family from Kentucky. Both parents, the hearing-impaired two-year-old, and a couple of brothers and sisters, drove down each week. I liked them immensely. They seemed so receptive to everything I said, so eager to do whatever I suggested. Yet, each week, when they returned, somehow nothing had ever been done. Always there were lots of excuses and always promises of doing better. Finally, I don't know what prompted me, but I said, "Look, you drive 180 miles each week to come here. You talk a good game, but you don't do anything. You're wasting your time and money to come and I'm wasting my time meeting with you. You all decide whether you want to stay in this program or get out." I did not tell my colleagues what I had said because I wondered if I had upset the parents so they wouldn't return. But they came back, regularly, for a long time. We worked hard, together, and their child made good progress.

Though I think words are important, even when we stumble around, and put our feet in our mouths, if parents sense that we care about them we are going to come out all right. I'm not interested in developing "techniques" for working with parents. I find it far more important to demonstrate genuine regard for them as people.

My colleague in our project tells of the time, soon after she began teaching in the Infant Program, a mother she was with began to cry. Cynthia got up and started toward the door, saying, "I'll go get Laura." The mother had the good sense to grab Cynthia by the arm and say, "Sit down. I don't know Laura. I want to talk to you!"

Sometimes, in the early years when I was with parents individually or in a group, I was so uncomfortable with silence, or so moved by their pain, or so eager to help, that I charged ahead talking about what I wanted to discuss. Or, offered unsolicited advice, and then felt a tad irritated later, when they didn't act on my suggestion. Occasionally, I even thought "This parent can't take it, or isn't ready to talk about this yet," so I moved to a "safer" topic. But I have learned that parents will not risk more than they are able to take. My assumptions more often indicated my own discomfort in the situation. All I needed to do in those moments was simply to be there. Be there, and listen.

Listening to another person is difficult. Listening, not just with my head, but with my heart, moving beyond the angry words to hear the message. Sometimes I still find it hard to listen without talking. Sometimes I talk without listening at all. And much of what I call listening is thinking about what I'm going to say as soon as the other person gets to a comma and I can jump in. But, when I am able to be quiet, to allow time to feel, and to reflect on what the parent has said, when I can resist the temptation to tell parents what to do or when I can ask one good question and then hush, I see parents begin to draw on some inner reserve and begin to find within themselves their own answers for what they want to do.

How do we enrich our relationship with parents? Madison Sarratt, beloved and almost legendary Dean of Students at Vanderbilt for many decades, told of visiting with an old woman up in the mountains of East Tennessee. After a while he said, "Mama Sally Lou, how come—without any formal education—you're so wise?" The old woman replied, "Little Madie, when you don't have no education, you have to use your head."

I have been fortunate to work with many parents who were patient and forgiving with my shortcomings. I have learned much from them about nobility of spirit, determination of purpose and the strength of compassion and love.

Now that I am very close to 60, I realize even more how precious, how fragile, life is. I am finally realizing how simple life can be when we don't complicate it. As a society we have developed the technology to kill everybody in the world three or four—how many?—times over. It seems to me that we have learned more about how to kill each other than about how to live together in peace and harmony. The Indians have a lovely word, *Namaste*—"I honor the light within you." What a lovely spot our homes and work places would be if we took the time, each day, to look for the light that dwells so surely in each person there. Because you occupy important positions in your field, you have remarkable opportunities to influence others. You set the tone for your organization by the way you treat the people there. What kind of atmosphere do you need, not just to survive, but to flourish? What enables you to develop more fully as a human being? Don't parents need the same?

Keep your eye on your dream!
Let your spirit soar!

Subject Index

(Page numbers in italics indicate material in figures or tables.)

Author Index

(Only the names of authors whose work is discussed in some detail are included in this index.)